Animal Behavior for Shelter Veterinarians and Staff

Animal Behavior for Shelter Veterinarians and Staff

Edited by

Brian A. DiGangi, DVM, MS, DABVP
Senior Director, Shelter Medicine
Shelter & Veterinary Services
ASPCA®
Gainesville, FL, USA

Victoria A. Cussen, PhD, CAAB
Senior Director, Applied Behavior Research
Behavioral Sciences Team
ASPCA®
Seattle, WA, USA

Pamela J. Reid, PhD, CAAB
Vice President
Behavioral Sciences Team
ASPCA®
Hendersonville, NC, USA

Kristen A. Collins, MS, ACAAB
Vice President, Behavioral Rehabilitation Services
ASPCA®
Mars Hill, NC, USA

Second Edition

WILEY Blackwell

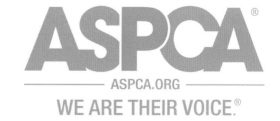

Registered Office
John Wiley & Sons, Inc., 111 River Street, Hoboken, NJ 07030, USA

Editorial Office
111 River Street, Hoboken, NJ 07030, USA

For details of our global editorial offices, customer services, and more information about Wiley products visit us at www.wiley.com.

Wiley also publishes its books in a variety of electronic formats and by print-on-demand. Some content that appears in standard print versions of this book may not be available in other formats.

Library of Congress Cataloging-in-Publication Data

Names: DiGangi, Brian A., 1980– editor. | Cussen, Victoria A., 1979– editor.
 | Reid, Pamela, 1960– editor. | Collins, Kristen A., 1976– editor.
Title: Animal behavior for shelter veterinarians and staff / editors, Brian A. DiGangi,
 Victoria A. Cussen, Pamela J. Reid, Kristen A. Collins.
Description: Second edition. | Hoboken, NJ : Wiley-Blackwell, 2022. |
 Preceded by: Animal behavior for shelter veterinarians and staff /
 editors, Emily Weiss, Heather Mohan-Gibbons, Stephen Zawistowski. 2015.
 | Includes bibliographical references and index.
Identifiers: LCCN 2022016280 (print) | LCCN 2022016281 (ebook) | ISBN
 9781119618478 (paperback) | ISBN 9781119618492 (adobe pdf) | ISBN
 9781119618508 (epub)
Subjects: MESH: Behavior, Animal–physiology | Veterinary Medicine–methods
 | Animal Welfare | Cats | Dogs | Human-Animal Interaction
Classification: LCC SF412.5 (print) | LCC SF412.5 (ebook) | NLM SF 756.7
 | DDC 636.088/7–dc23/eng/20220412
LC record available at https://lccn.loc.gov/2022016280
LC ebook record available at https://lccn.loc.gov/2022016281

Cover Design: Wiley
Cover Images: Courtesy of Brian A. DiGangi, Dana K. Trotta, Rachel Maso

Set in 9.5/12.5pt STIXTwoText by Straive, Pondicherry, India

Printed in Singapore
M100894_170522

Contents

List of Contributors

Julia D. Albright, MA, DVM, DACVB
Associate Professor of Veterinary Behavior
Department of Small Animal Clinical Sciences
University of Tennessee
Knoxville, TN, USA

Haleh Amanieh, MS
Graduate Student
Department of Psychology
West Virginia University
Morgantown, WV, USA

Chumkee Aziz, DVM, DABVP (Shelter Medicine Practice)
Outreach Veterinarian
University of California, Davis, USA
Koret Shelter Medicine Program
Houston, TX, USA

Sara L. Bennett, DVM, MS, DACVB
Clinical Assistant Professor of Veterinary Behavior
College of Veterinary Medicine
North Carolina State University
Raleigh, NC, USA

Jeannine Berger, DVM, DACVB, DACAW, CAWA
Senior VP Rescue and Welfare
San Francisco Society for the Prevention of Cruelty to Animals (SPCA)
San Francisco, CA, USA

Kelley Bollen, MS, CABC
Principal Consultant
Kelley Bollen Consulting, LLC
Reno, NV, USA

Janis Bradley, MA
Director of Communications & Publications
National Canine Research Council
Stanford, CA, USA

Christine Calder, DVM, DACVB
Clinical Veterinary Behaviorist
Calder Veterinary Behavior Services
Portland, OR, USA

Victoria A. Cussen, PhD, CAAB
Senior Director, Applied Behavior Research
Behavioral Sciences Team
ASPCA®
Seattle, WA, USA

Brian A. DiGangi, DVM, MS, DABVP (Canine & Feline Practice, Shelter Medicine Practice)
Senior Director, Shelter Medicine
Shelter & Veterinary Services
ASPCA®
Gainesville, FL, USA

Nicole R. Dorey, PhD, CAAB
Senior Lecturer
Department of Psychology
University of Florida
Gainesville, FL, USA

Seana Dowling-Guyer, MS
Associate Director, Center for Shelter Dogs
Tufts Center for Animals and Public Policy
Cummings School of Veterinary Medicine
at Tufts University
North Grafton, MA, USA

Erin Doyle, DVM, DABVP (Shelter Medicine Practice)
Senior Director, Shelter Medicine & Residency Programs
Shelter & Veterinary Services
ASPCA®
Needham, MA, USA

Jacklyn J. Ellis, MRes, PhD, CAAB
Director, Behaviour
Toronto Humane Society
Toronto, Ontario, Canada

Erica Feuerbacher, PhD, CAAB, CPDT-KA, BCBA-D
Associate Professor, Applied Animal Behavior & Welfare
Department of Animal and Poultry Science
Virginia Tech
Blacksburg, VA, USA

Elise Gingrich, DVM, MPH, MS, DACVPM, DABVP (Shelter Medicine Practice)
Senior Director, Shelter Medicine
Shelter & Veterinary Services
ASPCA®
Fort Collins, CO, USA

Brenda Griffin, DVM, MS, DACVIM, DABVP (Shelter Medicine Practice)
Adjunct Associate Professor
College of Veterinary Medicine
University of Florida
Gainesville, FL, USA

Lisa Gunter, PhD, CBCC-KA
Maddie's Fund Research Fellow
Department of Psychology
Arizona State University
Tempe, AZ, USA

Julie Hecht, MSc
PhD Candidate
Department of Psychology
The Graduate Center, CUNY
NY, USA

Alexandra Horowitz, PhD
Senior Research Fellow
Adjunct Associate Professor
Department of Psychology
Barnard College
NY, USA

Stephanie Janeczko, DVM, MS, DABVP (Canine & Feline Practice, Shelter Medicine Practice), CAWA
Vice President, Shelter Medicine Services
Shelter & Veterinary Services
ASPCA®
NY, USA

Colleen S. Koch, DVM, DACVB
Veterinary Behavior Consultant
Lincoln Land Animal Clinic, LTD, Animal Behavior Service
Jacksonville, IL, USA

Amy Learn, VMD
Chief of Clinical Behavioral Medicine
Animal Behavior Wellness Center
Richmond, VA, USA

Sue McDonnell, MA, PhD, CAAB
Adjunct Professor of Reproductive Behavior
Head, Equine Behavior Program
University of Pennsylvania School of Veterinary Medicine
Kennett Square, PN, USA

Trish McMillan, MSc, CPDT-KA, CDBC
Owner
McMillan Animal Behavior, LLC
Mars Hill, NC, USA

Lindsay R. Mehrkam, PhD, BCBA-D
Assistant Professor
Department of Psychology
Monmouth University
West Long Branch, NJ, USA

Katherine Miller, PhD, CAAB
Senior Director, Learning Lab
Policy, Response & Engagement
ASPCA®
Weaverville, NC, USA

Lila Miller, BS, DVM
Retired Vice President
ASPCA®
NY, USA

Gary J. Patronek, VMD, PhD
Adjunct Professor
Tufts Center for Animals and Public Policy
Cummings School of Veterinary Medicine at
Tufts University
North Grafton, MA, USA

Alexandra Protopopova, PhD
Assistant Professor, NSERC/BC SPCA Industrial
Research Chair in Animal Welfare
Animal Welfare Program
The University of British Columbia
Vancouver, Canada

**Tristan Rehner-Fleurant, MS, CPDT-KA,
CBCC-KA**
Senior Director, Behavior Rehabilitation
Policy, Response & Engagement
ASPCA®
Weaverville, NC, USA

Pamela J. Reid, PhD, CAAB
Vice President
Behavioral Sciences Team
ASPCA®
Hendersonville, NC, USA

Bridget Schoville, MS
Senior Director, Shelter Behavior Science
Behavioral Sciences Team
ASPCA®
Madison, WI, USA

Leslie Sinn, DVM, DACVB, CPDT-KA
Veterinary Behavior Clinician and
Consultant
Behavior Solutions, LLC
Ashburn, VA, USA

Margaret R. Slater, DVM, PhD
Senior Director, Research
Strategy & Research
ASPCA®
Northampton, MA, USA

Kristina Spaulding, PhD, CAAB
Educator, Behaviour Consultant, and Owner
Smart Dog Training and Behavior, LLC
Saratoga Springs, NY, USA

Wailani Sung, MS, PhD, DVM, DACVB
Director of Behavior and Welfare Programs
San Francisco SPCA
San Francisco, CA, USA

Valarie V. Tynes, DVM, DACVB, DACAW
Veterinary Services Specialist
Ceva Animal Health
Lenexa, KS, USA
Premier Veterinary Behavior Consulting
Sweetwater, TX, USA

Karen S. Walsh, CAWA, LVMT, CFE
Senior Director, Animal Relocation
Shelter & Veterinary Services
ASPCA®
Dunlap, TN, USA

Katie Watts, MAT
Former Senior Feline Behavior Counselor
ASPCA® Adoption Center
NY, USA

Stephen Zawistowski, PhD, CAAB Emeritus
Adjunct Professor
Hunter College
Chelsea, MI, USA

Foreword

The field of applied shelter animal welfare is undergoing rapid change, and it is an exciting time to witness the progress. Since we edited the first edition of *Animal Behavior for Shelter Veterinarians and Staff*, several developments drove rapid advancement in the field. In 2015, the first shelter medicine veterinary specialists were certified while we were writing the first edition. Once published, that textbook became required reading for their certification program. Those specialists, along with other scientists, have greatly expanded the literature on applied behavioral health of dogs and cats since then. Additionally, shelters are changing. The number of dogs and cats entering shelters continues to decline, and dogs and cats receiving behavioral interventions have increased. This is likely due to a shift in the population of animals coming into shelters, an increase in available resources (kennel space, staff, etc.) to support that population, as well as what you will see in this textbook: a growing sophistication of programs and processes to support the behavioral health of the shelter population.

The editors in this edition bring incredible depth and expertise to this book. All four editors have decades of experience working in animal welfare. Dr. Brian DiGangi is the Senior Director of Shelter Medicine at the ASPCA. Being dual board certified in Canine and Feline Practice and Shelter Medicine Practice allows him to bring a unique perspective and deep expertise to this body of work. Dr. Victoria Cussen is a Certified Applied Animal Behaviorist and Senior Director of Applied Behavior Research for the ASPCA's Behavioral Sciences Team. With expertise in comparative cognition and canine behavior, she has a deep understanding of the scientific literature on animal behavior topics. Dr. Pam Reid serves as Vice President of the ASPCA's Behavioral Sciences Team. She provides specialized behavioral services, expertise in humane animal handling, behavioral evaluations, placement, and euthanasia recommendations for cruelty cases. Kristen Collins is an Associate Certified Applied Animal Behaviorist, and as Vice President of the ASPCA Behavioral Rehabilitation Center, she oversees all programs and operations with drive and compassion. Together, this revision will be an exemplary contribution to the field of shelter medicine and animal behavior.

This textbook will be a key resource for shelter professionals. Like the first edition, this content was written and edited by top leaders in the field. There are several new topics tackled in this text that will have a positive impact on thousands of sheltering professionals, from science-driven guidance when making decisions regarding behavioral well-being, to best practices during transportation of animals, to a focus on behavioral health for dogs and cats that are victims of cruelty or disaster, and much more. We look forward to seeing this edition published and used.

Heather Mohan-Gibbons, RVT, MS, ACAAB
Emily Weiss, PhD

Acknowledgments

First, we would like to thank the authors and editors of the first edition of *Animal Behavior for Shelter Veterinarians and Staff*. Dr. Emily Weiss, Ms. Heather Mohan-Gibbons, and Dr. Stephen Zawistowski astutely recognized the need for and importance of a book like this to further the progression of animal sheltering, and their work has laid a solid foundation on which we were able to capitalize. Their enthusiasm and advice as they handed over the reins for the second edition were much appreciated.

We would also like to acknowledge the support and encouragement of our colleagues. Drs. Lila Miller, Stephanie Janeczko, Chumkee Aziz, Erin Doyle, and Elise Gingrich provided thoughtful input on content, played roles as guest editors, and, perhaps most invaluable, served as sounding boards throughout the process. Ms. Rachel Maso assisted in managing this project and enthusiastically took on the unenviable tasks of handling contracts and accounting. Ms. Laura Nelson assisted with preparation of figures, and Carey Parrack provided administrative support, allowing us to focus on content and manuscript preparation.

Finally, we would like to acknowledge the ASPCA's Executive Leadership Team, particularly Ms. Bert Troughton, Ms. Stacy Wolf, and our CEO, Mr. Matt Bershadker, for recognizing the value a project like this brings to the field of animal welfare at-large and allowing us to devote time to the effort.

Brian A. DiGangi
Victoria A. Cussen
Pamela J. Reid
Kristen A. Collins

About the Companion Website

This book is accompanied by a companion website:

www.wiley.com/go/digangi/animal

The website includes:

- Appendices – downloadable PDFs from the book
- Videos – demonstrations of concepts and techniques presented by the authors

Part I

Foundations in Behavioral Health

Introduction

"Everyone is on the behavior team." That is the philosophy of the ASPCA's Behavioral Rehabilitation Center, a purpose-built facility designed to house, care for, and treat dogs with extreme fear. However, this philosophy is also applicable outside a specialized rehabilitation facility, even when staffing structure, roles, and responsibilities vary. This approach recognizes that all shelter personnel have important insights and impacts on the behavior and welfare of animals. A collaborative approach to sheltering—from intake to outcome and everything in between—representing the perspectives of medical, behavior, and operations team members, can result in enhanced delivery of care and ultimately improve the entirety of the sheltering experience for the animals and humans involved.

The topics, contributors, and scope of content throughout this book have been chosen and designed to highlight the interplay of all animal care team members toward a shared goal of happy, healthy pets enriching the lives of their humans. The reader will find authors with expertise in animal training, applied behavior, operations and programs, veterinary behavior, shelter medicine, and research—and in many cases authors have been intentionally paired to present as broad a perspective as possible on each topic.

Building upon the foundations laid in the first edition, this volume has been divided into five sections intended to present an evidence-based approach to the current knowledge of animal behavior in animal shelters. **Section 1: Foundations in Behavioral Health** addresses fundamental concepts important for the application of the principles explored in the subsequent sections and features a new chapter to introduce the reader to learning theory (Chapter 3). **Section 2: Pets in the Community** describes the implications of community-wide programs on the behavioral health of shelter animals and features a timely new chapter on safety net programs to prevent pet relinquishment (Chapter 5). **Section 3: Dogs in the Shelter** and **Section 4: Cats in the Shelter** have each been expanded to accommodate the ever-growing knowledge base in topics that were presented together in the first edition. Chapters dedicated solely to advances in animal handling (Chapters 8 and 14), behavior assessment (Chapters 9 and 15), and housing (Chapter 10 and 16) for dogs and cats will focus on practical applications of both old and new concepts. In addition, Section 3 also features an entire chapter on the science and impact of play in dogs along with guidance for the successful, humane operation of playgroups (Chapter 13). **Section 5: Special Topics** encompasses a variety of timely and important topics with direct implications on animal health and welfare. New chapters feature frameworks for welfare

Animal Behavior for Shelter Veterinarians and Staff, Second Edition. Edited by Brian A. DiGangi, Victoria A. Cussen, Pamela J. Reid, and Kristen A. Collins.
© 2022 John Wiley & Sons, Inc. Published 2022 by John Wiley & Sons, Inc.
Companion website: www.wiley.com/go/digangi/animal

assessment and ethical decision-making (Chapter 19) and consider programming with particular impact on behavioral health such as animal relocation (Chapter 20) and the behavioral care of animals during disasters, cruelty cases, and long-term holds (Chapter 21). This section also includes an expanded discussion of behavioral pharmacology in animal shelters (Chapter 22) and introduces concepts in the care of small mammals (Chapter 23) and horses (Chapter 24).

The reader is encouraged to use all of the resources compiled to supplement the material in the text. Chapter appendices offer sample protocols and checklists that will help put new knowledge into practice. An online video library is available to demonstrate many of the conditions, concepts, and techniques presented by the authors. General appendices provide ethograms of common canine and feline behaviors as well as a summary of behavior professional credentialing requirements.

Read from cover to cover, consult a chapter before writing a new protocol, assign a staff member to present a chapter at a staff meeting, or build a volunteer training session using material gleaned from your favorite chapter—choose whichever means of applying this material will most enrich you, the animals, and the people in your circles. After all, there is bound to be something valuable for everyone, because everyone is on the behavior team!

1

Introduction to Dog Behavior
Julie Hecht and Alexandra Horowitz

1.1 Evolutionary History of the Species

The domestic dog, *Canis familiaris*, is a member of the Canidae family, genus *Canis*, which also includes wolves, coyotes, and jackals. *Canis lupus*, the present-day gray wolf, is the domestic dog's closest living ancestor (Vilà et al. 1997), and the divergence began more than 10,000 years ago, possibly with early hunter-gatherers and then in association with early agriculture (vonHoldt and Driscoll 2017). The dog is the only domesticated species of the genus: that is to say, the only canid for whom artificial selection (selective breeding) by humans has usurped natural selection as a major mover of the species.

Considering dog behavior in the context of their wild cousins can at times clarify some common dog behavior. Wolves living among family members approach and greet those returning from hunting by licking—"kissing"—their faces. Licks are prompts for the wolf to regurgitate some of the kill just ingested. Similarly, a dog's "kiss" is a greeting, but it is also a vestigial interest in whatever it was an owner might have consumed since leaving the house (Horowitz 2009b). A dog's propensity to sniff peoples' genital area could be viewed as intrusive or "impolite," yet it is analogous to canids' olfactory investigations of

the genital and anal areas of conspecifics, which contain information about the identification, and perhaps recent activities and health, of that individual (Sommerville and Broom 1998). At the same time, there are numerous differences between dogs and wolves, particularly regarding ecological niche and social organization (Marshall-Pescini et al. 2017), and analogies between the two should be made with caution. Instead, dogs' intimate association with humans has had a seminal impact on every aspect of their being.

1.2 Dogs and Humans

Canis familiaris and *Homo sapiens* share a special relationship. They engage in the seemingly mundane—walking side by side in a park—to the complex—running an agility course or alerting a hearing-impaired person to a ringing telephone. In recent years, cognitive, behavioral, and physiological studies have added clarity to this unique interspecific bond.

1.2.1 Dog Interspecific Social Cognition

Dogs display behaviors that can give people the feeling of a shared experience and mutual understanding. Dogs monitor human behavior closely, are sensitive to human actions and attentional states, and act in accordance with

Animal Behavior for Shelter Veterinarians and Staff, Second Edition. Edited by Brian A. DiGangi, Victoria A. Cussen, Pamela J. Reid, and Kristen A. Collins.

humans in coordinated and synchronized ways. For example, when unable to access a desired item, dogs may alternate their gaze between the item and a person to direct the person to retrieve it (Miklósi et al. 2000). Even as puppies, dogs readily respond to human communicative gestures, whether stemming from hands, the face, (e.g., the eyes), or other body parts (Reid 2009; Riedel et al. 2008). This propensity is even observed in some free-ranging dogs (Bhattacharjee et al. 2020), and personality, enculturation, and reinforcement history could also affect outcomes. Dogs take note of human attentional states from the eyes as well as head and body orientation—a dog being more likely to remove a muffin from a countertop if a person's back is turned or eyes are closed than if the person's eyes are open (Schwab and Huber 2006). Dogs discriminate human emotional expressions such as happy and angry faces (Müller et al. 2015). A number of dogs have proved extraordinarily attentive and responsive to human language (Kaminski et al. 2004; Pilley and Reid 2011). Not all dogs attend to verbal cues (Ramos and Mills 2019), and the emotional content, tone, and intonation of human vocalizations are particularly relevant. Behavioral synchronization—staying close to and moving in pace with a person—has been observed in owned dogs and, to a lesser extent, between shelter dogs and caretakers (Duranton and Gaunet 2018). Dogs and humans also play together, and these vastly different species can attend to each other's play signals; a dog's play bow—or a person's play lunge—is often responded to meaningfully (Rooney et al. 2001). People visiting a shelter searching for their new best friend may not be aware of the complex social exchanges underlying the dog-human relationship, but they may have experienced it with another dog and may even be seeking it out.

1.2.2 Dog-Human Relationships

Attachment theory initially described the affectionate bond relating to safety, security, and protection between a child and caregiver, and it has since been extended to and identified between dogs and their caretakers (Bowlby 1958; Topál et al. 1998). Attachment is displayed through particular behaviors such as proximity maintenance, approach, and gaze toward a caregiver when reunited. Similar to infants, dogs display the "secure base effect" by exploring and playing more in a novel environment when in the presence of an owner than a stranger (Horn et al. 2013). Like the child-parent relationship, dogs can display different attachment styles described broadly as secure (explore and also seek contact) or insecure (avoidant, ambivalent, or disorganized) (Solomon et al. 2019). Dog attachment style and owner caregiving strategies both contribute to the dyad's relationship (Rehn and Keeling 2016).

Early exposure to humans is important for normal dog social development, but attachment relationships can form later in life, multiple times, and toward multiple people. Gácsi et al. (2001) found that similar to owned dogs, shelter dogs displayed attachment behaviors toward a newly appointed "owner" (designated by three short interactions with the dog). Thielke and Udell (2020) found that, similar to owned dogs, dogs in foster care formed secure attachments, and leaving the shelter seems to further support relationship development. If adopters are concerned about shelter dogs forming bonds, these studies could provide comfort.

Biological mechanisms could also underpin the dog-human relationship. The neurohormone oxytocin is often highlighted for its role in bonding and affiliation, good feelings, and stress buffering. Studies find that pleasurable interactions such as gentle petting, light play, talking in a positive tone, greeting, and sharing gaze with a known person promote oxytocin release in both dogs and people (Kis et al. 2017; Powell et al. 2019b). Although oxytocin appears to contribute to the dog-human relationship, a positive oxytocin effect is not always observed (Powell et al. 2019a).

Researchers are also exploring whether administering oxytocin to dogs elicits affiliative and social behaviors. Findings to date are not straightforward. For example, Romero et al. (2014) found that oxytocin promoted affiliative behavior toward humans and other dogs, but Barrera et al. (2018) found that intranasal oxytocin did not improve reactions toward a stranger during a sociability test, as was expected. Additionally, administering oxytocin to dogs can be challenging, and Schaebs et al. (2020) found that a vaporizer mask—which requires training—administers oxytocin more reliably than the more commonly used intranasal spray. Regardless, unclear sex, neuter status, and breed differences have been identified, and outcomes are not always in the anticipated direction. In humans, for example, oxytocin has been linked to distrust of and preemptive aggression toward strangers (Sapolsky 2018). The utility and real-world use of oxytocin administration remains to be seen.

1.2.3 Relationships between Dogs

Dog relationships with conspecifics may differ from those formed with humans, and research in this area is in its infancy. Behavioral indicators of attachment toward the dam have been identified and, in some circumstances, the stress response can be reduced by the presence of a cohabitant dog (Mariti et al. 2014, 2017). Cimarelli et al. (2019) suggest that it is the individuals involved, not the species type, who impact the quality of the bond. They observed that while referencing/information seeking was more often found in dog-human relationships, both dog-dog and dog-human relationships shared similarities in terms of affiliation and stress alleviation (i.e., members of either species could provide more or less affiliation or stress alleviation). Taken together, dogs can have complex, amicable, and longstanding relationships with members of their own and other species. The potential for intra- and interspecies integration starts at the beginning of life.

1.3 Dog Behavioral Development

While genetics provide the blueprint for life, experiences—particularly those early in life—can impact dog behavioral development. Increased early life plasticity allows a growing dog to be affected by and responsive to environmental inputs, which in turn has the ability to affect immediate and future behavior. Understanding early life developmental periods goes hand in hand with identifying environments and experiences that support normal development and those associated with the development of pathological behaviors (behavior problems) and behaviors expressed out of context or excessive in terms of frequency, duration, or intensity (Dietz et al. 2018; Hammerle et al. 2015).

"Critical" or "sensitive" periods are specific weeks or months where behavior patterns emerge and environment, stimuli, and social exposure support development (Scott and Fuller 1965). Additionally, events during the prenatal period—such as in utero exposure to maternal stress—as well as subsequent dam care styles can influence puppy behavioral and cognitive development and later coping (Santos et al. 2020). While developmental periods have a clear progression (dogs will not play bow before opening their eyes), transitions between stages are more gradual than initially thought (Bateson 1979). The following periods are therefore guidelines—without hard-and-fast beginning and end points. Rates of development (heterochrony) can also differ among breeds. As well as among individuals.

1.3.1 Neonatal and Transitional Periods

In less than a month, pups move from complete dependence on the mother (zero to two weeks) to increasing autonomy (two to three weeks). Dogs enter the world without vision, hearing, or coordination, and they rely on tactile and simple olfactory sensations. They are unable to self-regulate temperature and spend most of their time sleeping, nursing, and in physical proximity to the dam and littermates. Newborns display "kneading" or "swimming" behavior directed at the teat or milk source to attain food, and the dam initiates elimination by tactile stimulation. If isolated they make high-pitched calls—whines or yelps—that indicate distress and are frequently described as care soliciting (Elliot and Scott 1961). These early vocalizations transform into high-pitched, high-frequency "alone barks" that are contextually similar and also elicit attention (Yin and McCowan 2004). At around two to three weeks, eyes and ears open, and characteristic "dog" qualities begin to emerge such as walking and tail wagging, rudimentary elements of play, and a startle response (Case 2005). An interest in solid food may begin, and anogenital licking is no longer required for elimination.

Dam maternal care styles throughout these early periods vary in quantity and quality and contribute to pup development (Dietz et al. 2018). Experiencing brief mild stressors beginning from birth—such as human handling and brief separations from conspecifics—could have long-term beneficial effects on stress resilience (Gazzano et al. 2008). Brief, gentle exposure to social (human and non-human animals) and asocial (auditory and visual) stimuli can further support physical and cognitive development.

1.3.2 Sensitive or Socialization Period

Week 3 to approximately week 12 is a time of immense growth, particularly for species-specific social behaviors and learning opportunities. Approach and avoidance emerge early in this period, followed by more coordinated motor patterns, such as play fighting with littermates. Pups increasingly send and receive intraspecific signals, and vocalizations become more complex and are incorporated into social situations. Dogs identify littermate and species members, and social learning from conspecifics and humans has been demonstrated in puppies as young as eight weeks of age (Fugazza et al. 2018;

Serpell et al. 2017). Pups also show attention to and interest in humans, and from an early age they can follow human communicative signals like gaze or pointing (Riedel et al. 2008). A period of interest and investigation can be followed by wariness or fearfulness, particularly after week 5 and culminating between weeks 8 and 10 (Case 2005). The presentation of fear could be modulated by factors such as genetics, individual coping styles, or early life experiences (Rooney et al. 2016).

Premature weaning and early separation from littermates are inadvisable. Separated dogs miss valuable social exchanges, both observational learning opportunities and feedback on their own behavior. Dogs vary in weaning time even within breed, and weaning prior to two months has been associated with subsequent behavior challenges such as increased destructive behavior and possessiveness, excessive barking, and fearfulness (Pierantoni et al. 2011).

As suggested, the socialization period is the time when dogs acquire "behavior patterns appropriate to the social environment in which [an individual will] live, allowing them to coexist/interact with other individuals" (Blackwell 2010). Dog interest and comfort with all that the human environment has to offer should not be assumed simply because dogs are "domestic." Instead, socialization involves short, repeated doses of enjoyable, varied experiences and exposing pups to social and non-social stimuli that will be part of *their* environment. Individual dog behavior should be closely monitored for indications of discomfort with consideration for under- as well as overstimulation (Howell et al. 2015). Pluijmakers et al. (2010) found that puppies between three and five weeks of age exposed to audiovisual playback—consisting of animate and inanimate objects and noises at normal volume—showed decreased fear of novel objects and unfamiliar settings compared to a control group who displayed increased stress-related behaviors.

Veterinary professionals recommend considering puppy socialization classes as early as seven to eight weeks and with a minimum of one set of vaccines (American Veterinary Society of Animal Behavior 2008). Early life restrictions can have profound effects on dogs. Numerous studies find that dogs raised in commercial breeding establishments (commonly known as "puppy mills" or "puppy farms") or purchased from pet stores displayed ongoing behavioral and emotional challenges such as increased fear and aggression and difficulty with separation when compared to dogs not raised in such environments (McMillan 2017).

1.3.3 Juvenile and Adolescent Periods

The periods from approximately three to six months and six months to one to two years (during which sexual maturity occurs) have received much less attention than other developmental periods. The juvenile period is sometimes described as the secondary socialization period because, like early in life, experiences can affect developing personality. Harvey et al. (2016) conducted behavior tests with dogs at five and eight months and found that some traits like jumping, barking, and low posture during greeting were stable, while others such as obedience, lip licking, and body shaking were not consistent between the two periods. A retrospective examination of guide dog development found that owner-directed aggression decreased in German shepherds, Labrador retrievers, golden retrievers, and golden × Labrador crosses from 6 to 12 months, but German shepherds showed an increase in stranger-directed aggression during this period (Serpell and Duffy 2016). Reductions in trainability and responsiveness to owner commands have also been documented during these periods (Asher et al. 2020). Although they have long since shed their puppy appearances, these dogs are still very much in a period of transition and

growth. The dog-human relationship could benefit if people set their expectations with this in mind.

1.3.4 Senior Dogs

Senior dogs are members of the shelter population, and identifying normal, successful aging versus cognitive dysfunction merits consideration. Factors like breed, size, and weight can affect how long dogs live, and as they age, they can display a number of normal age-related declines in physical and mental functioning (Chapagain et al. 2018). Changes in levels of play and responsiveness to commands, enthusiasm for food, and increases in fears and phobias can be part of normal, successful aging (Salvin et al. 2011). Older dogs also display less social interest, diminished learning and memory, and less interest in novelty compared to young dogs (Kubinyi and Iotchev 2020). Normal aging can also affect a dog's ability to cope with a social challenge such as a mild separation from an owner (Mongillo et al. 2013).

Canine cognitive dysfunction syndrome differs from normal aging and is summarized by the acronym DISHA: "Disorientation, altered Interactions with people or other pets, Sleep–wake cycle alterations, House-soiling and altered Activity level" (Landsberg et al. 2003). It parallels human dementia and Alzheimer's disease. Locomotion may be erratic or aimless, dogs may be less responsive to social isolation or interactions with people, and an increase in destructive behavior or house soiling may be observed (Chapagain et al. 2018). A therapeutic diet aimed at enhancing cognitive function as well as behavioral enrichment like participating in dog training activities are both promising interventions for delaying cognitive decline (Chapagain et al. 2018; Szabó et al. 2018). Awareness of the differences between normal aging and cognitive dysfunction can enhance care for older dogs entering the shelter.

1.4 Dog Communication

Dogs engage in visual, acoustic, and olfactory communication, and each contributes to intra- and interspecific communication. Studies complement—and at times clarify—existing interpretations of dog behavior and communication.

1.4.1 Visual Communication

Identifying expressive and meaningful body parts is integral to dog communication and emotional expression (see Figure 1.1; see General Appendix A for a canine body language ethogram). Meaning should not be obtained from any single body part or behavior in isolation. Instead, meaning takes shape when considering the totality of dog communicative behavior as well as environment and social contexts. To this point, observing and describing behavior precedes ascribing function, and individual differences in behavioral expression are commonly documented—even in response to the same stimulus or context.

Research-based resources provide background for visual communication descriptions (Beerda et al. 1998; Bradshaw and Rooney 2017; Miklósi 2015; Schenkel 1967), and visual representations of dog behavior and communication, such as Aloff (2005) and more recently Chin (2020), aid the study and recognition of visual signals.

Dog size and postural movements are observed by dogs and people alike. Unlike body size, posture can be modified to expand or contract, the former suggesting confidence or alertness and the latter conveying fear, prevention or reduction of conflict, or affiliation (Schenkel 1967). Dogs reduce size in multiple contexts and with different communicative meanings. A dog lying on the back in "passive submission," often with ears back, tail tucked, and the inguinal region exposed, deescalates conflict and inhibits attack. Dogs can also display a more inviting "belly-up" posture to solicit a belly rub. Alternatively, "active submission" may not be motivated by deference or a response to threat (Bradshaw and Rooney 2017). Instead, approach with low

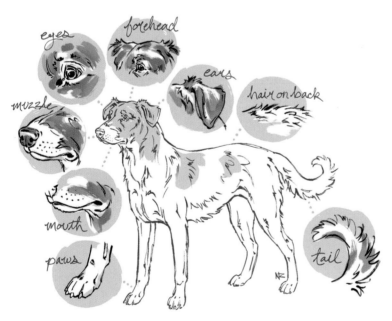

Figure 1.1 Body parts that contribute to canine visual communication. *Source:* Illustration created by and used with permission of Natalya Zahn.

posture, low wag, and muzzle (or mouth) licking is an affiliative display to gain food, greet, or maintain or restore social bonds.

In interspecific contexts—such as if a dog has done something an owner deems wrong—submissive displays can be misinterpreted as a dog's knowledge of wrongdoing. Instead, behaviors such as freezing, approaching or retreating with a depressed posture, low and quick wagging, ears back, or rolling onto the back or lifting a paw are best viewed along ethological lines as cohesive displays and non-threatening appeasement postures to keep the group together. Research finds these behaviors are not indicative of a dog's "knowledge" of misdeed or an admission of guilt (Horowitz 2009a).

Dog body posture can encourage "coming closer" (distance between individuals decreasing) or "backing up" (distance between individuals increasing), and a dog's body-weight distribution offers subtle yet valuable information. A dog with weight shifted forward and upper body pressed over the front legs shows forward momentum, interest, confidence, or alertness. If a dog leans forward toward another dog—and the receiver leans back, looks away, or moves away—the second is engaging in conflict avoidance or communicating the dog's desire to avoid closer interaction. If signals go unheeded, dogs may resort to defensive aggression over time and even fade out the use of distance-increasing signals.

Limbs are central to body-weight distribution and dog movement. While people may take note of limbs in the context of parlor tricks like "high five" or "give paw," these gestures bear no social meaning for dogs apart from possible food reward or human praise. Instead, "offering a paw" is a submissive or appeasing display and, for example, may be performed in response to an upset owner. Sweating paws could indicate acute stress, but these are difficult to interpret as they could be related to other factors, like temperature (Polgár et al. 2019).

Piloerection is a physical response outside a dog's control akin to getting goosebumps. This reflexive response can be seen in a dog's hackles, or erect hair. Hackles run from the base of the tail to the shoulders, and because raised hackles indicate arousal in general, piloerection should be evaluated in conjunction with ear, tail, mouth, and overall body posture to assess specifics of the aroused state.

Tails are integral to communicative signaling. They can assume a range of heights, movements, and speeds, and even the side-of-wag offers meaningful information. Observing the tail-base provides details as to whether the tail is being carried along the midline or is raised or tucked. Generally speaking, a high tail indicates excitement or arousal, and a high tail can be seen in a variety of approach-oriented contexts ranging from greeting and playing to fighting and threatening; lowered tails suggest fear, submission, or appeasement/affiliation (Kiley-Worthington 1976). To explore the value of tails within intraspecific communication, Leaver and Reimchen (2008) designed a study where dogs encountered a mechanical dog outfitted with tails of different lengths (long or short) that could move or remain still. Dogs were more likely to approach the mechanical dog when the tail was long and wagging as opposed to when it was long and still, suggesting that absent other communicative signals, dogs interpreted a wagging tail as "friendly." On the other hand, a short tail, whether still or wagging, was approached similarly, suggesting that short (or docked) tails might be more difficult to view or interpret. Tail absence or surgical shortening affects communication (Bennett and Perini 2003).

Probably the most noticeable component of the tail relates to movement. A tail wagging fluidly and loosely from side to side (usually at the level of the midline) is most readily associated with greeting or excitement. This "happy" tail might be accompanied by jumping, licking, running in circles, or other behaviors of arousal. A tail wagging low and quickly indicates nervousness or timidity. High, fast wags indicate arousal, and they should be viewed with some caution. Arousal can take different forms, such as general excitement, interest in interacting, or even aggression. There are further individual variations in wags—circling, going more counter- than clockwise, banging—whose significance has not been studied (and should not be assumed). Tails can also lack movement and be held in a stiff, still position at all heights, which could either be the dog's natural tail position or a postural display. Stillness is common in dog interactions: for example, play incorporates entire body pauses (including the tail) interspersed within fluid movements and play signals. Outside of play, a still tail should be evaluated along with the entire body to assess meaning.

While often imperceptible to the naked human eye, wags can be performed asymmetrically—more to the right or left of midline—and offer insight into stimulus perception or emotional valence due to brain lateralization hypotheses (Siniscalchi et al. 2021). For example, dogs wagged more to the right side when encountering an owner (suggesting positive valence), while the sight of an unknown, unfriendly dog, prompted more left-side wags (negative valence) (Quaranta et al. 2007). When observing other dogs wagging more to their left side (negative valence), the observer dogs displayed increased cardiac activity and more stress behaviors, suggesting dogs may assess tail asymmetries in their interactions with other dogs (Siniscalchi et al. 2013). Ultimately tails vary in appearance and position such as curled, tucked, or falling to one side, and tails should be evaluated in relation to a normal, relaxed position.

Dog facial expressions and head movements contribute to visual communication, and the mouth imparts numerous signals (Bradshaw and Rooney 2017). Observing whether the mouth is open versus shut is the first consideration, and further qualitative elements provide more detail. An open, relaxed mouth indicates a comfortable dog, while a "tight mouth" could indicate emotional or physical discomfort or fear. Yawns can indicate a soporific state, but context and other behaviors may also indicate a stress-related behavior. The corners of the mouth, or labial commissure, are also meaningful. A "long lip" describes when the commissure is pulled back toward the ear and is often seen in fear, distress, or appeasement displays. In a submissive grin, the lips are retracted, and the teeth are visible, but the eyes may be squinty and the forehead smooth as well as ears pulled back. A "short lip" is pushed forward, forming a tight forward-moving "c" shape of the mouth. This is part of an aggressive display: the top of the muzzle is wrinkled, and the eyes are open and "hard". Mouth positions may be fleeting and challenging to notice, and shelter staff and volunteers may benefit from concerted practice observing subtle dog mouth positions and their relation to other body positions.

Dog tongues hang generously from mouths during play, and a panting tongue in this context can be a sign of pleasure. Panting can also serve as an indicator of acute stress or physical discomfort (Beerda et al. 1998), especially when seen outside the contexts of activity or thermal stress. Oral behaviors, like mouth licking, are often—but not always—identified in situations of stress, pain, or uncertainty (Owczarczak-Garstecka et al. 2018), and they are also a component of appeasement and greetings/active submission. In one study, dogs viewing angry human faces displayed an increase in "mouth licking," suggesting that they may find angry facial expressions aversive (Albuquerque et al. 2018). "Tongue flick" or "tongue out" is described as the tip of the tongue extended and retracted quickly outside food or eating contexts, while "snout licking" describes the tongue moving along the upper lip possibly near the nose (Beerda et al. 1998). Dogs also use tongues socially to investigate substrates and surfaces.

Eye-tracking studies find that dogs attend quickly to the eye region of other dogs (Somppi et al. 2016). A "hard eye" can be present before or during a threat and include a direct and prolonged gaze, sometimes with dilated pupils. A stiff, unwavering body posture may accompany this type of eye presentation. Pupil dilation—caused by activation of the sympathetic nervous system—indicates arousal, but further contextual information is needed to determine whether it is distress or eustress (Polgár et al. 2019). Conversely, "whale eye" is a label applied when the sclera of the eye is visible; it can indicate discomfort or nervousness as it is most frequently caused by gaze aversion. Eyes can also assume an inviting softer, squintier, more almond-shaped appearance, which can be accompanied by a wrinkled brow.

Ears are varied in natural presentation and carriage. Some are permanently pricked, while others droop to the side. Ear carriage is best evaluated by looking at the base of the ear, and the pinna—the external part of the ear—can be assessed from "maximally backwards" to "maximally forward" (Schilder and van der Borg 2004). Even in long-eared breeds like basset hounds, "ears back" can be noted by paying attention to the base. Ears pressed back are generally associated with greater levels of fear, submission, retreat, or even defensive aggression. Alternatively, ears forward suggest interest, attention, alert, or approach.

The body parts that contribute to dog visual communication merit discussion because people can have difficulty attending to actual in situ dog behavior (Tami and Gallagher 2009; Mariti et al. 2012). People often make assumptions and personality assessments about dogs based on *appearance* rather than *behavior*. In one study, an image of a yellow dog was rated as more agreeable, conscientious, and possessing emotional stability as compared to an image of the same dog with black fur (Fratkin and Baker 2013). Surgical procedures like tail docking and ear cropping can also affect personality attributions, and modified dogs have been perceived less positively—more aggressive and dominant, and less playful and attractive—than their natural counterparts (Mills et al. 2016). Awareness of the potential to make assessments based on appearance rather than behavior, coupled with an understanding of where to look for dog visual signals, can help people in their interactions with dogs.

Additionally, artificial selection and dog morphological diversity can impede social signaling and visual communication (Bradshaw and Rooney 2017). For example, brachycephalic dogs lack the highly flexible and expressive faces of more lupine-type dogs, and hair or fur can prevent visible piloerection. Ultimately, some dogs may be physically unable to signal, or their signals may be difficult to notice, and dog behavior should be considered in light of what is physically possible for that dog.

1.4.2 Acoustic Communication

Social animals tend to have wider vocal repertoires than asocial animals, and dogs make a lot more noise than other canids, both in quality and quantity. Dogs whine, yelp, growl, howl, and bark (Lord et al. 2009) in addition to other less-described vocalizations such as pant-laughing and grunting, to name a few.

Howls and barks are loud and noisy. Howls carry for long distances, while barks are for shorter-range communication (Feddersen-Petersen 2000). Both attract attention and can be socially facilitated, although some dogs bark more than others even in the presence of the same stimulus. Barks vary in acoustic property and duration, but each is repetitive and loud. Barks performed in different contexts sound different from one another, so barks from a "stranger approaching," isolation, or play context will each sound distinct (Yin and McCowan 2004). Tonal and high-pitched barks indicate fear or desperation (e.g., "alone" bark), while low-pitched barks that are harsher with little amplitude modulation are described as aggressive (e.g., "stranger approaching" bark) (Pongrácz et al. 2006).

Barks are one of the lesser-appreciated vocalizations and are associated with dog relinquishment and "misbehavior" (Wells and Hepper 2000). Problems with barking can stem from bark quantity (frequency), quality (style or context), or even perceived annoyance (Pongrácz et al. 2016). Yet barking can be affected by altering its consequences, and positive reinforcement procedures have been found effective. Even pairing a neutral stimulus with a tasty treat has been found to decrease barking (Protopopova and Wynne 2015). Barking can be increased or decreased, and people can modulate barking if necessary.

Growls, too, are nuanced, and dogs attend to these differences. Growls can indicate growler size (Taylor et al. 2010), and they are performed in agonistic as well as play contexts. Faragó et al. (2010) recorded growls in three contexts: guarding a bone, growling at an approaching stranger, and during play. These growls were then played to dogs as they approached a bone that was sitting in front of a crate that, unbeknownst to them, had speakers concealed inside. Dogs were more likely to retreat when they heard the "my bone" growl than when they heard the "threatening stranger" growl. People may have more difficulty than dogs in evaluating growls, and people should attend to both dog behavior and context to infer meaning (Faragó et al. 2017).

1.4.3 Olfactory Communication

Dogs are known for their noses and with good reason. Compared to microsmatic, or "poor smelling," animals like humans, dogs have physiological structures that prioritize smelling and can detect and discriminate a large number of, what are for humans, imperceptible odors (Horowitz 2009b). Scent particles enter the dog's nose both by sniffing and regular breathing (Neuhaus 1981). These particles then enter the nasal cavity, where a mucus lining covers the olfactory epithelium and mediates olfaction—smelling (Furton and Myers 2001). Considerably more genes code for olfactory receptors in dogs than in humans (Quignon et al. 2003).

Compared to humans, dogs seek out and access a much wider set of contextual and social information through smell, and olfaction is a major part of dog intra- and interspecific social encounters. Dogs, like many mammals, have a secondary molecule-detection organ, the vomeronasal organ (VNO), that is directly involved in social communication and pheromone assessment (Adams and Wiekamp 1984). Distinct from the main olfactory epithelium, the VNO is located below the nasal cavity, and its receptors also carry information to the olfactory bulb. This chemosensory organ is ordinarily viewed as responsible for pheromone detection in urine, feces, and saliva as well as glands in the anogenital region, mouth, and face. Using odor cues, dogs can discriminate conspecifics as well as identify something unique about themselves compared to other odors (Bekoff 2001; Horowitz 2017). Horowitz (2020) also found that dogs can distinguish their owner's odor from that of a stranger. Additionally, dogs appear to take note of human odors associated with fear or happiness (D'Aniello et al. 2018).

Dog social encounters are marked by close olfactory inspection, particularly of the head and anogenital area. Body sniffing is common between dogs when they first meet, either on or off leash (Bradshaw and Lea 1992; Westgarth et al. 2010). Initial encounters are typically short, and dogs often explore the environment instead of furthering the interaction, a phenomenon that has been described in free-ranging dogs and at dog parks (Howse et al. 2018; Ward 2020). In the samples studied, often self-selected groups at dog parks or open spaces, post-greeting aggression and even play were relatively rare. Direct encounters between dogs at shelters may be rare, and dogs tend to be on leash (or in kennels), and interactions might be thwarted due to shelter operational protocols. Without the opportunity for direct olfactory investigation, these dogs might experience tension, restraint, or frustration upon seeing other dogs, which could affect subsequent intraspecific interactions.

Olfaction also plays a role in dog interactions with people. For example, the anogential and thigh areas of unfamiliar people are investigated more than those areas of the owner, who is already known to the dog (Filiatre et al. 1991). Unfortunately, humans may thwart olfactory investigation, for example, reaching out or descending a hand on top of a dog's head, instead of allowing the dog to approach and sniff.

Communication via scents is common by depositing secretions and excretions in the environment. Urination is more than waste expulsion; canids gain valuable social information by attending to these splatterings and pay considerable attention to unfamiliar urine (Lisberg and Snowdon 2009). Scent marking can even be performed differently between dogs of the same sex. Small male dogs have been found to mark higher than they are tall; hypotheses for why they do this have not yet been tested (McGuire et al. 2018). Depending on the surface, scent marks could be visual, olfactory, or even, possibly, auditory (Bekoff 1979).

Olfaction is essential to the dog *umwelt*, or perceptual world (Horowitz 2009b). Providing dogs with opportunities to actively use their noses—for instance, through nosework—can enhance well-being. Duranton and Horowitz (2019) found that dogs who participated in nosework for two weeks displayed a more optimistic outlook—measured via cognitive bias test—when compared to dogs who participated in heelwork practice. Engaging in sniffing is *good* for dogs. Humans' jobs, as their observers and caretakers, is to know that the dog's nose is constantly engaged, to actively provide them with smelling opportunities, and to not discourage them from using their nose in species-typical ways.

1.5 Complex Behaviors

Behavioral and physiological parameters help assess canine negative and positive affective states. This section focuses on the former, particularly multi-modal behavior patterns

relevant for dog welfare and well-being both in and out of the shelter.

Despite the good intentions of people and organizations, shelters are awash in stressors. While adaptive in that the stress response and fear prompt physiological and behavioral changes when something is perceived as frightening or indicative of danger (Boissy 1995), stressors (or the perception of such) can also be unrelenting. Persistent or chronic stress challenge short- and long-term well-being, and studies identify relationships between stress and a decrease in immune function (Glaser and Kiecolt-Glaser 2005), a decrease in lifespan (Dreschel 2010), and an increase in arousal, fear, and aggression (Dreschel and Granger 2005).

Stress-related behaviors summarized by Mariti et al. (2012) overlap with fear, anxiety, conflict, or appeasement. Snout/lip licking, yawning, whining, and panting are oral behaviors. Dogs may avoid eye contact, look away, or have their ears back. Trembling and body shaking are often indicators of high psychological stress and could be accompanied by a lowered body posture, cowering, and hiding. Dogs paw-lift in both social and asocial contexts, when alone and distressed, and also during social (inter- or intraspecific) conflict, confusion, or fear (e.g., of punishment). Periods of continual barking, whining, and howling suggest frustration or distress, although vocalization could also be socially mediated and serve other functions. Dogs with either low or high activity should be monitored for additional behaviors of anxiety. Dogs may also be excessive or under-consumers of food and water. Individual differences are common, and behaviors presented can be affected by stressor type, such as social or non-social context, as well as severity and duration. Overt indicators such as trembling and whining may be more recognizable than subtle behaviors, for example, turning away, yawning, and licking (Mariti et al. 2012).

Stress-related, fear, and aggressive behaviors can be connected. If pressed, dogs exhibiting fearful postures may freeze, continue to withdraw, flip onto their backs in a display of passive submission, or display a defensive attack. Defensive aggression differs from an offensive display in that the defensive dog's posture is pulled back, with ears back and tail tucked. Ultimately, the dog is attempting to increase distance from the fear-inducing stimulus but may come forward to bite prior to retreating. Alternatively, dogs displaying more offensive aggression may lean forward with a fixed stare, raised tail, and stiff or frozen body and present a "hard eye" with a closed mouth or offensive pucker, in a sense making themselves appear bigger.

Dog bites to people can occur in any context where dogs and humans overlap, such as situations where resources are present (like food or toys), on private property, in play, and during seemingly "normal" interactions (like petting or being in a dog's presence), as well as in occupational contexts such as those involving entering the dog's home environment, or veterinary or shelter work, among others. People are often familiar with the dog who bit them, and young children, who are often bitten on the face or upper body, constitute a large number of those bitten (Reisner et al. 2011). Breed, neuter status, age, and sex are often explored as contributory factors to bites, yet relationships between these factors and bites are not always clear and should be interpreted cautiously (Newman et al. 2017). Instead, the conditions under which a dog is reared, kept, or managed—such as lacking socialization experience or being left unsupervised with children—could increase bite risk. A UK survey found that numerous factors influence the presence of aggressive displays, and a dog who shows aggressive behavior in one context, such as outside the home, might not do so in another context, such as in the home (Casey et al. 2014). Dogs cannot be characterized as universally "safe" or universally "dangerous," as people might like.

Human behavior prior to a bite is an important piece of the puzzle. Owczarczak-Garstecka et al. (2018) analyzed dozens of bites from YouTube videos and found that human contact-related behaviors increased approximately 20 seconds prior to the bite. Petting, restraining, and "standing over" the dog were observed frequently. On the dog's part, behaviors such as low body position, head turning, and panting, as well as staring and stiffening, increased approximately 30 seconds prior to the bite. These findings are valuable: they suggest that bites are not "coming out of nowhere," highlight the value of the "ladder of aggression" theory (Shepherd 2009), and suggest that people could notice dog signals and respond in turn. The ladder of aggression suggests that dog responses to threatening or stressful stimuli (social, environmental, or other) tend to be graded. A dog is apt to yawn, lick, look away, or move away before growling, snapping, or biting. These cues, proceeding from subtle to overt, aim to increase distance, and while not all dogs will exhibit all signals, the ladder concept provides a general or average progression. These subtle behaviors demand attention because if ignored, dogs might learn that these behaviors are ineffectual and develop a lower threshold for more overt distance-increasing indicators, like growling, barking, baring teeth, lunging, and even biting.

Abnormal behaviors are also present in captive environments and suggest a negative affective state. While taken from the normal repertoire of the species, these behaviors are inappropriate in terms of the manner and context in which they are performed. They can be repetitive, unvarying, and seemingly without immediate goal or function (Mason 1991), or they can be goal directed but abnormally repeated or performed outside typical contexts (Dodman et al. 2010). Abnormal repetitive behaviors (ARBs) manifest differently between species, and in dogs, pacing, spinning or tail chasing, and bouncing off the wall are common. Dogs also chase shadows and perform oral motor patterns like enclosure biting, excessive licking, excessive drinking (polydipsia), flank sucking, feet chewing, snapping at the air (fly snapping), and/or excessive grooming. Studies have also found an increased incidence of certain ARBs in particular breeds, such as flank sucking in Dobermans, tail chasing in bull terriers, and shadow/light chasing in herding breeds (Tynes and Sinn 2014).

While ARBs can develop as a coping mechanism to poor environments, they can persist even after environmental improvement and even be present in highly enriched settings (Garner 2005). In poor environments, ARBs could offer a sort of "do-it-yourself" enrichment, and non-stereotyping individuals in poor environments could be in a worse state than stereotyping individuals (Mason and Latham 2004). Factors such as individual coping styles and kennel space could affect ARB presentation (Protopopova 2016). While ARBs could perseverate because of reinforcement, they are suggestive of an experience of chronic rather than acute stress, at some point (Polgár et al. 2019).

Overly generalized treatment plans are typically not recommended. Sequential behavior analysis of shelter dogs performing any form of ARB found that sequences ranged from highly repetitive to quite variable, suggesting ARBs necessitate personalized care strategies (Loftus et al. 2018). Abnormal behaviors can vary in underlying motivation and triggers (Hall et al. 2015), and thwarting behaviors could increase distress or the frequency of new deleterious behaviors. Underlying medical conditions or pain should also be considered.

Similar motor patterns can appear in both positive and negative affective contexts (Csoltova and Mehinagic 2020). For example, "nose lick" may appear in both frustration and positive anticipation contexts (Caeiro et al. 2017; Bremhorst et al. 2019). With this in mind, context and total motor patterns, as opposed to a single behavior in isolation, contribute to meaning. Motor patterns in line with wanting, seeking, or liking are suggestive of positive affect states (Yeates and Main 2008).

Young dogs may spend up to one-third of their awake life in object, social, or locomotor (movement) play; unlike most mammals, dogs continue playing regularly in adulthood (Horowitz 2002). Dogs not only play with one another but readily and often with humans and even other species. Since play appears to be pleasurable, it might seem non-functional, but in fact it is an integral part of dog social and physical development (Rooney and Bradshaw 2014). Cooperative behaviors such as turn taking and self-handicapping appear in social play, demonstrating that dogs are gauging their play partner's size and skill level (Horowitz 2009b). While play uses many behaviors that would be considered aggressive in other contexts—biting, jumping on, tackling, chasing—within play the intensity of the behaviors is moderated; rarely does play turn into aggression. Recognizing and giving space for play is important: play is not only rewarding for the dog and part of normal social life, it can be used as a reward in training, is suggestive of good welfare, and is thought to improve health and well-being (Sommerville et al. 2017). See Chapter 13 for information on play and playgroups in shelter dogs.

1.6 Influences on Dog Behavior

Ask a beagle to herd sheep and you will come face-to-face with a confused beagle as well as genetic influences on behavior. Though genetic influences can be strong and quite prominent in terms of appearance and behavior, they are *tendencies*, not inevitabilities. Additionally, genetics—often discussed at the breed or breeding-line level—is just one influence on behavior, and this section highlights other factors, such as sterilization and shelter environment, that also contribute to why dogs do what they do.

1.6.1 Breeds and Behavior

The result of just a few hundred years of specific breeding has made dogs as diverse in size and morphology as the Great Dane and the

Maltese. Appearance-based variations have driven the breeding of dogs with markedly different body sizes, head sizes and shape, nose lengths, weight, leg lengths, coats, tail lengths, and shape (Bateson 2010). As discussed earlier, changes in "communicative anatomy" can affect intraspecific social behavior (Horowitz and Hecht 2014). While dogs have existed as a separate species from wolves for thousands of years, for most of that time, there were not segregated, genetically isolated breeds. Ancient art and writing suggest that there were distinctive *types* of dogs, from mastiff-type dogs and saluki-shaped dogs, to small, terrier-like lapdogs. However, these were not "purebred" dogs as the word is used today. Dogs were selected for their function: for instance, for herding, guarding, hunting, and as companions (Grier 2006). Today, by contrast, there are an estimated 400 breeds as well as "mixed breeds." The word "breed" is now used to describe a genetically closed population of animals whose members share many physical and behavioral traits. While early dogs were the result of normal evolutionary processes and geographic segregation as well as some human selection, today's "purebred" dogs are entirely the result of artificial selection: that is, dogs are specifically bred with other dogs of the same genetic lineage (Serpell and Duffy 2014). Initially, dogs with desirable traits and appearance were mated with dogs of similarly desirable features, creating new named breeds: German shepherd, pug, golden retriever, Akita, and so on. Some breed members resemble the imagery of ancient dogs, but there is no evidence of a continuous link between the purebred mastiffs and salukis of today and the ancient versions. Shortly after the inception of a breed line, the line is genetically closed, and future pups must be bred exclusively from other members of the breed (Wayne and Ostrander 2007).

The rise of purebred dogs began in the late nineteenth century with the advent of dog breed clubs and dog shows, also known as "the dog fancy". In contrast with the function-based selection of early dogs, purebred dogs have been bred largely to have a particular appearance consistent with a breed "standard"—the description of the ideal appearance and temperament of members of a breed. Extreme breed standards for specific appearance can be physically damaging: to give just one instance, dogs with large heads, such as the Boston terrier and bulldog, must be birthed surgically since they cannot fit out the birth canal of their mothers (Bateson 2010; numerous other deleterious predispositions are described in Asher et al. 2009).

Distinct behavioral tendencies seen in various breeds can reflect genetic changes that often lead to the expression (or change the intensity) of certain behaviors, given an environment that supports that behavior. For instance, the border collie, often used and bred as a herding dog, performs behaviors like showing "eye" (fixing one's gaze at an animal), "stalking" (creeping toward the animal while maintaining eye), and chasing (Coppinger and Schneider 1995). A dog's predisposition to these actions can be molded, with training, into sheep-herding behavior. Other examples of breed tendencies abound: the pointer's tendency to "point" with his body toward game; the retriever's ability to fetch and retrieve game in water or on land; a hound's vocalizations while tracking an animal with his nose; and coursing dogs' running pursuit of game.

In J. P. Scott and J. L. Fuller's classic longitudinal studies of five breeds of dogs (sheltie, cocker spaniel, basenji, beagle, and fox terrier), they noticed distinct differences between the breeds on scales of emotional reactivity, trainability, problem-solving behavior, and other capacities (Scott and Fuller 1965). Subsequent studies continue to identify breed-based heritability of complex behavioral traits (MacLean et al. 2019). For instance, golden retrievers tend to rank highly on trainability, while the beagle ranks low; huskies rank low on attention-seeking, while dachshunds and toy poodles rank high (Serpell and Duffy 2014). At the same time, variance *within* breed is also observed (Mehrkam and Wynne 2014). A study of impulsiveness—the inability to inhibit behavior in the presence of particular cues—found differences between breeds but also within breed, particularly according to working, show, or pet lines (Fadel et al. 2016). While dog behavioral traits may have genetic influences, neither breed nor genetics will predict an individual dog's behavior.

For contemporary dogs who are not employed as working dogs, their behavioral tendencies may be more problematic than functional. For instance, a border collie without sheep to herd may take to stalking and chasing bicyclists and small children who are running. Pursuit of and nipping at the motion of feet in the dog's vicinity is typically an undesired behavior and may even be perceived as "aggressive." A guard dog's barking at legitimate guests may be considered inappropriately "dominant" or "territorial." Owners may wield ill-suited measures to try to fend off this perceived threat to their authority (Herron et al. 2009). In both cases, the tendencies that humans have bred into the dogs are recharacterized as "misbehavior" in a companion-dog context. Giving a new owner some understanding of the breed tendencies of a dog will assist the owner in working appropriately with what could otherwise be considered puzzling or disturbing dog behavior at home.

1.6.2 Spay and Neuter and Behavior

Sterilization—spaying and neutering, or desexing—is currently well established as normal, even preferable, for owned domestic dogs in the United States. Animal protection groups and humane societies advocate dog sterilization, and it is required for dog adoption from many animal shelters. A common argument for sterilization is that it improves the welfare of the individual animal. Another ostensible benefit of sterilization is reducing the population of unwanted animals; however, published evidence of the degree of such benefit in

reducing intake of shelter dogs is limited (Urfer and Kaeberlein 2019).

While state laws and advocacy groups often tout behavioral improvements that result from sterilization, such as reduced roaming behavior, reduced aggression, and fewer unwanted sexual behaviors, including mounting (Horowitz 2019), research is conflicting as to these claims. Studies gauging levels of aggression by male dogs, for instance, have found variously that aggression either decreased, remained at the same level, or even increased after neutering (Bain 2020). What is clear is that sterilized dogs have been "deprived of the ability to perform one of the most fundamental natural behaviours" (Rooney and Bradshaw 2014), which, with the health and behavioral effects still debated, may most robustly reflect a cultural aversion to canine sexual practices (Horowitz 2014). Similarly, it is also clear that early removal of the source of gonadal hormones has repercussions beyond the sexual: the hormones are implicated in functions as varied as bone growth, maintaining muscle mass, and learning and memory (Horowitz 2019). Ideally, considerations about sterilization should take into account the breed, age, and sex of the dog as well as the owner's circumstances and expectations for the dog. See Chapter 4 for further discussion of the physical and behavioral health impacts of spay and neuter.

1.6.3 Shelter Environment

Shelters can be characterized as novel environments, and while less neophobic than their wild relatives, novelty in its many forms can still act as a stressor for dogs. To support dog well-being, shelters increasingly consider individual dog perception of the shelter and use available resources to identify and address challenges posed by new sights, social encounters (both with conspecifics and people), "loud" smells and sounds, and general unpredictability.

1.6.3.1 Age

Puppies may be particularly challenged if there is an inundation of sensory information and lack of socialization opportunities that prepare for later-in-life experiences. Shelters can consider dam and littermate contact, prioritize early life socialization experiences, and explore real-world housing opportunities outside the shelter. Many dogs entering shelters are between one and three years of age and in the midst of social maturity; these dogs would benefit from many of the early life socialization considerations that younger dogs are afforded (Hammerle et al. 2015). Senior dogs may have difficulty coping with separation from an attachment figure as well as novelty. Considering behavioral differences between normal aging and cognitive dysfunction, as discussed earlier, would greatly assist this population. While collecting information on owner-relinquished dogs is valuable—for example, through owner report or behavior observation—so too is not over speculating about a dog's past or future. Owner reports do not always correlate with observed behaviors in shelters or subsequent homes (Stephen and Ledger 2007), and behavior may be modifiable.

1.6.3.2 Prior Kenneling

Prior experiences can affect dog perception of the shelter. Dogs with prior kenneling or sheltering showed a less-activated stress response when introduced to a new kennel environment, while dogs without showed elevated cortisol levels (Rooney et al. 2007). Similarly, dogs relinquished from homes who had not had prior exposure to a shelter showed an increased physiological stress response without adaptation during the first week; meanwhile, dogs marked as strays and returns showed a decreased physiological stress response during that time (Hiby et al. 2006). At the same time, length of stay, coupled with behavior issues—either from before or during a dog's shelter stay—can contribute to chronic stress and diminished well-being.

1.6.3.3 People

Numerous studies find that the mere presence of a human can buffer a dog's stress response to the innate challenges of the shelter environment, yet differences between dogs are also observed (Hennessy et al. 2020). Owner-relinquished dogs—who may be separated from a figure of attachment and lose social stability and predictability—may be particularly challenged; while petting interactions as short as 15 minutes have the potential to reduce physiological stress levels, this reduction was observed in strays, not owner-relinquished dogs (Willen et al. 2017). Additionally, peoples' individual characteristics as well as the nature of the interaction can affect dogs. Some studies find that dogs show more comfort with people who are identified as women than men. Hennessy et al. (1998) found that when men spoke more quietly and petted in a more soothing way, men were as effective as women in maintaining lower dog stress levels. All dog lovers entering shelters should remember that each dog has his own past experiences and may perceive new people as unfamiliar or be wary of their personal characteristics. Considering how physical contact may be interpreted by the dog, allowing dogs to initiate contact and prioritizing consent (Horowitz 2021) as well as modulating one's voice and avoiding direct eye contact can help support dogs in shelters.

1.6.3.4 Conspecifics

Pair or group housing of dogs is often recommended (Hetts et al. 1992). The presence of conspecifics can offer more social complexity—in terms of social interactions and even olfactory composition—which could decrease abnormal behaviors and mitigate stress (Taylor and Mills 2007). At the same time, social housing benefits could be confounded by increased space as well as environmental complexity. While a pilot study moving long-term kenneled dogs from solitary to pair housing identified considerable individual variation, behavior observations generally supported social housing (Grigg et al. 2017). Socially housed dogs showed less active vigilance and a trend toward a reduction in repetitive jumping and pacing as well as a reduction in barking. While aggression or fights are offered as reasons against group housing, these concerns have not been substantiated (Mertens and Unshelm 1996). At the same time, individual dog considerations—such as a history of or observed aggression—and shelter-level features—such as organizational philosophy, facility design, and operation and monitoring capabilities—also factor into social housing decisions.

1.6.3.5 Smells

Introduced odors have had varied effects on dogs. Dogs in the shelter exposed to diffused lavender and chamomile rested more and were less active than dogs exposed to no scent, rosemary, or peppermint (Graham et al. 2005). Introducing pheromones may also affect behavior. Dogs exposed to dog-appeasing pheromone (DAP)—a synthetic version of the pheromone secreted by lactating females after giving birth—for three hours daily on five consecutive days lay down more compared to a control group (Amaya et al. 2020). However, while some studies observe a reduction in stress-related behaviors when exposed to DAP, others have not (Tod et al. 2005; Hermiston et al. 2018). Cleaning products, or the husbandry activities associated with cleaning, could also act as stressors for dogs (Rooney et al. 2009).

1.6.3.6 Sounds

Shelter acoustics generally include husbandry-oriented noises, people talking at varying decibels, barking, and even loud music. Shelter noise levels are in the area of 85 to 120 db, comparable to a subway, jackhammer, or propeller aircraft (Coppola et al. 2006). Noises, depending on their regularity and acoustic properties, can promote acute or chronic stress. Benefits of the addition of human-centric noises, such as different types of music, is somewhat equivocal. Heavy metal music significantly increased dog body shaking, whereas classical music was associated with more resting behavior (Wells et al. 2002). At the same time, the effect of the same or inescapable music over extended periods of time has not been studied.

1.6.3.7 Lack of Predictability and Control

Lack of predictability and control over contingencies are known challenges to welfare (Taylor and Mills 2007). Dogs living on the streets or in homes build up expectations and associations in relation to known environments. The imposition of daily cleaning and feeding and walking schedules as well as consistent interactions can offer shelter dogs a sense of predictability. However, excessive monotony is a risk factor for dogs as well. Creating motivations for dogs to perform behaviors for particular rewards could enhance welfare, and positive affective states could be achieved as a result of self-directed problem solving (McGowan et al. 2014). Identifying potential shelter stressors provides an opportunity to ameliorate them and make them predictable, controllable, or decreased in terms of intensity, frequency, or duration. In shelters, control can be diminished by physical restriction, for example, in terms of space, that limits agency to flee or retreat. As a result, frustration or appetitive behaviors may appear as well as new, possibly undesirable behaviors.

1.7 Conclusions

Dogs have a unique worldview that differs from that of other companion animal species. Although dogs and humans have lived together for thousands of years, dogs maintain their own species-specific worldview, behaviors, and interests. Dogs have not become more "human-like" because some now have birthday parties or Instagram accounts. Dogs living on streets will scavenge, while dogs living in homes might be reprimanded for "exploring" the trash—same behavior, interpreted differently due to context. This chapter asks that people regard dogs on their terms, not ours, and pay direct attention to in situ behavior.

Acknowledgments

We thank Natalya Zahn for lending her artistic talents and eye for dogs to this project. Heaps of thanks to Merav Stein (first edition) and Molly Ball (second edition) for taking on the unenviable task of citation compilation and editing.

Please visit the companion website for video clips and downloadable resources associated with this chapter.

References

Adams, D.R. and Wiekamp, M.D. (1984). The canine vomeronasal organ. *J. Anat.* 138: 771–787.

Albuquerque, N., Guo, K., Wilkinson, A. et al. (2018). Mouth-licking by dogs as a response to emotional stimuli. *Behav. Process.* 146: 42–45.

Aloff, B. (2005). *Canine Body Language: A Photographic Guide Interpreting the Native Language of the Domestic Dog*. Wenatchee, WA: Dogwise Publishing.

Amaya, V., Paterson, M.B.A., and Phillips, C.J.C. (2020). Effects of olfactory and auditory enrichment on the behaviour of shelter dogs. *Animals* 10: 581.

American Veterinary Society of Animal Behavior. (2008). AVSAB Position Statement on Puppy Socialization. https://avsab.org/wp-content/uploads/2018/03/Puppy_Socialization_Position_Statement_Download_-_10-3-14.pdf (accessed 7 April 2021).

Asher, L., Diesel, G., Summers, J.F. et al. (2009). Inherited defects in pedigree dogs. Part 1: Disorders related to breed standards. *Vet. J.* 182: 402–411.

Asher, L., England, G.C.W., Sommerville, R., and Harvey, N.D. (2020). Teenage dogs? Evidence for adolescent-phase conflict behaviour and an association between attachment to humans and pubertal timing in the domestic dog. *Biol. Lett.* 16: 20200097.

Bain, M. (2020). Surgical and behavioral relationships with welfare. *Front. Vet. Sci.* 7: 519

Barrera, G., Dzik, V., Cavalli, C. et al. (2018). Effect of intranasal oxytocin administration on human-directed social behaviors in shelter and pet dogs. *Front. Psychol.* 9: 2227.

Bateson, P. (1979). How do sensitive periods arise and what are they for? *Anim. Behav.* 27: 470–486.

Bateson, P. (2010). Independent inquiry into dog breeding. University of Cambridge. Report.

Beerda, B., Schilder, M.B.H., van Hooff, J.A.R.A.M. et al. (1998). Behavioural, saliva cortisol and heart rate responses to different types of stimuli in dogs. *Appl. Anim. Behav. Sci.* 58: 365–381.

Bekoff, M. (1979). Ground scratching by male domestic dogs: A composite signal. *J. Mammal.* 60: 847–848.

Bekoff, M. (2001). Observations of scent-marking and discriminating self from others by a domestic dog (*Canis familiaris*): Tales of displaced yellow snow. *Behav. Process.* 55: 75–79.

Bennett, P.C. and Perini, E. (2003). Tail docking in dogs: A review of the issues. *Aust. Vet. J.* 81: 208–218.

Bhattacharjee, D., Mandal, S., Shit, P. et al. (2020). Free-ranging dogs are capable of utilizing complex human pointing cues. *Front. Psychol.* 10: 2818.

Blackwell, E. (2010). Socialization. In: *The Encyclopedia of Applied Animal Behaviour & Welfare* (eds. D.S. Mills et al.), 567–568. Wallingford, UK: CAB International.

Boissy, A. (1995). Fear and fearfulness in animals. *Q. Rev. Biol.* 70: 165–191.

Bowlby, J. (1958). The nature of the child's tie to his mother. *Int. J. Psychoanal.* 39: 350–373.

Bradshaw, J.W.S. and Lea, A.M. (1992). Dyadic interactions between domestic dogs. *Anthrozoös* 5: 245–253.

Bradshaw, J.W.S., Rooney, N. (2017). Dog social behavior and communication. In: *The Domestic Dog: Its Evolution, Behavior and*

Interactions with People (ed. J. Serpell), 133–159. Cambridge, UK: Cambridge University Press.

Bremhorst, A., Sutter, N.A., Würbel, H. et al. (2019). Differences in facial expressions during positive anticipation and frustration in dogs awaiting a reward. *Sci. Rep.* 9: 19312.

Caeiro, C., Guo, K. and Mills, D. (2017). Dogs and humans respond to emotionally competent stimuli by producing different facial actions. *Sci. Rep.* 7: 15525.

Case, L. (2005). *The Dog: Its Behavior, Nutrition, and Health*, 2nd ed. Ames, IA: Blackwell.

Casey, R.A., Loftus, B., Bolster, C. et al. (2014). Human directed aggression in domestic dogs (*Canis familiaris*): Occurrence in different contexts and risk factors. *Appl. Anim. Behav. Sci.* 152: 52–63.

Chapagain, D., Range, F., Huber, L. et al. (2018). Cognitive aging in dogs. *Gerontology* 64: 165–171.

Chin, L. (2020). *Doggie Language: A Dog Lover's Guide to Understanding Your Best Friend*. London: Summersdale Publishers Ltd.

Cimarelli, G., Marshall-Pescini, S., Range, F. et al. (2019). Pet dogs' relationships vary rather individually than according to partner's species. *Sci. Rep.* 9: 3437.

Coppinger, R. and Schneider, R. (1995). Evolution of working dogs. In: *The Domestic Dog: Its Evolution, Behaviour and Interactions with (eople* (ed. J. Serpell), 21–47. Cambridge, UK: Cambridge University Press.

Coppola, C.L., Enns, R.M., and Grandin, T. (2006). Noise in the animal shelter environment: Building design and the effects of daily noise exposure. *J. Appl. Anim. Welf. Sci.* 9: 1–7.

Csoltova, E. and Mehinagic, E. (2020). Where do we stand in the domestic dog (*Canis familiaris*) positive-emotion assessment: A state-of-the-art review and future directions. *Front. Psychol.* 11: 2131.

D'Aniello, B., Semin, G.R., Alterisio, A. et al. (2018). Interspecies transmission of emotional information via chemosignals: from humans to dogs (*Canis lupus familiaris*). *Anim. Cogn.* 21: 67–78.

Dietz, L., Arnold, A.K., Goerlich-Jansson, V.C. et al. (2018). The importance of early life experiences for the development of behavioural disorders in domestic dogs. *Behaviour* 155: 83–114.

Dodman, N.H., Karlsson, E.K., Moon-Fanelli, A. et al. (2010). A canine chromosome 7 locus confers compulsive disorder susceptibility. *Mol. Psychiatry* 15: 8–10.

Dreschel, N.A. (2010). The effects of fear and anxiety on health and lifespan in pet dogs. *Appl. Anim. Behav. Sci.* 125: 157–162.

Dreschel, N.A. and Granger, D.A. (2005). Physiological and behavioral reactivity to stress in thunderstorm-phobic dogs and their caregivers. *Appl. Anim. Behav, Sci.* 95: 153–168.

Duranton, C. and Gaunet, F. (2018). Behavioral synchronization and affiliation: Dogs exhibit human-like skills. *Learn. Behav.* 46: 364–373.

Duranton, C. and Horowitz, A. (2019). Let me sniff! Nosework induces positive judgement bias in pet dogs. *Appl. Anim. Behav. Sci.* 211: 61–66.

Elliot, O. and Scott, J.P. (1961). The development of emotional distress reactions to separation, in puppies. *J. Genet. Psychol.* 99: 3–22.

Fadel, F.R., Driscoll, P., Pilot, M. et al. (2016). Differences in trait impulsivity indicate diversification of dog breeds into working and show lines. *Sci. Rep.* 6: 22162.

Faragó, T., Pongrácz, P., Range, F. et al. (2010). "The bone is mine": Affective and referential aspects of dog growls. *Anim. Behav.* 79: 917–925.

Faragó, T., Takács, N., Miklósi, Á. et al. (2017). Dog growls express various contextual and affective content for human listeners. *R. Soc. Open Sci.* 4: 170134.

Feddersen-Petersen, D.U. (2000). Vocalisation of European wolves (*Canis lupus lupus* L.) and various dog breeds (*Canis lupus f. familiaris*). *Arch. Tierz.* 43: 387–397.

Filiatre, J.C., Millot, J.L., and Eckerlin, A. (1991). Behavioural variability of olfactory exploration of the pet dog in relation to human adults. *Appl. Anim. Behav. Sci.* 30: 341–350.

Fratkin, J.L. and Baker, S.C. (2013). The role of coat color and ear shape on the perception of personality in dogs. *Anthrozoös* 26: 125–133.

Fugazza, C., Moesta, A., Pogány, A. et al. (2018). Social learning from conspecifics and humans in dog puppies. *Sci. Rep.* 8: 9257.

Furton, K.G. and Myers, L.J. (2001). The scientific foundation and efficacy of the use of canines as chemical detectors for explosives. *Talanta* 54: 487–500.

Gácsi, M., Topál, J., Miklósi, Á. et al. (2001). Attachment behavior of adult dogs (*Canis familiaris*) living at rescue centers: Forming new bonds. *J. Comp. Psychol.* 115: 423–431.

Garner, J.P. (2005). Stereotypies and other abnormal repetitive behaviors: Potential impact on validity, reliability, and replicability of scientific outcomes. *ILAR J.* 46: 106–117.

Gazzano, A., Mariti, C., Notari, L. et al. (2008). Effects of early gentling and early environment on emotional development of puppies. *Appl. Anim. Behav. Sci.* 110: 294–304.

Glaser, R. and Kiecolt-Glaser, J.K. (2005). Stress-induced immune dysfunction: Implications for health. *Nat. Rev. Immunol.* 5: 243–251.

Graham, L., Wells, D.L., and Hepper, P.G. (2005). The influence of olfactory stimulation on the behaviour of dogs housed in a rescue shelter. *Appl. Anim. Behav. Sci.* 91: 143–153.

Grier, K.C. (2006). *Pets in America: A History.* Orlando, FL: Harcourt.

Grigg, E.K., Nibblett, B.M., Robinson, J.Q. et al. (2017). Evaluating pair versus solitary housing in kennelled domestic dogs (*Canis familiaris*) using behaviour and hair cortisol: A pilot study. *Vet. Rec. Open* 4: e000193.

Hall, N.J., Protopopova, A., and Wynne, C.D.L. (2015). The role of environmental and owner-provided consequences in canine stereotypy and compulsive behavior. *J. Vet. Behav.* 10: 24–35.

Hammerle, M., Horst, C., Levine, E. et al. (2015). AAHA canine and feline behavior management guidelines. *J. Am. Anim. Hosp. Assoc.* 51: 205–221.

Harvey, N.D., Craigon, P.J., Sommerville, R. et al. (2016). Test-retest reliability and predictive validity of a juvenile guide dog behavior test. *J. Vet. Behav.* 11: 65–76.

Hennessy, M.B., Willen, R.M., and Schiml, P.A. (2020). Psychological stress, its reduction, and long-term consequences: What studies with laboratory animals might teach us about life in the dog shelter. *Animals* 10: 2061.

Hennessy, M.B., Williams, M.T., Miller, D.D. et al. (1998). Influence of male and female petters on plasma cortisol and behaviour: Can human interaction reduce the stress of dogs in a public animal shelter? *Appl. Anim. Behav. Sci.* 61: 63–77.

Hermiston, C., Montrose, V.T., and Taylor, S. (2018). The effects of dog-appeasing pheromone spray upon canine vocalizations and stress-related behaviors in a rescue shelter. *J. Vet. Behav.* 26: 11–16.

Herron, M.E., Shofer, F.S., and Reisner, I.R. (2009). Survey of the use and outcome of confrontational and non-confrontational training methods in client-owned dogs showing undesired behaviors. *Appl. Anim. Behav. Sci.* 117: 47–54.

Hetts, S., Derrell C., Calpin, J.P. et al. (1992). Influence of housing conditions on beagle behaviour. *Appl. Anim. Behav. Sci.* 34: 137–155.

Hiby, E.F., Rooney, N.J., and Bradshaw, J.W.S. (2006). Behavioural and physiological responses of dogs entering re-homing kennels. *Physiol. Behav.* 89: 385–391.

Horn, L., Huber, L., and Range, F. (2013). The importance of the secure base effect for domestic dogs—Evidence from a manipulative problem-solving task. *PLOS ONE* 8: e65296.

Horowitz, A. (2002). The behaviors of theories of mind, and a case study of dogs at play. PhD dissertation. University of California—San Diego.

Horowitz, A. (2009a). Disambiguating the "guilty look": Salient prompts to a familiar dog behaviour. *Behav. Process.* 81: 447–452.

Horowitz, A. (2009b). *Inside of a Dog: What Dogs See, Smell, and Know*. New York: Scribner.

Horowitz, A. (2014). *Canis familiaris*: Companion and captive. In: *The Ethics of Captivity* (ed. L. Gruen), 7–21. Oxford, UK: Oxford University Press.

Horowitz, A. (2017). Smelling themselves: Dogs investigate their own odours longer when modified in an "olfactory mirror" test. *Behav. Process.* 143: 17–24.

Horowitz, A. (2019). *Our Dogs, Ourselves: The Story of a Singular Bond*. New York: Scribner.

Horowitz, A. (2020). Discrimination of person odor by owned domestic dogs. *Int. J. Comp. Psychol.* 33: 1–8.

Horowitz, A. (2021). Considering the "dog" in dog-human interaction. *Front. Vet. Sci.* https://doi.org/10.3389/fvets.2021.642821.

Horowitz, A. and Hecht, J. (2014). Looking at dogs: Moving from anthropocentrism to canid umwelt. In: *Domestic Dog Cognition and Behavior* (ed. A. Horowitz), 201–219. Berlin: Springer-Verlag.

Howell, T.J., King, T., and Bennett, P.C. (2015). Puppy parties and beyond: The role of early age socialization practices on adult dog behavior. *Vet. Med. Res. Rep.* 6: 143–153.

Howse, M.S., Anderson, R.E., and Walsh, C.J. (2018). Social behaviour of domestic dogs (*Canis familiaris*) in a public off-leash dog park. *Behav. Process.* 157: 691–701.

Kaminski, J., Call, J., and Fischer, J. (2004). Word learning in a domestic dog: Evidence for "fast mapping." *Science* 304: 1682–1683.

Kiley-Worthington, M. (1976). The tail movements of ungulates, canids and felids with particular reference to their causation and function as displays. *Behaviour* 56: 69–115.

Kis, A., Ciobica, A., and Topàl, J. (2017). The effect of oxytocin on human-directed social behaviour in dogs (*Canis familiaris*). *Horm. Behav.* 94: 40–52.

Kubinyi, E. and Iotchev, I.B. (2020). A preliminary study toward a rapid assessment of age-related behavioral differences in family dogs. *Animals* 10: 1222.

Landsberg, G.M., Hunthasuen, W.L., and Ackerman, L.J. (2003). The effects of aging on the behavior of senior pets. In: *Handbook of Behavior Problems of the Dog and Cat*, 2nd ed. (eds. G.M. Landsberg, W.L. Hunthausen, and L. Ackerman), 269–304. Edinburgh: Elsevier.

Leaver, S.D.A. and Reimchen, T.E. (2008). Behavioural responses of *Canis familiaris* to different tail lengths of a remotely-controlled life-size dog replica. *Behaviour* 145: 377–390.

Lisberg, A.E. and Snowdon, C.T. (2009). The effects of sex, gonadectomy and status on investigation patterns of unfamiliar conspecific urine in domestic dogs, *Canis familiaris. Anim. Behav.* 77: 1147–1154.

Loftus, B.A., Asher, L., and Casey, R.A. (2018). Sequential analysis to quantify variability in canine abnormal repetitive behaviour. *Proceedings of the 11th International Conference on Methods and Techniques in Behavioral Research*, Manchester, United Kingdom (6–8 June 2018). Manchester, UK: Measuring Behavior 2018.

Lord, K., Feinstein, M., and Coppinger, R. (2009). Barking and mobbing. *Behav. Process.* 81: 358–368.

MacLean, E. L., Snyder-Mackler, N., vonHoldt, B. M. et al. (2019). Highly heritable and functionally relevant breed differences in dog behaviour. *Proc. R. Soc. B.* 286: 20190716.

Mariti, C., Carlone, B., Ricci, E. et al. (2014). Intraspecific attachment in adult domestic dogs (*Canis familiaris*): Preliminary results. *Appl. Anim. Behav. Sci.* 152: 64–72.

Mariti, C., Carlone, B., Votta, E. et al. (2017). Intraspecific relationships in adult domestic dogs (*Canis familiaris*) living in the same household: A comparison of the relationship with the mother and an unrelated older female dog. *Appl. Anim. Behav. Sci.* 194: 62–66.

Mariti, C., Gazzano, A., Moore, J.L. et al. (2012). Perception of dogs' stress by their owners. *J. Vet. Behav.* 7: 213–219.

Marshall-Pescini, S., Cafazzo, S., Virányi, Z. et al. (2017). Integrating social ecology in explanations of wolf-dog behavioral differences. *Curr. Opin. Behav. Sci.* 16: 80–86.

Mason, G.J. (1991). Stereotypies: A critical review. *Anim. Behav.* 41: 1015–1037.

Mason, G.J. and Latham, N.R. (2004). Can't stop, won't stop: Is stereotypy a reliable animal welfare indicator? *Anim. Welf.* 13: S57–S69.

McGowan, R.T.S., Rehn, T., Norling, Y. et al. (2014). Positive affect and learning: Exploring the "Eureka Effect" in dogs. *Anim. Cog.* 17: 577–587.

McGuire, B., Olsen, B., Bemis, K.E. et al. (2018). Urine marking in male domestic dogs: Honest or dishonest? *J. Zool.* 306: 163–170.

McMillan, F.D. (2017). Behavioral and psychological outcomes for dogs sold as puppies through pet stores and/or born in commercial breeding establishments: Current knowledge and putative causes. *J. Vet. Behav.* 19: 14–26.

Mehrkam, L.R and Wynne, C.D.L. (2014). Behavioral differences among breeds of domestic dogs (*Canis lupus familiaris*): Current status of the science. *Appl. Anim. Behav. Sci.* 155: 12–27.

Mertens, P.A. and Unshelm, J. (1996). Effects of group and individual housing on the behavior of kennelled dogs in animal shelters. *Anthrozoös* 9: 40–51.

Miklósi, Á. (2015). Affiliative and agonistic social relationships. In: *Dog Behaviour, Evolution and Cognition*, 2nd ed., 223–251. Oxford, UK: Oxford University Press.

Miklósi, Á., Polgárdi, R., Topál, J. et al. (2000). Intentional behaviour in dog-human communication: An experimental analysis of "showing" behaviour in the dog. *Anim. Cog.* 3: 159–166.

Mills, K.E., Robbins, J., and von Keyserlingk, M.A.G. (2016). Tail docking and ear cropping dogs: Public awareness and perceptions. *PLOS ONE* 11: e0158131.

Mongillo, P., Pitteri, E., Carnier, P. et al. (2013). Does the attachment system towards owners change in aged dogs? *Physiol. Behav.* 120: 64–69.

Müller, C.A., Schmitt, K., Barber, A.L.A., et al. (2015). Dogs can discriminate emotional expressions of human faces. *Curr. Biol.* 25: 601–605.

Neuhaus, V.W. (1981). The importance of sniffing to the olfaction of the dog. *Z. Saugetierkd.* 46: 301–310.

Newman, J., Christley, R.M., Westgarth, C. (2017). Risk factors for dog bites—An epidemiological perspective. In: *Dog Bites: A Multidisciplinary Perspective* (eds. D.S. Mills and C. Westgarth), 133–158. Sheffield, UK: 5m Publishing.

Owczarczak-Garstecka, S.C., Watkins, F., Christley, R. et al. (2018). Online videos indicate human and dog behaviour preceding dog bites and the context in which bites occur. *Sci. Rep.* 8: 7147.

Pierantoni, L., Albertini, M., and Pirrone, F. (2011). Prevalence of owner-reported behaviours in dogs separated from the litter at two different ages. *Vet. Rec.* 169: 468–473.

Pilley, J. W. and Reid, A. K. (2011). Border collie comprehends object names as verbal referents. *Behav. Processes* 86: 184–195.

Pluijmakers, J.J.T.M., Appleby, D.L., and Bradshaw, J.W.S. (2010). Exposure to video images between 3 and 5 weeks of age decreases neophobia in domestic dogs. *Appl. Anim. Behav. Sci.* 126: 51–58.

Polgár, Z., Blackwell, E.J., and Rooney, N.J. (2019). Assessing the welfare of kennelled dogs—A review of animal-based measures. *Appl. Anim. Behav. Sci.* 213: 1–13.

Pongrácz, P., Czinege, N., Haynes, T.M.P. et al. (2016). The communicative relevance of auditory nuisance barks that are connected to negative inner states in dogs can predict annoyance level in humans. *Interaction* 17: 19–40.

Pongrácz, P., Molnár, C., and Miklósi, Á. (2006). Acoustic parameters of dog barks carry emotional information for humans. *Appl. Anim. Behav. Sci.* 100: 228–240.

Powell, L., Edwards, K.M., Bauman, A. et al (2019a). Canine endogenous oxytocin responses to dog-walking and affiliative human-dog interactions. *Animals* 9: 51.

Powell, L., Guastella, A.J., McGreevy, P. et al. (2019b). The physiological function of oxytocin in humans and its acute response to human-dog interactions: A review of the literature. *J. Vet. Behav.* 30: 25–32.

Protopopova, A. (2016). Effects of sheltering on physiology, immune function, behavior, and the welfare of dogs. *Physiol. Behav.* 159: 95–103.

Protopopova, A. and Wynne, C.D.L. (2015). Improving in-kennel presentation of shelter dogs through response-dependent and response-independent treat delivery. *J. Appl. Behav. Anal.* 48: 590–601.

Quaranta, A., Sinischalchi, M., and Vallortigara, G. (2007). Asymmetric tail-wagging responses by dogs to different emotive stimuli. *Curr. Biol.* 17: R199–R201.

Quignon, P., Kirkness, E., Cadieu, E. et al. (2003). Comparison of the canine and human olfactory receptor gene repertoires. *Genome Biol.* 4: 80.1–80.9.

Ramos, D. and Mills, D.S. (2019). Limitations in the learning of verbal content by dogs during the training of OBJECT and ACTION commands. *J. Vet. Behav.* 31: 92–99.

Rehn, T. and Keeling, L.J. (2016). Measuring dog-owner relationships: Crossing boundaries between animal behaviour and human psychology. *Appl. Anim. Behav. Sci.* 183: 1–9.

Reid, P.J. (2009). Adapting to the human world: Dogs' responsiveness to our social cues. *Behav. Process.* 80: 325–333.

Reisner, I.R., Nance, M.L., Zeller, J.S. et al. (2011). Behavioural characteristics associated with dog bites to children presenting to an urban trauma centre. *Inj. Prev.* 17: 348–353.

Riedel, J., Schumann, K., Kaminski, J. et al. (2008). The early ontogeny of human-dog communication. *Anim. Behav.* 75: 1003–1014.

Romero, T., Nagasawa, M., Mogi, K. et al. (2014). Oxytocin promotes social bonding in dogs. *Proc. Natl. Acad. Sci. U.S.A.* 111: 9085–9090.

Rooney, N.J. and Bradshaw, J.W.S. (2014). Canine welfare science: An antidote to sentiment and myth. In: *Domestic Dog Cognition and Behavior* (ed. A. Horowitz), 241–274. Heidelberg, Germany: Springer-Verlag.

Rooney, N.J., Bradshaw, J.W.S., and Robinson, I.H. (2001). Do dogs respond to play signals given by humans? *Anim. Behav.* 61: 715–722.

Rooney, N.J., Clark, C.C.A., and Casey, R. A. (2016). Minimizing fear and anxiety in working dogs: A review. *J. Vet. Behav.* 16: 53–64.

Rooney, N.J., Gaines, S.A., and Bradshaw, J.W.S. (2007). Behavioural and glucocorticoid responses of dogs (*Canis familiaris*) to kenneling: Investigating mitigation of stress by prior habituation. *Physiol. Behav.* 92: 847–854.

Rooney, N.J., Gaines, S., and Hiby, E. (2009). A practitioner's guide to working dog welfare. *J. Vet. Behav.* 4: 127–134.

Salvin, H.E., McGreevy, P.D., Sachdev, P.S. et al. (2011). Growing old gracefully—Behavioral changes associated with "successful aging" in the dog, *Canis familiaris*. *J. Vet. Behav.* 6: 313–320.

Santos, N.R., Beck, A., and Fontbonne, A. (2020). A review of maternal behaviour in dogs and potential areas for further research. *J. Small Anim. Pract.* 61: 85–92.

Sapolsky, R.M. (2018). Double-edged swords in the biology of conflict. *Front. Psychol.* 9: 2625.

Schaebs, F.S., Deschner, T., Range, F. et al. (2020). Consistency and efficacy of two methods of intranasal oxytocin application in dogs. *Domest. Anim. Endocrinol.* 72: 106436.

Schenkel, R. (1967). Submission: Its features and function in the wolf and dog. *Am. Zool.* 7: 319–329.

Schilder, M.B.H. and van der Borg, J.A.M. (2004). Training dogs with help of the shock collar: Short and long term behavioural effects. *Appl. Anim. Behav. Sci.* 85: 319–334.

Schwab, C. and Huber, L. (2006). Obey or not obey? Dogs (*Canis familiaris*) behave differently in response to attentional states of their owners. *J. Comp. Psychol.* 120: 169–175.

Scott, J.P. and Fuller, J.L. (1965). *Genetics and the Social Behavior of the Dog*. Chicago: University of Chicago Press.

Serpell, J.A. and Duffy, D.L. (2014). Dog breeds and their behavior. In: *Domestic Dog Cognition and Behavior: The Scientific Study of* Canis familiaris (ed. A. Horowitz), 31–57. Heidelberg, Germany: Springer-Verlag.

Serpell, J.A. and Duffy, D.L. (2016). Aspects of juvenile and adolescent environment predict aggression and fear in 12-month-old guide dogs. *Front. Vet. Sci.* 3: 49.

Serpell, J.A., Duffy, D.L., and Jagoe, A. (2017). Becoming a dog: Early experience and the development of behavior. In: *The Domestic Dog, Its Evolution, Behaviour and Interactions with People* (ed. J. Serpell), 93–117. Cambridge, UK: Cambridge University Press.

Shepherd, K. (2009). Ladder of aggression. In: *BSAVA Manual of Canine and Feline Behavioural Medicine*, 2nd ed. (eds. D.F. Horwitz and D.S. Mills), 13–16. Gloucester, UK: British Small Animal Veterinary Association.

Sinischalchi, M., d'Ingeo, S., and Quaranta, A. (2021). Lateralized emotional functioning in domestic animals. *Appl. Anim. Behav. Sci.* 237: 105282.

Siniscalchi, M., Lusito, R., Vallortigara, G. et al. (2013). Seeing left- or right-asymmetric tail wagging produces different emotional responses in dogs. *Curr. Biol.* 23: 2279–2282.

Solomon, J., Beetz, A., Schöberl, I. et al. (2019). Attachment security in companion dogs: Adaptation of Ainsworth's strange situation and classification procedures to dogs and their human caregivers. *Attach. Hum. Dev.* 21: 389–417.

Sommerville, B.A. and Broom, D.M. (1998). Olfactory awareness. *Appl. Anim. Behav. Sci.* 57: 269–286.

Sommerville, R., O'Conner, E.A., and Asher, L. (2017). Why do dogs play? Function and welfare implications of play in the domestic dog. *Appl. Anim. Behav. Sci.* 197: 1–8.

Somppi, S., Törnqvist, H., Kujala, M.V. et al. (2016). Dogs evaluate threatening facial expressions by their biological validity— Evidence from gazing patterns. *PLOS ONE* 11 (1): e0143047.

Stephen, J. and Ledger, R. (2007). Relinquishing dog owners' ability to predict behavioural problems in shelter dogs post adoption. *Appl. Anim. Behav. Sci.* 107: 88–99.

Szabó, D., Miklósi, Á., and Kubinyi, E. (2018). Owner reported sensory impairments affect behavioural signs associated with cognitive decline in dogs. *Behav. Process.* 157: 354–360.

Tami, G. and Gallagher, A. (2009). Description of the behaviour of domestic dog (*Canis familiaris*) by experienced and inexperienced people. *Appl. Anim. Behav. Sci.* 120: 159–169.

Taylor, A.M., Reby D., and McComb K. (2010). Size communication in domestic dog, *Canis familiaris*, growls. *Anim. Behav.* 79: 205–210.

Taylor, K.D. and Mills, D.S. (2007). The effect of the kennel environment on canine welfare: A critical review of experimental studies. *Anim. Welf.* 16: 435–447.

Thielke, L.E. and Udell, M.A.R. (2020). Characterizing human-dog attachment relationships in foster and shelter environments as a potential mechanism for achieving mutual wellbeing and success. *Animals* 10: 67.

Tod, E., Brander, D., and Waran, N. (2005). Efficacy of dog appeasing pheromone in reducing stress and fear related behaviour in shelter dogs. *Appl. Anim. Behav. Sci.* 93: 295–308.

Topál, J., Miklósi, Á., Csányi, V. et al. (1998). Attachment behavior in dogs (*Canis familiaris*): A new application of Ainsworth's (1969) Strange Situation Test. *J. Comp. Psychol.* 112: 219–229.

Tynes, V.V. and Sinn, L. (2014). Abnormal repetitive behaviors in dogs and cats: A guide for practitioners. *Vet. Clin. N. Am. Small Anim. Pract.* 44: 543–564.

Urfer, S.R. and Kaeberlein, M. (2019). Desexing dogs: A review of the current literature. *Animals* 9: 1086.

Vilà, C., Savolainen, P., Maldonado, J.E. et al. (1997). Multiple and ancient origins of the domestic dog. *Science* 276: 1687–1689.

vonHoldt, B.B. and Driscoll, C.A. (2017). Origins of the dog: Genetic insights into dog domestication. In: *The Domestic Dog: Its Evolution, Behavior and Interactions with People* (ed. J. Serpell), 22–41. Cambridge, UK: Cambridge University Press.

Ward, C. (2020). Greeting behavior between dogs in a dog park. *Pet Behav. Sci.* 10: 1–14.

Wayne, R.K. and Ostrander, E.A. (2007). Lessons learned from the dog genome. *Trends Genet.* 23: 557–567.

Wells, D.L., Graham, L., and Hepper, P.G. (2002). The influence of auditory stimulation on the behaviour of dogs housed in a rescue shelter. *Anim. Welf.* 11: 385–393.

Wells, D.L. and Hepper, P.G. (2000). Prevalence of behaviour problems reported by owners of dogs purchased from an animal rescue shelter. *Appl. Anim. Behav. Sci.* 69: 55–65.

Westgarth, C., Christley, R.M., Pinchbeck, G.L. et al. (2010). Dog behaviour on walks and the effect of use of the leash. *Appl. Anim. Behav. Sci.* 125: 38–46.

Willen, R.M., Mutwill, A., MacDonald, L.J. et al. (2017). Factors determining the effects of human interaction on the cortisol levels of shelter dogs. *Appl. Anim. Behav. Sci.* 186: 41–48.

Yeates, J.W. and Main, D.C.J. (2008). Assessment of positive welfare: A review. *Vet. J.* 175: 293–300.

Yin, S. and McCowan, B. (2004.) Barking in domestic dogs: Context specificity and individual identification. *Anim. Behav.* 68: 343–355.

2

Introduction to Cat Behavior

Julia D. Albright, Christine Calder, and Amy Learn

2.1 Introduction

The domestic cat (*Felis silvestris catus*) remains one of the most popular pets in the United States and throughout much of Europe. Recent survey statistics show that approximately 31.9 million households in the United States are home to more than 58 million cats, with an average of 1.8 cats in each cat-owning home (American Veterinary Medical Association 2018). These data do not capture the millions of community or feral cats that may live amongst people, yet no one claims to own. The ubiquity of the domestic cat may be rooted in its ability to adapt to almost any environment and human perception of the cat as an affectionate yet self-sustaining household pet (Bradshaw et al. 2012). Despite their popularity, many aspects of the cat's normal behavior and cognitive abilities have yet to be explored. Fortunately, the last few decades have seen a rapid rise in research related to human-cat social interactions, cognitive abilities, and factors that may improve welfare or reduce behavior problems within human homes.

2.2 Domestication

Cats and humans have a long and somewhat complicated history. Mitochondrial DNA evidence suggests the *Felis* genus of small cats diverged from other larger members of the Felidae family about 6.2 million years ago. The domestication of cats likely started as a commensal process around the Fertile Crescent approximately 10,000 years ago (Driscoll, Macdonald et al. 2009). Stores of grain created by early agricultural villages attracted mice, which in turn provided an excellent source of food for wildcats (Hu et al. 2014). Individuals with minimal fear of humans would have best survived in close contact with villages, placing more confident cats in proximity to breed and produce offspring with a genetic predisposition for bolder temperaments (Driscoll, Clutton-Brock et al. 2009; Driscoll, Macdonald et al. 2009).

The practice of taming individuals of various *Felis* wildcat species, presumably for their usefulness as rodent hunters, appears to have been commonplace throughout many cultures prior to domestication of the cat (Hu et al. 2014; Serpell 2014). The first archeological evidence of a cat-human relationship dates back almost 10,000 years to a cat skeleton in a Cypriot human grave (Vigne et al. 2016). The success of cats in human cultures, however, cannot be solely attributed to their mousing skills. Appealing juvenile traits like large eyes and a small mouth also likely enticed humans to keep cats as objects of affection, gaining an advantage over other animals, such as those in the weasel family, that were arguably even more efficient vermin exterminators (Serpell 2014). Although many *Felis* species seemed to be feasible candidates for domestication, genetic evidence clearly indicates the sole ancestral species is *Felis silvestrus lybica,* or the African wildcat subspecies (Driscoll, Macdonald et al. 2009).

The perception of cats in human culture has had its highs and lows over the centuries. Cats were revered by some ancient cultures and then demonized in parts of Christian-dominated Europe due to this association with paganism starting in the Middle Ages. The negative connotations spread to the United States, and even today we can see lingering effects, particularly with black cats, in superstitious folklore and literature. Although many countries and cultures never lost their respect for the cat and its usefulness in agrarian society, a more affectionate outlook toward the cat began starting in the eighteenth century. Many consider domestication of the cat as fully achieved during Victorian England, at which time humans began purposefully breeding cats for specific physical traits rather than behavior or function (Montague et al. 2014). The past 150 years has seen the recognition of approximately 50 different cat breeds (Cat Fanciers Association 2020), although purebred cats make up only 6–8% of the total US cat population today (Bradshaw et al. 2012).

2.3 Sensory Perception

The sensory systems of the domestic cat, which are almost identical to other *Felis* wildcats, have evolved to allow these species to become efficient hunters under a variety of environmental conditions. Perception also dictates the manner by which cats communicate with one another and with humans (Brown and Bradshaw 2013).

2.3.1 Vision

Small rodents are typically active at dawn and dusk, and cats have evolved features to enhance low-light vision for crepuscular hunting. Cats have large eyes, and their pupils greatly expand in dark conditions, allowing increased light transmission to the retina. The pupil can narrow to a very thin slit to protect the retina in bright lighting. The tapetum is a reflective layer of tissue in the choroid of the eye. In addition to creating the "eye shine" observed when passing a light across the eyes of a cat (and many other species) at night, this structure also allows any light entering the eye to be reflected and amplified (Houpt 2018). The cat's retina contains about three times more rods than cones. Rods are photoreceptor cells responsible for night vision, but the sacrifice in cone density results in lower visual acuity and color perception. Cats probably have a dichromatic spectrum of mainly blues and greens (Bradshaw et al. 2012). Color is unlikely to be an important factor in a cat's sensory world. Cats have binocular vision but may not be able to focus well on an object within a foot from the eyes. Caged cats are nearsighted compared to outdoor cats (Belkin et al. 1977). Excellent motion detection due to specialized neurocircuitry in the visual cortex is yet another sensory capability that greatly enhances predatory success.

2.3.2 Hearing

Cats are able to detect sounds between 45 and 64,000 Hz, including 10.5 octaves, which is one of the broadest hearing ranges of any mammalian species (Fay and Popper 1994). The high-frequency, even ultrasonic sound perception is likely helpful for the detection of prey and possibly kitten communication, but the evolutionary function for detecting very low-frequency sounds remains a mystery (Bradshaw et al. 2012). The pinnae, or external parts of the ear, are highly moveable, amplify sounds, and allow the cat to more easily pinpoint the location of the source. Additionally, the pinnae position can be used to visually communicate emotional information to a conspecific (Leyhausen 1979; Overall 2013).

2.3.3 Olfaction

The importance of olfactory signals in hunting and conspecific communication has not been well studied. Cats seem to rely less on smell to locate prey compared to dogs (Montague et al. 2014); nevertheless, cats have a relatively robust sense of smell based on the numbers of olfactory receptors (Shreve and Udell 2017). Olfaction in cats, as in most non-human animals, is composed of both the main and accessory systems. The main olfactory system is responsible for scent detection, whereas the distinct secondary system identifies socially relevant chemicals, such as pheromones. At the center of the accessory system is the vomeronasal organ, a cluster of specialized sensory cells that sit above the nasopalatine bone and connect to both oral and nasal passages, allowing evaluation of both airborne and fluid-borne molecules (Brown and Bradshaw 2013). The information is relayed to the emotional centers of the brain, which can permit the animal to physiologically and behaviorally prepare for the appropriate action, usually without any conscious awareness (Mills 2005). A cat using the accessory olfactory system can be observed holding the mouth slightly agape, during which the flicking tongue draws salient molecules into the incisive duct, then up to the vomeronasal organ. The flehmen or "gaping" behavior is most commonly seen when a cat smells a strange cat's urine (Hart and Leedy 1987; Houpt 2018).

2.3.4 Taste

Cats are obligate carnivores and must consume prey animals to obtain essential compounds (Montague et al. 2014). Cats have relatively few taste buds and no ability to taste sweet substances, perhaps because cats have little need to detect plant-based sugars as an energy source. Recent research has shown that cats do have bitter taste receptors, which may provide a means of toxin detection and avoidance (Lei et al. 2015).

2.3.5 Touch and Balance

Balance is due to an integration of information from the visual, vestibular, central, and peripheral nervous systems. Cats are famous for the ability to right themselves during a fall by reflexively twisting the head and spine to land on their feet. This righting reflex relies primarily on the fluid in the bony labyrinth and semicircular canals of the vestibular system (Cremieux et al. 1984).

Whiskers, or vibrissae, are richly innervated specialized hairs with follicles originating from deep in the subcutaneous skin layer on the face, head, and carpi of a cat (Dyce et al. 2010). Mechanical stimulation of the whiskers transmits information to the sensory cortex of the brain and allows the cat to gain information about environmental conditions and objects within close range. Most notably, whiskers provide important information about the movement of prey, kittens, and other social partners immediately adjacent to the cat. Touch becomes the primary sense at close range due to poor visual acuity at this distance (Bradshaw et al. 2012). The cat's canine teeth and claws also have pressure receptors to aid in preventing the escape of prey once captured (Byers and Dong 1989).

At rest cat facial whiskers are positioned slightly backward, but when moving or aroused, whiskers move forward and away from the head to prepare for gathering information (Beaver 2003). Therefore, whisker position can be a form of conspecific visual communication as well.

2.4 Communication

2.4.1 Vocalization

Conspecific vocal communication is only heard during agonistic, sexual, or mother-kitten encounters (Kiley-Worthington 1984). Cats vocalize much more frequently to humans, primarily through the open-mouthed meow (or miaow) sound, which functions as attention seeking with a learned component. Close-range affiliative communications include the purr and the trill. The purr is a care-soliciting behavior heard from kittens when nursing, during friendly interactions, or when the cat is mildly anxious or ill (Crowell-Davis et al. 2004; Overall 2013). The chirr or trill is a modified, mostly closed-mouth meow sound used in greeting. The estrus call is also a closed-mouth vocalization heard from females during courtship and can be similar in character to a type of agonistic male cat call (Overall 2013; Wolski 1982). However, aggressive intercat vocalizations are usually open-mouthed and include the hiss, spit, growl, snarl, growl, yowl, and shriek (Crowell-Davis et al. 2004).

2.4.2 Scent

Urination, defecation, and scratching are behaviors used to disseminate olfactory information (Brown and Bradshaw 2013). Urine, feces, and sebaceous glands, predominantly located on the head, perianal area, and between the digits of the paws, are rich in information about an individual and,

therefore, effective forms of olfactory communication. Head rubbing of objects or social targets leaves olfactory signals from sebaceous glands located on the temporal region of the head, under the chin, and around the lips. This head bunting behavior is often accompanied by purring (Crowell-Davis et al. 2004). Pheromones have been identified from the cheek sebaceous glands (Pageat and Gaultier 2003) and are thought to be a form of conspecific social signaling.

2.4.3 Visual Signals

Body postures and facial expressions communicate intent and emotional state at a particular moment. Specific behaviors and body positions can have multiple meanings; thus, assessing the entire body, other signals (e.g., vocalizations), and the context is critical when humans are trying to interpret a cat's emotional state.

The vertical "tail up" is one of the most important visual signals (see Figure 2.1). It largely signals the desire to interact amicably. The cat receiving a "tail up" signal may reciprocate with an approach, followed by touching

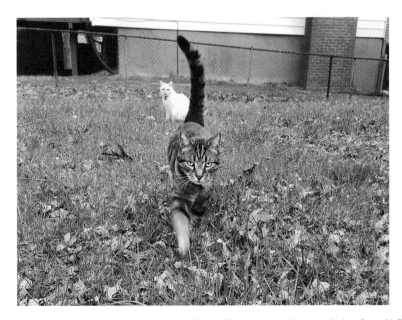

Figure 2.1 Tail up greeting display. *Source:* Reproduced with permission from N. Drain. © Natasha Drain.

noses; rubbing of the head, neck, and body along the body of another cat; and tail twining (Cafazzo and Natoli 2009). A similar approach and rubbing behavior sequence may be displayed toward an individual of another species, especially human, or an object near the intended receiver (Turner 2017). A stiff, lashing tail indicates aggression, and a tail tucked under the body signifies fear in a non-resting cat. Piloerection, or hairs stiffened and standing away from the body, indicates strong arousal and is usually accompanied by an upright or arched body, but the tail may be erect or low. A tail wrapped around the body of a sitting cat is thought to communicate ambivalence—the cat is unlikely to show aggression but is not enthusiastic about the interaction (Leyhausen 1979).

Facial expressions are associated with a range of emotions. A distressed cat's eyes may blink and pupils dilate, ears lower or flatten to the head, and whiskers move forward. These expressions may be accompanied by hissing or other defensive vocalizations (see Figure 2.2). A very relaxed cat is often lying lateral with the eyes, pupils, and ears in a neutral position. A cat resting in a sternal or sphinx-like position, often with the tail wrapped around the body, may be slightly more anxious or vigilant about the surroundings (Leyhausen 1979; Bennett et al. 2017; Gourkow et al. 2014).

General Appendix B describes common feline body language characteristics.

2.5 Behavioral Development

As a species, cats are extremely adaptable to various environments, but the degree of plasticity is determined by a combination of genetics, prenatal environment, and postnatal experiences, especially those occurring during the socialization development period. Born blind, deaf, and completely dependent on the queen for nourishment, the neurological, musculoskeletal, and cognitive maturation of a kitten from birth to adulthood is a short but complex process.

2.5.1 Genetics

Comparative genetics studies have revealed the domestic cat varies from wildcats at 13 chromosomal loci, many of which code for genes related to neurodevelopment or neurotransmitters known to affect various emotional or motivational states, perhaps revealing the genetic basis for tameness

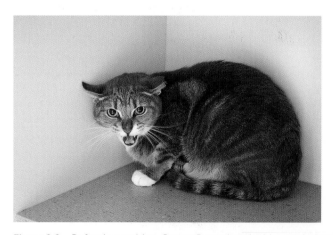

Figure 2.2 Defensive position. *Source:* Reproduced with permission from K. Watts. © Katie Watts.

(Montague et al. 2014). Humans have a long history of enhancing certain traits through genetic selection, and this is most evident in the domestic dog, the species with the greatest morphologic diversity on earth. Humans have a much shorter history of selectively breeding domestic cats, and the primary objective has been advancement of desired physical, not functional, traits. Nevertheless, consistent breed predispositions for certain behavioral characteristics seem to exist. Several observational and survey studies have identified differences among purebred cats in terms of aggression, propensity to elimination outside the litterbox, playfulness, shyness, and activity level (Mendl and Harcourt 2000; Wilhelmy et al. 2016; Salonen et al. 2019). Many people believe that coat color and certain personality traits are linked. For example, calico or tortoiseshell color cats are often thought to be more aggressive and anxious (Stelow et al. 2015). While the owner-queried survey results of Stelow et al. (2015) did indicate some minor increases in aggressive behavior within sex-linked orange color cats, Wilhelmy et al. (2016) found that differences in behavior among purebred cat coat colors were largely explained by breed alone.

Cat personalities seem to be stable and vary along several dimensions of confidence, nervousness, sociability, and activity (Lowe and Bradshaw 2001; Karsten et al. 2017; Litchfield et al. 2017). Personality, like most behavioral phenotypes, is a confluence of environmental and genetic influences. Kittens sired by males with outgoing and friendly personalities were found to show more approach and affiliative behaviors to people, be less stressed by the approach of unfamiliar people, and be more likely to spend time near a novel object (McCune 1995; Reisner et al. 1994). However, handling and socialization provided a protective effect against some fearful and defensive behaviors. Friendly sired but unsocialized kittens behaved in a similar manner to unfriendly sired socialized kittens (McCune 1995).

2.5.2 Sensitive Periods of Development

2.5.2.1 Prenatal

The nutritional status of a dam and her exposure to certain stimuli during the 63-day gestation period can influence postnatal behavior of her offspring. For instance, kittens show a preference for certain flavors fed to their queen during the prenatal period (Becques et al. 2009). Queens placed on protein- or calorie-restricted diets can produce offspring with elevated emotional reactivity and impairments in social interactions, environmental exploration, and learning (Gallo et al. 1980). Even food restriction limited to the second half of gestation can result in abnormal physical and emotional traits (Smith and Jansen 1977). Studies from other mammalian species indicate offspring born to dams exposed to excessive environmental stressors, such as unpredictable noise stimuli, may suffer from impaired cognitive and neurologic development (Schneider and Moore 2000). Kittens exposed to significant prenatal stress may suffer similar developmental dysfunction.

2.5.2.2 Neonatal (0–14 days)

The neonatal period consists of the first two postnatal weeks. The queen encircles the kittens with her body and legs immediately after the birth of all of the kittens. The kittens are suckling within an hour of birth, and a loose teat order is established by 12 hours postparturition (Ewer 1960; Houpt 2018). The kittens engage in little other than suckling and sleeping during the neonatal stage. Waste elimination is initiated by the queen via grooming of the perineal region. Neonate kittens do not have the ability to thermoregulate, and thus body temperature is maintained by huddling with their littermates and mother (Jensen et al. 1980; Olmstead et al. 1979). Tactile, thermal, and olfactory stimuli help the kitten orient to the queen and littermates, as the eyes and ears are closed during much of the neonatal period. Orienting to the queen's abdomen and suckling are highly reflexive behaviors

(Raihani et al. 2009), although nursing is largely initiated by the queen during the first two weeks. Purring is observed in nursing kittens and may serve to communicate active suckling to the mother (Bradshaw 2017). The first set of teeth erupt between 2 and 5 weeks of age with adult teeth erupting at approximately 12 weeks. Movement at this age occurs by limb paddling or pulling of the body by the front limbs due to weaker neuromusculature of the hindlimbs in this early stage.

Kittens are usually able to hear by the fifth day of life, although the external pinnae do not become erect and the ear canal does not open for another few days. Eyes open during the second week, and several factors can influence the exact timing. The eyes of kittens born to younger mothers tend to open earlier than kittens born to older mothers, female kittens' eyes are more likely to open prior to males, and excessively dark conditions hasten eye opening. The timing of eye opening is also heritable (Braastad and Heggelund 1984). Vision becomes the kitten's dominant sensory guide once the eyes are open.

Early maternal care is another important environmental factor in healthy kitten behavioral development. Kittens separated from their mother and hand reared by humans from two weeks of age were more fearful and aggressive toward people and other cats, more sensitive to novel stimuli, developed poor social and parenting skills, and did not learn as well as kittens raised by their mother (Mellen 1992).

Scruffing is a maternal behavior of grasping the kitten's loose skin around the neck and shoulders with her teeth. The kitten reflexively goes limp and quiet. This allows the queen to move her kittens to new dens with a lower risk of detection from predators. In free-roaming situations, a queen typically moves den sites multiple times prior to weaning of the litter. Some cats may retain this limp or trance-like state reflex into adulthood, but many do not, and scruffing by a human during handling usually induces distress (Moody et al. 2020).

2.5.2.3 Socialization (Two–Seven Weeks)

First described by Bateson (1979), kittens have an important "sensitive" period when individual life experiences can have lasting effects on behavioral, neurological, and sensory development. The sensitive period for socialization to humans is thought to occur between the ages of two and seven weeks of age in kittens. In one series of studies, kittens handled by humans between the ages of 3 and 14 weeks were more likely to approach humans and accept human handling for a longer duration than kittens who were handled after 7 weeks or never handled before 14 weeks of age. Withholding handling until 7 weeks of age resulted in kittens who seemed unafraid of humans but did not choose to remain in proximity to humans after initial contact (Karsh and Turner 1988). Another study found that even if handling is delayed to 5 weeks of age, kittens can catch up by 6 months of age in terms of sociability with humans to those kittens for whom handling began several weeks earlier (Lowe and Bradshaw 2001, 2002). These studies indicate that exposure to gentle handling from humans by 7 weeks of age is critical for a cat to enjoy human contact.

Other studies have focused on the quality of human exposure during the sensitive socialization period. Kittens housed at rescue centers demonstrated significantly fewer signs of fear toward humans when handled for two and five minutes daily from birth to 45 days compared to those kittens who experienced only passive exposure to humans during basic husbandry, such as cage cleaning (Casey and Bradshaw 2008). Kittens handled five minutes daily from birth to 45 days of age were more likely to approach strange toys and unfamiliar people as well as slower to learn avoidance tasks (Wilson et al. 1965). The end of the socialization period (seven weeks) corresponds with further development of the emotional system and fear of novel stimuli. Intraspecific social development has received little research attention, but the timeline presumably parallels that of cat-human social development (Bradshaw 2017).

The socialization development period also corresponds to a time of exponential physical development. Kittens begin running around five weeks of age and have full coordination by seven weeks (Peters 1983). Air righting, or the ability of cats to land on their feet after falling, is first observed between the third and sixth week of life. Kittens produce ultrasonic vocalizations, and the pitch becomes lower with age. Expansion of the vocalization repertoire and avoidance of agonistic vocalizations begins around four weeks of age. Interestingly, the vocalizations of deaf kittens are louder but otherwise almost identical to those of kittens with normal hearing (Houpt 2018).

Visual acuity and binocular vision continue to develop during this stage. Cats have been used extensively as models for research into the neurodevelopment of the mammalian visual system. From this research, we know proper sensory development requires environmental stimulation. Deprivation of certain visual stimuli during development creates permanent alterations and deficiencies in the visual cortex. For instance, cats raised in environments with only horizontal lines did not respond to vertical stripes because of degeneration of the neurons responsible for recognizing vertical edges (Blakemore and Cooper 1971). Kittens not allowed to visualize their front paws due to placement in dark conditions or in an Elizabethan collar did not develop fine motor skills needed for placement of the paws (Hein and Held 1967).

2.5.2.4 Juvenile (Seven Weeks–Sexual Maturity)

Socialization with humans may continue to improve into the juvenile period, provided the kitten received some handling from humans in the preceding weeks (Lowe and Bradshaw 2001; McCune 1995). This is assumed to be the case with intercat socialization as well (Bateson 2014).

Rapid physical development allows the kitten to become fully independent from the mother during this period. Kittens have well-developed senses, thermoregulation, movement, and detection of danger by this stage. The weaning process is completed during the juvenile stage, and kittens are fully functioning predators by the early part of the juvenile period. The mother cat initiates weaning by bringing dead prey to the kittens around four weeks of age. As the kittens become more successful at killing prey, she later releases increasingly more mobile prey items near the kittens. Kittens continue to initiate suckling, but the queen gradually decreases the duration of nursing bouts to keep the kittens hungry enough to encourage exploration and hunting behavior. As their motor skills develop, the kittens also follow the dam on hunting trips. Eventually the dam only allows short suckling bouts, presumably for bonding purposes, and weaning of the kittens is usually complete by seven weeks (Bateson 2014).

Weaning age appears to have broader impacts on social and abnormal oral behaviors according to a recent survey study (Ahola et al. 2017). Owners of cats weaned before 8 weeks of age were more likely to report behavior problems than owners of cats weaned in the 12–15-week range. Kittens weaned before 8 weeks were more likely to show aggressive behaviors than those weaned later. Later weaning was a protective factor against aggression toward other cats as well as familiar and unfamiliar people. The prevalence of abnormal oral behaviors like excessive grooming and wool sucking as well as shyness toward novel objects decreased in the kittens weaned after 14 weeks as well (Ahola et al. 2017; Houpt 2018). Overall, owners of cats weaned before 8 weeks of age were more likely to report behavior problems than those weaned in the 12–13-week range. Aggression, abnormal oral behaviors, and shyness toward novel objects were shown to be inversely correlated to the age of weaning as well (Ahola et al. 2017).

2.5.2.5 Adult (Sexual and Social Maturity)

The juvenile period ends with sexual maturity. In female cats, this correlates with the first sign of estrus, which can be as early as 3 to 4 months and as late as 12 months of age. Environmental factors such as the time of year born, exposure to mature tomcats, the presence of other female cats in estrus, and increasing periods of light all influence the age of estrus onset. Male domestic cats reach sexual maturity between 9 and 12 months. In free-ranging cat colonies, however, a male may not become reproductively active until two or three years of age, when full integration into a colony is achieved (Hart and Hart 2014a). Social maturity is the stage of final transition into adult behaviors such as territoriality and aggression and in domestic cats is thought to occur between 36 and 48 months of age (Landsberg et al. 2013).

2.6 Maintenance Behaviors

2.6.1 Play

Play is ubiquitous amongst many genera of animals, and cats are no exception. Domestic cat play behaviors are classified as social, locomotor, predatory, or object play (Delgado and Hecht 2019). It has been widely assumed that play is neuromuscular, social, and cognitive preparation for critical adult behaviors (Burghardt 2005). However, research of kittens raised in barren environments provided evidence that play does not seem to be a required precursor for many behaviors, particularly those like predation that are related to survival (Thomas and Schaller 1954). Early experiences can impact the timing and character of play behaviors. Genetics, sex, learning, and characteristics of the queen, litter, and target of play can alter the development of play behaviors in cats (Delgado and Hecht 2019).

Social interactions begin around 2 to 3 weeks of age in kittens, and social play is apparent by 4 weeks, peaking around 9 to 14 weeks. Social play progresses from chasing and running to stalking and wrestling. Play solicitation behaviors include exposing the belly, pouncing, raising the front paws up, and side stepping (West 1974). As the kitten ages, interest switches from social partners to objects. The first instances of object play coincide with the queen's provision of prey items to her kittens. Object play is very prevalent by 7 weeks, or the end of weaning, but does not peak until around 18 to 21 weeks of age (Mendoza and Ramirez 1987). Object play in older kittens and adults resembles predatory behaviors such as batting, scooping, pouncing, grasping and biting. Singleton kittens, those weaned early, and those under food restriction tend to display more object play (Guyot et al. 1980; Bateson and Young 1981) (see Figure 2.3).

As most cat owners can attest, object play continues into adulthood (Mendoza and Ramirez 1987). Although there are no studies

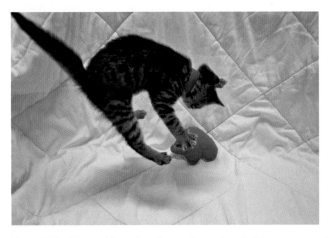

Figure 2.3   Kitten object play. *Source:* Reproduced with permission from M. Allison. © Meg Allison.

documenting any long-term benefits of play in cats, object play is frequently recommended by veterinarians and behaviorists as a tool to provide aerobic exercise and environmental enrichment to cats. Toys that mimic features of a mouse—small, furry, moving in quick motions like prey—seem to elicit the most interest and predatory play response from cats (Hall et al. 2002; Vitale Shreve and Udell 2015). Movement of an object away from the cat elicits a stronger chase reaction (Leyhausen 1979). Repeated interactions with an object can result in habituation, or a loss of interest in that item. Novelty in color, shape, and odor can reduce habituation. Hall et al. (2002) suggest toys that somehow change in shape help maintain a cat's interest in the toy.

2.6.2 Hunting

Cats are highly motivated to hunt. In fact, hunger and recent feeding behavior may reduce consumption and time spent hunting but not the motivation to stalk and capture prey (Fitzgerald and Turner 2000). Cats may even stop eating if the opportunity to hunt and kill presents itself during a meal. A cat may eat 10 to 20 small meals throughout a 24-hour period, although this may be concentrated to crepuscular periods in free-roaming cats but spread throughout the day for housecats. In general, cats living in human homes tend to take on a more diurnal pattern like humans (Overall et al. 2005). Although hunting is a reflexive behavioral pattern displayed even if a cat is raised in isolation, maternal influence and early experience can shape hunting behavior and food preference (Kuo 1930, 1938). Cats are less likely to predate on small mammals if raised with these potential prey species from a young age, preferably starting during the two to seven weeks of age socialization period (Kuo 1938).

2.6.3 Ingestive Behavior

Cats are obligate carnivores and have specific dietary requirements best met through animal-based diets. Several essential compounds cannot be autosynthesized by cats and, therefore, must be obtained from the environment. Animal products contain sulfur-rich amino acids (methionine, cysteine, taurine), vitamins (niacin and thiamine), essential fatty acids, and high-protein content necessary for basic feline metabolic functions. Moreover, cats are limited in their ability to process plant-derived foods (Zoran and Buffington 2011).

Cats can be picky eaters, developing a strong preference for only a few foods while refusing to eat others (Overall et al. 2005; Stasiak 2002). Food preference or aversion can be mitigated if food items with a variety of textures and flavors are presented to kittens at a young age. Cats may develop a learned aversion if a certain food becomes associated with nausea, force feeding, or medication administration (Stasiak 2001).

Obesity is the most prevalent form of malnutrition in cats living in developed countries. In the United States, an estimated 60% of cats have a body condition score above the ideal range, and 34% of cats are classified as obese (Association for Pet Obesity Prevention 2019). Free-roaming cats tend to eat many small meals, and the unnatural practice of feeding housecats one or two larger meals may be a risk factor for obesity. Therefore, offering cats ad libitum food may trigger more natural feeding behavior and intake regulation, but this practice is complicated by competition in multi-cat homes. The optimal feeding routine in a home setting appears to be mimicking natural hunting and feeding strategies by providing opportunities for a cat to seek out food and manipulate food-dispensing objects throughout the day (Rochlitz 2005; Dantas et al. 2016). An alternative could include using food as a reward during behavior training sessions instead of bowl feeding. Such environmental enrichment has been shown to be an effective therapy for stress-related conditions like chronic feline lower urinary tract disease (Buffington et al. 2006) and may also be a means of increasing activity and possibly reducing obesity (Dantas et al. 2016). Indoor cats are at a higher risk for both conditions and enrichment is of particular importance for this population (Rodan and Heath 2015).

Some cats display unacceptable or abnormal oral behaviors. Chewing or ingesting non-food materials (pica) such as plants, fabric, plastic, rubber, cords, or string has been reported by some cat owners (Houpt 2018). Plant or grass eating seems to be a normal behavior, although anecdotally the practice has been linked to gastrointestinal purging (Hart and Hart 2014a). Discomfort due to dental or abdominal pain as well as any metabolic, organ, or neurologic disease should be ruled out or addressed as potential factors in abnormal oral behaviors. Hunger may trigger chewing of unacceptable targets, and some instances of pica may occur during predatory play or predation misdirected toward an object. Chewing can become a learned attention-seeking or stress-displacement behavior in some cats, but excessive pica may be consistent with a compulsive disorder. A behavior can be classified as a compulsive disorder when it is repetitive, occurs outside of the normal context, and, once established, often occurs unrelated to any obvious trigger and interferes with basic functioning. Stress or emotional conflict is thought to be an initiating factor in compulsive disorders. Wool and other fabrics are the most common targets in cats diagnosed with a compulsive pica behavior (Landsberg et al. 2013). Recent studies suggest compulsive pica in cats may be associated with gastric dysregulation (Demontigny-Bédard et al. 2019). In addition to a complete medical assessment, treatment includes restricting access to objects (e.g., blocking access to certain rooms, covering of rubber/plastic cords with PVC piping), enrichment, and potentially psychoactive medications (Landsberg et al. 2013).

2.6.4 Elimination

Basic feline elimination behavior consists of searching for a quiet and secluded area, digging a small depression in an acceptable substrate, and covering the waste after elimination (Heath 2019). On closer inspection, the sequence is actually quite complex and may include up to 39 individual behaviors (McGowan et al. 2017). Cats are known to be fastidious, traveling to specific latrine areas located away from sleeping or feeding sites to eliminate. This limits the odor and reduces the risk of disease and parasite transmission (Hart and Hart 2014a).

Failure to provide an indoor cat with a litterbox environment that sufficiently mimics natural conditions can result in elimination outside of a designated box. Eliminations also serve a communication function, and waste found outside the litterboxes or latrine areas may be an indication of social or environmental stress. Several terms for elimination issues can be found in the literature. Broad descriptors that do not give any indication of the underlying motivation include inappropriate urination, housesoiling, and periuria (if specific to urination) (Barcelos et al. 2018; Borns-Weil 2019). Some have recently argued for replacing the term "inappropriate" with "unacceptable" when referring to feline eliminations outside of designated areas because the cats are behaving normally in most instances, but the human caretakers have provided suboptimal conditions (Heath 2019). The physiologic need to empty the bladder or colon is referred to as toileting or elimination. Urine marking/spraying and middening are depositing urine or feces, respectively, outside of the box for communicative purposes. Risk factors for unacceptable elimination include living in a multi-cat household, suboptimal litterbox facilities, stress and anxiety, and detection of unfamiliar outdoor cats (Borns-Weil 2019; Heath 2019). Research findings warn against using any single factor to diagnose toileting or marking behavior (Barcelos et al. 2018).

Housesoiling is often a life-threatening condition in cats due to the high risk of relinquishment or euthanasia of these cats. Proper diagnosis of medical problems, toileting, or marking begins with obtaining a thorough history, physical examination, blood work, urinalysis, and fecal analysis. Many cats with urinary toileting issues often have an underlying medical component such as bacterial infection or feline interstitial cystitis (Westropp et al. 2019). The substrate and location of the soiled area may be consistent or seem random but is usually a horizontal surface. Cats tend to prefer large, uncovered boxes with fine-grained clumping litter and once-daily cleaning (Guy et al. 2014; Landsberg et al. 2013). However, recent studies isolating individual factors bring into question some of these clinical impressions (Barcelos et al. 2018; Ellis et al. 2017; Grigg et al. 2012). Boxes located in areas that are too noisy or require a cat to come into contact with an aversive stimulus (e.g., stairs for arthritic cat, another aggressive cat) are common triggers for toileting away from the litterbox as well.

Marking cats often spray urine on vertical surfaces in socially prominent areas. Less commonly, marking is on a horizontal surface. Use of the litterbox to toilet usually remains consistent. Often social conflict with other cats, people, or animals in the home results in marking behavior. Some cats will mark near windows and walls, suggesting the presence of an outdoor cat. Treatment for marking focuses on alleviating the stress and anxiety experienced by the cat as well as maintaining a proper litterbox environment. Psychoactive medications are a primary therapy for marking and may be helpful in toileting cases that involve stressors as well (Mills et al. 2011). Cleaning of soiled areas with an enzyme-based cleaner is a treatment for any form of unwanted elimination due to the cat's natural inclination to gravitate toward previous soiled areas for elimination. All cats in the home with spraying cats have evidence of increased stress levels, and a global approach to reducing stress and anxiety should be undertaken (Ramos et al. 2020).

2.6.5 Scratching

Newborn kittens are able to withdraw their claws at four weeks of age, and they begin adult-like scratching behavior by the fifth week (Mengoli et al. 2013). Scratching on surfaces serves to maintain claw health by aiding in removal of aging nail sheaths and sharpening claws (Hart and Hart 2014a). Although claw health is theoretically vital for successful hunting and long-term survival, declawed cats are reportedly efficient hunters (Landsberg 1991). By depositing chemical signals originating from interdigital glands, scratching also disseminates olfactory signals. The act of scratching and slashes resulting from scratching may also convey a visual marker (Feldman 1994). Indoor cats may scratch to gain attention from humans or as a stress-displacement behavior (Mengoli et al. 2013).

Scratching is a normal and necessary part of the feline behavioral repertoire, and attempts to stop a cat from scratching completely will not only be unsuccessful but can diminish the cat's welfare. Suggested parameters for the ideal object designated for scratching (scratcher) include a vertical post more than 3 ft. in height or of sufficient length for full forelimb extension and a stable base width between 1 and 3 ft. (Wilson et al. 2016; Zhang and McGlone 2020). There may be some preference for vertical compared to longitudinal orientation of the scratcher in adult cats. Cats in a controlled study seemed to use scratchers covered in sisal rope or cardboard more often than posts with carpet or fabric (Zhang and McGlone 2020), though cat owners frequently reported their cats scratch furniture or flooring covered with soft material (Moesta et al. 2018). An important factor that may help explain these inconsistent findings is the location of the scratcher. The optimal placement of scratchers is in prominent social areas (Mengoli et al. 2013; Moesta et al. 2018). Studies suggest that synthetic interdigital chemicals (Cozzi et al. 2013) and plant-based attractants (silver vine and catnip) can increase the use of scratching posts (Zhang and McGlone 2020).

Up to 50% of cats exhibit inappropriate scratching behavior, and it is a commonly reported factor in relinquishment (Wilson et al. 2016). Therefore, several methods have been proposed to diminish damage caused to homes by cat scratching behavior. In addition to posts with attractive attributes, outdoor access, deterrents from unacceptable objects, and nail-altering procedures have been suggested. These procedures range from basic nail trimming and covering to removal of the distal portion of the phalanges (Moesta et al. 2018). Onychectomy, or declawing, is still widely performed in the United States and Canada (Lockhart et al. 2014).

Onychectomy is controversial because it involves removal of the distal phalanges and has the potential for complications including hemorrhage and pain, claw regrowth, chronic draining tracts, radial nerve paralysis, infection, wound dehiscence or incomplete healing, protrusion or loss of the adjacent phalanx, and persistent lameness. Force plate analysis of cats following onychectomy has demonstrated abnormal gaits for at least 12 days post-surgery, making appropriate anesthesia and analgesia imperative (Romans et al. 2005; Lockhart et al. 2014). Evidence of inadequate surgical technique was common in one study population (Martell-Moran et al. 2017). The same study also strongly suggested that declawed cats are more likely to display other behavioral problems such as increased aggression, biting, and housesoiling.

2.6.6 Reproduction

Reproductive behaviors of the female cat, or queen, vary depending on the stage of her estrous cycle. High levels of estrogen are necessary for ovulation and initiation of estrus, or "heat" phase. As estrogen levels start to rise early in the cycle (proestrus), the queen shows courtship behaviors, such as increased activity and the appearance of a distinct estrus call vocalization. She also displays frequent rubbing of cheeks, head, flank, and back on various substrates as well as rolling and spraying urine to advertise her estrus status. Another defining queen behavior displayed during courtship is the lordosis posture—crouching with perineal area lifted vertically and back

legs treading. Estrus behaviors occur regardless of a male cat's presence. In the proestrus phase, the queen displays courtship behaviors but acts aggressively if the male (tom) cat tries to mount. She only becomes immobile and allows mounting and biting of the neck as she enters the estrus phase and estrogen levels rise. Felids are induced ovulators, meaning physical stimulation of the vagina is needed to trigger release of an egg from the ovary (Hart and Hart 2014b).

Tomcats are drawn to the estrus female via olfactory cues. His courtship behavior is a sequence of genital sniffing, displaying the gaping or flehmen response, and then using teeth to grasp the nape of the queen's neck before mounting. The tom also treads his back legs during mounting and intercourse. The female reacts strongly at the time of intromission, likely a result of hyperstimulation or discomfort from the tomcat penile spines. She produces a loud shriek accompanied by dilated pupils and darting away from the male (Houpt 2018).

Natural mating behavior consists of frequent copulations (approximately every 10 minutes for several hours) of less than 1 minute. In a free-ranging cat environment, this mating strategy provides an opportunity for multiple males to mate with a queen during estrus. Numerous toms surround the queen and try to displace each other during or between copulation. Thus, multiple paternity within litters is common. Estrus ends about two days post-ovulation, but an unbred cat will cycle approximately every three weeks throughout the breeding season, which is January through October in the Northern Hemisphere (Houpt 2018).

2.7 Sociality

2.7.1 Intraspecific

Domestication involves morphological changes as well as alterations to physiology, emotional systems, and social behavior (Coppinger and

Smith 1983). Considering the domestic cat's ancestral species as well as all other living members of the *Felis* genus are solitary and territorial individuals, the degree of intra- and interspecific social behavior displayed by the cat is extensive. Nevertheless, domestic cats tend to be solitary hunters in settings with sparse food sources. To allow cats to take full advantage of concentrated food niches provided by humans, feline social signaling and the ability to deescalate territorial tensions had to evolve (Bradshaw 2016). The social framework of feline colonies is matrilineal, meaning related females often form stable groups and are intolerant of unrelated females. In addition, females within a group often cooperatively raise kittens through group nursing and sharing of captured prey (Macdonald et al. 2000). Moreover, the basis of all affiliative cat social behavior seems to be maternal care. Many friendly behaviors observed between cats, such as allogrooming and allorubbing, as well as the purr and kneading behavior, are first seen between kittens and their dam (Bradshaw et al. 2012). Physical contact provided through mutual grooming and rubbing probably maintains group cohesion through both olfactory and tactile cues (Bradshaw 2016). The vertically raised tail is one of the most notable body postures for signaling friendly intentions from a distance.

Proximity, particularly with non-group members, inevitably leads to some degree of conflict, prompting cats to communicate the intent to avoid conflict or willingness to fight by means of ritualized interactions (Bradshaw 2016). Threat behaviors convey a cat's desire to maintain personal space or access to a resource. A confident cat conveying a threat may stare at and/or move without hesitation toward the intended receiver. The body posture is usually upright and ear pinnae turned to the side. The tail may be low but curved up at the level of the hocks with tail lashing occurring with higher-arousal encounters. Firm head bunting and urine spraying can be threatening behaviors that incorporate tactile and/or olfactory

signals without overt aggression. A confident cat rarely vocalizes during a threat. The cat receiving these signals may respond by moving away, typically with a lowered tail, body posture, and ear pinnae. Body posture becomes increasingly crouched, with the tail tucked under the body, ears flattened, and pupils dilated with elevated distress or fear. A roll onto the back is often observed in extreme situations as well. Although a roll may be seen during some friendly interactions, in this situation the cat is maneuvering to use the claws defensively if necessary (Leyhausen 1979). Vocalizations like hissing and yowling increase with the level of distress and threat perception as well. Although scratching and biting are possible, avoidance and appeasement behaviors are much more common, thereby reducing the risk of injury that may incur during a physical altercation (Dantas et al. 2011). The aggressor is not always confident, and a mix of fear and threat behaviors is often seen in both parties during an agonistic encounter. Aggression may become more prevalent in heavily populated and physically constrained colonies (Knowles et al. 2004).

2.7.2 Interspecific

Millions of cats interact with humans in various housed or free-roaming environments, and the field of feline social cognition is uncovering what most cat owners already know—cats are capable of forming strong bonds with humans (Turner 2017). Geering (1986) found that food may be an initial attractant for a cat, but affiliative behaviors such as stroking are needed to maintain contact with a person. More recent studies have suggested that once a cat has bonded with a human, the cat shows a preference for contact from this person compared to others and feels more comfortable in exploring surroundings with familiar people present (Edwards et al. 2007). Cats tend to look for cues from a familiar person in the presence of a frightening stimulus (Merola et al. 2015) but, unlike dogs, may not necessarily seek human guidance when solving spatial tasks (Miklósi et al. 2005). Cats can both recognize the voice of familiar humans (Saito and Shinozuka 2013) and alter vocalizations directed toward humans. Cats emit the meow (Yeon et al. 2011) and modified purrs (McComb et al. 2009) almost exclusively toward humans when seeking resources such as food and affection, although similar sounds may be heard in the queen-kitten context. Most affiliative behaviors displayed by cats toward humans—kneading with the forepaws, purring, allorubbing, and allogrooming—mirror conspecific behavior. Human scratching and stroking are likely perceived as reciprocation and maintenance of the bond. Human personality and perception of the cat as a social partner have been shown to influence the characteristic of both the specific human-cat interaction and a cat's general behaviors in the home (Wedl et al. 2011; Kotrschal et al. 2014). Arguably the most important factor in the degree of sociability of any cat is early life experiences with humans or any other social partner.

2.7.3 Aggression

Aggressive behavior is often a normal reaction to a stressful social situation, such as the presence of an unfamiliar cat or unwanted attention from a human. Cats tend to avoid conflict as much as possible, but physical constraints or limited resources may force a cat into proximity of the concerning human or cat, triggering aggression. Learning can shape emotions and behavioral responses. Negative emotional associations between individuals result from aversive experiences, and aggressive behavior may be reinforced as the most effective tactic to end unwanted interactions.

2.7.3.1 Play Aggression

Play often involves predatory-like stalking, chasing, pouncing, scratching, and biting. This is considered a normal behavior in kittens and some adults, but aggressive play may be

abnormal or warrant intervention if the biting and scratching are intense or the target of play attacks is vulnerable (e.g., child or senior person, geriatric cat). Kittens and cats who were hand raised, separated from littermates at a young age, or singleton kittens are more likely to display more frequent and intense play aggression (Mendl 1988).

Play is a normal aspect of development, and suppression of play may lead to long-term problems. Aversive punishment is likely to create lasting associations of fear and frustration. The most appropriate methods for reducing play aggression are providing ample opportunities for play with appropriate toys, eliminating use of human hands or feet for play, and managing the environment to reduce exposure to inappropriate targets. For example, a family may keep a basket of toys handy and toss one of the objects in the opposite direction for a cat that tends to stalk and bite the ankles of people walking past a certain doorway.

2.7.3.2 Territorial Aggression

Cats are territorial creatures and, while overt aggression within a group tends to be low, aggression to outsiders can be intense. Defense of territories is normal in free-living colonies, especially during breeding season (Turner 2014). Even though most housecats are sexually altered, they are still very likely to hiss and yowl at outside cats. This is a common trigger for urine spraying as well. Cats within a multi-cat household are prone to territorial (and fear) aggression toward one another when first introduced, particularly if the cats are not slowly introduced using positive associations (Levine et al. 2005). In many situations, cats do form a social bond or at least largely tolerate the presence of the other cat. Cats, however, do not associate with each other randomly, and the expectation of a harmonious multi-cat home is not a given outcome. Aggression to unfamiliar people is typically a result of fear, but territorial aggression is possible (Landsberg et al. 2013). The problem is often complicated by the inability of the cat to escape and other underlying fears or anxieties.

2.7.3.3   Fear-Related Aggression

A cat may show fear-related aggression whenever feeling threatened or afraid. A fearful cat can be identified by certain body postures (e.g., crouched, eyes dilated) and vocalizations (e.g., hiss). Similar to territorial aggression, a cat may be compelled to show aggression instead of fleeing when there is no opportunity to escape. Learning can shape and reinforce the behavior.

2.7.3.4   Redirected Aggression

It is not uncommon for cats to redirect aggression to a nearby animal or human when the primary target of aggression cannot be accessed. This may occur regardless of the motivation, although fear, frustration, and/or territoriality are the most commonly recognized factors. Unfortunately, arousal levels often escalate quickly, associative learning can be strong and long-lasting, and relationships between household cats or people that have lived together for years can be damaged due to redirected aggression.

2.7.3.5   Treatment for Aggression

Treatment plans for aggression motivated by a negative emotional state, such as fear, territoriality, and redirection, have basic commonalities. Avoidance of triggers outside of any behavior modification session is critical and may include minimizing human petting or holding of the cat, blocking the view of outdoor cats, or providing adequate space in a multi-cat household. Space can be created by providing areas for hiding, elevated spaces, or other physical barriers (e.g., completely separate rooms or gates). A social relationship or association with another target can be improved through close-proximity feeding, play, or training sessions using high-value treats. Most cats can easily be taught behaviors to be used as alternative responses to fleeing or aggression. A cat showing low-level signs of

distress or aggression can be cued to move to a distant location like a bed or cat tree. Calming medications or adjunctive treatments may be helpful as well.

2.7.4   Fears, Phobias, and Anxiety

Fear is a normal, often adaptive emotion experienced in the presence of a threat, whereas phobia is an extreme and non-adaptive fear response. Anxiety is the anticipation of a negative event, whether real or imagined, and can be become chronic and debilitating in some cats. These emotions can produce a range of responses, broadly referred to as Fight, Flight, Freeze, or Fidget (Landsberg et al. 2013). As previously discussed, escape, avoidance, or motionless behaviors are the most common feline responses for minimizing danger, but fear-related aggression can occur when a cat cannot escape and/or learns aggression is the most successful tactic. Treatment for fear without aggression follows similar protocols to fear-related aggression: avoidance, behavior modification intended to change the behavioral and emotional response to the trigger, and antianxiety therapies.

Noises can be triggers for anxious or phobic responses. This may be most noticeable with sharp, sudden sounds like thunder or alarms but also with novel stimuli such as visitors or a new baby. In fact, most sources of fear in the home are primarily related to social stress with another cat, dog, or human. However, hyper-attachment, typically to human family member(s), is also possible and can lead to separation-related distress. Excessive vocalization, eliminations outside the litterbox, or destruction are behaviors reported to occur in these cats when the family is absent or around their arrival or departure times. Some cats do not show signs of fear or distress at the time of a stressful event but develop chronic anxiety, which tends to manifest as displacement behaviors ("fidget") including overgrooming, pacing, changes in social behavior, and vague sicknesses like vomiting, diarrhea, and chronic urinary tract disease. Treatment involves creating pleasant associations to separation from the family (Schwartz 2002).

Unfortunately, fear of the veterinary clinic and handling for procedures is ubiquitous in cats. One study indicated feline distress reduces a cat owner's willingness to take the cat to the vet, and this, in turn, could have a deleterious effect on overall feline health and well-being (Volk et al. 2011). There are several initiatives to help veterinarians and shelter staff create a less stressful experience through a reduction in noise and exposure to unfamiliar people and animals, low-stress restraint, and antianxiety medications when appropriate (Fear Free Pets 2020; Low Stress Handling 2020). Behavior modification used to create pleasant associations with the carrier, restraint, and procedures such as nail trims and oral medication administration is an important aspect of fear reduction in the veterinary clinic and proper care at home. See Chapter 14 for more information about applying these concepts to shelter cats.

Just as early experiences have strong influences on the development of cognitive abilities, age-related degeneration can create significant behavior changes. Cognitive dysfunction syndrome (CDS) refers to sensory degeneration, impairments in memory and decision-making abilities, and emotional dysregulation. An aging cat may display disorientation, changes in social interactions, sleep-wake cycle alterations, house-soiling, changes in activity, excessive vocalization, appetite changes, and decreased self-hygiene (Landsberg et al. 2010). Most of these issues could be due to a primary medical cause; therefore, CDS is an antemortem diagnosis of exclusion, although postmortem histology reveals neurotoxic amyloid-beta accumulation, similar to CDS in dogs and Alzheimer's disease in human patients. As in other species, there is no definitive treatment, although antioxidant diets or supplements in addition to environmental enrichment may improve cognitive signs and quality of life for aging cats.

2.8 Learning and Cognition

Cats, like all species, are constantly learning and potentially changing their behavior as they navigate their environment. Learning and memory are aspects of feline cognition, or the manner by which a cat perceives, processes, and acts on environmental information (Shettleworth 2001). Sensory capabilities, working memory, understanding of the physical world (e.g., object permanence or manipulation of objects to achieve a resource), problem solving, and social communication are specific domains often assessed in cognitive research. However, some investigators have recently suggested that many previous studies have likely undervalued the cognitive capacity of cats due to the use of protocols originally aimed at assessing primate or canine cognitive abilities (Vitale Shreve and Udell 2015).

2.9 Conclusions

Cats are unique amongst domestic species in that they have evolved from a solitary ancestral species to become one of the most beloved household pets today. Interestingly the cat's physical appearance and sensory systems remain almost identical to their wild counterparts. Recognition of the perceptual parameters allows us to better understand how the domestic cat responds to environment and communicates with social partners. Sociality is unequivocally the aspect of feline life most affected by the domestication process. Cats can display a wide range of social behaviors, and evidence indicates that early exposure to a variety of social and environmental stimuli is the most important postnatal factor for a well-adjusted life in a domestic setting and resiliency to basic stressors. In addition, a moderate amount of handling and enrichment will ensure shelter staff improves the future welfare of kittens in their care and increases adoptability. It is imperative that shelter staff gain an understanding of feline natural behavior, communication, learning, and cognition to provide cats with an ideal environment, change

unwanted behaviors, and improve the welfare of our cats.

Please visit the companion website for video clips and downloadable resources associated with this chapter.

References

Ahola, M.K., Vapalahti, K., and Lohi, H. (2017). Early weaning increases aggression and stereotypic behaviour in cats. *Sci. Rep.* 7 (1): 10412–10419.

American Veterinary Medical Association. (2018). *2018 U.S. Pet Ownership and Demographics Sourcebook*. Schamburg, IL: AVMA.

Association for Pet Obesity Prevention (2019). 2018 Pet Obesity Survey Results. www.petobesityprevention.org/2018 (accessed 18 July 2020).

Barcelos, A.M., McPeake, K., Affenzeller, N. et al. (2018). Common risk factors for urinary house soiling (periuria) in cats and its differentiation: the sensitivity and specificity of common diagnostic signs. *Front. Vet. Sci.* 5: 335–312.

Bateson, P. (1979). How do sensitive periods arise and what are they for? *Anim. Behav.* 27 (2): 470–486.

Bateson, P. (2014). Behavioural development in the cat. In: *The Domestic Cat: The Biology of Its Behaviour*, 3rd ed. (eds D.C. Turner and P. Bateson), 11–26. Cambridge, UK: Cambridge University Press.

Bateson, P. and Young, M. (1981). Separation from the mother and the development of play in cats. *Anim. Behav.* 29: 173–180.

Beaver, B.V. (2003). *Feline Behavior: A Guide for Veterinarians*. St. Louis: Elsevier Science.

Becques, A., Larose, C., Gouat, P. et al. (2009). Effects of pre- and postnatal olfactogustatory experience on early preferences at birth and dietary selection at weaning in kittens. *Chem. Senses* 35 (1): 41–45.

Belkin, M., Yinon, U., Rose, L. et al. (1977). Effect of visual environment on refractive error of cats. *Doc. Ophthalmol.* 42: 433–437.

Bennett, V., Gourkow, N., and Mills, D.S. (2017). Facial correlates of emotional behaviour in the domestic cat (*Felis catus*). *Behav Processes* 141: 342–350.

Blakemore, C. and Cooper, G.F. (1971). Modification of the visual cortex by experience. *Brain Res. Rev.* 31 (2): 366.

Borns-Weil, S. (2019). Inappropriate urination. *Vet. Clin. North Am. Small Anim. Pract.* 49 (2): 141–155.

Braastad, B.O. and Heggelund, P. (1984). Eye-opening in kittens: Effects of light and some biologic factors. *Dev. Psychobiol.* 17: 675–681.

Bradshaw, J.W.S. (2016). Sociality in cats: A comparative review. *J. Vet. Behav.* 11: 113–124.

Bradshaw, J.W.S. (2017). Behaviour of cats. In: *The Ethology of Domestic Animals* (ed. P. Jensen), 1–254. Boston: CABI.

Bradshaw, J.W.S., Casey, R.A., and Brown, S.L. (2012). Behavioural development. In: *The Behaviour of the Domestic Cat*, 2nd ed. (eds J.W.S. Bradshaw, R.A. Casey, and S.L. Brown), 63–112. Boston: CABI.

Brown, S.L. and Bradshaw, J.W.S. (2013). Communication in the domestic cat: Within- and between-species. In: *The Domestic Cat: The Biology of Its Behavior*, 3rd ed. (eds. D.C. Turner and P. Bateson), 37–62. Cambridge, UK: Cambridge University Press.

Buffington, C., Westropp, J., Chew, D. et al. (2006). Clinical evaluation of multimodal environmental modification (MEMO) in the management of cats with idiopathic cystitis. *J. Fel. Med. Surg.* 8 (4): 261–268.

Burghardt, G.M. (2005). *The Genesis of Animal Play: Testing the Limits.* Cambridge, MA: Massachusetts Institute of Technology.

Byers, M.R. and Dong, W.K. (1989). Comparison of trigeminal receptor location and structure in the periodontal ligament of different types of teeth from the rat, cat, and monkey. *J. Comp. Neurol.* 279 (1): 117–127.

Cafazzo, S. and Natoli, E. (2009). The social function of tail up in the domestic cat (*Felis silvestris catus*). *Behav. Processes* 80 (1): 60–66.

Casey, R.A. and Bradshaw, J.W.S. (2008). The effects of additional socialisation for kittens in a rescue centre on their behaviour and suitability as a pet. *Appl. Anim. Behav. Sci.* 114 (1–2): 196–205.

Cat Fanciers' Association, Inc. (2020). CFA Breeds. https://cfa.org/breeds/ (accessed 19 July 2020).

Coppinger R.P. and Smith C.K. (1983) The domestication of evolution. *Environ. Conserv.* 10: 283–292.

Cozzi, A., Lecuelle, C.L., Monneret, P. et al. (2013). Induction of scratching behaviour in cats: Efficacy of synthetic feline interdigital semiochemical. *J. Fel. Med. Surg.* 15: 872–878.

Cremieux, J., Veraart, C., and Wanet, M. (1984). Development of the air righting reflex in cats visually deprived since birth. *Exp. Brain Res.* 54: 564–566.

Crowell-Davis, S.L., Curtis, T.M., and Knowles, R.J. (2004). Social organization in the cat: A modern understanding. *J. Fel. Med. Surg.* https://doi.org/10.1016/j.jfms.2003.09.013.

Dantas, L.M.S., Crowell-Davis, S.L., Alford, K. et al. (2011). Agonistic behavior and environmental enrichment of cats communally housed in a shelter. *J. Am. Vet. Med. Assoc.* 239 (6): 796–802.

Dantas, L.M.S., Delgado, M.M., Johnson, I. et al. (2016). Food puzzles for cats: Feeding for physical and emotional wellbeing. *J. Fel. Med. Surg.* 18 (9): 723–732.

Delgado, M. and Hecht, J. (2019). A review of the development and functions of cat play, and future research considerations. *Appl. Anim. Behav. Sci.* 214: 1–17.

Demontigny-Bédard, I., Bélanger, M.-C., Hélie, P., et al (2019). Medical and behavioral evaluation of 8 cats presenting with fabric ingestion: An exploratory pilot study. *Can. Vet. J.* 60 (10): 1081–1088.

Driscoll, C.A., Clutton-Brock, J., Kitchener, A.C. et al. (2009). The taming of the cat: Genetic and archaeological findings hint that wildcats became housecats earlier—and in a different place—than previously thought. *Sci. Am.* 300 (6): 68–75.

Driscoll, C.A., Macdonald, D.W., and O'Brien, S.J. (2009). From wild animals to domestic pets, an evolutionary view of domestication. *Proc. Natl. Acad. Sci. U.S.A.* 106 Suppl 1: 9971–9978.

Dyce, K.M., Sack., W.O., and Wensing, C.J.G. (2010). *Textbook of Veterinary Anatomy*, 4th ed. Philadelphia: W.B Saunders.

Edwards, C., Heiblum, M., Tejeda, A., and Galindo, F. (2007). Experimental evaluation of attachment behaviors in owned cats. *J. Vet. Behav.* 2: 119–125.

Ellis, J.J., McGowan, R.T.S., and Martin, F. (2017). Does previous use affect litter box appeal in multi-cat households? *Behav. Processes* 141: 284–290.

Ewer, R. F. (1960). Suckling behaviour in kittens. *Behaviour* 15 (1–2): 146–162.

Fay, R. and Popper, A. (1994). *Comparative Hearing: Mammals.* Springer Handbook of Auditory Research Series. New York: Springer-Verlag.

Fear Free Pets. (2020). www.fearfreepets.com (accessed 19 July 2020).

Feldman, H. (1994). Methods of scent marking in the domestic cat. *Can. J. Zool.* 72 (6): 1093–1099.

Fitzgerald, B.M. and Turner, D.C. (2000). Hunting behaviour of domestic cats and their impact on prey populations. In: *The Domestic Cat: The Biology of Its Behaviour*, 2nd ed. (eds. D.C. Turner and P. Bateson), 151–176. Cambridge, UK: Cambridge University Press.

Gallo, P.V., Werboff, J., and Knox, K. (1980). Protein restriction during gestation and lactation: Development of attachment behavior in cats. *Behav. Neural Biol.* 29 (2): 216–223.

Geering, K. (1986). Der Einfluss der Fütterung auf die Katze-Mensch-Beziehung. Master's thesis. University of Zurich (Zoology Inst.).

Gourkow, N., LaVoy, A., Dean, G.A. et al. (2014). Associations of behaviour with secretory immunoglobulin A and cortisol in domestic cats during their first week in an animal shelter. *Appl. Anim. Behav. Sci.* 150: 55–64.

Grigg, E.K., Pick, L., and Nibblett, B. (2012). Litter box preference in domestic cats: Covered versus uncovered. *J. Fel. Med. Surg.* 15 (4): 280–284.

Guy, N.C., Hopson, M., and Vanderstichel, R. (2014). Litterbox size preference in domestic cats (*Felis catus*). *J. Vet. Behav.* 9 (2): 78–82.

Guyot, G.W., Bennett, T.L., and Cross, H.A. (1980). The effects of social isolation on the behavior of juvenile domestic cats. *Dev. Psychobiol.* 13: 317–329.

Hall, S.L., Bradshaw, J.W.S., and Robinson, I.H. (2002). Object play in adult domestic cats: The roles of habituation and disinhibition. *Appl. Anim. Behav. Sci.* 79: 263–271.

Hart, B.L. and Hart, L.A. (2014a). Feline behavioural problems and solutions. In: *The Domestic Cat: The Biology of Its Behaviour*, 3rd ed. (eds. D.C. Turner and P. Bateson), 201–214. Cambridge, UK: Cambridge University Press.

Hart, B.L. and Hart, L.A. (2014b). Normal and problematic reproductive behaviour in the domestic cat. In: *The Domestic Cat: The Biology of Its Behaviour*, 3rd ed. (eds. D.C. Turner and P. Bateson), 179–190. Cambridge, UK: Cambridge University Press.

Hart, B.L. and Leedy, M.G. (1987). Stimulus and hormonal determinants of flehmen behavior in cats. *Horm. Behav.* 21 (1): 44–52.

Heath, S. (2019). Common feline problem behaviours: Unacceptable indoor elimination. *J. Fel. Med. Surg.* 21 (3): 199–208.

Hein, A. and Held, R. (1967). Dissociation of the visual placing response into elicited and guided components. *Science* 158 (3799): 390–392.

Houpt, K.A. (2018). *Domestic Animal Behavior for Veterinarians and Animal Scientists*, 6th ed. Hoboken, NJ: Wiley Blackwell.

Hu, Y., Hu, S., Wang, W. et al. (2014). Earliest evidence for commensal processes of cat domestication. *Proc. Natl. Acad. Sci. U.S.A.* 111 (1): 116–120.

Jensen, R.A., Davis, J.L., and Shnerson, A. (1980). Early experience facilitates the development of temperature regulation in the cat. *Dev. Psychobiol.* 13: 1–6.

Karsh, E.B. and Turner, D.C. (1988). The human-cat relationship. In: *The Domestic Cat: The Biology of Its Behaviour* (eds. D.C. Turner and P. Bateson), 67–81. Cambridge, UK: Cambridge University Press.

Karsten, C.L., Wagner, D.C., Kass, P.H. et al. (2017). An observational study of the relationship between Capacity for Care as an animal shelter management model and cat health, adoption and death in three animal shelters. *Vet. J.* 227: 15–22.

Kiley-Worthington, M. (1984). Animal language? Vocal communication of some ungulates, canids and felids with particular reference to their causation and function as displays. *Acta Zool. Fenn.* 171: 83–88.

Knowles, R.J., Curtis, T.M., and Crowell-Davis, S.L. (2004). Correlation of dominance as determined by agonistic interactions with feeding order in cats. *Am. J. Vet. Res.* 65 (11): 1548–1556.

Kotrschal, K., Day, J., McCune, S., and Wedl, M. (2014). Human and cat personalities: Building the bond from both sides. In: *The Domestic Cat: The Biology of Its Behaviour*, 3rd ed. (eds. D.C. Turner and P. Bateson), 113–129. Cambridge, UK: Cambridge University Press.

Kuo, Z.Y. (1930). The genesis of the cat's responses to the rat. *J. Comp. Psychol.* 11 (1): 1.

Kuo, Z.Y. (1938). Further study of the behavior of the cat toward the rat. *J. Comp. Psychol.* 25 (1): 1.

Landsberg, G.M. (1991). Cat owner' attitudes towards declawing. *Anthrozoös.* 4 (3):192–197.

Landsberg, G.M., Denenberg, S., and Araujo, J.A. (2010). Cognitive dysfunction in cats: A syndrome we used to dismiss as "old age." *J. Fel. Med. Surg.* 12 (11): 837–848.

Landsberg, G.M., Hunthausen, W.L., and Ackerman, L.J. (2013). *Behavior Problems of the Dog and Cat*. Amsterdam: Elsevier.

Lei, W., Ravoninjohary, A., Li, X. et al. (2015). Functional analyses of bitter taste receptors in domestic cats (*Felis catus*). *PLOS ONE* 10 (10): e0139670–12.

Levine, E., Perry, P., Scarlett, J. et al. (2005). Intercat aggression in households following the introduction of a new cat. *Appl. Anim. Behav. Sci.* 90 (3–4): 325–336.

Leyhausen, P. (1979). *Cat Behavior*. New York: Garland STPM Press.

Litchfield, C.A., Quinton, G., Tindle, H. et al. (2017). The "Feline Five": An exploration of personality in pet cats (*Felis catus*). *PLOS ONE* 12 (8): e0183455–17.

Lockhart, L.E., Motsinger-Reif, A.A., Simpson, W.M. et al. (2014). Prevalence of onychectomy in cats presented for veterinary care near Raleigh, NC and educational attitudes toward the procedure. *Vet. Anaesth. Analg.* 41 (1): 48–53.

Low Stress Handling®. (2020). www. lowstresshandling.com (accessed 19 July 2020).

Lowe, S.E. and Bradshaw, J.W.S. (2001). Ontogeny of individuality in the domestic cat in the home environment. *Anim. Behav.* 61 (1): 231–237.

Lowe, S.E. and Bradshaw, J.W.S. (2002). Responses of pet cats to being held by an unfamiliar person, from weaning to three years of age. *Anthrozoös* 15 (1): 69–79.

Macdonald, D.W., Yamaguchi, N., and Kerby, G. (2000). Group-living in the domestic cat: Its sociobiology and epidemiology. In: *The Domestic Cat: The Biology of Its Behaviour*, 2nd ed. (eds. D.C. Turner and P. Bateson), 95–115. Cambridge, UK: Cambridge University Press.

Martell-Moran, N.K., Solano, M., and Townsend, H.G. (2017). Pain and adverse behavior in declawed cats. *J. Fel. Med. Surg.* 55: 1098612X17705044.

McComb, K., Taylor, A.M., Wilson, C. et al. (2009). The cry embedded within the purr. *Curr. Biol.* 19 (13): R507–R508.

McCune, S. (1995). The impact of paternity and early socialisation on the development of cats' behaviour to people and novel objects. *Appl. Anim. Behav. Sci.* 45: 109–124.

McGowan, R.T.S., Ellis, J.J., Bensky, M.K. et al. (2017). The ins and outs of the litter box: A detailed ethogram of cat elimination behavior in two contrasting environments. *Appl. Anim. Behav. Sci.* 194: 67–78.

Mellen, J.D. (1992). Effects of early rearing experience on subsequent adult sexual behavior using domestic cats (*Felis catus*) as a model for exotic small felids. *Zoo Biol.* 11 (1): 17–32.

Mendl, M. (1988). The effects of litter-size variation on the development of play behaviour in the domestic cat: Litters of one and two. *Anim. Behav.* 36 (1): 20–34.

Mendl, M. and Harcourt, R. (2000). Individuality in the domestic cat: Origins, development and stability. In: *The Domestic Cat: The Biology of Its Behaviour*, 2nd ed. (eds. D.C. Turner and P. Bateson), 47–64. Cambridge, UK: Cambridge University Press.

Mendoza, D.L. and Ramirez, J.M. (1987). Play in kittens (*Felis domesticus*) and its association with cohesion and aggression. *Psychon. Bull. Rev.* 25: 27–30.

Mengoli, M., Mariti, C., Cozzi, A. et al. (2013). Scratching behaviour and its features: A questionnaire-based study in an Italian sample of domestic cats. *J. Fel. Med. Surg.* 15 (10): 886–892.

Merola, I., Lazzaroni, M., Marshall-Pescini, S. et al. (2015). Social referencing and cat-human communication. *Anim. Cogn.* 18 (3): 639–648.

Miklósi, Á., Pongrácz, P., Lakatos, G. et al. (2005). A comparative study of the use of visual communicative signals in interactions between dogs (*Canis familiaris*) and humans and cats (*Felis catus*) and humans. *J. Comp. Psychol.* 119 (2): 179–186.

Mills, D.S. (2005). Pheromonatherapy: Theory and applications. *In Pract.* 27: 368–373.

Mills, D.S., Redgate, S.E., and Landsberg, G.M. (2011). A meta-analysis of studies of treatments for feline urine spraying. *PLOS ONE* 6 (4): e18448.

Moesta, A., Keys, D., and Crowell-Davis, S. (2018). Survey of cat owners on features of, and preventative measures for, feline scratching of inappropriate objects: A pilot study. *J. Fel. Med. Surg.* 20 (10): 891–899.

Montague, M.J., Li, G., Gandolfi, B. et al. (2014). Comparative analysis of the domestic cat genome reveals genetic signatures underlying feline biology and domestication. *Proc. Natl. Acad. Sci. U. S.A.* 201410083.

Moody, C.M., Mason, G.J., Dewey, C.E. et al. (2020). Getting a grip: Cats respond negatively to scruffing and clips. *Vet. Rec.* 186 (12): 385.

Olmstead, C.E., Villablanca, J.R., Torbiner, M. et al. (1979). Development of thermoregulation in the kitten. *Physiol. Behav.* 23: 489–495.

Overall, K.L. (2013). *Manual of Clinical Behavioral Medicine for Dogs and Cats*. St. Louis: Mosby.

Overall, K.L., Rodan, I., Beaver, B. et al. (2005). Feline behavior guidelines from the American Association of Feline Practitioners. *J. Am. Vet. Med. Assoc.* 227 (1): 70–84.

Pageat, P. and Gaultier, E. (2003). Current research in canine and feline pheromones. *Vet. Clin. North Am. Small Anim. Pract.* 33 (2): 187–211.

Peters, S.E. (1983). Postnatal development of gait behaviour and functional allometry in the domestic cat (*Felis catus*). *J. Zool.* 199 (4): 461–486.

Raihani, G., González, D., Arteaga, L. et al. (2009). Olfactory guidance of nipple attachment and suckling in kittens of the domestic cat: Inborn and learned responses. *Dev. Psychobiol.* 51 (8): 662–671.

Ramos, D., Reche-Junior, A., Luzia Fragoso, P. et al. (2020). A case-controlled comparison of behavioural arousal levels in urine spraying and latrining cats. *Animals* 10 (1): 117.

Reisner, I.R., Houpt, K.A., Erb, H.N. et al. (1994). Friendliness to humans and defensive aggression in cats: The influence of handling and paternity. *Physiol. Behav.* 55 (6): 1119–1124.

Rochlitz, I. (2005). A review of the housing requirements of domestic cats (*Felis silvestris catus*) kept in the home. *Appl. Anim. Behav. Sci.* 93 (1–2): 97–109.

Rodan, I. and Heath, S. (2015). *Feline Behavioral Health and Welfare*. St Louis: Elsevier Health Sciences.

Romans, C.W., Gordon, W.J., Robinson, D.A. et al. (2005). Effect of postoperative analgesic protocol on limb function following onychectomy in cats. *J. Am. Vet. Med. Assoc.* 227 (1): 89–93.

Saito, A. and Shinozuka, K. (2013). Vocal recognition of owners by domestic cats (*Felis catus*). *Anim. Cogn.* 16 (4): 685–690.

Salonen, M., Vapalahti, K., Tiira, K. et al. (2019). Breed differences of heritable behaviour traits in cats. *Sci. Rep.* 9 (1): 7949.

Schneider, M.L. and Moore, C.F. (2000). Effect of prenatal stress on development: A nonhuman primate model. In: *Minnesota Symposia on Child Psychology*, vol. 31, 201–244. Mahwah, NJ: Lawrence Erlbaum Associates.

Schwartz, S. (2002). Separation anxiety syndrome in cats: 136 cases (1991–2000). *J. Am. Vet. Med. Assoc.* 220 (7): 1028–1033.

Serpell, J.A. (2014). Domestication and history of the cat. In: *The Domestic Cat: The Biology of Its Behaviour*, 3rd ed. (eds. D.C. Turner and P. Bateson), 83–100. Cambridge, UK: Cambridge University Press.

Shettleworth, S.J. (2001). Animal cognition and animal behaviour. *Anim. Behav.* 61: 277–286.

Shreve, K.R.V. and Udell, M.A.R. (2017). Stress, security, and scent: The influence of chemical signals on the social lives of domestic cats and implications for applied settings. *Appl. Anim. Behav Sci.* 187: 69–76.

Smith, B.A. and Jansen, G.R. (1977). Maternal undernutrition in the feline: Behavioral sequelae. *Nutr. Rep. Int.* 16: 513–526.

Stasiak, M. (2001). The effect of early specific feeding on food conditioning in cats. *Dev. Psychobiol.* 39 (3): 207–215.

Stasiak, M. (2002). The development of food preferences in cats: The new direction. *Nutr. Neurosci.* 5: 221–228.

Stelow, E.A., Bain, M.J., and Kass, P. H. (2015). The relationship between coat color and aggressive behaviors in the domestic cat. *J. Appl. Anim. Welf. Sci.* 19 (1): 1–15.

Thomas, E. and Schaller, F. (1954). Das Spiel der optisch isolierten, jungen Kaspar-Hauser-Katze. *Naturwissenschaften* 41: 557–558.

Turner, D.C. (2014). Social organisation and behavioural ecology of free-ranging domestic cats. In: *The Domestic Cat: The Biology of Its Behaviour*, 3rd ed. (eds. D.C. Turner and P. Bateson), 63–70. Cambridge, UK: Cambridge University Press.

Turner, D.C. (2017). A review of over three decades of research on cat-human and human-cat interactions and relationships. *Behav. Processes* 141 (part 3): 297–304.

Vigne, J.D., Evin, A., Cucchi, T. et al. (2016). Earliest "domestic" cats in china identified as leopard cat (*Prionailurus bengalensis*). *PLOS ONE* 11 (1): e0147295–11.

Vitale Shreve, K.R. and Udell, M.A.R. (2015). What's inside your cat's head? A review of cat (*Felis silvestris catus*) cognition research past, present and future. *Anim. Cogn.* 18 (6): 1195–1206.

Volk, J.O., Felsted, K.E., Thomas, J.G. et al. (2011). Executive summary of phase 2 of the Bayer veterinary care usage study. *J. Am. Vet. Med. Assoc.* 239 (10): 1311–1316.

Wedl, M., Bauer, B., Gracey, D. et al. (2011). Factors influencing the temporal patterns of dyadic behaviours and interactions between domestic cats and their owners. *Behav. Processes* 86 (1): 58–67.

West, M. (1974). Social play in the domestic cat. *Am. Zool.* 14: 427–436.

Westropp, J.L., Delgado, M., and Buffington, C.A.T. (2019). Chronic lower urinary tract signs in cats. *Vet. Clin. North Am. Small Anim. Pract.* 49 (2): 187–209.

Wilhelmy, J., Serpell, J., Brown, D. et al. (2016). Behavioral associations with breed, coat type, and eye color in single-breed cats. *J. Vet. Behav.* 13: 1–8.

Wilson, C., Bain, M., DePorter, T., Beck, A., Grassi, V. and Landsberg, G. (2016). Owner observations regarding cat scratching behavior: An internet-based survey. *J. Fel. Med. Surg.* 18 (10): 791–797.

Wilson, M., Warren, J.M., and Abbott, L. (1965). Infantile stimulation, activity and learning in cats. *Child Dev.* 36: 843–853.

Wolski, T. (1982). Social behavior of the cat. *Vet. Clin. North Am. Small Anim. Pract.* 12 (4): 693–706.

Yeon, S.C., Kim, Y.K., Park, S.J. et al. (2011). Differences between vocalization evoked by social stimuli in feral cats and house cats. *Behav. Processes* 87 (2): 183–189.

Zhang, L. and McGlone, J.J. (2020). Scratcher preferences of adult in-home cats and effects of olfactory supplements on cat scratching, *Appl. Anim. Behav. Sci.* 227: 1–33.

Zoran, D.L. and Buffington, C.A.T. (2011). Effects of nutrition choices and lifestyle changes on the well-being of cats, a carnivore that has moved indoors. *J Am Vet Med Assoc.* 239 (5): 596–606.

3

How Animals Learn

Haleh Amanieh and Nicole R. Dorey

3.1 Introduction: What Is Learning?

Working with animals daily allows us a great advantage—getting to know their behavior. We get to know their likes, their dislikes, and how they tend to act in certain circumstances. Knowledge about an animal's motivations to engage in or avoid certain behaviors and consequences that follow those behaviors gives us the opportunity to deeply understand the animal. The first step toward understanding animal behavior is understanding behavior in general. Behavior is anything an organism does as it interacts with its environment. From playing catch to reacting to human emotional states, animals exhibit a large variety of behavior, all of which can be analyzed.

It is apparent that each animal has a unique set of highly probable behaviors. Some dogs jump when someone new walks in, while others might hide. These differences are due to their individual experiences, also known as their *learning history*. Learning occurs when an animal's behavior changes as a result of its experiences. Learning is much more than just the formal acquisition of a new behavior. As long as an animal is experiencing its environment, it is learning. Animals are learning all the time, meaning that their behavior is constantly changing,

even if just a little bit. Knowing how easily and often behavior can change raises the question: How do animals learn? Answers to that question can help us effectively teach new behaviors or address behaviors that can be problematic.

Learning can be broken up into two categories: associative and non-associative learning. Just like in its name, associative learning takes place when two or more events become associated with or related to each other. Events that can be paired may be two environmental stimuli, such as the sound of a can opener with the smell of food, or a behavior and a consequence, such as pawing a food bowl and the addition of more food. On the flip side, non-associative learning does not involve a relationship between two events. This type of learning takes place with repeated exposure to a stimulus that occurs unrelated to any other stimulus. Depending upon the salience and timing of the stimulus, this exposure might cause the animal to pay less or more attention, exhibiting habituation and sensitization, respectively.

3.2 Non-associative Learning

Habituation is a type of non-associative learning in which an animal stops or reduces its response to a stimulus after repeated exposure

Animal Behavior for Shelter Veterinarians and Staff, Second Edition. Edited by Brian A. DiGangi, Victoria A. Cussen, Pamela J. Reid, and Kristen A. Collins.

to that stimulus. Consider Brutus, a terrier who barks at the sound of a lawn mower buzzing outside. As soon as the lawn mower turns on, Brutus barks wildly at the new sound. However, after a few minutes of the lawn mower continuously buzzing, Brutus calms down. In this example, the lawn mower buzz is the stimulus that elicits the response of barking. The response eventually stops even though the stimulus is still present in the animal's environment. Brutus habituates to the buzzing. Essentially, he gets used to it. Habituation to the sound occurred without any other stimulus present in Brutus's environment. The process of habituation is used widely to reduce animals' fear response to harmless stimuli.

Sensitization is the opposite of habituation in that repeated exposure to a stimulus increases an animal's response to the stimulus. As a new dog owner, Ruth had no idea that dogs can be so deathly terrified of fireworks. She naively took her Lhasa apso, Scruffy, to see fireworks to celebrate the New Year. When the fireworks started, Scruffy started to nervously pace around and pant heavily. Even though Ruth tried to calm her down by petting her and holding her close, it was no use. As the fireworks continued, she became increasingly nervous. After just a few minutes, Scruffy somehow got out of her collar and ran away into the crowd (Ruth found Scruffy shortly after, of course). Ruth expected Scruffy to habituate to the sound, but instead, she became sensitized to it. The presence of other stimuli was not relevant to Scruffy learning to become more and more sensitized to the noise. Her response to the stimulus became more intense as the stimulus continued to be present in her environment.

3.3 Associative Learning

3.3.1 Respondent Conditioning

One way that associative learning takes place is when a stimulus gets paired with another stimulus, a process called classical or respondent conditioning. Pavlov famously demonstrated this process in the early 1900s. While researching the physiology of digestion in dogs, Pavlov observed that dogs salivated in the presence of food. This was no surprise because Pavlov knew that salivation was a reflex elicited by the presence of food. However, Pavlov was puzzled when he noticed that the dogs began to salivate in the presence of the technician who normally fed the dogs. Pavlov began an experiment based on his serendipitous findings to uncover the process that he informally observed. In his experiment, he presented the sound of a metronome (commonly misreported as having been a "bell") right before giving the dogs food. By itself, the metronome did not elicit salivation. However, after several pairings of the metronome followed by food, the metronome became associated with food and elicited salivation by itself!

The process of classical conditioning can be easily understood if we divide it into three phases: before conditioning, during conditioning, and after conditioning. Before conditioning, a stimulus automatically elicits an unlearned behavior (i.e., produces an involuntary response). This is the *unconditioned stimulus* because it automatically triggers a response. For similar reasons, the response that is naturally triggered by the stimulus is the *unconditioned response*. The food in Pavlov's experiment served as the unconditioned stimulus and the salivation as the unconditioned response. Initially, the metronome was a *neutral stimulus* because it did not produce a response (yet!).

During conditioning, the neutral stimulus and the unconditioned stimulus are repeatedly presented together. The most effective method by which classical conditioning takes place is when the neutral stimulus precedes the unconditioned stimulus. The association occurs less effectively if the neutral stimulus occurs after or during the unconditioned stimulus, or if there is a long period of time between their presentations. During this phase, the metronome and food were repeatedly paired. This is the phase in which associative learning takes place; the metronome and food become related and the animal learns to salivate in the presence of the metronome.

After conditioning, the neutral stimulus becomes a *conditioned stimulus* and can reliably elicit the response by itself. When a conditioned stimulus elicits the response, the response is called a *conditioned response*. The conditioned response and unconditioned response are the same response; the difference is in what stimulus caused the response to happen. The associative learning is demonstrated in this phase when the metronome can produce salivation by itself. The metronome is now a conditioned stimulus and salivation produced by the metronome is the conditioned response. This example is a common one, but it can be hard to translate processes discovered in a laboratory to the real world. Instead, let's look at an example you may have witnessed yourself.

When a caregiver enters the kennel area to feed, from a dog's perspective the person makes a lot of noise, and these sounds are distinct. An animal that is naive to the shelter environment might not notice these sounds. Thus, the sound of the first run door opening is a *neutral stimulus*: one that elicits no response and thus has no meaning. Food is the *unconditioned stimulus*. It requires no conditioning to elicit a response (in this case, salivation). The animal's salivation is the *unconditioned response,* because if caregivers present the animal with food, it will salivate automatically (without training). After multiple pairings of the first door opening with the daily feeding, the once-neutral stimulus (the sound of the door opening) is now the conditioned stimulus and causes a conditioned response (salivating at the sound of the run door opening). See another example in Box 3.1 and try to label the neutral stimulus, unconditioned stimulus, unconditioned response, conditioned response, and the conditioned stimulus yourself.

3.3.2 Operant Conditioning

A second form of associative learning occurs when a behavior is paired with a consequence, a process called operant conditioning. Though B. F. Skinner originated the term operant conditioning (also known as instrumental conditioning), his approach to studying animal behavior was largely based on the work of Edward L. Thorndike. As a graduate student, Edward Thorndike studied how success and failure affect behavior (i.e., trial and error

---

Box 3.1   Understanding Respondent Conditioning

Can you identify the *neutral stimulus, unconditioned stimulus,* and *unconditioned response* in this example?

Nail trimming is essential to the well-being of animals, but it could be an unpleasant experience if the owner is inexperienced at trimming nails. During a dog's first experience with nail trimming, the dog might react calmly as his owner approaches him with the nail clippers. However, if the nail is trimmed too short, the dog could wince in pain. From then on, just the sight of the nail clippers can cause the dog to wince.

Do you think you labeled them correctly? Here is the answer:

The nail clippers are the *neutral stimulus* because it had no meaning to the dog prior to the trim. The *unconditioned stimulus* is getting the nails clipped. The *unconditioned response* is the pain the animal felt when the nail was trimmed too short because there is no conditioning required to make an animal react to pain. After pairing the nail clippers with the pain (conditioning), the once-neutral stimulus becomes the conditioned stimulus and causes a conditioned response (just seeing the nail clippers can cause the animal to wince).

learning) by putting cats (among other species) inside a "puzzle box." The cats had incentive to leave the box; they were hungry and there was food outside of the box that entrapped them. The box could be opened from the inside, but only if the cat pressed a lever, pulled a string, and lifted a latch. Naturally, a cat with no experience would struggle haphazardly to get out of the box. During its struggle, it would accidentally press the lever, pull the string, and lift the latch, and voila! the door would open. At first, the cats were slow and unsystematic when trying to open the box. However, Thorndike observed that the cats opened the box faster with more practice. Based on these observations, Thorndike developed the "law of effect," which states that behaviors resulting in a pleasant consequence are likely to be repeated, and those resulting in an unpleasant consequence are likely to stop.

B. F. Skinner found Thorndike's experimental setup to be lacking, mainly because he had to place the cat in the puzzle box after every successful escape. Thus, he looked to create new equipment. The apparatus he made was an *operant chamber*, a box in which a pigeon could peck an illuminated disk or a rat could press a lever to earn food (see Figure 3.1). With this apparatus, Skinner was able to control exactly when the animals would be rewarded

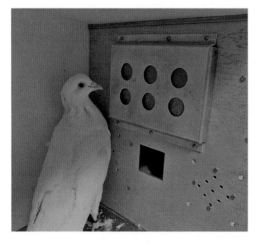

Figure 3.1 A pigeon in a modern, touch-screen-equipped operant chamber.

and didn't have to take the animal out after every trial. Furthermore, data from the operant chamber were collected electronically on a device called a cumulative recorder. He ran a series of experiments in which he tested how an animal's response rate increased or decreased as a result of the frequency of reward. Skinner differentiated between the behaviors in his operant chamber from reflexes by using the term *operant behavior*.

Unlike responses learned through respondent conditioning, operant behaviors are those that "operate" or act on their environment to produce consequences. A key distinction between respondent behaviors and operant behaviors is that operant behaviors are strengthened and weakened by consequences. For example, if the key is turned then the car starts; if the tail is pulled then the dog bites; if the target is touched then food is delivered; if a leash is pulled then the dog is choked; if the electric fence is touched then the animal is shocked. With operant conditioning, the consequence only occurs if the animal engages in a particular behavior; the consequence impacts the likelihood that the behavior occurs again.

Through his research, Skinner demonstrated the effects of *reinforcement* and *punishment*. He found that behavior can be changed by its consequences and went on to distinguish between two types of consequences based on how they affect behavior. Behaviors that are followed by reinforcement are strengthened and more likely to occur again in the future. Thorndike's cat that pressed the lever, pulled a string, and lifted a latch to leave the box was likely to repeat that sequence and even get faster at it because there was food available after escaping. On the other hand, behaviors that are followed by punishment are weakened and less likely to occur again. If instead of getting food after escaping the cat experienced an electric shock, the cat is less likely to repeat the sequence needed to escape the box. It is important to note that reinforcement and punishment are defined *functionally*. This means that it doesn't matter what the consequence is, it could be food, a sound, or

Table 3.1 The four contingencies in operant conditioning.

	Increases behavior (reinforcement)	Decreases behavior (punishment)
Stimulus is added (positive)	Positive reinforcement	Positive punishment
Stimulus is removed (negative)	Negative reinforcement	Negative punishment

an object. As long as a stimulus increases behavior, it is reinforcement, and as long as it decreases behavior, it is punishment.

Skinner (1938, 1953) identified four basic arrangements by which operant conditioning occurs (see Table 3.1). In this context, the words "positive" and "negative" are related to mathematical terms; "positive" means *adding* a stimulus to the situation, and "negative" means *taking away* a stimulus. Adding or removing a stimulus can increase or decrease behavior, depending on the situation. To train a dog to sit, a trainer might offer a dog a treat after she sits down. This would be an instance of *positive reinforcement* because the consequence consisted of a treat *added* to the dog's environment resulting in an *increased* likelihood of sitting in the future. A cat owner might describe using a spray bottle to reduce furniture scratching. This would be an instance of *positive punishment* because the consequence—the water spray—was *added* to the cat's environment and *decreased* scratching.

In *negative reinforcement*, a response results in the removal of an aversive event, and the response increases. The negative reinforcer is ordinarily something the animal tries to avoid or escape, such as a shock from an electric fence. For example, consider training a dog to sit. Instead of offering the dog a treat, a trainer might put pressure on the dog's bottom to get the dog to sit and then release the pressure once the dog is sitting. Assuming the behavior of sitting increases, the behavior of sitting was negatively reinforced. The response (sitting) results in the removal of an event (pressure from the trainer's hand) and the likelihood of the response increases (sitting when hand is on their bottom). A second example of negative

reinforcement is a guard dog barking at a fence as a person walks by. If that person leaves the dog's sight, the dog is likely to bark at the next person that comes to the fence. The response (barking) results in the removal of an event (seeing a person) and the likelihood of the response increases (barking when a person walks by).

The last basic arrangement is *negative punishment*. In this case, the removal of a stimulus decreases the target behavior. For example, if a dog jumps on their owner to get the person's attention, the owner might remove that attention by walking away or turning their back to the dog in an attempt to decrease the behavior. If the jumping up behavior decreases when attention is removed, this is an example of negative punishment. Negative punishment occurs when a behavior results in the removal of a pleasant stimulus, causing a decrease in the behavior's occurrence in the future.

3.4 Effectiveness of Consequences

There are two major factors that can determine the effectiveness of reinforcement and punishment: when and how often the consequences occur. Remember that operant conditioning takes place when a behavior is paired or associated with a consequence. It becomes increasingly difficult for an association to take place if the consequence is delayed from the moment behavior occurs (Wilkenfield et al. 1992). Therefore, *timing* (the *when*) is one important factor for the effectiveness of consequences during the acquisition of new behaviors.

Browne et al. (2013) demonstrated the importance of timing by attempting to teach dogs to sniff the inside of one of two containers with either an immediately delivered reinforcer or a reinforcer delayed by 1 second. Most dogs (86%) were able to learn the behavior within 20 minutes when treats were delivered immediately. In contrast, only 40% of dogs learned the behavior when treats were delayed by 1 second. In fact, if a consequence is delayed from the moment of the target behavior, then it is possible that other behaviors get associated with the consequence instead.

The problem of timing is a common one with pet owners. The following scenario might be familiar: Many dog owners come home to find that their dog has rummaged through the trash. In an attempt to punish trash-rummaging behavior, the owner scolds the dog, perhaps by yelling or confining the dog to a crate. The problem, though, is that it is likely the dog rummaged through the trash hours before the owner came home. Then, even though the dog was peacefully chewing on its dog bone upon the owner's return, it experienced an aversive consequence. Subsequently, the scolding was associated with appropriate behavior instead of the trash-rummaging behavior that the owner attempted to punish. Timing, or more specifically, immediacy, is crucial for the development of a behavior-consequence association.

The second major factor that determines the effectiveness of a reinforcer or punisher in establishing a new or eliminating an unwanted behavior is *how often* the behavior is followed by the consequence. Formally, how often a consequence follows a behavior is called a schedule. If a consequence follows every instance of behavior, then the consequence is on a *continuous* schedule. In contrast, if a consequence does not follow every time a behavior occurs, then the consequence is on an *intermittent* schedule. For a strong association between a behavior and a consequence to develop, the consequence needs to follow the behavior every time it occurs. This is especially true when attempting to teach a new behavior with reinforcement or when attempting to reduce

an unwanted behavior with punishment (Zimmerman and Ferster 1963).

Schedules of consequence deliveries are usually referred to as reinforcement schedules, though they are relevant to punishment as well. Schedules of reinforcement can differ in two ways. First, they can differ based on whether the reinforcer is delivered after a certain number of responses or after some amount of time passed. In *ratio* schedules, reinforcement is delivered following a particular number of responses. *Interval* schedules are set to deliver reinforcement when one response is made after some amount of time has passed. Continuous and intermittent consequence deliveries can be broken down into four schedules: fixed ratio, variable ratio, fixed interval, and variable interval (see Table 3.2).

In *fixed* schedules, the number of responses needed to obtain reinforcement or the amount of time that needs to pass is the same every time. With *fixed ratio* schedules, the number of responses that need to occur for reinforcement to be delivered stays the same after each delivery. The number of responses can be 1, 10, or more. Regardless, the same number of responses is required for reinforcement to occur. For example, in scent detection dogs might not get reinforced with the target scent until the 10th bag they smell. With *fixed interval* schedules, the amount of time that must pass before a response is reinforced is the same across deliveries. Whether the interval is one minute or one hour, the same amount of time must pass before a response is reinforced. For example, a dog begging at the table will not be reinforced for the begging behavior until after the owner is done with dinner and gives the dog a handout.

In *variable* schedules, the number of responses or the interval duration for reinforcement changes around some average. A *variable ratio* schedule requires a different number of responses each time reinforcement occurs. That is, the number of responses can change from one reinforcement to the next (e.g., 5 responses may occur prior to one

Table 3.2 Reinforcement schedules.

Reinforcement schedule	Definition	Example
Fixed interval	Reinforcement is delivered at a predictable time interval	Letting animals out in the play yard: every morning at 9 a.m. the animal caregiver opens the enclosure door, but the animal's behavior of checking the door to go outside isn't reinforced until it checks the door after 9 a.m.
Variable interval	Response is reinforced after an interval of time that varies but centers around some average amount of time	Animal feedings: the time of feeding an animal may vary from day to day, but on average a caregiver provides food every eight hours. Therefore, the animal's response to checking the bowl will not be reinforced until an average of eight hours has passed.
Fixed ratio	Response is reinforced only after a specified number of responses	Multiple repetitions: a trainer wants an animal to do multiple repetitions of the same behavior. Therefore, the trainer delivers reinforcement after every two correct responses.
Variable ratio	Response is reinforced after an average number of responses	Opening the door: an animal might paw at the door several times to be let through. The owner lets the animal in after the animal paws on average five times.

reinforcement, while 10 may occur prior to the next reinforcement, but overall the average number of responses to reinforcement is, for instance, 6). Similarly, with a *variable interval* schedule, the amount of time between reinforcements changes. For instance, on a variable interval schedule of five seconds, reinforcement might be delivered when the animal responds after two seconds has passed this time and not until nine seconds has passed the next time. Box 3.2 explores some examples of variable schedule reinforcement in the shelter.

Though intermittent schedules don't work as well as continuous reinforcement for establishing a new behavior, they work really well in *maintaining* an already established behavior (Jenkins and Stanley 1950). Typically, after a dog is trained to sit, trainers reduce the number of reinforcers she receives for sitting. The trainer gradually transitions the continuous schedule of reinforcement to an intermittent schedule. As long as the dog receives a treat once in a while, she reliably sits on cue.

Changing a continuous schedule of reinforcement to an intermittent one is often called "schedule thinning." This procedure is beneficial for trainers because not only does it reduce the number of reinforcers needed to maintain behavior, but it also causes the animal to perform consistently. Intermittent schedules result in unpredictable deliveries of reinforcers that essentially teach the animal to be a devoted "gambler." Without knowing when a response will be reinforced, the animal performs the behavior consistently and reliably! Based on laboratory research, once a behavior is maintained intermittently, it can be very hard to eliminate (Harper and McLean 1992).

The effects of intermittent reinforcement are commonly found in the shelter. Food-dispensing toys are often provided to facilitate an enriching environment. Caregivers might vary the type of food or switch between food or scent. However, the dog has a preference for food enrichment over the scent enrichment, and after some experience getting the toy with food on some occasions and getting the toy

---

Box 3.2   Variable Schedule Reinforcement in the Shelter

Training Dogs to Sit Using Variable Ratio Reinforcement

An animal trainer is training dogs in the shelter to sit when someone walks by their kennel. The trainer decides to deliver food on a variable ratio 5 (written as VR 5). This means that on average, every fifth response will receive a food reward when someone walks by. The dog might receive a piece of food on the first response (sitting when the first person walks by), sixth response, second response, eighth response, fifth response, eighth response, and so on. If that same dog was trained the same behavior with a fixed ratio 5 (FR 5), then it would receive a piece of hotdog after every fifth response since the number of required responses is *fixed* at five.

Training Dogs Not to Bark Using Variable Interval Reinforcement

An example of an interval schedule would be an animal trainer training dogs in a shelter not to bark when someone enters the kennels. During this training the trainer walks by and randomly rewards a quiet dog. The dog could be quiet for 30 seconds or 10 seconds, but on average the dog will get rewarded for being quiet every 30 seconds, thus this results in a variable interval schedule of reinforcement (VI 30 sec).

---

with scent on others, whether or not the toy contains food is a mystery to the dog! The effect of the intermittent presence of food is evident in the dog's behavior: the dog is likely to check the toy every time it is placed into its enclosure. The behavior of *checking* the toy is on an intermittent schedule of reinforcement, leading the behavior to occur reliably when the toy is present (even though the food reinforcer only occurs sometimes).

Trainers often take advantage of intermittent schedules of reinforcement to facilitate the persistence of behavior in dog training programs (Hall 2017). For example, detection dogs are trained to search for a target item, like drugs or explosives, for long periods of time. As soon as the dogs detect the item, they are trained to notify the handler. In other words, detecting the item is a cue to engage in a different behavior (notifying the handler). The dogs are then given reinforcement for correctly notifying their handler about the found item. Because reinforcers are delivered only after the dog finds an item, it can be tricky to train the dog to continue to persist in searching behavior since no reinforcement is

delivered during that time. To examine the behavior further, Thrailkil et al. (2016) demonstrated how an intermittent schedule of reinforcement can be used to increase the persistence of behavior in a rat model of detection dog training. In their experiment, rats were trained to pull a chain that served as an analog for search behavior. Successfully pulling the chain resulted in the production of a lever that was analogous to finding a target item. The lever presentation cued a lever press, which was then reinforced with food. Pressing the lever was analogous to notifying the handler about the found item. All rats were first trained to pull the chain on a *continuous reinforcement schedule*, meaning that each chain pull gave the rats the opportunity to press the lever. Later, for some rats, the schedule of reinforcement was slowly faded to an *intermittent schedule* so that pulling the chain produced the lever only one-third of the time. For other rats, the schedule of reinforcement remained continuous such that every chain pull produced the lever. To test how the two groups of rats would behave when reinforcement is no longer available, the researchers stopped providing the lever altogether. The rats that underwent intermittent reinforcement persisted in the chain-pulling behavior for a much longer period of time than rats that received continuous reinforcement. This is good news for those dogs working in the field—as long as they find the target item every now and then and get reinforcement, their searching behavior should maintain for long durations.

3.4.1 Conditioned Reinforcement and Conditioned Punishment

When using reinforcement in animal training, we often think of using food, like meat-flavored treats. Food is a biologically based reinforcer, along with others such as water, shelter, and mating, and these are all called primary or unconditioned reinforcers. The same goes for punishers. Some stimuli are unconditioned and function as punishers because of their inherent aversiveness, such as a painful electric shock.

It is obvious, especially when analyzing human behavior, that most of what influences behavior is not a piece of food or access to a mate. Instead, human behavior is often influenced by stimuli that are more complex. For example, students study to get good grades, employees work for money, and children draw silly cartoons for their parent's approval. These stimuli (i.e., grades, money, and approval) get their reinforcing efficacy through the individual's prior learning experience. Without an associative learning history, a good grade or a dollar bill are unlikely to produce any behavior changes. In this respect, they begin as neutral stimuli. Neutral stimuli acquire reinforcing function by being paired with an already established reinforcer. After repeated pairings of the neutral stimulus and a reinforcer, the neutral stimulus becomes a conditioned reinforcer. This should sound familiar! The classical conditioning process of stimulus-stimulus pairings results in the capacity for neutral stimuli to become conditioned reinforcers or conditioned punishers (Williams 1994).

Conditioned reinforcement has been thoroughly investigated in the behavioral laboratory. In the laboratory, when pigeons earn food reinforcers by pecking a key, a grain dispenser, also called a food hopper, is made accessible for a certain period of time so that the pigeon can consume the primary reinforcer (grain). When the food hopper activates, it produces a distinct sound. After repeated pairings of the sound and food, the sound itself becomes a conditioned reinforcer and thus can strengthen behavior (Kelleher 1961). This means that the pigeon will peck at the key just to produce the hopper sound!

Conditioned reinforcers have been shown not only to be effective in strengthening or maintaining behavior, but they can also establish new behavior (Alfernik et al. 1973). A dog is not born wanting to play with toys, but when that toy is paired with primary reinforcers such as social interaction, the toy itself can reinforce a response. The toy can be used to reinforce behaviors the dog already knows as well as behaviors that the dog is learning.

Although conditioned reinforcers can maintain learned responses and establish new ones, they are at risk of losing their reinforcing value if they aren't periodically paired with the unconditioned reinforcer. If the pigeon's key pecks produced only the sound of the hopper but no food, after a while the pigeon would stop pecking. The sound will only function as a reinforcer if it is occasionally paired with food. Similarly, money maintains its reinforcing value because it can be exchanged for goods and services. If someone tried to use Canadian dollars in the United States, the Canadian dollars will lose their reinforcing value quickly because they are no longer paired with other reinforcers.

The same concepts that apply to conditioned reinforcers also apply to conditioned punishers. For example, some dog owners use invisible fencing systems to keep their dogs within the boundaries of their yard. When the dog approaches a boundary, the dog's collar emits a tone and then shortly thereafter a shock. After some experience hearing the tone and then experiencing the shock, the tone alone is aversive to the dog, and the dog refrains from approaching the boundaries. Once a stimulus becomes a conditioned punisher, it can successfully diminish behaviors beyond the context in which they were first paired. That same collar tone could be used to suppress barking, jumping, or potentially any other operant behavior. However, the punishing effects of the tone will eventually wear off if the shock no longer accompanies it. For a conditioned punisher to maintain its suppressive effects, it too must occasionally precede the unconditioned punisher.

Readers experienced in animal training may wonder why we don't discuss clickers in this section. For those non-animal trainers, *clickers* are hand-held devices that, when pressed, make a clicking sound. Clickers and similar devices (such as whistles) are discussed by animal trainers as conditioned reinforcers because they are paired with food. However, this function has been questioned (Dorey and Cox 2018), and more research needs to be conducted to make this claim.

3.4.2 Extinction and Shaping

Behaviors maintained by consistent and predictable reinforcement are highly sensitive to discontinuing reinforcement (Williams 1994). For example, if someone pressed an elevator button, but it didn't light up to indicate that an elevator was on its way, what would the person do? Most people would press the button again, maybe a few more times in rapid succession, or hold the button down harder and longer than usual. After a few attempts, most people would eventually just take the stairs. The process by which a response stops occurring when reinforcement no longer follows the behavior is termed *extinction*.

Extinction can be both a process and a procedure. Extinction as a *procedure* entails withholding the reinforcer that previously maintained a response. Extinction as a *process* involves the decrease and eventual elimination of a response. It is important to note this difference because for extinction as a process to successfully occur, the reinforcer that is maintaining the response must be identified. Sometimes we assume that a behavior is maintained by a certain reinforcer, but relying on assumptions can lead us astray when trying to implement extinction to decrease behavior.

The discovery of extinction as a behavioral process in operant conditioning was completely serendipitous (Skinner 1956). Skinner was running an experiment in which a rat pressed a lever for food. Unbeknownst to Skinner, the pellet dispenser jammed at some point during the session. Therefore, presses on the lever no longer produced reinforcement and underwent extinction. The rat didn't immediately stop pressing the lever; instead, there was a gradual reduction in the number of lever presses before the behavior finally stopped. Skinner's accidental demonstration of extinction highlights an important feature of the process: the behavior under extinction diminishes gradually, not in an all-or-none fashion. How quickly behavior decreases during extinction is a function of the schedule of reinforcement that maintained the behavior, the length of time the behavior has been in the animal's repertoire, and whether conditioned reinforcers are delivered during extinction.

At the beginning of the extinction process, an increase in frequency or intensity of the behavior, called an extinction burst, may occur. Extinction bursts can make the use of extinction difficult when the intention is to reduce behavior. Many pet owners are familiar with a dog who persistently begs during dinner time. She might sit politely by the dining table waiting for the usual handout. The dog has a long history of reinforcement for begging at the table and has learned some methods that might increase the odds of her getting a snack. When she is ignored, she might escalate to whining. When that doesn't work, she might start to bark. The barking can be pretty annoying, making it really difficult to continue ignoring her. If the owner gives the dog food at that point, he or she would have been relieved of the dog's barking temporarily but would have also reinforced barking as a way to get food. In addition, it teaches the dog to be further resistant to extinction because the owner has effectively thinned the reinforcement schedule. Using an extinction procedure can take a long time, and owners must wait for the extinction burst to subside before the begging behavior is completely extinguished. When begging no longer occurs, the association between begging at the dinner table and getting food is overridden by the new learning that begging does not result in food.

Extinction and reinforcement are used in combination to teach new behaviors through a technique called *shaping*. In shaping, a behavior is trained by reinforcing responses with forms that are closer and closer to a final desired behavior. In the laboratory, a common scenario is for a rat to press a lever for food. However, when a rat is put in the operant chamber for the very first time, it is highly unlikely that he would press the lever since the lever-press response and the reinforcer have yet to be associated. Experimenters must first shape the lever-press response before they can run their experiments. As the rat sniffs around the operant chamber and looks in the direction of the lever, the experimenter delivers a food pellet. As the rat moves progressively closer, each approach is reinforced with a food pellet. The experimenter might then wait for the rat to place his paw on the lever before delivering food. And finally, the rat presses down on the

lever, exhibiting the final desired behavior. As *successive approximations* to a lever press are reinforced, previous responses that had formerly been reinforced are extinguished.

3.4.3 Stimulus Control

An important aspect of learning is emitting certain behaviors at certain times or in certain contexts. Otherwise, energy and time are wasted emitting behaviors when the desired consequence is unlikely to happen. We answer the phone when it rings, a cat runs to the sound of the can opener, a trained scent detection dog sits when they smell the target scent, and drivers stop at intersections when the light is red. A stimulus that precedes operant behavior, called an *antecedent*, can become correlated with the consequences that follow behavior. When an antecedent stimulus exerts control over whether or not a behavior occurs, it is said that behavior is under *stimulus control*. Stimulus control explains why animals don't engage in random behavior all the time—an antecedent stimulus that an animal experiences at any given moment signals the animal to behave in ways that are likely to produce reinforcement and avoid behaving in ways that are likely to result in punishment or extinction. In other words, the antecedent stimulus "controls" the occurrence of behavior because it signals that the behavior will be reinforced, punished, or extinguished. A thorough analysis of behavior in terms of operant conditioning usually entails looking at the ABCs: antecedents, behaviors, and consequences (see Table 3.3).

Table 3.3 The ABCs of behavior analysis.

	Description	Example
Antecedent	A stimulus that precedes a response	Mailperson walks down the street
Behavior	The organism's response to the antecedent	The dog barks
Consequence	The stimulus change that follows the behavior (addition or removal of a stimulus)	The mailperson crosses the street and thereby reinforces the dog's barking behavior

In technical terms, if the presentation of a stimulus reliably evokes an operant response, the stimulus is called a "discriminative stimulus." In application, a discriminative stimulus is often called a "cue." For a stimulus to reliably function as a discriminative stimulus, the same rules for creating strong associations apply. The cue needs to reliably and consistently signal a certain consequence if a behavior occurs. Naive trainers sometimes attempt to train their pet to sit by repeatedly saying "sit." After saying "sit" a dozen times, the pet sits and gets a treat. Unfortunately, "sit" never becomes a reliable cue because the pet did not sit most of the time the cue was presented. However, after a few pairings of the trainer saying "sit" once and the dog sits, and the dog is unlikely to sit when the trainer refrains from saying "sit," then the behavior can be said to be under stimulus control.

Antecedent stimuli can reliably evoke behavior after being correlated with reinforcement. Antecedent stimuli can also reliably inhibit behavior by signaling that there is no chance that reinforcement will occur following a behavior (i.e., extinction). A stimulus that signals extinction is termed *s-delta*. Stimuli that signal whether a behavior will be reinforced or not are ubiquitous and very effective in guiding behavior. An "Out of Order" sign on a vending machine tells us that using the machine will not yield us any goodies. In animal behavior, research has found that dogs don't beg from people who aren't looking at them (Udell et al. 2011). A person not looking at the dog is effectively an "Out of Order" sign to the dog that means if the dog begs, it is highly unlikely that she will get food. If the person is making eye contact with the dog, it is more likely that food will be given.

One area of training in which "tight" stimulus control is desired is landmine detection. A non-profit organization called Anti-Persoonsmijnen Ontmijnende Product Ontwikkeling (APOPO) employed the use of giant pouched rats to help with de-mining areas of Africa (Poling et al. 2010). The rats are given extensive training on detecting the odor of a landmine and emitting a behavior to indicate that they found an explosive. So that each landmine is identified and removed safely, it is imperative that the explosives have perfect stimulus control over the indicator behavior. That is, the behavior must occur each time a landmine is found, it must never occur when there is no landmine present, it must never occur in response to a different stimulus, and no other behavior should occur in the presence of the landmine (Pryor 1999). Otherwise, it would be a waste of resources to dig for a landmine that isn't there and would put lives at risk if a landmine is missed.

3.4.3.1 Discrimination and Generalization

After some experience learning a target behavior with one person, a dog might respond to a discriminative stimulus (such as "sit") from other people. Responding to the same cue from a different person is an instance of *generalization*. Conversely, if the dog does *not* respond to a cue by that different person, then the dog is said to *discriminate* between cues (the cue given by the trainer versus the cue given by the new person). To put it simply, stimulus generalization occurs when an animal responds *similarly* to different stimuli, whereas stimulus discrimination occurs when an animal responds *differently* to different stimuli. The extent to which an organism generalizes or discriminates between stimuli is indicative of varying degrees of stimulus control (Cooper et al. 2007).

Animals can learn to discriminate or generalize very subtle features of a stimulus. Nagasawa et al. (2011) demonstrated this aspect of discrimination and generalization with dogs. In their study, dogs were presented two pictures: one of their owner's smiling face and one of their owner's neutral face. Touching the smiling picture resulted in a reinforcer, whereas touching the neutral face did not. The dogs learned to choose the smiling picture of their owner most often, meaning that they learned to *discriminate* between the two pictures. When presented with a smiling and neutral picture of an unfamiliar person, dogs responded similarly in that they chose the smiling face most of the time. The dogs *generalized* to pictures of novel individuals. Interestingly, though, the dogs were only successful in generalizing their responses to pictures of novel individuals of the same sex as their owner. Since they only learned the discrimination task with one sex, they discriminated between sexes.

The processes of discrimination and generalization are complex; *generalization* more readily occurs when two stimuli are *similar*, whereas *discrimination* readily occurs when two stimuli are very *different*. In Nagasawa et al.'s (2011) study, the pictures of the smiling face and neutral face were very different, which helped the dogs learn to discriminate between them. The pictures of their owner and another person of the same sex were similar enough that the dogs were able to generalize

across those stimuli and choose the smiling face. However, the pictures of their owner and another person of a different sex were distinct enough that generalization did not occur.

3.5 Conclusions

Though learning might seem like a complex topic, understanding the processes that take place when an animal learns helps us to develop tools to modify behavior. Observing changes in an animal's behavior in response to changes in its environment allows us the opportunity to gain insight into the learning history and make changes to the animal's behavior. Animals are responding to their environment constantly, and often, the environment responds back in one form or another. This interaction between environment and behavior can be understood through the processes of associative and nonassociative learning.

References

Alferink, L.A., Crossman, E.K., and Cheney, C.D. (1973). Control of responding by a conditioned reinforcer in the presence of free food. *Learn. Behav.* 1 (1), 38–40. https://doi.org/10.3758/BF03198996.

Browne, C.M., Starkey, N.J., Foster, T.M. et al. (2013). Delayed reinforcement—Does it affect learning? *J. Vet. Behav.* 8 (4): e37–e38. https://doi.org/10.1016/j.jveb.2013.04.039.

Cooper J.O., Heron T.E., and Heward W.L. (2007). *Applied Behavior Analysis*. Upper Saddle River, NJ: Pearson.

Dorey, N.R. and Cox, D.J. (2018). Function matters: A review of terminological differences in applied and basic clicker training research. *Peer J.* 6: e5621. https://doi.org/10.7717/peerj.5621.

Hall, N.J. (2017). Persistence and resistance to extinction in the domestic dog: Basic research and applications to canine training. *Behav.*

Process. 141 (1): 67–74. https://doi.org/10.1016/j.beproc.2017.04.001.

Harper, D.N. and McLean, A.P. (1992). Resistance to change and the law of effect. *J. Exp. Anal. Behav.* 57 (3): 317–337. https://doi.org/10.1901/jeab.1992.57-317.

Jenkins, H.M. and Stanley, J.C. (1950). Partial reinforcement: A review and critique. *Psychol. Bull.* 47: 193–234. https://doi.org/10.1037/h0060772.

Kelleher, R.T. (1961). Schedules of conditioned reinforcement during experimental extinction. *J. Exp. Anal. Behav.* 4 (1): 1–5. https://doi.org/10.1901/jeab.1961.4-1.

Nagasawa, M., Murai, K., Mogi, K. et al. (2011). Dogs can discriminate human smiling faces from blank expressions. *Anim. Cogn.* 14 (4): 525–533. https://doi.org/10.1007/s10071-011-0386-5.

Poling, A., Weetjens, B.J., Cox, C. et al. (2010). Teaching giant African pouched rats to find landmines: Operant conditioning with real consequences. *Behav. Anal. Pract.* 3 (2): 19–25. https://doi.org/10.1007/BF03391761.

Pryor, K. (1999) *Don't Shoot the Fog*. New York: Random House.

Skinner, B.F. (1938). *The Behavior of Organisms: An Experimental Analysis*. New York: Appleton-Century-Crofts.

Skinner, B.F. (1953). *Science and Human Behavior*. New York: Macmillan.

Skinner, B.F. (1956). A case history in scientific method. *Am. Psychol.* 11 (5): 221–233.

Thrailkil, E.A., Kacelnik, A., Porritt, F. et al. (2016). Increasing the persistence of a heterogeneous behavior chain: Studies of extinction in a rat model of search behavior of working dogs. *Behav. Process.* 129: 44–53. https://doi.org/10.1016/j.beproc.2016.05.009.

Udell, M.A.R., Dorey, N.R., and Wynne, C.D.L. (2011). Can your dog read your mind? Understanding the causes of canine perspective taking. *Learn. Behav.* 39 (4): 289–302. https://doi.org/10.3758/s13420-011-0034-6

Wilkenfield, J., Nickel, M., Blakely, E. et al. (1992). Acquisition of lever-press responding in rats with delayed reinforcement: A comparison of three procedures. *J. Exp. Anal. Behav.* 58 (3): 431–443. https://doi.org/10.1901/jeab.1992.58-431.

Williams, B.A. (1994). Conditioned reinforcement: Experimental and theoretical issues. *Behav. Anal.* 17: 261–285. https://doi.org/10.1007/bf03392675.

Zimmerman, J. and Ferster, C.B. (1963). Intermittent punishment of S^Δ responding in matching-to-sample. *J. Exp. Anal. Behav.* 6: 349–356. https://doi.org/10.1901/jeab.1963.6-349.

4

The Relationship between Physiology and Behavior in Dogs and Cats

Valarie V. Tynes, Colleen S. Koch, and Leslie Sinn

4.1 Introduction

Behavior can change as a result of medical problems or physiological changes. If shelter operations, behavior, and/or medical staff identify behaviors that may have an underlying medical cause, they can be addressed immediately, relieving suffering and increasing the adoptability of the animal. Conversely, if medical conditions that cause or exacerbate problematic behaviors are missed, time may be wasted on training or attempted behavior modification, thus prolonging suffering and time spent in the shelter. At the same time, a complex relationship can exist between physical conditions or disease and behavior, so careful attention must be given to how the two systems (mind and body) affect each other.

4.2 General Concepts of the Relationship between Medical and Behavioral Issues

To provide optimal medical care for any animal, it is imperative that we first move beyond the paradigm where we attempt to separate "medical" conditions from "behavioral" conditions. All medical conditions will result in some behavioral change (American Psychiatric Association 2013). Many of these are the most basic of signs and symptoms that all veterinarians are taught to look for, such as the lethargy and anorexia associated with many illnesses. In addition, every behavior is a result of neurochemical action at the molecular level in the nervous system and thus cannot ever be completely separated from the physiological (see Figure 4.1). While some behavioral changes can be associated with organic diseases, such as space-occupying masses in the central nervous system or the changes that occur as a result of infection and/or inflammation, other behaviors can result from dysregulation at the neurophysiological or neurochemical level—problems that we still have much to learn about. It is hoped that with advancing technology, our understanding of the neurophysiologic basis of behavior will continue to improve.

Using a medical model approach to problem behaviors can improve communications between caregivers, shelter staff, and the rest of the health care team. This approach broadly categorizes behavior problems using terminology similar to that used in human mental health. However, these categories are purely descriptive and often attempt to assign a motivation to the unwanted behavior. This terminology does not necessarily reflect a knowledge of the cause, mechanism, or

Animal Behavior for Shelter Veterinarians and Staff, Second Edition. Edited by Brian A. DiGangi, Victoria A. Cussen, Pamela J. Reid, and Kristen A. Collins.
© 2022 John Wiley & Sons, Inc. Published 2022 by John Wiley & Sons, Inc.
Companion website: www.wiley.com/go/digangi/animal

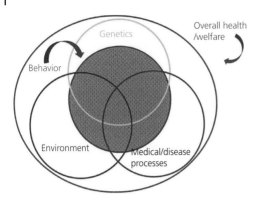

Figure 4.1 This diagram depicts how genetics, the environment, and medical conditions/disease processes all contribute to behavior. The relationship and interconnectedness of all of these components will be reflected in the overall health and welfare of the individual.

neurobiology underlying the behavior (American Psychiatric Association 2013). Some behaviors may reflect a dysregulation or disruption of the neurological system and may thus be considered truly malfunctional, as the medical model suggests. Other behaviors may represent an animal's attempt to adapt to an environment to which adaption is not completely possible and should be considered maladaptive (Mills 2003). Having a thorough understanding of normal species-typical behaviors for the animal in question is critical to developing a management and/or treatment plan for the individual exhibiting maladaptive or malfunctional behaviors. A third category that will not be covered in this chapter is the normal adaptive behaviors of animals that are simply inconvenient or problematic for their caretakers. See Chapters 12 and 18 for more information on training and behavior modification.

A variety of different disease processes can cause and/or contribute to the worsening of both maladaptive and malfunctional behaviors. Many individuals will simply differ in how readily they react to stimuli, the degree to which they respond, and how long they stay emotionally aroused. These differences often represent normal individual variations in temperament and are also affected by an individual's experience during development.

4.3 Recognizing the Behavior of the Sick Animal

It is well understood that dogs and cats continue to express many of the behavioral patterns expressed by their wild ancestors. The behaviors typical of sick animals represent a highly adaptive behavioral strategy, so it is not surprising that many of these behaviors have been retained in spite of domestication. Initially, most sick animals will display varying degrees of lethargy and anorexia. In many cases, this occurs due to the development of a febrile response. These behaviors, often viewed by caretakers as abnormal, are in fact normal and serve a beneficial purpose for the affected animal (see Box 4.1). Fever has the effect of assisting the animal to combat infectious disease by potentiating numerous immunologic responses (Hart 2010; Hart 2011). It also produces a body temperature that is inappropriate for the growth of most pathogenic organisms. The same physiologic response that produces the fever results in anorexia, and the animal, with no desire to move about in search of food or water, will save energy needed to make up for the increased metabolic cost of the fever.

Due to the fact that febrile animals feel cold, they are likely to lie curled up. This reduces the body surface area and decreases

---

Box 4.1 General Behavioral Responses to Illness in Dogs and Cats

Reduced activity
Reduced appetite
Decreased water intake
Increased sleep
Decreased interest in social interaction
Decreased play behavior
Decreased grooming behavior

heat loss by convection and radiation. Piloerection is also likely in sick animals, as it provides some increased insulating ability (Hart 2010). The lethargic, ill animal will spend less time grooming, so a coat that appears dirtier or oilier than normal may be an indication of illness. Grooming requires movement and thus expenditure of energy, and oral grooming can lead to a significant amount of water loss, especially critical to a febrile animal attempting to conserve water, energy, and body heat.

There will be some variation in how rapidly these behavioral changes set in and in the degree to which they appear, depending upon the pathogen involved. Some diseases will cause a rapid and severe onset of lethargy and anorexia, while others may develop more slowly, and the behavioral signs may be less obvious. The status of each individual's immune system may also affect the degree of illness experienced and thus the degree of behavioral change.

An animal's coat can provide important clues regarding its health status. Grooming behavior has evolved in mammals to serve a variety of purposes, depending upon the species. These behaviors may spread natural body oils throughout the coat, contributing to coat health and thermoregulation, as well as effectively decreasing ectoparasite loads (Hart 2011). Saliva contains a variety of anti-bacterial and wound-healing substances, so that the predisposition for animals to lick body parts and wounds is likely an evolved behavioral tool for decreasing the incidence of infection (Hart 2011). When animals fail to practice normal self-grooming behavior, it should serve as a warning sign that something is wrong.

4.3.1 Cats

Some dogs can be adept at hiding their ill-nesses, but cats are even better at it. This may be due to the cat's unusual position of being both predator and prey, depending upon the environment. Anorexia is often the first sign noted by caretakers of sick cats. The fastidious nature of the cat contributes to the ability to mask signs of disease. For example, if cats have diarrhea, they are likely to clean themselves, removing all signs of the mess, until they become too ill to do so. The more sedentary and nocturnal nature of the cat may also cause caretakers to overlook inactivity due to illness until it becomes severe. Unkempt hair coat in a cat should be immediately noted and a possible cause investigated because the cat must be either ill, injured, or otherwise impaired in its movement in order for it to stop grooming itself.

A variety of different studies have suggested that monitoring sickness behaviors in the cat may be an excellent means of evaluating feline welfare and that cats' behavior is a more reliable indicator of their level of stress than their physiological responses (Stella et al. 2013). One study demonstrated that the presence of unusual external events is enough to increase the risk of sickness behaviors in cats (Stella et al. 2011). When cats are exposed to multiple unpredictable stressors, including exposure to unfamiliar caretakers, an inconsistent husbandry schedule, and discontinuation of play time, socialization, food treats, and auditory enrichment, they demonstrate a higher incidence of sickness behaviors (Stella et al. 2013). These behaviors include increased vomiting (Stella et al. 2013), decreased food intake, avoidance of elimination for 24 hours, and elimination outside the litterbox (Stella et al. 2011).

4.4 The Role of Stress

Nowhere else is the interplay between behavioral and physical health more apparent than when looking at the impact that stress plays on every aspect of health. Increasingly, science is uncovering the myriad of different ways in which stress affects living organisms at every stage of development. Much controversy exists about how to define stress, so for the purpose of this chapter, stress (or stressors) is defined as anything that disturbs or threatens homeostasis. These stressful forces may be physical, chemical, or emotional and typically result in physiological or behavioral responses as the organism attempts to restore homeostasis. The physiological events that occur during an acutely stressful event are intended to be adaptive, and, in most cases, they do succeed in helping an organism maintain homeostasis by adapting to the stressor. When stress is chronic and unremitting, or the individual cannot successfully act in such a way as to decrease the stressors, a variety of physiological events can conspire to damage the overall health and well-being of the organism. Thus, in the long term, the stress response can be maladaptive.

There are two primary components of the stress response, involving two different endocrine systems. The first is the sympathetic nervous system response. Within seconds of perceiving a stressor, the sympathetic nervous system begins secreting norepinephrine, and the adrenal medullae begin secreting epinephrine. This begins to prepare the body for "fight or flight." The second system is the hypothalamic-pituitary-adrenal (HPA) axis, generally believed to be the body's primary stress-responsive physiological system (Hennessy 2013). When the HPA axis is triggered, the hypothalamus releases corticotrophin-releasing factor that triggers the release of adrenocorticotropic hormone from the pituitary gland. This hormone then stimulates the release of glucocorticoids from the adrenal cortex. Several other hormones, including prolactin, glucagon, thyroid hormones, and vasopressin, are secreted from various other endocrine organs. The overall effect of these circulating hormones is to increase the immediate availability of energy, increase oxygen intake, decrease blood flow to areas not critical for movement, and inhibit digestion, growth, immune function, reproduction, and pain perception. In addition, memory and sensory functions are enhanced. Essentially, the goals of all of this physiological activity are to make more energy available for immediate use and to put on hold any and all processes that are not involved in immediate survival.

Acute stress has been shown to enhance the memory of an event that is threatening (McEwen 2000). This is clearly adaptive if it allows the organism to form strong associations, enabling it to avoid dangerous things in the future. Knowing this should increase animal handlers' awareness of the important and lasting impact that their behavior and actions can have on an animal. An unpleasant handling experience may have long-term, negative effects on the animal's behavior, ultimately making that animal less adoptable.

If the stress response continues, for whatever reason, cardiovascular, metabolic, reproductive, digestive, immune, and anabolic processes can all be pathologically affected. The results can include myopathy, fatigue, hypertension, decreased growth rates, gastrointestinal distress, and suppressed immune functioning with subsequent impaired disease resistance. Chronic stress can even lead to structural and functional changes in the brain, and when extreme conditions persist, permanent damage can result (McEwen 2000). It is believed that when dealing with chronic stress, the HPA axis becomes dysregulated, and the various components of the system may no longer respond in the predicted fashion. For example, in some cases, chronic stress results in adrenal hypertrophy and elevated levels of glucocorticoids, while adrenocortical-stimulating hormone (ACTH) levels remain unchanged. At this point, the dysregulation results in an HPA axis that is no longer able to respond appropriately to future stressful events, and measurements of glucocorticoid levels may become less meaningful (Hennessy 2013).

Stress can arise from a variety of different sources, both physiological and psychological. Physical stress can be caused by hunger, thirst, pain, exposure to extreme temperatures, disease, illness, and sleep deprivation. Psychological stress can result from exposure to novelty, unpredictable environments, social conflict, and constant exposure to fear- or anxiety-provoking stimuli as well as any other situation that leads to chronic frustration or conflict. A lack or loss of control is another important psychological stressor. In fact, novelty, withholding of reward, and the anticipation of punishment (not the punishment itself) have been found to be the most potent of all psychological stressors (McEwen 2000).

A variety of different means have been used in an attempt to measure physiological stress, including but not limited to measuring glucocorticoids and their metabolites in hair, urine, feces, blood, and saliva. Glucocorticoids in blood and saliva do appear to measure the condition of the animal at that moment, whereas glucocorticoids in urine, feces, and hair reflect the condition of the animal over a longer time frame (Hennessy 2013). ACTH and luteinizing hormone-releasing hormone stimulation tests have also been used to measure adrenal and pituitary sensitivities, respectively, and one study demonstrated increased HPA responsiveness and reduced pituitary sensitivity occurring in the face of chronic stress (Carlstead et al. 1993). The altered responsiveness was suggestive of HPA dysfunction. A decrease in peripheral lymphocyte numbers and an increase in neutrophil numbers, along with an increased neutrophil:lymphocyte ratio, is another well-documented response to glucocorticoid release and has been proposed as another reliable method for evaluating the stress an animal may be experiencing (Davis et al. 2008).

Studies have shown that the average shelter dog does have higher levels of circulating cortisol than pet dogs that were sampled in their homes (Hennessy et al. 1997). Some studies of shelter dogs have found that circulating levels of cortisol return to normal within days to weeks, but others have found that HPA axis dysregulation develops in some dogs (Hennessy 2013).

Any single individual's response to stress will vary as a result of several different factors such as genetics, temperament, experience, environment, and learning. For example, cats not socialized to people have been shown to be more likely to experience high levels of stress when exposed to people in a shelter

setting (Kessler and Turner 1999a). Experiences during the first weeks of life have been shown to have profound effects on an animal's ultimate ability to cope with stress (Foyer et al. 2013). The importance of the role of maternal stress on the developing offspring during the prenatal period is receiving an increasing amount of attention (Jensen 2014). Research in numerous species has demonstrated that when the gestating mother experiences stress, it can alter her behavior and affect the behavioral development of her young (Braastad et al. 1998; Chapillon et al. 2002; Champagne et al. 2006). Subsequently, her offspring often show a decreased ability to deal with stress: they may have some learning impairment and they may be more susceptible to the conditioning of fearful responses, especially to auditory stimuli (Ross et al. 2017). The individual's perception of stress, which will also vary based on experience, is ultimately the most important factor that influences the effect of stress. Many potential stressors exist for the sheltered dog and cat. Table 4.1 provides a summary of common shelter stressors and behavioral signs of stress.

4.4.1 Cats

Several studies have evaluated the stressors impacting shelter and laboratory cats. Shelter cats exhibiting higher stress scores are at higher risk of developing upper respiratory tract infections (Tanaka et al. 2012). One study reported that feigned sleep may be a coping mechanism seen in stressed shelter cats (Dinnage 2006). An increased need for restorative sleep has been demonstrated in both humans and animals exposed to physiological or biological stress (Rampin et al. 1991; Rushen 2000). These data suggest that while cats may appear to be the most relaxed of animals, they may, in fact, suffer the highest levels of stress.

The stress level of most kenneled cats will decrease over the first few days to weeks. One study demonstrated that two-thirds of cats will adjust well within the first two weeks (Kessler

Table 4.1 Common Stressors and Behavioral Signs of Stress in Shelter Dogs and Cats (Jones and Josephs 2006; Horváth et al. 2008; Beerda et al. 1998, 1999; Carlstead et al. 1993; Kessler and Turner 1999b; Tanaka et al. 2012; Kessler and Turner 1997; Dinnage 2006).

Common stressors	Behavioral signs of stress
Dogs	
Separation from familiar social figures	Trembling
Loud noises	Crouching
Restraint and unpredictable handling	Oral behaviors (e.g., snout licking, swallowing, smacking)
Confinement	
Elimination on unfamiliar surfaces and/or in living space	Yawning
	Restlessness
Sounds and odors associated with the stress and aggressive behavior of other dogs	Lowered body posture
	Increased autogrooming
Altered routines	Paw lifting
Immersion in novel environment, surrounded by novel stimuli	Vocalizing
	Repetitive behavior
	Coprophagy
Cats	
Unpredictable handling and husbandry routines	Decreased food intake and weight loss
Increased density of group-housing	Less play and active exploratory behaviors
Inability to hide	More time awake and alert
	Attempting to hide
	Behavioral apathy
	Vocalization
	Escape behaviors
	Aggressive behavior
	Feigned sleep

and Turner 1997). The same study demonstrated that about 4% of cats maintained a high level of stress for the entire study period, suggesting that for a small segment of the feline population, housing in the shelter for any extended period may not be in the best interest of that individual (Kessler and Turner 1997).

4.5 The Behavior of Pain

Recognizing the behavioral signs of pain in nonverbal species is challenging. Because animals can't tell us when they experience pain, it is critical to train shelter staff to recognize their nonverbal signs if we are to ensure good welfare. A number of problem behaviors can occur in dogs and cats in response to pain. These can include irritability (increased sensitivity and reactivity to

stimuli), aggressiveness, restlessness, excessive vocalization, changes in activity level, and an increase in anxiety-related behaviors. In an animal that was previously behaviorally stable, any abrupt changes in behavior can signal pain, but they are especially noteworthy when occurring in a middle-aged or geriatric animal.

Pain in the shelter animal may be even more difficult to identify since caretakers may not be familiar enough with an individual to determine what is normal or abnormal for that animal. To further complicate matters, physiologic responses to pain and stress can be similar, and because animals entering a shelter are likely to experience stress, this may make differentiating the two very difficult. In addition, it is normal for most animals to try to mask their pain, and they may be even more likely to do this when placed in a stressful situation.

The objective signs of medical problems that typically result in pain cannot always be identified with a physical exam, radiographs, laboratory work, and so forth. Therefore, it is generally accepted that behavioral rather than physiological signs are the most important parameters we should attend to when evaluating pain in animals (Epstein et al. 2015). We should also always keep in mind that if a procedure, injury, or illness causes pain in humans, then it would be wise to assume that it causes pain in dogs and cats as well.

Different animals will manifest pain differently, and there is no single behavior that can be considered pathognomonic for pain. Neither does the absence of certain behaviors always indicate the absence of pain. Many behaviors considered to be indicative of pain can also occur due to anxiety or fear in both dogs and cats. In addition, the presence of other diseases can change the appearance of pain behaviors. Several studies have found that subjective behavioral measures can be used successfully to identify pain in animals and subsequently evaluate the efficacy of treatment (Holton et al. 1998; Cloutier et al. 2005; Bennett and Morton 2009). However, more research is needed to refine and validate some of the current methods. Because some diagnostic capabilities may be limited in a shelter situation, anecdotal information suggests that when in doubt, a course of treatment with analgesics and/or anti-inflammatories may be warranted if a painful condition is suspected. Failure to recognize pain is a significant welfare concern. Training shelter staff is a crucial task for shelter management to ensure that staff can reliably and consistently recognize even the most subtle signs of pain in animals. Table 4.2 provides a summary of behavioral signs of pain in dogs and cats.

4.5.1 Cats

Improving our ability to identify pain in cats is important for many reasons. Degenerative joint disease (DJD) is more common in cats than previously believed (Perry 2014). Although some cats will appear pain free and still have joint abnormalities visible on radiographs (Monteiro and Steagall 2019), several studies have shown that signs of pain and discomfort associated with DJD commonly occur prior to the appearance of radiographic signs (Hardie et al. 2002; Clarke and Bennett 2006). Overt lameness is much less common in cats than dogs (Clarke and Bennett 2006). In addition, while palpation may be effective at determining when and where dogs experience pain, cats often resist palpation under normal circumstances; therefore, response to palpation is unlikely to be diagnostic for pain or discomfort. Osteoarthritis is not the only cause of chronic pain in the cat; pain secondary to cancer and dental disease (e.g., feline orofacial pain syndrome [FOPS]) should also be of concern.

4.5.2 Neuropathic Pain

When evaluating dogs and cats for pain, it is also important to be aware that there are different kinds of pain and altered sensation. Neuropathic pain has been defined as "pain arising as a direct consequence of a lesion or disease affecting the somatosensory system" (Shilo and Pascoe 2014). It is considered a chronic pain state that results from peripheral or central nerve injury and can be due to acute events such as amputation or systemic disease such as diabetes. As opposed to functional pain, neuropathic pain is believed to serve no purpose. Nociceptors are not involved, and the mechanisms underlying the syndrome are unclear. The relief of neuropathic pain is generally considered extremely challenging.

The possibility of phantom limb pain, where the patient perceives pain in a limb that is no longer present, should also be considered as a possible outcome of amputation (Shilo and Pascoe 2014). Since animals cannot report what they are experiencing verbally, and limited diagnostic capabilities may prevent us from being able to clearly recognize these conditions in animals, it will be even more incumbent upon the caretaker to be extremely observant for signs of pain in animals.

Table 4.2 Behavioral signs of pain in dogs and cats (Mills et al. 2020; Bacon et al. 2019; Godfrey 2005; Bennett and Morton 2009; Slingerland et al. 2011).

Dogs	Cats
More common	*General signs*
Anorexia	Avoidance or flight behavior
Avoidance behaviors	Restlessness or agitation
Hiding	Hunched posture
Aggression	Squinting eyes
Hunched body posture	Reluctance to move
Whining or howling	Vocalization (including purring)
Decreased social interactions	Gait changes
Changes in activity level	Decreased appetite
Changes in temperament or mood	Changes in grooming behavior
Reluctance to move or change position when recumbent *or*	Tail flicking
Increased restlessness and frequent changes in position	Changes in interactions with people
Tense facial muscles with ears pulled back from the face and a grimace	Decreased tolerance to handling
May attempt to bite at or lick a painful area	Aggression when certain body parts are manipulated
May rub painful areas against walls, doors, or other objects	Aggression when attempting to move or lift
Increased heart rate, respiratory rate, and/or blood pressure	
Less common	*Signs of pain associated with degenerative joint disease*
Pica	Decreased walking, running, jumping, or climbing
Housesoiling	Increased sleep
Noise sensitivity	Decreased play
Clinginess	Stiff movement or a shuffling gait
Excessive licking	Appearance of weakness
	Difficulty jumping
	Altered temperament
	Inappropriate elimination

4.6 Common Medical Conditions Resulting in Behavioral Signs

4.6.1 Anxiety Disorders

Anxiety is the emotional response that occurs when there is the anticipation of future danger. What is critical for animal caretakers to be aware of is that the danger does not have to be real; it may be unknown or imagined. Equally important is that when animals perceive something to be dangerous or threatening, that is what they will respond to emotionally. The physiological responses to feelings of anxiety are similar to the responses that are seen with fear (see Box 4.2). Many of these behaviors can also be seen associated with particular medical conditions, further complicating some diagnoses.

In addition, it appears that some individuals have behavioral dysfunction due to pathological anxiety, and this results in maladaptive

Box 4.2   Behavioral Signs of Anxiety
Panting
Pacing
Trembling
Salivating
Increased blood pressure
Increased heart rate
Increased respiratory rate
Dilated pupils
Avoidance behaviors such as hiding
Hypervigilance
General behavioral arousal
Irritability
Restlessness
Freezing or tonic immobility response
Increased aggression or threatening behaviors
Sleep-wake cycle disturbances
Lowered body posture (crouching)
Lowered ears
Tucked tail
Repeated lip or snout licking
Yawning

behavior. A definition for pathological anxiety has been proposed: "Pathological anxiety is a persistent, uncontrollable, excessive, inappropriate and generalized dysfunctional and aversive emotion, triggering physiological and behavioural responses lacking adaptive value. Pathological anxiety-related behaviour is a response to the exaggerated anticipation or perception of threats, which is incommensurate with the actual situation" (Ohl et al. 2008).

Differentiating pathological anxiety from the situational anxiety that might be expected in an animal that has recently been introduced into a shelter situation will not be easy as the line between normal and abnormal is often vague. However, caretakers should remain aware that some animals will not adapt well to the shelter environment due to preexisting behavioral pathology. In addition, the behavioral pathology may predispose these animals to illness and poor welfare due to the chronic stimulation of the HPA axis and the animal's

inability to adapt to the changing environment. Lastly, anxiety can occur as a result of any disease process, pain, or discomfort, especially if it remains unidentified by caretakers and thus untreated.

4.6.2   Neurological Disorders

A variety of different neurological disorders have the capability of affecting behavior in a variety of different ways. While many neurological disorders are steadily progressive and, thus, will eventually present additional non-behavioral signs, in many cases, behavioral changes will precede the appearance of other more severe neurological signs by weeks or even months. Storage diseases, neoplasia, inflammatory conditions, degenerative conditions, toxicosis, malformations, ischemia, and infections can all lead to changes in behavior.

The location of a brain lesion will dictate the associated behavior changes. The limbic system, whose structures lie deep within the brain, functions to control memory, emotions, and basic drives such as sexual activity, anxiety, and feelings of pleasure. Damage to the limbic system can result in personality changes, including increases in fearfulness and aggressive behavior. In other cases, seizures may result. The forebrain, including the prefrontal area, is the part of the brain associated with cognitive behavior, motor planning, thought, and perception. Forebrain lesions can lead to changes in temperament, loss of previously learned behaviors, and failure to recognize or respond appropriately to environmental stimuli. Lesions of the brain stem or forebrain may lead to changes in awareness or consciousness and mentation. Animals with brain stem lesions may demonstrate altered responses to stimuli, dullness, and stupor and may become comatose (Lorenz et al. 2011).

4.6.2.1   Neoplasia

Intracranial neoplasia can be either primary or secondary, and, depending on the location within the brain and the character of the tumor, brain neoplasia can result in several different behavioral changes. Primary brain tumors originate from cells within the brain and meninges and are more likely to result in insidious, slowly progressive effects, whereas secondary tumors resulting from metastatic disease will usually result in acute changes.

Seizures, while the most recognizable, are not always the most common sign of a brain tumor. Other early behavioral and clinical signs of a brain tumor such as changes in behavior and mentation, visual deficits, circling, ataxia, head tilt, and cervical spinal hyperesthesia are often not appreciated. Reluctance to climb stairs, pacing, standing in corners, stumbling over objects, housesoiling, and agitation may also be seen.

4.6.2.1.1 Dogs

Primary brain tumors in the dog may include meningioma, astrocytoma, neuroblastoma, oligodendroglioma, and ependymoma, to name a few. Dogs with brain tumors are usually presented with concurrent neurologic deficits, but one study found that when brain tumors developed in the rostral cerebrum, behavioral changes commonly occurred prior to the appearance of other neurologic deficits (Foster et al. 1998). These changes were described as dementia, aggression, and alteration in established habits. Many of the dogs in the study, but not all, also had seizures, but 72% of them had no neurological deficits on presentation. Neurological deficits eventually appeared in all cases, with some taking up to three months to appear (Foster et al. 1998). Meningiomas, the most common primary brain tumor in dogs, usually occur in dogs more than seven years of age but have been seen in dogs as young as 11 weeks. Behavioral signs may include increases in aggression, head pressing, circling, housesoiling, pacing and panting (common signs of agitation), vocalizations, seizures, and changes in mentation.

While neoplasia in dogs younger than six months occurs less often, the brain is the second most common site for it to develop, so age alone cannot always rule out the possibility of a brain tumor. However, brain tumors occur most often in dogs more than five years of age.

4.6.2.1.2 Cats

Meningiomas are also the most common tumor of the feline brain and have been documented in cats as young as one year of age. Geriatric cats with meningioma have been presented to their veterinarian with the owner complaint of "just not being themselves" (Sessums and Mariani 2009). Clinical signs that have been reported include reluctance to play, episodic lethargy, and aggression. One owner reported apparent pain when she touched her cat's head, three months prior to presentation with other clinical signs (Karli et al. 2013).

4.6.2.2 Seizures

Generalized seizures in dogs and cats are characterized by the animal falling into a laterally recumbent position with limbs rigid and paddling. They may or may not evacuate their bladder or bowels, they may vocalize, and they will usually fail to respond if spoken to or touched. Focal seizures, however, are involuntary movements that may be localized to a single limb or part of the face. The animal experiencing a focal seizure may be somewhat responsive to other stimuli, but an aura and pre- and postictal phases may be present. These types of seizures can result in unusual behavioral presentations and can be difficult to diagnose.

Focal seizures may be divided into motor and sensory-type seizures. While motor seizures involve involuntary movement of one part of the body, sensory focal seizures may result in abnormal sensations such as tingling, pain, or visual hallucinations. Fly-biting or fly-snapping behaviors in some dogs may occur as a result of focal seizures with visual hallucinations. However, evidence linking these and similar behaviors to gastrointestinal distress confirms the possibility of multiple etiologies that can be associated with this non-specific behavioral sign (Frank 2012; Mills et al. 2020). Complex focal seizures (formerly known as psychomotor seizures) are focal seizures with alterations in awareness. Affected dogs may exhibit repetitive motor activities such as head pressing, vocalizing, or aimless walking or running (Berendt and Gram 1999). In some cases, complex focal seizures manifest as impaired consciousness and bizarre behavior, such as unprovoked aggression or extreme, irrational fear (Dodman et al. 1992, 1996).

Seizures are just one type of involuntary movement disorder in dogs and cats. Other forms of involuntary movements can occur and will need to be differentiated from seizures and primary behavioral disorders. Movements seen during periods of inactivity can be confirmed as movement disorders rather than behavioral disorders. However, involuntary movement disorders such as those associated with cerebellar diseases will occur during periods of activity. Some metabolic diseases and peripheral nervous system and musculoskeletal disorders may also result in involuntary movements. Involuntary movements limited to facial or head movements are likely to be caused by a seizure disorder.

4.6.2.2.1 Cats

Cats with acute onset of partial seizure involving orofacial movements, such as salivation, facial twitching, lip smacking, chewing, licking, or swallowing, along with other behavioral changes, such as sitting and staring while motionless and/or acting confused, have been diagnosed with a form of hippocampal necrosis (Pakozdy et al. 2011). The majority of these cats exhibited other neurological abnormalities on their first presentation. Seizures in cats may also be associated with metabolic disease such as diabetes mellitus, hepatic encephalopathy, neoplasia, or meningoencephalitis (Barnes et al. 2004).

4.6.2.3 Toxicosis

Toxins may lead to personality changes in animals. Animals that have been intoxicated may present with central nervous system signs such as ataxia, stupor, seizures, or death. When signs are acute, a history of exposure is usually present. Shelter staff will be unlikely to encounter these scenarios since once the animal is in the shelter, opportunities to access toxic substances will be limited.

4.6.2.4 Degenerative Conditions

Most degenerative conditions of the neurologic system are heritable and will appear within the first few weeks to months of life. They include such conditions as cerebellar abiotrophy and lysosomal storage diseases.

Cerebellar abiotrophy can be minimal to rapidly progressive and varies to some degree by the breed affected. The condition has been reported in many breeds, including the Kerry blue terrier, rough-coated collie, beagle, Samoyed, Irish setter, Gordon setter, Airedale, Finnish harrier, Bernese mountain dog, Labrador and golden retriever, cocker spaniel, cairn terrier, and Great Dane. Most puppies will be normal at birth. At two to nine weeks of age, they begin to show signs of cerebellar damage, including ataxia, intention tremors, swaying, hypermetria, a head tilt, and a broad-based stance. At the extreme, pups may demonstrate opisthotonos with extensor rigidity of the forelimbs and flexed hindlimbs, the typical decerebellate posture. While the age of onset is prior to four months in most cases, some animals may not show signs of disease until two to two-and-a-half years of age. In some cases where the disease progression is minimal or very slow, some animals can learn to compensate for their disabilities. Cerebellar abiotrophy can develop in the cat but has been less well documented. A single case report has described adult-onset cerebellar cortical abiotrophy with retinal degeneration in a domestic shorthaired cat (Joseph 2011). If observed and examined carefully, the clinical signs associated with cerebellar degeneration should be readily differentiated from primary behavioral problems.

Lysosomal storage diseases are relatively rare genetic defects that are characterized by progressive neuronal degeneration. They are most likely to occur in purebred animals with a history of inbreeding in the affected line. Animals born with lysosomal storage diseases are normal at birth, with clinical signs usually developing during the first year of life. Neuronal ceroid lipofuscinosis is one of the storage diseases that can appear in adult animals. Case reports of dachshunds with this condition have reported dogs developing the signs at three, five, and seven years of age (Cummings and de LaHunta 1977; Vandevelde and Fatzer 1980). Early signs may include ataxia, disorientation, weakness, and behavioral changes, but, with time, affected individuals will suffer vision loss, progressive motor and cognitive decline, and seizures.

4.6.2.5   Inflammatory Conditions

Clinical signs will vary with the site of the brain inflammation and may be acute or chronic. A progressive, acute disease process is most typical. Neurological deficits seen with inflammation may be diffuse, focal, or multifocal. Encephalitis or parenchymal central nervous inflammation may present with depression, stupor, coma, or other types of altered consciousness. Blindness, ataxia, seizures, and other behavioral changes may also be seen. Box 4.3 lists some of the more common infectious and parasitic causes of central nervous system signs in dogs and cats.

4.6.3   Urogenital Disorders

Inappropriate elimination is a common behavioral complaint for pet owners, but it is also often a primary sign of a medical condition. Distinguishing the two and/or recognizing when a medical condition exists at the same time as learned behavior (or a failure of house training) can be challenging but will be critical to solving the problem. Box 4.4 lists some of the more common reasons for dogs and cats to soil the house with urine. Regardless of the species, the first challenge is to observe the animal and attempt to determine if it has voluntary control over urination some of the time, all of the time, or none of the time, as this will help narrow down the list of differential diagnoses.

> **Box 4.3   Infectious and Parasitic Causes of Central Nervous System Signs in Dogs and Cats**
>
> Feline infectious peritonitis
> Feline leukemia virus
> Toxoplasmosis
> Canine distemper virus
> Rabies
> Fungal infections
> Protozoal infections
> - *Encephalitozoon cuniculi*
> Parasite migrations
> - Dirofilariasis
> - Ascarid larval migrans
> - Cuterebriasis

4.6.3.1   Urinary Incontinence

Incontinence is the failure of voluntary control of micturition (urination), with either a constant or intermittent, unconscious passage of urine. Several different medical conditions can result in urinary incontinence. Disorders of micturition are generally divided into two types: neurogenic and non-neurogenic. Some animals can experience urinary incontinence some of the time and still have voluntary control of urination at other times. This is most likely to occur with non-neurogenic conditions.

Behaviorally, incontinence can appear differently, ranging from constant dribbling, leaking during activities with abdominal push (getting up from lying down, jumping up, stretching, changing positions), leaking only when sleeping, intermittent dribbling while maintaining the ability to signal and void, and/or sometimes appearing to be under conscious control. Diagnosis may require a complete history, comprehensive physical examination including palpation of the distended and empty urinary bladder, a digital rectal examination, a neurologic examination, and a urinalysis. Obtaining a complete history in the shelter setting can be difficult or impossible, especially if the relinquishing owner is not forthcoming about the pet not

---

**Box 4.4   Medical Causes of Urinary
Housesoiling in Dogs and Cats**

Increased volume (polyuria)
- Renal disease, hepatic disease, hypercal-
  cemia, pyometra, Cushing's disease,
  diabetes mellitus, or insipidus

Increased frequency of urination (pollakiuria)
- Urinary tract infection, urinary calculi,
  bladder tumors

Painful urination (dysuria)
- Arthritis, urinary tract infection, urinary
  calculi, prostatitis

Reduced control (incontinence)
- Neurologic damage; spinal or peripheral
  nerve
- Sphincter incompetence or impairment
- Cranial/impairment of central control
  (tumors, infections, etc.)

Sensory decline

Cognitive dysfunction syndrome

Altered mobility
- Neuromuscular, orthopedic disease

Medications
- Steroids, diuretics

Marking
- Increased anxiety due to endocrinopathy
- Hormonal (e.g., androgen-producing tumors)

---

being house trained or litterbox trained, fearing that the information may prevent adoption and/or result in euthanasia. Observation of the pet for postural changes during urination can be helpful in identifying the etiology of the problem. If an animal assumes the postures associated with elimination (squatting, lowering of pelvic limbs, tail position, ear position, etc.) then one can assume that the elimination is conscious. It is important to remember that these elimination processes do not always occur alone, and there may be several etiologies underlying a problem behavior. There may be neurological, infectious, anatomical, and/or behavioral components contributing to the

incontinence. When this is the case, treating only one etiology is not likely to result in a discontinuation of the incontinence. Each will need to be addressed separately for the best results.

4.6.3.3.1 Dogs

One of the most common non-neurogenic disorders seen in dogs is hormone-responsive incontinence. Older studies have suggested that this condition may affect more than 20% of gonadectomized female dogs (Arnold 1992; Thrusfield et al. 1998). However, more recent studies have not found incidence rates that high. Specifically, the condition appears to occur secondary to urethral sphincter mechanism incompetence (USMI) and results in incontinence most often when the animal is relaxed or asleep. Neutering appears to increase the risk of urethral incompetence in large dogs (>20 kg), and neutering prior to three months of age may increase the risk of urinary incontinence in female dogs (Spain et al. 2004), but additional studies have not consistently supported this finding (see Section 4.8.4). Other conditions that can lead to USMI and the occasional dribbling of urine are urinary tract infection (UTI), inflammation, prostatic disease, or a history of prostate surgery. Animals with these problems should still have voluntary control of urination some of the time, but at other times the urethral incompetence allows urine to dribble out, and the animal cannot voluntarily stop the flow.

Urinary bladder storage dysfunction can also result in frequent leakage of small amounts of urine. This can occur due to detrusor muscle instability, UTIs, chronic inflammatory disorders, infiltrative neoplastic lesions, external compression, and chronic partial outlet obstruction. These animals, too, will have voluntary control over urination some of the time.

Continuous dribbling of urine with the ability to urinate voluntarily can also occur in cases of ectopic ureters. Ectopic ureters are a congenital anomaly of the urinary system and are most commonly seen in juvenile female dogs. Some dog breeds, including golden retrievers, Labrador retrievers, Siberian huskies, Newfoundlands, miniature and toy poodles, and some terriers appear to be predisposed (Berent 2011). However, there appear to be regional differences in breed prevalence. The condition occurs infrequently in cats. Affected dogs will display urinary incontinence from birth and may have problems with chronic UTIs. Diagnosing the condition will require imaging such as cystoscopy, ultrasonography, contrast urography, or cystourethrovaginoscopy. Surgery is required to correct the condition.

Dogs may also urinate due to excitement, fear, or conflict. This is an involuntary action that can occur due to fear-inducing or social stimuli. It typically occurs as the dog lowers its pelvic limbs, with the ears held back and tail tucked. The tail may be stiff, and the tip may be wagged rapidly if the dog is more conflicted rather than fearful. The dog may also roll over and then urinate while demonstrating the same ear and tail posture. It is critical that the dog not be punished for this behavior. Even acting upset or frustrated with the dog may increase their fear, anxiety, and conflict and, thus, make the problem worse. The problem is more likely to occur in young dogs and may be exacerbated by the presence of a full bladder during exciting or fear-inducing events. Young female puppies may be particularly prone to this problem due to poor sphincter control. Ideally, these dogs should be greeted only after first being allowed outside to eliminate to ensure that they have an empty bladder. People should avoid leaning over these dogs when greeting. If all people who interact with the dog greet the dog in a calm, non-threatening manner, the problem will usually improve with age.

When an animal is experiencing continuous dribbling of urine, without the ability to voluntarily control urination, it is most likely a result of a neurogenic disorder such as lower motor neuron bladder. However, the presence of uroliths often have a similar presentation. These conditions occur as a result of a lesion in the spinal cord and have a guarded to poor prognosis, depending on the cause of the lesion (e.g., trauma, neoplasia, intervertebral disc disease). Lesions of the cerebellum or cerebral micturition center can also result in frequent, involuntary urination or leakage of small amounts of urine.

When faced with a dog that is urinating inappropriately and the urination appears to be conscious rather than unconscious, consider that the dog may have been incompletely house trained or may have a medical condition resulting in polyuria and polydipsia or an inflammatory disease leading to an increased urgency and frequency of urination. Dogs with cognitive decline may begin housesoiling simply due to a loss of previously learned behaviors. Canine cognitive decline is an irreversible, neurodegenerative condition of aging dogs (and cats) and is a diagnosis of exclusion. In addition to housesoiling, pets with cognitive decline may also act disoriented, seem less interested in social interactions, have altered sleep-wake cycles, and appear anxious or apathetic.

Aged dogs may need a more complete medical workup to rule out the large number of conditions that could be contributing to the behavior. For example, anything leading to musculoskeletal pain or weakness can result in incomplete elimination, where a dog postures to eliminate but cannot maintain the posture until she has completely voided the bladder or bowels. The dog may then return indoors and need to eliminate shortly thereafter, resulting in housesoiling. Good observation skills are necessary to recognize this problem in a case where the cause may not be readily identified with radiographs.

Urine marking is another potential cause for housesoiling in the dog. Urine-marking behavior is a normal form of communication. Intact male dogs urine mark more than castrated or female dogs but all dogs may urine mark. When neutered animals mark indoors, it is often due to situations involving conflict, frustration, or anxiety. However, this may also simply reflect incomplete house training. Regardless of the posture used for urination, medical conditions will need to be ruled out.

4.6.3.2 Cats

There are a variety of medical causes that may contribute to housesoiling in the cat, and housesoiling is likely one of the more common reasons for cats to be relinquished to shelters. If cats are placed in a cage in a shelter, they are likely to begin using the litterbox due to the lack of other preferable surfaces. However, some cats develop preferences for soft, absorbent substrates, so they may choose to eliminate on any bedding that is placed in their cages. If the cat has an aversion to the litterbox or the substrate offered in the box, it may eliminate on newspaper or other surfaces in the cage.

Cats housed in groups in rooms within the shelter may be more likely to eliminate outside the litterbox, and due to the presence of multiple cats, it may be challenging to determine which cat is not using the box. Fear or stress associated with interactions with unfamiliar cats may lead to urine-marking behavior and possibly even feline interstitial cystitis, also known as feline idiopathic cystitis (FIC). If other cats block access to boxes (either overtly or covertly), or a cat is simply too afraid to approach a box out of fear that it may be ambushed by another cat, elimination outside the box may occur. However, any elimination outside the box should prompt exploration for an underlying medical condition first, before making the determination that it is purely a behavioral problem. Any medical condition resulting in polyuria, polydipsia, incontinence, constipation, diarrhea, pain associated with elimination, increased frequency and/or urgency to eliminate, orthopedic disease making it difficult or painful to climb into a box, and declining sensory capabilities making it difficult to locate the box can all lead to elimination outside the box. Caretakers should also be aware that an aversion to the litterbox may

still exist long after the medical condition that promoted it is treated and eliminated.

Feline lower urinary tract disease (FLUTD) is a relatively common syndrome in the cat and often leads to the deposition of urine outside the box. FLUTD refers to disorders affecting the urethra and/or urinary bladder. Stranguria, dysuria, pollakiuria, hematuria, and urination outside the box are all signs that are consistent with FLUTD, but numerous underlying etiologies are possible. Common etiologies include UTI, uroliths, urethral plugs, idiopathic cystitis, bladder neoplasia, malformations, trauma, and urinary incontinence.

UTIs should first be ruled out with a urinalysis, preferably using urine collected by cystocentesis. One study demonstrated that clinical signs are, in fact, a poor predictor of UTI in cats and recommended urine culture as the best method for confirming the presence or absence of bacterial infections (Martinez-Rustafa et al. 2012). The same study found that the best predictive factor for the presence of UTI was urinary incontinence (Martinez- Rustafa et al. 2012). UTIs are often associated with other underlying medical conditions and are rarely a primary disorder in cats. Good antibiotic stewardship requires that we avoid treating cats presumptively with antibiotics since the likelihood of infection in young cats is small.

FIC has been shown to be the most common cause of signs of FLUTD in the cat (Lekcharoensuk et al. 2001; Gerber et al. 2005; Saevik et al. 2011). However, FIC is a diagnosis of exclusion. FIC describes recurring cystitis when no underlying cause for signs can be identified; a variety of different causative factors are suspected. Cats with FIC appear to have altered bladder permeability, and several studies have documented its association with stress (Buffington et al. 2002; Westropp et al. 2006; Stella et al. 2013). Cats with FIC appear to have increased sympathetic activity (Buffington and Pacak 2001; Buffington et al. 2002), to be more sensitive to environmental stress, and to have a decreased ability to cope with changes in their environment. Research continues to support the hypothesis that stress is associated with the development of FIC. One study, published by Cameron et al. (2004), found that cats with FIC were more likely to live in multi-cat households and to experience conflict with another cat in the household. Clearly, a shelter environment has the potential to negatively affect the welfare of cats that are prone to FIC, and appropriate treatment will involve the treatment of symptoms as well as an attempt to identify and reduce the stressors that may be affecting the cat.

Several different treatments for FIC have been investigated, and no single medication has been found to be consistently effective at treating the signs. Since FIC is likely a condition with a multifactorial etiology, it is likely that treatment will be multifactorial as well. One study that evaluated multi-modal environmental modification (MEMO) in the management of cats with interstitial cystitis found that with MEMO there was a significant reduction in lower urinary tract signs, fearfulness, and nervousness (Buffington et al. 2006). MEMO was defined as changing the cat's environment to decrease stress. Examples of these changes included avoidance of punishment, diet changes, techniques for increasing water consumption, changing to unscented clumping litter, improved litterbox management, provision of more structures for climbing and perches for resting and viewing, scratching posts, audio and visual stimuli when the owner was absent, increased client interactions with the cat, and identification and resolution of inter-cat conflict in the household. See Chapters 16 and 17 for more information on feline housing and enrichment.

4.6.4 Gastrointestinal Disorders

The nervous system of the gastrointestinal (GI) tract and the central nervous system are linked in a bidirectional manner by the sympathetic and parasympathetic pathways, resulting in what is referred to as the brain–gut axis. Due to this interrelationship, chronic stress can have profound effects on the enteric nervous system

(ENS). Severe life stressors have been associated with several GI tract conditions in humans (Bhatia and Tandon 2005), and the effects in animals are just now being explored. Chronic stress has been demonstrated to decrease gastric emptying, increase intestinal contractility, increase gut permeability, reduce water absorption in the gut, disrupt normal electrolyte absorption, and increase the colonic inflammatory response (Bhatia and Tandon 2005). Many gastrointestinal conditions such as chronic diarrhea and vomiting may be closely associated with stress. However, when presented with an animal with GI signs, the possibility of internal parasites and infectious organisms must also be ruled out. Newer polymerase chain reaction (PCR) tests can be helpful in ruling out some of these conditions. It is important to always keep in mind that nothing precludes an animal from having GI distress from multiple etiologies; therefore, both infectious causes and stress may need to be addressed.

Disruptions in the microbiome have been shown to play a role in anxiety and depression in many species (Foster and Neufeld 2013). In addition, studies in laboratory animals have shown that when young developing animals do not have normal gut microbiomes, they develop an exaggerated stress response and a dysregulated HPA axis (Sudo et al. 2004). Minimal work has been done on the role of the gut microbiome on behavior in dogs, but some limited research suggests that dogs demonstrating aggressive behavior may have distinctly different populations of gut bacteria compared to dogs that do not show aggression (Kirchoff et al. 2019; Mondo et al. 2020). More research is needed to identify what constitutes a healthy gut microbiome and how to adjust an "unhealthy" gut before we can apply what we have learned to companion animal care. Once again, the impact of stress on normal development and general health is clear and reminds us that it must not be overlooked.

Behavioral signs that may be associated with gastrointestinal disease include polyphagia, hyperphagia, polydipsia, coprophagia, and grass and plant eating. Oral behaviors such as frequent licking of surfaces (not self-licking), sucking, pica, gulping, and lip-smacking behaviors may all be associated with gastrointestinal disorders. However, some partial motor seizures may also be associated with similar behaviors. Many gastrointestinal disorders can manifest with unusual behavioral signs. In one recent study where 19 dogs were examined due to frequent surface-licking behaviors, 14 of the dogs were determined to have some form of gastrointestinal disease (Bécuwe-Bonnet et al. 2012). These included conditions such as delayed gastric emptying, irritable bowel syndrome, gastric foreign body, pancreatitis, and giardiasis, to name a few. The unusual behavior of fly biting, considered by some to be a compulsive disorder, has even been found to be associated with gastrointestinal conditions such as gastroesophageal reflux (Frank et al. 2012).

4.6.4.1 Pica

Pica is the consumption of non-nutritive items such as fabric, paper, and plastic. There is little research available involving companion animals and pica. However, a literature search for pica as a clinical sign links it to a variety of disease processes, including portal caval shunts, iron-deficiency anemia, pyruvate kinase deficiency, ehrlichiosis, gastrointestinal disorders, neurologic damage, feline infectious peritonitis (FIP), and other medical conditions (Thomas et al. 1976; Black 1994; Goldman et al. 1998; Marioni-Henry et al. 2004; Kohn et al. 2006; Kohn and Fumi 2008; Bécuwe-Bonnet et al. 2012; Berset-Istratescu et al. 2014). Both cats and dogs can be affected. Pica has also been described in horses, cattle, sheep, and other domestic species (Houpt 2011). In rats and mice, pica has been associated with gastrointestinal disturbances and may be an adaptive mechanism used to cope with gastrointestinal upset (Takeda et al. 1993; Yamamoto et al. 2002). In a recent case report, a 5.5-year-old dog with a 4.5-year history of pica (eating rocks) resolved when diagnosed and treated for mild hip dysplasia (Mills et al. 2020).

There is some indication in the literature that oriental cat breeds (Burmese and Siamese) may be represented in numbers higher than the general hospital population, suggesting the possibility of an underlying genetic predisposition for pica (Blackshaw 1991; Bradshaw et al. 1997; Overall and Dunham 2002; Bamberger and Houpt 2006). To date, the evidence for a genetic basis is purely correlative.

Underlying medical causes for pica should always be investigated and ruled out through appropriate diagnostics. A behavioral diagnosis of an abnormal repetitive disorder is made by excluding all possible medical conditions. If financial constraints limit testing, a clinical trial with appropriate gastrointestinal protectant drugs is indicated prior to using any kind of psychoactive substance. Behavioral enrichment is indicated, and behavior modification can be attempted (Blackshaw 1991). There is a single documented case study that successfully used behavior modification to diminish the occurrence of pica in a cat (Mongillo et al. 2012).

4.6.5 Dermatological Disease

In humans, the relationship between skin disease and mental health has received much attention in the past decade. The skin and the central nervous system are both derived from the embryonic ectoderm, and they share many of the same hormones, neuropeptides, and receptors. Many of these substances are involved in neurogenic inflammation, pruritus, and pain sensation, and stress can alter their release. A substantial number of chronic dermatoses in humans are heavily influenced by stress. It has been estimated that in as many as one-third of the humans with skin disease, the condition is complicated by significant psychosocial and psychiatric morbidity. Patients with atopic skin disorders also have a higher prevalence of anxiety, depression, excitability, and suicidal ideation and a decreased ability to cope with stress.

While many of these emotions may be impossible to confirm in our non-verbal patients, it is logical to assume that stress has the potential to cause similar pathophysiologic responses that perpetuate the itch-scratch cycle. Cases of dogs with pyoderma and pruritic skin disease associated with psychogenic factors have been reported (Nagata et al. 2002; Nagata and Shibata 2004). Newer research supports the likelihood that chronic skin disease, especially that which causes pruritis, can lead to stress and subsequent behavior change (Harvey et al. 2019; Yeom et al. 2020; McAuliffe et al. accepted for publication). Harvey et al. (2019) found that dogs with chronic atopic dermatitis demonstrated problematic behaviors such as mounting, chewing, hyperactivity, coprophagia, begging for and stealing food, attention seeking, excitability, excessive grooming, and reduced trainability. The frequency of unwanted behaviors increased when the degree of pruritis was more severe. In another study (data not yet published), dogs with higher levels of pruritis were found to have significantly higher levels of aggression, fear, separation-related problems, attention-seeking behaviors, excitability, and sensitivity to touch (McAuliffe et al. accepted for publication). While the exact relationship between these problem behaviors and atopy have not yet been determined, chronic atopy and pruritis is known to result in reduced quality of life; therefore, the potential for chronic anxiety and stress is clear. For that reason, the clinician should remain aware of two important things. First, many skin conditions may be exacerbated in the stressed shelter animal. Second, animals with chronic skin conditions may be more likely to exhibit problem behaviors—and these behaviors might be reduced by treatment that improves their skin condition.

4.6.5.1 Overgrooming

When placed in situations of frustration or conflict, some animals will show displacement behaviors, and grooming is commonly seen as a displacement behavior in many species. Psychogenic alopecia is a term often used to refer to a skin condition of cats in which irregular patches of hair are removed, presumably by licking and chewing. Some have suggested that oriental cat breeds (Siamese, Burmese, Abyssinian) may be at higher risk of developing this problem (Sawyer et al. 1999). Hair may be missing over the flanks, abdomen, front legs, or virtually anywhere on the body. This condition may occur secondary to anxiety or environmental stress but is a diagnosis of exclusion because many pathophysiological conditions can contribute to feline overgrooming. One case series that examined cats with a presumptive diagnosis of psychogenic alopecia found that 76% of the cats had medical conditions causing pruritus (Waisglass et al. 2006). A painful sensation may cause cats to overgroom as well, so radiographs may be helpful in some cases. Regrowth of hair and resolution of the overgrooming, after treatment with pain medication, is suggestive of pain as an underlying cause for the behavior.

While less common, dogs can also overgroom areas of their body due to environmental stress or anxiety, although, as is the case with cats, painful sensations may also lead to overgrooming in the dog. When overgrooming behavior occurs primarily as a response to anxiety or conflict, it has the potential to develop into a repetitive disorder, generalize, and eventually occur even in the absence of the original stressors. Some have referred to this as a compulsive disorder. Regardless of the terminology applied, if the animal is believed to be overgrooming due to stress or anxiety, the primary treatment approach must be aimed at relieving the anxiety through a combination of environmental management, behavioral modification, and anxiety-relieving medications.

4.6.5.2 Acral Lick Dermatitis

Acral lick dermatitis (ALD), also sometimes referred to as acral lick granuloma, is primarily a dermatological syndrome that is a result of self-trauma. While some individuals may begin licking a leg to excess due to anxiety, frustration, or conflict, studies have found that many other underlying causes for these lesions are possible (Denerolle et al. 2007). Pruritus due to allergies, orthopedic pain, trauma, neoplasia, bacterial pyoderma, and fungal infections are just a few possibilities.

Once a dog begins to lick and causes an open lesion, the dog will continue to lick it, no matter the original cause. When presented with a patient with ALD, a complete medical workup aimed at identifying the underlying cause is ideal. Long-term treatment with appropriate antibiotics will almost always be required. Treatment may also include ancillary medications to break the itch-scratch cycle (e.g., glucocorticoids, antihistamines). Physically preventing the dog from licking the lesion may be necessary to ensure resolution. This may be accomplished with the use of e-collars, bandages, socks, body suits, or leggings, depending on what the individual patient tolerates.

Once the lesion is completely healed, attention will need to be paid to the patient to determine if they continue to lick at the legs. In the experience of these authors, ALD is rarely a primary behavioral problem. If that is suspected, then the patient needs to be fully evaluated for other signs of fears or anxieties, such as noise sensitivities or phobias, barrier frustration, or separation anxiety, as it is unlikely that ALD would exist as a primary behavioral problem without one of these comorbid conditions. Grooming is a common displacement behavior, and the dog who is anxious about the strange sights, sounds, and smells of the shelter, as well as the sudden change in its living arrangement and separation from familiar people, may be inclined to exhibit displacement grooming to the extent that it develops or worsens an existing ALD.

4.6.5.3 Feline Hyperesthesia

Feline hyperesthesia is a poorly understood syndrome, known by a variety of different names, including rolling skin syndrome, twitchy skin syndrome, and feline neurodermatitis, to name a few. It is characterized by short episodes of thoracolumbar skin rolling or rippling, and, in some cases, epaxial muscle spasms. Cats may appear anxious or agitated and demonstrate exaggerated tail movements, running, vocalizations, or self-directed aggression. The self-directed aggression may be the extreme end of a spectrum that includes excessive licking, plucking, biting, and/or chewing directed at the tail, lumbar, flank, or anal area. In some cases, the increased motor activity, exaggerated rolling, crouching, and elevation of the perineal area may be confused with the behavior typically shown by an estrus female.

Feline hyperesthesia is referred to as idiopathic in most textbooks because no single causal factor has been elucidated. It has been hypothesized that the behaviors are a result of focal seizures, sensory neuropathies, and dermatologic disease resulting in pruritus. As is the case with other skin conditions, it is likely that environmental and social stressors play a role in this condition. Systemic diseases such as toxoplasmosis and hyperthyroidism should be ruled out, as well as painful spinal or skin conditions, severe pruritus, FLUTD, anal sacculitis, and myositis, as they may all contribute to the behavior. Any disease condition that affects the central nervous system or alters reactivity to stimuli will need to be ruled out if the clinician is presented with a cat showing signs similar to feline hyperesthesia (Ciribassi 2009).

After ruling out and treating any underlying medical problems causing pain or pruritus, feline hyperesthesia may be treated empirically as a partial seizure disorder. Both phenobarbital and primidone have been used to treat the condition (Aronson 1998), as well as clomipramine and fluoxetine (Overall 1998). Ultimately, treatment of every individual animal will need to reflect the putative etiological basis of that particular case. Attention will need to be paid to identifying and, if possible, removing the environmental stressors that may be contributing to the problem.

4.6.5.4 Self-Injurious Behaviors

Pathologic self-mutilation has been studied much more in humans and non-human primates than in domestic animals. In non-human primates, it is believed by many to be a maladaptive coping mechanism. Rearing in a suboptimal environment, and specifically social isolation, is considered a risk factor (Dellinger-Ness and Handler 2006). Stressors such as relocation have also been known to lead to self-injurious behavior (SIB) in some primates (Davenport et al. 2008). SIB in dogs and cats is often but not always associated with tail chasing, circling, and subsequent tail tip mutilation. Self-mutilation is most likely to be associated with pain, dysesthesia, or paresthesia. One case has been documented of a 30-month-old Labrador retriever that presented with acute onset tail mutilation (Zulch et al. 2012). Radiographs of the tail revealed some soft-tissue swelling and a mineralized ossicle in one intervertebral space that may have caused discomfort. Administration of analgesics led to complete resolution of the behavior. Self-mutilation has been documented in several other species secondary to nerve injury, pain, and altered sensation, so self-mutilation behaviors should always lead to a thorough physical exam and imaging, if possible, to rule out underlying medical causes. Empirical treatment with analgesics or anti-inflammatories may be warranted in some patients before determining that self-mutilation is a primary behavioral problem. Box 4.5 lists some of the most important medical rule-outs for common repetitive behaviors (often referred to as compulsive disorders) in dogs and cats.

4.6.6 Endocrine Disease

Endocrine imbalances have the potential to change many aspects of an animal's behavior because they usually result in altered motivation for meeting particular bodily needs (see Table 4.3). For example, an animal with diabetes mellitus will demonstrate increased thirst and hunger. The subsequent drive to acquire more food or water can lead to unusual behaviors such as attempting to drink water left on the floor during cleaning procedures.

4.6.6.1 Dogs

Hypothyroidism is one of the endocrinopathies most often mentioned as being associated with behavioral changes in dogs. However, there are minimal data supporting any causal association between hypothyroidism and aggression. One study compared the analytes commonly used to evaluate thyroid function between dogs with and without aggression toward people and found no difference between the two groups (Radosta et al. 2012). A double-blind placebo-controlled trial evaluated the effect of six weeks of thyroid replacement on owner-directed aggression in 29 normal dogs with borderline low thyroid values and found no difference between the treatment and control groups (Dodman et al. 2013). In another study of 20 hypothyroid dogs without diagnosed behavior problems, treatment with levothyroxine resulted in no behavioral change other than increased activity levels (Hrovat et al. 2018). Serotonin and prolactin levels were also measured prior to, at six weeks, and six months after the initiation of levothyroxine therapy, and no significant changes in levels were noted (Hrovat et al. 2018). Thus, at this time, there are no data to support the proposal that thyroid supplementation may benefit behavioral therapy in dogs.

4.6.6.2 Cats

Hypothyroidism rarely occurs naturally in cats but is a common sequela to treatment for hyperthyroidism. Clinical signs are similar to those seen in dogs with hypothyroidism. Congenital

---

Box 4.5   Medical Conditions That May Result in Repetitive Behaviors

Tail chasing
- Intervertebral disc disease
- Injury of the tail
- Anal sac disease
- Spinal cord disease including neoplasia
- Cauda equina syndrome
- Focal seizures
- Flea allergy

Fly snapping
- Viral diseases such as distemper
- Tick-borne diseases such as Lyme, ehrlichiosis, and Rocky Mountain spotted fever
- Focal seizures
- Central nervous system neoplastic disease
- Gastroesophageal reflux
- Lymphocytic, eosinophilic, or plasmacytic enteritis
- Delayed gastric emptying
- Chiari malformation
- Chorioretinitis or other ocular abnormalities

Acral lick dermatitis
- Allergic dermatitis
- Peripheral neuropathy
- Orthopedic disease or arthropathy
- Osteosarcoma or other neoplasia
- Foreign body (retained pin, grass awns)
- Infection: bacterial, fungal, or parasitic
- Trauma (laceration)
- Endocrinopathies

Pica
- Pyruvate kinase deficiency and other blood abnormalities
- Feline infectious peritonitis
- Lead poisoning
- Portosystemic shunts and other forms of liver disease
- Gastrointestinal infections (*Campylobacter, Clostridium*)
- Ehrlichia
- Iron-deficiency anemia

Psychogenic alopecia in cats
- Allergies including atopy, food-based and hypersensitivity reactions
- Bacterial, fungal, or parasitic skin infections
- Hyperthyroidism
- Pain (from multiple causes and multiple sources)

Table 4.3 Endocrinological disorders that may lead to behavioral changes.

Conditions	Possible behavioral changes
Dogs	
Hyperadrenocorticism	Polyuria, polydipsia, polyphagia, increased panting, lethargy; the signs can be easily confused with signs of anxiety
Diabetes mellitus	Polyuria, polydipsia, polyphagia; if ketoacidotic may be lethargic, depressed, and anorexic
Hypoadrenocorticism	Lethargy, anorexia
Hypothyroidism	Weight gain, lethargy, weakness and exercise intolerance
Hyperthyroidism	Polyuria, polydipsia, polyphagia, weight loss, panting, irritability, and restlessness (uncommon in dogs)
Cats	
Hyperadrenocorticism	Polyuria, polydipsia, polyphagia, lethargy (dullness); excess sex hormones can also result in sexual behavior, including urine marking and intraspecific aggression; females may exhibit signs similar to those seen in estrous queens
Diabetes mellitus	Polyuria, polydipsia, polyphagia, lethargy, depression, and anorexia; diabetic neuropathy has the potential to result in discomfort when being touched or petted; may be irritable or aloof
Hypoadrenocorticism	Lethargy, anorexia
Hypothyroidism	Lethargy, mental dullness (rare in cats)
Hyperthyroidism	Polyuria, polydipsia, polyphagia, increased vocalization, irritability, and restlessness

hypothyroidism, while also rare, has been well documented in cats, as it is the most common cause of disproportional dwarfism (Jones et al. 1992). While the physical changes associated with congenital hypothyroidism are numerous, mental dullness and lethargy are the most commonly mentioned behavioral changes.

Hyperthyroidism is the most common endocrine disease of cats, and clinical signs reflect the overall increase in metabolism. These cats are often restless and have been described as hyperactive, polyphagic, irritable, and even aggressive. They may be more vocal, appear anxious, and urine mark.

4.7 Medical Conditions That Have Breed Tendencies and Their Associated Behavior Changes

Diseases that have a breed tendency can be due to morphologic extremes or to an inherited condition (Rooney 2009). Examples of morphologic extremes include characteristics like dome-shaped heads in Cavalier King Charles spaniels and corkscrew tails in bulldogs. Inherited conditions are numerous, and, at last count, 312 non-conformation-linked inherited disorders had been identified in the top 50 breeds of registered dogs (Summers et al. 2010).

Selecting for breed standards and specific characteristics leads to inbreeding, reducing variation and causing an increased likelihood of concentrating genes that may have undesired effects. In addition, the incidence of these diseases in mixed-breed and shelter dog populations has never been studied and is, therefore, unknown.

Recent research has attempted to divide diseases with breed tendencies into (i) disorders related to breed standards and (ii) inherited defects (Asher et al. 2009; Summers et al. 2010). In addition, a Genetic Illness Severity Index for Dogs (GISID) was developed to rank these conditions in terms of their impact on the welfare of the dog (Asher et al. 2009). In general, these diseases affect welfare by compromising a particular body system, often causing pain and discomfort (Yeates 2012). In addition, some of these conditions may further impact welfare by preventing normal expressions of behavior, either due to pain or associated with anatomical alterations such as ear, tail, and body conformation (Rooney 2009).

Although the cat genome has been mapped, not as much progress has been made in identifying genetic diseases in cats. Purebred cats make up only a small portion of the overall cat population (estimates show that about 8% of cats are purebred) (American Pet Products Association 2013). Compared to the multitude of genetic tests available for dogs, there are only 20 that have been developed for cats (Slutsky et al. 2013).

A database developed by the University of Pennsylvania allows users to search for available genetic tests in both cats and dogs (Slutsky et al. 2013):

https://www.vet.upenn.edu/research/academic-departments/clinical-sciences-advanced-medicine/research-labs-centers/penngen/tests-worldwide.

4.8 Behavior and/or Medical Conditions Seen in Intact versus Neutered Dogs

4.8.1 Female Canine

The normal reproductive cycle of the bitch consists of four phases that include proestrus, estrus, diestrus, and anestrus. Most breeds reach puberty and begin to cycle between 4 and 15 months of age. Generally, smaller breeds will come into heat sooner than larger breeds, although there is variation both within and among breeds. The domestic dog is a nonseasonal breeder and typically has two estrus cycles per year.

The female undergoes several changes during the estrus cycle. During the proestrus stage, the bitch's vulva becomes swollen and firm. There may be a slight discharge that ranges in color from clear to bloody. At this stage, males will be interested in her, although she will not be interested in them. The behavior at this time mimics play, including play bows, running together, and playful chasing. The female may briefly stand for the male and then move away. The bitch may also quickly turn and growl, snap, or bite an unwelcome suitor. Generally, her ears are held back, and her tail is tucked between her legs. While tail tucking is typically associated with fear, in this instance, it is an evasive behavior preventing intromission should a male become too insistent.

Behaviorally, estrus is the stage in which the female is receptive (allows copulatory mounting) to the male. During this time, her vulva is still enlarged, although it may be somewhat softer. The discharge may still be present and ranges from a clear to slightly serosanguinous fluid. The initial courtship behavior may still mimic play. The behavior may progress to more intense sniffing of genitalia. Instead of the female moving away, she will stand in a braced position with her back feet base wide and deviate her tail to the side if touched near her vulva. If the male is inexperienced, the female may mount him, or she may actively solicit the male by backing into him with her tail flagged to the side. An estrus bitch will urinate a small amount frequently, similar to a dog with a UTI. Dogs have a tremendous sense of smell, and the hormonal changes in the female's urine attract males over a large area (Bradshaw and Nott 1995). This results in the intact male roaming in search of the female.

The proestrus and estrus stages can last anywhere from a couple of days to four weeks. Behaviorally, diestrus is the first day the female is no longer receptive to the male. The vulva decreases in size, and the female may display aggressive threats as she defends herself from males. The diestrus period is the time from ovulation to either parturition or anestrus.

Initially, there are very few behavioral changes between a gravid and non-pregnant female. During the last two weeks of gestation, the pregnant bitch's abdomen starts to enlarge, her nipples and mammary glands continue to develop, and, at times, milk may even leak from her glands. She may prefer to eat smaller portions and may also be polydipsic and polyphagic. The enlarged uterus filled with growing feti places increasingly greater pressure on the stomach. Small frequent meals allow the bitch to ingest enough nutrients to support herself and the growing feti and to produce milk. Milk production also requires an increase in water consumption. The enlarging mammary glands may cause discomfort, resulting in increased licking of the uncomfortable area. Depending on the size of her litter and her body condition, she may also move more slowly. The change in hormones that occur during impending parturition may result in some bitches becoming anorectic and having looser feces. This may result in an evacuated gastrointestinal system, allowing for a more sanitary birthing process because general abdominal pressure may result in fecal expulsion.

Bitches, whether bred or not, may build a nest and act pregnant. Some will become very destructive in their nest building and dig up or destroy bedding, furniture, or other household items. In addition, they may also drag items from other parts of the house or yard to construct their nest. Some bitches will regard certain toys or objects as puppies and bring them to the nest. Others may carry the "pup" around with them. Some individuals may become very protective of their "surrogate litter."

Parturition occurs approximately 63 days after ovulation. Plasma progesterone drops to less than 2 ng/dl (Concannon et al. 1978), followed 10–14 hours later by a drop in rectal temperature. Twenty-four hours prior to parturition, many bitches' rectal temperature drops below 100° F for a short period of time and then returns to normal. During this time, the bitch may seem restless and uncomfortable, pant, and nest build. These behaviors may also occur intermittently during the last week or two prior to parturition, with an increase in frequency as parturition becomes imminent.

Anestrus is the time from parturition until the next estrus cycle. During this time, a bitch's behavior should be similar to that of a spayed female or unneutered male.

4.8.1.1 Pseudopregnancy (Pseudocyesis, False Pregnancy)

After estrus, the uterus undergoes the same changes whether the bitch is bred or open. Pseudopregnancy is just as it sounds. The bitch is in diestrus, and her body acts as though it is pregnant even though she is not. As described above, she may build a nest, become protective of toys, and exhibit mammary development. She may become restless, irritable, and/or lethargic. She may undergo contractions and have a liquid discharge. Pseudopregnancy is self-limiting and generally does not require treatment. If treatment is necessary, the type will depend on many factors: gonadal status of the dog, duration and severity of signs, and the types of signs (physical or behavioral). Treatment regimens have not been well described, and more research is needed on this problem.

Pseudopregnancy can occur in any breed and has been known to occur in bitches as young as 7 months of age and those as old as 10 years of age (Johnston 1986). The incidence of pseudopregnancy is unknown but estimated to be as high as 50–75% by one author (Johnston 1980). In a survey study in the United Kingdom, veterinarians reported seeing 10 cases per year on average (Root et al. 2018). Of greatest concern, 96% reported behavioral changes in these patients without noteworthy physical changes, and 97% reported aggression as one of the behavioral signs (Root et al. 2018). Pseudopregnancy may occur in a gonadectomized bitch three to four days after her ovariohysterectomy (Johnston 1986) if the surgery was performed during the diestrus phase of her cycle and not the anestrus phase. The implications of this, combined with the data from the Root study, should not be ignored. Collecting a vaginal swab for cytology is not difficult or time-consuming, and many resources exist for aiding in the analysis. Vaginal cytology is routinely used for determining stage of estrous. Performing ovariohysterectomy on female dogs in the shelter without knowing their stage of estrous could result in behavioral changes that are hormonally related. Similarly, if aggression is seen in a recently spayed female with an unknown history, an awareness that it could be related to hormonal changes may affect behavior assessments and any planned interventions, including behavior modification.

4.8.1.2 Mastitis

Mastitis is an infection of the mammary glands seen most commonly in intact bitches postparturition or post-pseudopregnancy. In most cases, it is not a life-threatening condition and generally only affects one or two glands. The bitch is typically pacing and restless, lying down and getting back up. She will often lick and/or chew the infected gland. The infected gland appears enlarged, firm, and erythematous, and it is likely painful to the touch. Suckling by the puppies may elicit an aggressive response, such as growling, lip lifting, snapping, or biting. The bitch may also move away from the puppies and avoid staying with them, as nursing is painful. This leaves the puppies hungry, so they initially cry more, but if they are not fed, they become lethargic, their cries become weaker, and their suckle response decreases.

4.8.1.3 Eclampsia

Eclampsia is an acute condition of the pregnant bitch where the blood levels of calcium fall to dangerously low levels. This hypocalcemic condition may occur pre- or postpartum and is most often seen in small breeds, although it can occur in any breed. Initial signs include restlessness, whining, and pacing that progresses to a stiff gait. The signs progress very quickly to lateral recumbency with extensor rigidity and impending death without treatment (Pathan et al. 2011). Upon physical exam, the bitch is generally hyperthermic due to muscle rigidity.

4.8.1.4 Metritis

Metritis is an infection of the uterus postpartum. Bitches with metritis are thin, lethargic, and have a purulent vaginal discharge. Initially, the bitch may spend an excessive amount of time licking and grooming the vulvar area. As the disease progresses, she may not feel well enough to expend the energy to clean herself. Often, the bitch will become anorectic, and because of the decreased caloric intake, her milk production may decrease. This will result in increased vocalization of the puppies, whose nutritional needs are not met. Any dog with puppies that suddenly begins avoiding her pups or acting aggressively toward them should be thoroughly examined for eclampsia, mastitis, and metritis, as her change in behavior may be a result of pain and discomfort.

4.8.1.5 Pyometra

Pyometra is an infection of the uterus that occurs when the uterus is under the influence of progesterone (Nelson and Feldman 1986). It is common in intact female dogs, but actual risk has been difficult to confirm in North America due to the high incidence of gonadectomy. Pyometra should be viewed as an important risk to the intact female dog.

Typical signs of pyometra include polydipsia and weight loss. Many bitches show depression, a slightly decreased appetite, increased panting (likely due to endotoxemia and their febrile state), and lethargy. Others may seem relatively normal except for polydipsia and excessive licking or grooming of the perineum and hindquarters. They may also have urinary "accidents" in the house; this is generally secondary to polydipsia and pressure on the bladder from the increased size of the uterus.

4.8.1.6 Mammary Tumors

Mammary gland tumors are the most common neoplasia of female dogs (Moulton 1978; Brodey et al. 1983; Moe 2001; Merlo et al. 2008; Dobson 2013; Sorenmo et al. 2013) and can occur in both intact and spayed bitches. In general, they do not change the behavior of the dog unless the tumor ruptures and drains, in which case it will result in excessive licking or grooming of the area. If the tumor is sufficiently large, it may alter the dog's gait or the way the dog lies down. Excessive licking of the mammary gland, often a sign of pain and discomfort, may be the first sign noted.

4.8.1.7 Ovarian Tumors

Ovarian tumors only occur in the intact bitch. Those that have had an ovariectomy or ovariohysterectomy have had their ovaries removed, thus completely eliminating the risk of ovarian cancer (Greenlee and Patnaik 1985; Klein 2001).

Some ovarian tumors will secrete excessive hormones. Those secreting estrogen may result in the bitch showing signs similar to estrus, including the development of an enlarged vulva and solicitation of male attention (McEntee 2002). If estrogen levels continue to rise, bone marrow suppression (Sontas et al. 2009) and/or hair loss may occur (Mecklenburg et al. 2009). Bone marrow suppression may lead to lethargy, anorexia, and epistaxis.

Most ovarian tumors, however, result in non-specific clinical and behavioral signs (McEntee 2002). These signs may include a painful abdomen, which may be due to ascites, pressure from the tumor on other organs, and/or discomfort if the tumor is large. The bitch may also be anorectic, appear constipated, urinate frequently, or show signs of discomfort when lying down due to the physical size of the tumor putting pressure on other organs.

4.8.1.8 Ovarian Remnant

Ovarian remnant syndrome occurs when some ovarian tissue is inadvertently left behind during ovariohysterectomy or ovariectomy and is characterized by signs typical of an animal that still has ovarian function (Miller 1995; Ball et al. 2010). Behaviorally, signs of estrus may be seen, as mentioned previously. In addition, signs of pyometritis may be present (Ball et al. 2010).

4.8.2 Male Canine

4.8.2.1 Prostatic Disease

The prostate is an accessory sex gland in the male dog. Its primary purpose is to produce fluids to transport and support sperm. It is located caudal to the bladder and generally can be palpated rectally on the pelvic floor if it is not enlarged. There are many diseases that affect the prostate, and most can result in the behavioral changes mentioned below. The most common of these diseases include benign prostatic hyperplasia (BPH), prostatic cysts, and prostatic tumors.

When the prostate is enlarged, regardless of etiology, its location can result in several behavioral changes. A slight increase in size may put pressure on the colon, resulting in tenesmus. This may be confused with constipation or diarrhea because the consistency of the feces may vary. As the prostate continues to enlarge, it may also put pressure on the urethra, resulting in incomplete bladder emptying. Dogs may strain to urinate, urinate frequently, or have a smaller stream of urine. They may also be uncomfortable lifting their leg to urinate, and thus may assume the typical male puppy stance for urination: standing in a sawhorse position with the hips lowered and the rear legs extended caudally. The urine may have some blood in it as well. In addition, the abdomen may be painful, causing the dog to be very uncomfortable. He may show reluctance to lie down or lie down cautiously, similar to a dog with painful joints. Depending on the etiology, if there is a discharge, the dog may lick his prepuce more often.

4.8.2.2 Cryptorchid Testis

The testicles in dogs typically descend into the scrotal sac before six months of age (Gier and Marion 1970), prior to closure of the inguinal ring (Kustritz 2009). Some males will have one (unilateral or mono cryptorchid) or both testicles (bilateral cryptorchid) that have not descended into the scrotal sac. The retained testicle still produces testosterone, but because it is located internally, the sperm are commonly non-viable. Some may mistake these males for being neutered (Reif et al. 1979). However, because they are still under the influence of testosterone, their behaviors are similar to those of any other intact male dog. There is a significantly higher risk of testicular tumors in dogs with retained testicles that have not been neutered (Hayes et al. 1985; Hayes and Pendergrass 1976).

4.8.2.3 Testicular Tumors

Testicular tumors may result in scrotal, inguinal, or abdominal enlargement, depending on the location of the testes. The size of the mass and the location will dictate any behavior changes that occur. Signs may include a stilted gait with the rear legs, difficulty sitting or reluctance to sit, and discomfort lying down. If the tumor is large enough where the testicle touches the ground when sitting or lying, it may become abraded, resulting in excessive licking to the area. Likewise, if the increase in size causes discomfort, excessive licking is a likely consequence.

Sertoli cell tumors are common in older dogs (Weaver 1983) and result in several behavioral and medical changes (Lipowitz et al. 1973). These tumors tend to secrete estrogen, so male dogs will undergo feminization. Externally, changes include mammary development, alopecia, and testicular and penile atrophy. Internally, there may be bone marrow suppression (Sherding et al. 1981). Behaviorally, Sertoli cell tumors are characterized by decreased libido and the compromised bone marrow results in an increase in infections, fever, anemia, weakness, and lethargy. These signs in a supposedly castrated male may indicate that he was a cryptorchid that was not bilaterally castrated.

Interstitial cell tumors and seminomas also affect the testes, although their resultant change in behavior is generally related to the size of the tumor, as described earlier. Excessive licking of the perianal area (due to the development of perianal adenomas) or enlargement of the inguinal area may be associated with hormonal imbalance.

4.8.3 Normal Sex-Related Behaviors

4.8.3.1 Marking

Urine marking is a natural behavior for both male and female dogs. Intact males typically mark more than intact females (Pal 2003). Neutering males has been shown to significantly decrease marking in most males (Neilson et al. 1997). Intact and spayed females appear to mark at about the same frequency (Wirant et al. 2004). The intact male will preferentially mark over the urine of an estrus female more than any other urine (Lisberg and Snowdon 2011).

When female dogs urine mark, they may squat, slightly elevate a rear leg while squatting, or alternate between legs while squatting. Just as leg lifting for urination can be a normal variation for female dogs, the squatting position is a normal variation of urination behavior for some male dogs. All of these are normal postures. When a urinary stance is atypical for a particular sex, it is not necessarily reflective of any disease, dysfunction, or abnormality. However, if the urinary stance is atypical for that *individual*, further investigation to identify underlying medical problems is indicated.

4.8.3.2 Non-copulatory Mounting

Non-copulatory mounting is a normal behavior for both male and female dogs. Young dogs often mount during play. In adults, it is more common in the intact male. The behavior in neutered animals is more likely to be a sign of anxiety or conflict (Luescher and Reisner 2008) than sexual in nature. However, anxiety due to other causes may be involved in some cases. If mounting behavior is increasing in the shelter situation, it is important to identify specific triggers and/or motivation if possible. Assessing the anxiety level of the animal being mounted is critical as well, as some dogs respond aggressively to this behavior. A dog that is frequently mounted by other dogs, regardless of the reason, may suffer poor welfare.

4.8.3.3 Masturbation

Masturbation is a normal behavior of both male and female, neutered, and sexually intact animals. It becomes pathological when the behavior is performed to the exclusion of other normal behaviors, such as eating, drinking, and environmental investigation. Frequent masturbation can also lead to an increased incidence of infection or trauma to the prepuce, penis, or vulva.

4.8.4 Effects of Gonadectomy on the Behavior of Dogs

The behavior of gonadectomized male dogs is similar to that of an anestrus female. Early studies indicated that castration of male dogs results in a reduction of sexually dimorphic behaviors, such as mounting, urine marking, roaming, and aggression directed toward other intact male dogs (Hopkins et al. 1976; Neilson et al. 1997). However, it should be noted that in these two studies the behaviors were only reduced in some dogs; none of the objectionable behaviors were completely eliminated. A more recent survey that included more than 9,000 dogs found that urine marking was the only behavior less likely to occur in the castrated dog (McGreevy et al. 2018). This study also found that behaviors relating to fear and aggression were less likely to occur the longer the dog remained intact prior to castration (McGreevy et al. 2018). Several other studies have demonstrated that there is no difference in aggression after gonadectomy (Maarschalkerweerd et al.1997), while other studies suggest that aggression in males may increase after gonadectomy (Guy et al. 2001; Spain et al. 2004; Reisner et al. 2005).

Conflicting results have also been found when attempting to determine if castration prior to six months of age has any effect on the development of certain behavioral problems.

One study found male puppies castrated prior to five-and-a-half months of age demonstrated increased aggression toward family members and were more likely to bark at visitors (Spain et al. 2004). However, in another study comparing puppies castrated prior to 24 weeks of age, no increased incidence of behavior problems was identified (Howe et al. 2001). Vizslas castrated prior to six months of age were found to have an increase in behaviors related to fear and anxiety (Zink et al. 2016).

A minimal amount of research has been performed examining the effects of gonadectomy on female dogs. One study (O'Farrell and Peachey 1990) suggested that if female dogs were already showing some aggression and gonadectomy was performed prior to one year of age, the risk of aggression increased after surgery. Other females in the study who were gonadectomized after one year of age did not show an increased likelihood of aggression. In another, more recent study that included 8,981 dogs who were gonadectomized prior to 10 years of age, fearful and aggressive behaviors were associated with a decreased lifetime exposure to gonadal hormones. In other words, the longer female dogs were left intact, the lower the incidence of several unwanted behaviors (Starling et al. 2019).

A 2018 survey study that included more than 13,000 dogs of both sexes found no evidence to suggest that gonadectomy at any age alters aggressive behavior directed toward people or dogs, but dogs that were gonadectomized prior to 12 months of age had a significant increase in the odds of demonstrating aggression toward strangers (Farhoody et al. 2018). The apparently conflicting nature of these data demonstrates the complex and multifactorial elements surrounding the development of behavior. A variety of different confounding factors may have influenced the results of the data in these studies, and much more prospective research is needed on this issue. Until we have that, all we can say is that gonadectomy may help to decrease behaviors that are strongly influenced by gonadal hormones.

An important concern not adequately addressed in any of the aforementioned studies is the possible role that a traumatic experience may have on the development of the aggressive behaviors that are described in some gonadecto-mized dogs. If dogs have a surgical procedure performed prior to 6 or 12 months of age (the most common time frames for dogs in the United States to be neutered), the fact that the surgery may be performed during a sensitive period of development needs to be taken into consideration. Dogs who experience a traumatic event, such as a frightening and/or painful experience in the veterinary hospital or shelter during the sensitive period, may be at a greater risk for developing fear- or anxiety-related prob-lems. This may artificially bias studies to sug-gest that it is the gonadectomy that leads to aggression, rather than the actual experience in the clinic or shelter. It is critical not to ignore the role that early experience plays in the develop-ment of behavior problems in dogs and cats.

When possible, special consideration should be given to intact dogs who enter the shelter already showing high levels of fear and anxi-ety. This can be challenging since the shelter is inherently a scary place for many dogs, and postponing surgery is impractical. To prevent the exacerbation of fear as much as possible, extra attention must be given to relieving their anxiety with medication prior to, during, and immediately after neuter surgery. Increased attention to low-stress handling and teaching staff to read canine body language, both strate-gies suggested by the Fear Free™ initiative, have the potential to decrease the likelihood of a traumatic experience associated with early gonadectomy that could profoundly affect the future behavior of companion animals. See Chapters 8 and 14 for more information about low-stress handling for dogs and cats.

All that we can really conclude at this time from the conflicting data regarding gonadec-tomy and the "ideal" age for gonadectomy is that there are, and always will be, certain risks and benefits to performing gonadectomy on any animal. Due to the variety of different methods used in studies thus far, the varying ways in which "early gonadectomy" is defined, and the differing definitions or descriptions used to identify behaviors in assorted studies, it is difficult to even compare data from one study to the next. In addition, due to the vary-ing populations used for the studies, we cannot automatically assume that all of the data can be extrapolated and applied equally to all other populations of dogs. Due to the important role that genetics and environment can play in so many of the discussed conditions, one can never assume that a population of dogs in one country will respond to any intervention in an identical way as the population of dogs in another country. The same can be said of the few breed-specific studies in the literature. The results among the studied breeds vary, so it is to be expected that other breeds as yet unstud-ied will reveal different findings. What we *do* know is that gonadectomy appears to be asso-ciated with a longer lifespan in dogs (Reichler 2009; Houlihan 2017), and more intact animals are returned to the shelter than neutered animals (Patronek et al. 1996; New et al. 2000), which has a more immediate impact on long-term health due to premature euthanasia. The benefit of early sterilization for animals in shelters and humane societies likely outweighs all of the other risks.

4.9 Behavior and/or Medical Conditions Seen in Intact versus Neutered Cats

4.9.1 Female Feline

The normal reproductive cycle of the queen is very different from the bitch. Unlike the bitch, the queen is an induced or reflex ovulator and is seasonally polyestrous, having more than one estrous cycle during the breeding season (Houpt 2005). Queens only ovulate in response to cervical stimulation. The queen's cycle con-sists of four phases that include proestrus,

estrus, metestrus (diestrus and interestrus), and anestrus (Griffin 2001). Metestrus is the time between two estrus cycles if breeding has not occurred. If breeding does not occur, the queen may return to proestrus with the next follicular wave, which is typically between one to three weeks but has been reported from three days to seven weeks in some cases (Feldman and Nelson 1996; Root et al. 1995). Anestrus is the time between breeding seasons. The age kittens begin to cycle is dependent on when they were born relative to the breeding season, typically anywhere from 6 to 10 months.

The female will undergo several behavioral changes during the estrus cycle. During the proestrus stage, the queen is often very affectionate, rubbing her head on any object, both animate and inanimate, and seeming friendlier, although some females will not show any signs during proestrus. This behavior is consistent with scent marking to notify other cats that there is a female coming into estrus. There may be a slight increase in vocalization and rolling, as well as stretching and lying in lateral recumbency while kneading with the paws. Toms may show some interest in the queen at this time, although she will not be interested in them and may act very aggressively: slapping, hissing, chasing, and/or biting the tom. The vulva may be slightly enlarged, but this generally goes unnoticed because of its anatomical location and relatively small size to begin with. Additionally, there may also be a discharge; this is not commonly observed due to the fastidious grooming behavior of most cats. However, one might notice that the queen is grooming her perineal area more often.

Estrus is the period in which the female is receptive (allows copulatory mounting) to the male. The queen often vocalizes loudly and constantly during this phase; indoor queens may run from window to window while vocalizing. The estrus queen may roll more vigorously. During petting, she will often lower her chest and raise her pelvis. She may also tread with her back legs and deviate her tail to the side. Excessive and persistent vocalization is alarming to some, and those unfamiliar with normal feline reproductive behavior may believe the cat is ill or in severe pain. The estrus queen also urinates more often, a sign that mimics a UTI, and may spray urine as well (Beaver 2003). Her excessive activity may result in decreased appetite and resultant weight loss. The proestrus and estrus stage can last anywhere from 9 to 10 days if the queen remains unbred and approximately 4 days if bred (Banks 1986; Root et al. 1995; Houpt 2005).

The length of metestrus varies from one to two days to several months, averaging seven to nine days for a non-bred queen (Banks 1986). If a queen is bred, she will generally return to estrus approximately one to two weeks after weaning during the breeding season, otherwise she will cycle again the next season. There have been reports of bred queens coming into estrus while pregnant. If the queen is bred during the pregnant estrus cycle, the resultant kittens will be immature. When she gives birth, there will be both full-term and immature kittens; this is known as superfetation (Hunt 1919). Some lactating queens will come into estrus 7 to 10 days after parturition (Schmidt 1985).

Feline breeding may be described as a violent act. The male and female call back and forth to each other. Multiple males fight, while the female watches at a distance. Once the female has decided on a mate, she allows him to mount, and he bites the back of her neck. The queen emits a piercing howl, which is thought to be the result of the spines on the male penis contacting the cervix after ejaculation (Banks 1986). After the cry, the queen almost immediately jumps away and actively rejects the male. This may include hissing, spitting, and striking at him. She then rolls, stretches, and vigorously grooms her vulva. The time between copulations is variable, from 20 minutes to several hours, and is determined by the queen.

A pregnant queen initially does not display many physical or behavioral changes compared to an anestrus cat. During the last three weeks of gestation, the physiological changes typical of pregnant animals begin to occur, including distension of the abdomen as well as reddening and slight swelling of the nipples. Because of the enlarged abdomen and change in center of gravity, the queen may not be as agile and therefore may not jump up as much. The enlarging uterus puts pressure on the internal organs. This results in the queen preferring small, frequent meals. She may also demonstrate increased frequency of urination and possible difficulty having bowel movements. The increased pressure and discomfort may result in increased grooming of painful areas.

The gestation lasts between 63 and 65 days on average. Since the queen breeds multiple times and is an induced ovulator, it is difficult to know the exact day of conception. Many queens become more docile and may nest build as they get closer to parturition. Nest building by queens is not reported to be as destructive as the same behavior by bitches. They tend to seek closets and other dark, secluded areas. Unlike dogs, a drop in rectal temperature is not a reliable predictor of impending parturition. Milk and colostrum may be present up to a week prior to parturition. Many queens become less active as their discomfort level increases, but some may seem more agitated or restless as they search for a place to deliver.

Queens in a colony setting will often cooperatively raise and nurse the kittens. In a shelter situation, this may be helpful, as a queen with a recent litter may willingly foster other kittens. Cooperatively nursed kittens grow faster and are weaned sooner, and, consequently, the queens return to estrus sooner than non-cooperatively nursing queens. If free to do so, queens will move kittens approximately every three weeks. This is not due to fouling of the nest but is thought to be a way to hide from predators. This suggests that if a queen with kittens in a shelter setting is unable to hide her kittens as she wishes, she may experience some degree of stress. Placement in a foster home, if possible, may be best for the welfare of the queen and kittens. When this is not an option, a quiet and secluded location in the shelter should be identified. Stress from a variety of different causes has been demonstrated to cause permanent changes in the neurophysiological development of offspring, and this can have far-reaching effects on the suitability of kittens as pets.

Anestrus in the queen is usually seasonal, although one study reported that only 90% of the longhaired queens and 40% of the short-haired queens in the study population entered anestrus (Jemmett and Evans 1977). Therefore, it would not be uncommon for a female cat to exhibit estrus-type behavior year-round.

4.9.1.1 Pseudopregnancy (Pseudocyesis, False Pregnancy)

Pseudopregnancy does not occur as often in the queen as it does in the bitch. Typically, if a queen does have a pseudopregnancy, it is secondary to non-fertile ovulation or miscarriage. The signs are usually minimal and may go unnoticed. However, the queen may produce milk and adopt inanimate objects as surrogate kittens. Treatment is unnecessary, and the queen will start her estrus cycle within 30–44 days (Hart and Eckstein 1997).

4.9.1.2 Mastitis

Mastitis is rarely seen in the cat. When it does occur, the first sign noted is often kitten death. Examination of the mammary gland reveals a red, erythematous gland that often produces a purulent discharge. Initially, one might notice that the kittens are more vocal, and the queen may avoid them and become more restless as her mammary gland becomes more uncomfortable. The queen may lick and groom the area more frequently, and she may growl as she grooms. As the infection progresses and the queen becomes more febrile, she will be anorectic, depressed, and adipsic. This will further decrease milk production, resulting in increased vocalization of the hungry kittens. Lack of milk will result in hypothermia, hypoglycemia, and premature death of the kittens.

Early identification and treatment can prevent degeneration of the mammary gland to gangrenous mastitis (Gruffydd-Jones 1980).

4.9.1.3 Eclampsia

Eclampsia is not common in cats; however, it has been reported (Bjerkas 1974). When it occurs, it is generally associated with queens who have had multiple litters in a short period of time on a substandard diet. A queen with eclampsia will become ataxic, which is followed by an increased respiratory rate, possibly open-mouth breathing, and then tonic spasms of the limbs. Following an eclampsic event, the queen may also become hypoglycemic. Eclampsia is life-threatening.

4.9.1.4 Pyometra

Pyometra is an infection of the uterus that occurs when the uterus is under the influence of progesterone. Pyometra in the cat generally occurs in queens between 3 and 14 years of age and is most common in nulliparous queens more than 5 years of age. This condition is also life-threatening.

Typical signs for pyometra include polydipsia, weight loss, and foul-smelling discharge in some cases. Many queens will be depressed, have a slightly decreased appetite, have an increased respiratory rate, and be lethargic. Some will seem relatively normal except for polydipsia and excessive licking or grooming of the hindquarters. Caretakers might notice that the urine in the litterbox has a bloody or mucoid consistency.

4.9.1.5 Metritis

Metritis is an infection of the uterus postpartum. In the queen, metritis is most often associated with the presence of a retained fetal membrane or fetus. Typically, the queen is anorectic, depressed, lethargic, and neglects her kittens. The decreased milk production results in inadequate nutrition for the kittens. Consequently, they become more vocal. The queen often has a copious, malodorous discharge. In her depressed condition, she may not groom herself, making the discharge even more apparent. Her febrile state results in a rapid respiratory rate.

4.9.1.6 Mammary Tumors

Mammary tumors in the cat are more likely to be malignant than benign by a ratio of 9:1 (Hayes et al. 1981; Morris 2013). Siamese queens are more likely to develop mammary tumors than other breeds (Hayes et al. 1981). In one study, queens spayed prior to six months of age had a 91% reduction in risk of mammary adenocarcinoma than intact cats (Overley et al. 2005). Mammary gland tumors do not change the behavior of the cat, unless they are large enough to alter the cat's gait, balance, or ability to rest. Excessive grooming with resultant alopecia of the area may be noted if the tumor grows rapidly, has ruptured, is draining, or is causing discomfort.

The lungs, iliac lymph nodes, and abdominal organs are the most common areas of metastasis (Morris 2013). A cat with a mammary tumor may have difficulty breathing while at rest, have an abnormal gait in the rear legs, be reluctant to jump up on things, be less active, or have gastrointestinal disturbances. If performed prior to a year of age, ovariohysterectomy results in an 86% reduction in the risk of mammary tumors (Overley et al. 2005).

4.9.1.7 Ovarian Tumors

Ovarian tumors are uncommon and only occur in the intact queen (Klein 2001). They are typically unilateral, metastasis is uncommon, and they become quite large before they are detected. Some ovarian tumors will secrete estrogen, resulting in a prolonged estrus. Unlike in the bitch, hyperestrogenism in the cat is not likely to result in alopecia (Mecklenburg et al. 2009).

Most of the ovarian tumors result in nonspecific clinical and behavioral signs. These signs include a distended abdomen due to tumor size or ascites. The queen may also vomit, be anorectic, appear constipated, urinate frequently, have an increased respiratory rate, or show signs of discomfort when lying down due to the physical size of the tumor putting pressure on other organs.

4.9.1.8 Ovarian Remnant

Ovarian remnant syndrome, as it is in the bitch, is characterized by signs typical of an animal who still has ovarian function after removal of the ovaries. In the queen, if parts of the ovary are left behind, they will revascularize when reattached to the mesentery after ovariohysterectomy and have follicular development (DeNardo et al. 2001). Cats that show signs of estrus following ovariohysterectomy should be evaluated for an ovarian remnant.

4.9.2 Male Feline

4.9.2.1 Cryptorchid

The male kitten is born with both testicles descended. He usually reaches puberty and can breed at six to eight months of age. There is a very low incidence of cryptorchidism in cats. Cryptorchid males will behave as a tom cat, showing a higher rate of spraying, increased incidence of abscesses secondary to inter-cat aggression, and sexual behaviors. A cat under the influence of testosterone will have spines on his penis. This is a relatively non-invasive method to discern older neutered cats from cryptorchids and potentially partially neutered cats.

4.9.2.2 Castration or Orchiectomy

Removal of the testicles is called castration or orchiectomy. The behavior of neutered male cats is very similar to an anestrus female. Castration results in a significant reduction in sexually dimorphic behaviors, such as mounting, urine marking or spraying, roaming, and fighting in cats (Spain et al. 2004). Gonadectomy to eliminate or decrease these problems tends to be more effective in cats than in dogs (Hart and Barrett 1973). After castration, male cats also have a decreased incidence of abscesses due to bite wounds.

4.9.3 Normal Sex-Related Behaviors

4.9.3.1 Marking

Urine marking or spraying is a natural behavior for both males and females and has a different underlying motivation than urination (or elimination) due to a full bladder. It is used primarily as a method of communication between cats. It occurs most commonly in intact males; however, gonadectomized males also mark. While it is somewhat less common, it is not rare for a gonadectomized female cat to urine mark. When gonadectomized animals urine mark inside the home, it is usually believed to be a result of anxiety or distress in response to the agonistic conflict between cats in the home or the presence of cats outside the home.

4.9.3.2 Non-copulatory Mounting

This is a normal behavior primarily of intact males but will occasionally occur in intact females (Houpt 2005). It is more common in the young intact male housed with other young males (Beaver 1989). If mounting behavior is increasing in the shelter, it is important to attempt to recognize specific triggers and/or motivation for the behavior so that the situation can be avoided or the environment changed as necessary to prevent excessive mounting. This may mean either removing the animal performing the mounting or the animal who is repeatedly mounted. Any change in the social grouping may affect the behavior.

4.9.3.3 Masturbation

Masturbation is not reported as a problem in the cat as frequently as in the dog, although owners are more likely to report it in castrated male cats (Beaver 1989). Female cats under the influence of prolonged estrogen, such as a cat with an ovarian remnant, ovarian tumors, or exposure to human estrogen creams, are more likely to masturbate (Kling et al. 1969). Females who masturbate rub their anogenital area against the floor. They may also vocalize and groom their genital area.

Masturbation in the intact male cat is most common in the laboratory setting. Masturbating male cats rub their perineal area on a surface or manipulate the area with their paws. The behavior becomes pathological when an animal performs it to the exclusion of normal behaviors, such as eating, drinking, and environmental investigation. Masturbation can lead to increased infection or trauma of the prepuce, penis, or vulva.

4.9.4 Effects of Gonadectomy on the Behavior of Cats

As with the dog, there are some concerns that early age neutering in the cat may have some long-term negative consequences, but far fewer studies have examined the risks and benefits of neutering at different ages in the cat. What is known is that more intact animals are returned to the shelter than neutered animals, so delaying gonadectomy could have an immediate impact on long-term health due to premature euthanasia. In the animal shelter situation, where the risk of owner non-compliance with sterilization policy (Alexander and Shane 1994) further increases the burden on shelters and rescue groups, early sterilization of cats remains important.

4.10 Side Effects of Common Medications

Many medications have the potential to affect behavior. When using any medication, its potential side effects must always be kept in mind, and the ways in which those side effects might change behavior should be considered. For example, medications that have the side effect of increasing thirst may result in increased drinking and lead to housesoiling because the animal suddenly needs to urinate more frequently.

Corticosteroids are one of the most commonly used drugs in veterinary medicine. They have a high likelihood of affecting behavior, and despite well-described behavioral effects in humans, very little research has examined the possibility of behavioral changes associated with the administration of corticosteroids in animals. In studies performed by Notari and Mills (2011; Notari et al. 2015) several behavioral changes were noted in dogs after the administration of corticosteroids. These included nervousness or restlessness, fearfulness, startling, barking, food-guarding behavior, and irritable aggression. In addition, they were also often less playful and more withdrawn from people and situations. Until more research is performed, reasonable precautions should be used when handling animals who are being treated with corticosteroids. See Chapter 22 for more information about behavioral pharmacology.

4.11 Conclusions

Changes in behavior are likely the first signs of stress, disease, and poor welfare in any animal. The changes that an animal experiences when relinquished or abandoned and in need of sheltering inevitably lead to a certain amount of stress. The important role of stress in the development of disease and many problem behaviors has been well documented. An awareness of the complex interrelationship between stress and physical and mental health is necessary for animal caretakers in shelters to ensure animals' best health and welfare. Recognizing that an animal's emotional health is equally as important as their physical health is the first critical step toward maintaining emotional and physical health in the shelter environment. Only by safeguarding both physical and emotional health can we improve overall quality of life for animals in our care, facilitate their placement in homes, and help prevent their return to the shelter.

Please visit the companion website for video clips and downloadable resources associated with this chapter.

References

Alexander, S.A. and Shane, S.M. (1994) Characteristics of animals adopted from an animal control center whose owners complied with a spaying/neutering program. *J. Am. Vet. Med. Assoc.* 205 (3): 472–476.

American Pet Products Association. (2013). *APPA National Pet Owners Survey 2013–2014*. Greenwich, CT: American Pet Products Association. Report.

American Psychiatric Association. (2013). *DSM 5*. Washington, DC: American Psychiatric Association.

Arnold, S. (1992). Relationship of incontinence to neutering. In: *Current Veterinary Therapy XI* (eds. R.W. Kirk and J.D. Bonagura), 857–877. Philadelphia: W.B. Saunders.

Aronson, L.P. (1998). Systemic causes of aggression and their treatment. In: *Psychopharmacology of Animal Behavior Disorders* (eds. N.H. Dodman and L. Shuster), 64–102. Malden, MA: Blackwell Science.

Asher, L., Diesel, G., Summers, J.F. et al. (2009). Inherited defects in pedigree dogs. Part 1: Disorders related to breed standards. *Vet. J.* 182: 402–411.

Bacon, H.J., Walters, H. Vancia, V. et al. (2019). The recognition of canine pain behaviours, and potentially hazardous catch-neuter-trap return practices by animal care professionals. *Anim. Welf.* 28: 299–306.

Ball, R.L., Birchard, S.J., May, L.R. et al. (2010). Ovarian remnant syndrome in dogs and cats: 21 cases (2000–2007). *J. Am. Vet. Assoc.* 236 (5): 548–553.

Bamberger, M. and Houpt, K.A. (2006). Signalment factors, comorbidity, and trends in behavior diagnoses in cats: 736 cases (1991–2001). *J. Am. Vet. Med. Assoc.* 229: 1602–1606.

Banks, D.R. (1986). Physiology and endocrinology of the feline estrous cycle. In: *Current Therapy in Theriogenology* (ed. D.E. Morrow), 795. Philadelphia: W.B. Saunders.

Barnes, H.L., Chrisman, C.L., Mariani, C.L. et al. (2004). Clinical signs, underlying cause, and outcome in cats with seizures: 17 cases (1997–2002). *J. Am. Vet. Med. Assoc.* 225: 1723–1726.

Beaver, B.V. (1989). Feline behavioral problems other than housesoiling. *J. Am. Anim. Hosp. Assoc.* 25: 465–468.

Beaver, B.V. (2003). Female feline sexual behavior. In: *Feline Behavior: A Guide for Veterinarians* (ed. B.V. Beaver), 182–204. St. Louis: Elsevier Science.

Bécuwe-Bonnet, V., Bélanger, M., Frank, D. et al. (2012). Gastrointestinal disorders in dogs with excessive licking of surfaces. *J. Vet. Behav.* 7: 194–204.

Beerda, B., Schilder, M.B.H., van Hoff, J.A.R.A.M. et al. (1998). Behavioural, saliva cortisol and heart rate responses to different types of stimuli in dogs. *Appl. Anim. Behav. Sci.* 58: 365–381.

Beerda, B., Schilder, M.B.H., van Hoff, J.A.R.A.M. et al. (1999). Chronic stress in dogs subjected to social and spatial restriction: I. Behavioral responses. *Physiol. Behav.* 66: 233–242.

Bennett, D. and Morton, C. (2009). A study of owner observed behavioural and lifestyle changes in cats with musculoskeletal disease before and after analgesic therapy. *J. Fel. Med. Surg.* 11: 997–1004.

Berendt, M. and Gram, L. (1999). Epilepsy and seizure classification in 63 dogs: A reappraisal of veterinary epilepsy terminology. *J. Vet. Int. Med.* 13: 14–20.

Berent, A.C. (2011). Ectopic ureter. In: *Blackwell's Five-Minute Veterinary Consult— Canine and Feline*, 5th ed. (eds. L.P. Tilley and F.W.K. Smith), 403. Chichester, UK: Wiley-Blackwell.

Berset-Istratescu, C.M., Glardon, O.J., Magouras, I. et al. (2014). Follow-up of 100 dogs with acute diarrhea in a primary care practice. *Vet. J.* 199: 188–190.

Bhatia, T. and Tandon, R.K. (2005). Stress and the gastrointestinal tract. *J. Gastroenterol. Hepatol.* 20: 332–339.

Bjerkas, E. (1974). Eclampsia in the cat. *J. Small Anim. Pract.* 15: 411–414.

Black, A.M. (1994). The pathophysiology and laboratory diagnosis of congenital portosystemic shunts in dogs. *N. Z. Vet. J.* 42: 75–75.

Blackshaw, J.K. (1991). Management of orally based problems and aggression in cats. *Aust. Vet. Pract.* 21 (3): 122–125.

Braastad, B.O. (1998). Effects of prenatal stress on behaviour of offspring of laboratory and farmed mammals. *Appl. Anim. Behav. Sci.* 61 :159–180.

Bradshaw, J.W.S., Neville, P.F., and Sawyer, D. (1997). Factors affecting pica in the domestic cat. *Appl. Anim. Behav. Sci.* 52: 373–379.

Bradshaw, J.W. and Nott, H.M. (1995). Social and communication behaviour of companion dogs. In: *The Domestic Dog: Its Evolution, Behaviour and Interactions with People* (ed. J. Serpell), 115–130. Cambridge, UK: Cambridge University Press.

Brodey, R.S., Goldschmidt, M.H., and Roszel, J.R. (1983). Canine mammary neoplasm. *J. Am. Anim. Hosp. Assoc.* 19: 61–90.

Buffington, C.A.T. and Pacak, K. (2001). Increased plasma norepinephrine concentration in cats with interstitial cystitis. *J. Urol.* 165: 2051–2054.

Buffington, C.A.T., Teng, B. and Somogyi, G.T. (2002). Norepinephrine content and adrenoceptor function in the bladder of cats with feline interstitial cystitis. *J. Urol.* 167: 1876–1880.

Buffington, C.A.T., Westropp, J.L., Chew, D.J. et al. (2006). Clinical evaluation of multimodal environmental modification (MEMO) in the management of cats with idiopathic cystitis. *J. Fel. Med. Surg.* 8: 261–268.

Cameron, M.E., Casey, R.A., Bradshaw, J.W.S. et al. (2004). A study of environmental and behavioural factors that may be associated with feline idiopathic cystitis. *J. Small Anim. Pract.* 45: 144–147.

Carlstead, K., Brown, J.L., and Strawn, W. (1993). Behavioral and physiological correlates of stress in laboratory cats. *Appl. Anim. Behav. Sci.* 38: 143–158.

Champagne, F.A., Weaver, I.C.G., Diorio, J. et al. (2006). Maternal care associated with methylation of the estrogen receptor alpha 1b promoter and estrogen receptor-alpha expression in the medial preoptic area of female offspring. *Endocrinology* 147 (6): 2909–2915.

Chapillon, P., Patin, V., Roy, V. et al. (2002). Effects of pre- and postnatal stimulation on developmental, emotional, and cognitive aspects in rodents: A review. *Dev. Psychobiol.* 41: 373–387.

Ciribassi, J. (2009). Feline hyperesthesia syndrome. *Compend. Contin. Educ. Vet.* 31 (6): 254.

Clarke, S.P. and Bennett, D. (2006). Feline osteoarthritis: A prospective study of 28 cases. *J. Small Anim. Pract.* 47 (8): 439–445.

Cloutier, S., Newberry, R.C., Cambridge, A.J. et al. (2005). Behavioural signs of postoperative pain in cats following onychectomy or tenectomy surgery. *Appl. Anim. Behav. Sci.* 92: 325–335.

Concannon, P.W., Butler, W.R., Hansel, W. et al. (1978). Parturition and lactation in the bitch: Serum progesterone, cortisol and prolactin. *Biol. Reprod.* 19: 1113–1118.

Cummings, J.F. and de Lahunta, A. (1977). An adult case of canine neuronal ceroid lipofuscinosis. *Acta Neuropathol.* 39: 43–51.

Davenport, M.D., Lutz, C.K., Tiefenbacher, S. et al. (2008). A rhesus monkey model of self-injury: Effects of relocation stress on behavior and neuroendocrine function. *Biol. Psychiatry* 63: 990–996.

Davis, A.K., Maney, D.L., and Maerz, J.C. (2008). The use of leukocyte profiles to measure stress in vertebrates: A review for ecologists. *Funct. Ecol.* 22 (5): 760–772.

Dellinger-Ness, L.A. and Handler, L. (2006). Self-injurious behavior in human and non-human primates. *Clin. Psychol. Rev.* 26: 503–514.

DeNardo, G., Becker, K., and Brown, N. (2001). Ovarian remnant syndrome: Revascularization of free-floating ovarian tissue in the feline abdominal cavity. *J. Am. Anim. Hosp. Assoc.* 37: 290–296.

Denerolle, P., White, S.D., Taylor, T.S. et al. (2007). Organic diseases mimicking acral lick dermatitis in six dogs. *J. Am. Anim. Hosp. Assoc.* 43 (4): 215–220.

Dinnage, J.D. (2006). *Measuring and assessing stress in shelter cats*. North American Veterinary Conference, Orlando, FL.

Dobson, J.M, (2013). Breed-predispositions to cancer in pedigree dogs. *ISRN Vet. Sci.* 2013: 941275.

Dodman, N. H., Aronson, L., Cottam, N. et al. (2013). The effect of thyroid replacement in dogs with suboptimal thyroid function on owner-directed aggression: A randomized, double-blind, placebo-controlled clinical trial. *J. Vet. Behav.* 8: 225–230.

Dodman, N.H., Knowles, K.E., Shuster, L. et al. (1996). Behavioral changes associated with suspected complex partial seizures in bull terriers. *J. Am. Vet. Med. Assoc.* 208: 688–689.

Dodman, N.H., Miczek, K.A., Knowles, K. et al. (1992). Phenobarbital-responsive episodic dyscontrol (rage) in dogs. *J. Am. Vet. Med. Assoc.* 201: 1580–1583.

Epstein, M.E., Rodan, I., Griffenhagen, G. et al. (2015). 2015 AAHA/AAFP pain management guidelines for dogs and cats. *J. Fel. Med. Surg.* 17: 251–272.

Farhoody, P., Mallawaarachchi, I., Tarwater, P.M., et al. (2018). Aggression toward familiar people, strangers, and conspecifics in gonadectomized and intact dogs. *Front. Vet. Sci.* 5 (18): 1–13.

Feldman, E.C. and Nelson, R.W. (1996). Ovarian cycle and vaginal cytology. In: *Canine and Feline Endocrinology and Reproduction*, 3rd ed. (ed. R. Nelson), 526–546. St. Louis: Saunders.

Foster, E.S., Carillo, J.M., and Patnik, A.K. (1998). Clinical signs of tumors affecting the rostral cerebrum in 43 dogs. *J. Vet. Intern. Med.* 2: 71–74.

Foster, J.A. and Neufeld, K.M. (2013). Gut-brain axis: How the microbiome influences anxiety and depression. *Trends Neurosci.* 36 (5): 305–312.

Foyer, P., Willsson, E., Wright, D. et al. (2013). Early experiences modulate stress coping in a population of German shepherd dogs. *Appl. Anim. Behav. Sci.* 146: 79–87.

Frank, D., Bélanger, M., Bécuwe-Bonnet, V. et al. (2012). Prospective medical evaluation of 7 dogs presented with fly biting. *Can. Vet. J.* 53 (12): 1279.

Gerber, B., Boretti, F.S., Kley, S. et al. (2005). Evaluation of clinical signs and causes of lower urinary tract disease in European cats. *J. Small Anim. Pract.* 46: 571–577.

Gier, H.T. and Marion, G.B. (1970). Development of the mammalian testis. In: *The Testis* (eds. A.D. Johnson, W.R. Gomes, and N.L. Vanemark), 1–45. New York: Academic Press.

Godfrey, D.R. (2005). Osteoarthritis in cats: A retrospective radiological study. *J. Small Anim. Pract.* 46: 425–429.

Goldman, E.E., Breitschwerdt, E.B., Grindem, C.B. et al. (1998). Granulocytic ehrlichiosis in dogs from North Carolina and Virginia. *J. Vet. Intern. Med.* 12 (2): 61–70.

Greenlee, P.G. and Patnaik, A.K. (1985). Canine ovarian tumors of germ cell origin. *Vet. Clin. Pathol.* 22 (2): 117–122.

Griffin, B. (2001). Prolific cats: The estrous cycle. *Compend. Contin. Educ. Vet.* 23 (12): 1049–1057.

Gruffydd-Jones, T.J. (1980). Acute mastitis in a cat. *Feline Pract.* 10 (6): 41–42.

Guy, N.C., Luescher, U.A., Dohoo, S.E. et al. (2001). Demographic and aggressive characteristics of dogs in a general veterinary caseload. *Appl. Anim. Behav. Sci.* 74: 15–28.

Hardie, E.M., Roe, S.C. and Martin, F.R. (2002). Radiographic evidence of degenerative joint disease in geriatric cats: 100 cases (1994–1997). *J. Am. Vet. Med. Assoc.* 220: 628–632.

Hart, B.L. (2010). Beyond fever: Comparative perspectives on sickness behavior. In: *Encyclopedia of Animal Behavior*, Vol. 1 (eds. M. Breed and J. Moore), 205–210. Oxford, UK: Academic Press.

Hart, B.L. (2011). Behavioural defences in animals against pathogens and parasites: Parallels with the pillars of medicine in humans. *Philos. Trans. R. Soc.* 366: 3406–3417.

Hart, B.L. and Barrett, R.E. (1973). Effects of castration on fighting, roaming, and urine spraying in adult male cats. *J. Am. Vet. Med. Assoc.* 163 (3): 290.

Hart, B.L. and Eckstein, R.A. (1997). The role of gonadal hormones in the occurrence of objectionable behaviours in dogs and cats. *Appl. Anim. Behav. Sci.* 52 (3): 331–344.

Harvey, N.D, Craigon, P.J., Shaw, S.C. et al. (2019). Behavioural differences in dogs with atopic dermatitis suggest stress could be a significant problem associated with chronic pruritus. *Animals* 9 (10): 813.

Hayes, H.M., Milne, K.L., and Mandell, C.P. (1981). Epidemiological features of feline mammary carcinoma. *Vet. Rec.* 108 (22): 476–479.

Hayes, H.M. and Pendergrass, T.W. (1976). Canine testicular tumors: Epidemiologic features of 410 dogs. *Int. J. Cancer* 18 (4): 482–487.

Hayes, H.M., Wilson, G.P., Pendergrass, T.W. et al. (1985). Canine cryptorchism and subsequent testicular neoplasia: Case-control study with epidemiologic update. *Teratology* 32 (1): 51–56.

Hennessy, M.B. (2013). Using hypothalamic–pituitary–adrenal measures for assessing and reducing the stress of dogs in shelters: A review. *Appl. Anim. Behav. Sci.* 149 (1–4): 1–12.

Hennessy, M.B., Davis, H.N., Williams, M.T. et al. (1997). Plasma cortisol levels of dogs at a public animal shelter. *Physiol. Behav.* 62: 485–490.

Holton, L.L., Scot, E.M., Nolan, A.M. et al. (1998). Comparison of three methods used for assessment of pain in dogs. *J. Am. Vet. Med. Assoc.* 212: 61–66.

Hopkins, S.G., Schubert, T.A., Hart, B.L. (1976). Castration of adult male dogs: Effects on roaming, aggression, urine marking and mounting. *J. Am. Vet. Med. Assoc.* 168: 1108–1110.

Horváth, Z., Dóka, A., and Miklósi, Á. (2008). Affiliative and disciplinary behavior of human handlers during play with their dog affects cortisol in opposite directions. *Horm. Behav.* 54: 107–114.

Houlihan, K.E. (2017). A literature review on the welfare implications of gonadectomy of dogs. *J. Am. Vet. Med. Assoc.* 250: 1155–1166.

Houpt, K.A. (2005). *Domestic Animal Behavior for Veterinarians and Animal Scientists*, 4th ed. Oxford, UK: Blackwell.

Houpt, K.A. (2011). *Domestic Animal Behavior for Veterinarians and Animal Scientists*, 5th ed. Hoboken, NJ: Wiley Blackwell.

Howe, L.M., Slater, M.R., Boothe, H.W. et al. (2001). Long-term outcome of gonadectomy performed at an early age or traditional age in dogs. *J. Am. Vet. Med. Assoc.* 218 (2): 217–221.

Hrovat, A., De Keuster T., Koostra, H.S. et al. (2018). Behavior in dogs with spontaneous hypothyroidism during treatment with levothyroxine. *J. Vet. Intern. Med.* 33: 64–71.

Hunt, H.R. (1919). Birth of two unequally developed cat fetuses (*Felis domestica*). *Anat. Rec.* 16 (6): 371–378.

Jemmett, J.E. and Evans, J.M. (1977). A survey of sexual behaviour and reproduction of female cats. *J. Small Anim. Pract.* 18 (1): 31–37.

Jensen, P. (2014). Behaviour epigenetics—The connection between environment, stress and welfare. *Appl. Anim. Behav. Sci.* 157: 1–7.

Johnston, S.D. (1980). False pregnancy in the bitch. In: *Current Theory in Theriogenology* (ed. D.A. Morrow), 623–662. Philadelphia: W.B. Saunders.

Johnston, S.D. (1986). Pseudopregnancy in the bitch. In: *Current Theory in Theriogenology*, 2nd ed. (ed. D.A. Morrow), 490–491. Philadelphia: W.B. Saunders.

Jones, A. and Josephs, R.A. (2006). Interspecies hormonal interactions between man and the domestic dog (*Canis familiaris*). *Horm. Behav.* 50: 393–400.

Jones, B.R., Gruffydd-Jones, T.J., Sparkes, A.H. et al. (1992). Preliminary studies on congenital hypothyroidism in a family of Abyssinian cats. *Vet. Rec.* 131: 145–148.

Joseph, R.J. (2011). Cerebellar degeneration. In: *Blackwell's Five-Minute Veterinary Consult—Canine and Feline*, 5th ed. (eds. L.P. Tilley and F.W.K. Smith), 227. Chichester, UK: Wiley Blackwell.

Karli, P., Gorgas, D., Oevermann, A. et al. (2013). Extracranial expansion of a feline meningioma. *J. Fel. Med. Surg.* 15: 749–753.

Kessler, M.R. and Turner, D.C. (1997). Stress and adaptation of cats (*Felis silvestris catus*) housed singly, in pairs and in groups in boarding catteries. *Anim. Welf.* 6 (3): 243–254.

Kessler, M.R. and Turner, D.C. (1999a). Socialization and stress in cats (*Felis silvestris catus*) housed singly and in groups in animal shelters. *Anim. Welf.* 8: 15–26.

Kessler, M.R. and Turner, D.C. (1999b). Effects of density and cage size on stress in domestic cats (*Felis silvestris catus*) housed in animal shelters and boarding catteries. *Anim. Welf.* 8: 259–267.

Kirchoff, N.S., Udell, M.A.R., and Sharpton, T.J. (2019). The gut microbiome correlates with conspecific aggression in a small population of rescued dogs (*Canis familiaris*). *Peer J.* http://doi.org/10.7717/peerj.6103.

Klein, M.K. (2001). Tumors of the female reproductive system. In: *Small Animal Clinical Oncology* (eds. S.J. Withrom and D.M. Vail), 610–618. St. Louis: Saunders.

Kling, A., Kovach, J.K., and Tucker, T.J. (1969). The behaviour of cats. In: *The Behaviour of Domestic Animals*, 2nd ed. (ed. E.S.E. Hafez), 482–512. Baltimore: Williams and Wilkins.

Kohn, B. and Fumi, C. (2008). Clinical course of pyruvate kinase deficiency in Abyssinian and Somali cats. *J. Fel. Med. Surg.* 10: 145–153.

Kohn, B., Weingart, C., Eckmann, V. et al. (2006). Primary immune-mediated hemolytic anemia in 19 cats: Diagnosis, therapy, and outcome (1998–2004). *J. Vet. Intern. Med.* 20: 159–166.

Kustritz, M.V.R. (2009). Canine reproductive physiology. In: *Clinical Canine and Feline Reproduction: Evidence-Based Answers*. (ed. M.V.R. Kustritz), 121. Hoboken, NJ: Wiley.

Lekcharoensuk, C., Osborne, C.A., and Lulich, J.P. (2001). Epidemiologic study of risk factors for lower urinary tract diseases in cats. *J. Am. Vet. Med. Assoc.* 218: 1429–1435.

Lipowitz, A.J., Schwartz, A., Wilson, G.P. et al. (1973). Testicular neoplasms and concomitant clinical changes in the dog. *J. Am. Vet. Med. Assoc.* 163 (12): 1364–1368.

Lisberg, A.E. and Snowdon, C.T. (2011). Effects of sex, social status and gonadectomy on countermarking by domestic dogs, *Canis familiaris. Anim. Behav.* 81 (4): 757–764.

Lorenz, M.D., Coates, J., and Kent, M. (2011). *Handbook of Veterinary Neurology*, 5th ed., 438–440. St. Louis: Elsevier Saunders.

Luescher, A.U. and Reisner, I.R. (2008). Canine aggression toward familiar people: A new look at an old problem. *Vet. Clin. N. Am. Small Anim. Pract.* 38 (5): 1107–1130.

Maarschalkerweerd, R.J., Endenburg, N., Kirpensteijn, J. et al. (1997). Influence of orchiectomy on canine behaviour. *Vet. Rec.* 140: 617–619.

Marioni-Henry, K., Vite, C.H., Newton, A.L. et al. (2004). Prevalence of diseases of the spinal cord of cats. *J. Vet. Intern. Med.* 18 (6): 851–858.

Martinez-Rustafa, I., Kruger, J.M., Miller, R. et al. (2012). Clinical features and risk factors for development of urinary tract infections in cats. *J. Fel. Med. Surg.* 14: 729–740.

McAuliffe, L., Koch, C., Serpell, J. et al. (accepted for publication). Associations between atopic dermatitis and anxiety, aggression and fear-based behaviors in dogs. *J. Am. Anim. Hosp. Assoc.*

McEntee, M.C. (2002). Reproductive oncology. *Clin. Tech. Small Anim. Pract.* 17 (3): 133–149.

McEwen, B.S. (2000). The neurobiology of stress: From serendipity to clinical relevance. *Brain Res.* 886: 172–189.

McGreevy, P.D., Wilson, B., Starling, M.J. et al. (2018). Behavioural risks in male dogs with minimal lifetime exposure to gonadal hormones may complicate population control benefits of desexing, *PLOS ONE* 13 (5): e0196284.

Mecklenburg, L., Linek, M. and Tobin, D.J. (2009). *Hair Loss Disorders in Domestic Animals*. Ames, IA: Wiley.

Merlo, D.F., Rossi, L., Pellegrino, C. et al. (2008). Cancer incidence in pet dogs: Findings of the Animal Tumor Registry of Genoa Italy. *J. Vet. Intern. Med.* 22: 976–984.

Miller, D.M. (1995). Ovarian remnant syndrome in dogs and cats: 46 cases (1988–1992). *J. Vet. Diagn. Invest.* 7 (4): 572–574.

Mills, D.S. (2003). Medical paradigms for the study of problem behaviour: A critical review. *Appl. Anim. Behav. Sci.* 81: 265–277.

Mills, D.S., Demontigny-Bedard, I., Gruen, M. et al. (2020). Pain and problem behavior in cats and dogs. *Animals.* https://doi.org/10.3390/ani10020318.

Moe, L. (2001) Population-based incidence of mammary tumours in some dog breeds. *J. Reprod. Fertil. [Suppl.]* 57: 439–443.

Mondo, E., Barone, M., Soverini, M. et al. (2020). Gut microbiome structure and adrenocortical activity in dogs with aggressive and phobic behavioral disorders. *Heliyon* 6: e03311.

Mongillo, P., Adamelli, S., Bernardini, M. et al. (2012). Successful treatment of abnormal feeding behavior in a cat. *J. Vet. Behav.* 7: 390–393.

Montiero, B.P. and Steagall, P.V. (2019). Chronic pain in cats—Recent advances in clinical assessment. *J. Fel. Med. Surg.* 21: 601–614.

Morris, J. (2013). Mammary tumours in the cat: Size matters, so early intervention saves lives. *J. Fel. Med. Surg.* 15 (5): 391–400.

Moulton, J.E. (1978). Tumors of the mammary gland. In: *Tumours in Domestic Animals*, 2nd ed. (ed. J.E. Moulton), 346–371. Berkley: University of California Press.

Nagata, M. and Shibata, K. (2004). Importance of psychogenic factors in canine recurrent pyoderma. *Vet. Dermatol.* 15 (Suppl. 1): 42.

Nagata, M., Shibata, K., Irimajiri, M. et al. (2002). Importance of psychogenic dermatoses in dogs with pruritic behavior. *Vet. Dermatol.* 13: 211–229.

Neilson, J.C., Eckstein, R.A., and Hart, B.L. (1997). Effects of castration on problem behaviors in male dogs with reference to age and duration of behavior. *J. Am. Vet. Med. Assoc.* 211 (2): 180–182.

Nelson, R.W. and Feldman, E.C. (1986). Pyometra in the bitch. In: *Current Therapy in Theriogenology*, 2nd ed. (ed. D.A. Morrow), 484–489. St. Louis: Saunders.

New, J.C., Jr., Salman, M.D., King, M. et al. (2000). Characteristics of shelter-relinquished animals and their owners compared with animals and their owners in US pet-owning households. *J. Appl. Anim. Welf. Sci.* 3 (3): 179–201.

Notari, L., Burman, O., and Mills, D. (2015). Behavioural changes in dogs treated with corticosteroids. *Physiol. Behav.* 151: 609–616.

Notari, L. and Mills, D. (2011). Possible behavioral effects of exogenous corticosteroids on dog behavior: A preliminary investigation. *J. Vet. Behav.* 6: 321–327.

O'Farrell, V.O. and Peachey, E. (1990). Behavioural effects of ovariohysterectomy on bitches. *J. Small Anim. Pract.* 31: 595–598.

Ohl, F., Arndt, S.S., and van der Staay, F.J. (2008). Pathological anxiety in animals. *Vet. J.* 175: 18–26.

Overall, K.L. (1998). Self-injurious behavior and obsessive compulsive disorder in domestic animals. In: *Psychopharmacology of Animal Behavior Disorders* (eds. N.H. Dodman and L. Shuster), 222–252. Malden, MA: Blackwell Science.

Overall, K.L. and Dunham, A.E. (2002). Clinical features and outcome in dogs and cats with obsessive-compulsive disorder: 126 cases (1989–2000). *J. Am. Vet. Med. Assoc.* 221: 1445–1452.

Overley, B., Shofer, F.S., Goldschmidt, M.H. et al. (2005). Association between ovariohysterectomy and feline mammary carcinoma. *J. Vet. Intern. Med.* 19 (4): 560–563.

Pakozdy, A., Gruber, A., Kneissl, S. et al. (2011). Complex partial cluster seizures in cats with orofacial involvement. *J. Fel. Med. Surg.* 13: 687–693.

Pal, S.K. (2003). Urine marking by free-ranging dogs (*Canis familiaris*) in relation to sex, season, place and posture. *Appl. Anim. Behav. Sci.* 80: 45–59.

Pathan, M.M., Sidiqquee, G.M., Latif, A. et al. (2011). Eclampsia in the dog: An overview. *Vet. World* 4 (1): 45–47.

Patronek, G.J., Glickman, L.T., Beck, A.M. et al. (1996). Risk factors for relinquishment of dogs to an animal shelter. *J. Am. Vet. Med. Assoc.* 209 (3): 572–581.

Perry, K. L. (2014). The lame cat: The challenge of degenerative joint disease. *Companion Animal* 19 (11): 582–590.

Radosta, A., Shofer, F.S., and Reisner, I.R. (2012). Comparison of thyroid analytes in dogs aggressive to familiar people and in non-aggressive dogs. *Vet. J.* 192: 472–475.

Rampin, C., Cepuglio, R.C.N., and Jouvet, M. (1991). Immobilization stress induced a paradoxical sleep rebound in rats. *Neuroscience Lett.* 126: 113–118.

Reichler, I.M. (2009). Gonadectomy in cats and dogs: A review of risks and benefits. *Reprod. Domest. Anim.* 44 (2): 29–35.

Reif, J.S., Maguire, T.G., Kenney, R.M. et al. (1979). A cohort study of canine testicular neoplasia. *J. Am. Vet. Med. Assoc.* 175 (7): 719–723.

Reisner, I.R., Houpt, K.A., and Shofer, F.S. (2005). National survey of owner-directed aggression in English springer spaniels. *J. Am. Vet. Med. Assoc.* 227: 1594–1603.

Rooney, N.J. (2009). The welfare of pedigree dogs: Cause for concern. *J. Vet. Behav.* 4: 180–186.

Root, M.V., Johnston, S.D., and Olson, P.N. (1995). Estrous length, pregnancy rate, gestation and parturition lengths, litter size, and juvenile mortality in the domestic cat. *J. Am. Anim. Hosp. Assoc.* 31 (5): 429–433.

Root, A.L., Parkin, T.D., Hutchison, P. et al. (2018). Canine pseudopregnancy: An evaluation of prevalence and current treatment protocols in the UK. *BMC Vet. Res.* https://doi.org/10.1186/s12917-018-1493-1.

Ross, D.A., Arbuckle, M.R., Travis, M.J. et al. (2017). An integrated neuroscience perspective on formulation and treatment planning for posttraumatic stress disorder: An educational review. *JAMA Psychiatry* 74 (4): 407–415.

Rushen, J. (2000). Some issues in the interpretation of behavioural responses to stress. In: *The Biology of Animal Stress: Basic Principles and Implications for Animal Welfare* (eds. G. Modberg and J.A. Mench), 23–42. Wallingford, UK: CABI Publishing.

Saevik, B.K., Trangerud, C., Ottesen, N. et al. (2011). Causes of lower urinary tract disease in Norwegian cats. *J. Fel. Med. Surg.* 13: 410–417.

Sawyer, L.S., Moon-Fanelli, A.A., and Dodman, N.H. (1999). Psychogenic alopecia in cats: 11 cases (1993–1996). *J. Am. Vet. Med. Assoc.* 214: 71–74.

Schmidt, P.M. (1985). Ovarian activity, circulating hormones and sexual behavior in the cat: Relationships during pregnancy, parturition, lactation and the postpartum estrus. Master's thesis. Texas A&M University.

Sessums, K. and Mariani, C. (2009). Intracranial meningioma in dogs and cats: A comparative review. *Compend. Contin. Educ. Vet.* 31: 330–339.

Sherding, R.G., Wilson, G.P., and Kociba, G.J. (1981). Bone marrow hypoplasia in eight dogs with Sertoli cell tumor. *J. Am. Vet. Med. Assoc.* 178 (5): 497–501.

Shilo, Y. and Pascoe, P.J. (2014). Anatomy, physiology and pathophysiology of pain. In: *Pain Management in Veterinary Practice* (eds. C.M. Egger, L. Love, and T. Doherty), 9–28. Ames, IA: Wiley Blackwell.

Slingerland, L.I., Hazewinkel, H.A.W., Meij, B.P., Picavet, P., and Voorhout, G. (2011). Cross-sectional study of the prevalence and clinical features of osteoarthritis in 100 cats. *Vet. J.* 187: 304–309.

Slutsky, J., Raj, K., Yuhnke, S. et al. (2013). A web resource on DNA tests for canine and feline hereditary diseases. *Vet. J.* 197 (2): 182–187.

Sontas, H.B., Dokuzeylu, B., Turna, O. et al. (2009). Estrogen-induced myelotoxicity in dogs: A review. *Can. Vet. J.* 50 (10): 1054.

Sorenmo, K.U., Worley, D.R., and Goldschmidt, M.H. (2013). Tumor of the mammary gland. In: *Withrow and McEwens Small Animal Oncology* (eds. S.J. Withrow, D.M. Vail, and R.L. Page), 538–556. St. Louis: Elsevier.

Spain, C.V., Scarlett, J.M., and Houpt, K.A. (2004). Long-term risks and benefits of early-age gonadectomy in cats. *J. Am. Vet. Med. Assoc.* 224 (3): 372–379.

Starling, M, Fawcett, A., Wilson, B.M. et al. (2019). Behavioural risks in female dogs with minimal lifetime exposure to gonadal hormones. *PLOS ONE* 14 (12): e0223709.

Stella, J.L., Croney, C., and Buffington, C.A.T. (2013). Effects of stressors on the behavior and physiology of domestic cats. *Appl. Anim. Behav. Sci.* 143: 157–163.

Stella, J.L., Lord, L.K., and Buffington, C.A.T. (2011). Sickness behaviors in response to unusual external events in healthy cats and cats with feline interstitial cystitis. *J. Am. Vet. Med. Assoc.* 238: 67–73.

Sudo, N. et al. (2004). Postnatal microbial colonization programs the hypothalamic-pituitary-adrenal system for stress response in mice. *J. Physiol.* 558: 263–275.

Summers, J.F., Diesel, G., Asher, L. et al. (2010). Inherited defects in pedigree dogs. Part 2: Disorders that are not related to breed standards. *Vet. J.* 183: 39–45.

Takeda, N., Hasegawa, S., Morita, M. et al. (1993). Pica in rats is analogous to emesis: An animal model in emesis research. *Pharmacol. Biochem. Behav.* 45 (4): 817–821.

Tanaka, A., Wagner, D.C., Kass, P.H. et al. (2012). Associations among weight loss, stress, and upper respiratory tract infection in shelter cats. *J. Am. Vet. Med. Assoc.* 240: 570–576.

Thomas, C.W., Rising, J.L., and Moore, J.K. (1976). Blood lead concentrations of children and dogs from 83 Illinois families. *J. Am. Vet. Med. Assoc.* 169: 1237–1240.

Thrusfield, M.V., Holt, P.E., and Muirhead, R.H. (1998). Acquired urinary incontinence in bitches: Its incidence and relationship to neutering practices. *J. Small Anim. Pract.* 39: 559–566.

Vandevelde, M. and Fatzer, R. (1980). Neuronal ceroid-lipofuscinosis in older dachshunds. *Vet. Pathol.* 17: 686–692.

Waisglass, S.E., Landsberg, G.M., Yager, J.A. et al. (2006). Underlying medical conditions in cats with presumptive psychogenic alopecia. *J. Am. Vet. Med. Assoc.* 228: 1705–1709.

Weaver, A.D. (1983). Survey with follow-up of 67 dogs with testicular Sertoli cell tumours. *Vet. Rec.* 113 (5): 105–107.

Westropp, J.L., Kass, P.H., and Buffington, C.A.T. (2006). Evaluation of the effects of stress in cats with idiopathic cystitis. *Am. J. Vet. Res.* 67: 731–736.

Wirant, S.C., McGuire, B. (2004). Urinary behavior of female domestic dogs (*Canis familiaris*): Influence of reproductive status, location and age. *Appl. Anim. Behav. Sci.* 85: 335–348.

Yamamoto, K., Matsunaga, S., Matsui, M. et al. (2002). Pica in mice as a new model for the study of emesis. *Methods Find. Exp. Clin. Pharmacol.* 24 (3): 135–138.

Yeates, J.W. (2012). Maximizing canine welfare in veterinary practice and research: A review. *Vet. J.* 192: 272–278.

Yeom, M., Ahn, S., Oh, J.Y. et al. (2020). Atopic dermatitis induces anxiety- and depressive-like behaviors with concomitant neuronal adaptations in brain reward circuits in mice. *Prog. Neuro-Psychopharmacol. Biol. Psychiatry.* https://doi.org/10.1016/j.pnpbp.2019.109818.

Zink, M.C., Farhoody, P., Elser, S.E. et al. (2014). Evaluation of the risk and age of onset of cancer and behavioral disorders in gonadectomized Vizslas. *J. Am. Vet. Med. Assoc.* 244: 309–319.

Zulch, H.E., Mills, D.S., Lambert, R. et al. (2012). The use of tramadol in a Labrador retriever presenting with self-mutilation of the tail. *J. Vet. Behav.* 7 (4): 252–258.

Part II

Pets in the Community

5

Safety Net Programs

Erin Doyle and Seana Dowling-Guyer

5.1 Introduction

Shelter relinquishment is closely linked to behavioral health in companion animals. Behavioral challenges are a major risk factor for pet relinquishment (Dolan et al. 2015; Weiss et al. 2014). In addition, relinquishment represents an inherent challenge to the behavioral well-being of a surrendered pet, disrupting routine and security for the pet and exposing the animal to the stressors of a shelter environment (Hennessy 2013). (See Chapter 6 for more information on behavioral risks for relinquishment.) Safety net programs include any program or service that reduces risk factors for relinquishment (Weiss 2015). They include intake diversion programs administered at the time of a potential relinquishment and proactive outreach into the community. All safety net programs operate with the common goal of supporting pet ownership and strengthening the human-animal bond. This chapter will present an overview of the impact and benefits of safety net programs, program types, and guidelines for program selection, implementation, and evaluation.

5.2 Benefits of Safety Net Programs

Safety net programs come in a variety of formats, but all have the same goal of facilitating pet retention. Their impact is the direct effect or outcome of the program—that is, increased pet retention. Benefits, on the other hand, are broader, positive effects that contribute to an improvement in the pet-owning environment. A safety net program's impact on the goal of reducing pet relinquishment should be a measurable effect, while a program's benefits may extend beyond the immediate goal of keeping pets in homes to broader positive changes for the pet, owner, sheltering organization, and community.

Pets derive direct benefits from safety net programs through accessible resources necessary for their welfare, such as basic needs, veterinary care, and behavioral support. Provisioning these resources and services directly improves an animal's health and welfare while reducing the risk of relinquishment. Keeping animals out of shelters through programs that support pet ownership also eliminates the stress of transition and inherent stressors of a shelter environment on the animal.

Animal Behavior for Shelter Veterinarians and Staff, Second Edition. Edited by Brian A. DiGangi, Victoria A. Cussen, Pamela J. Reid, and Kristen A. Collins.
© 2022 John Wiley & Sons, Inc. Published 2022 by John Wiley & Sons, Inc.
Companion website: www.wiley.com/go/digangi/animal

Pet owners also benefit from safety net programs. Programs that support pet ownership facilitate pet retention, decrease the stress related to an inability to meet the needs of the pet, and eliminate the need for a difficult relinquishment decision. Continued pet ownership may also allow owners to enjoy the benefits of improved physical and mental health (McCune et al. 2014; Wells 2019). In addition, safety net programs provide support services that can enhance the owner-pet relationship. Informational resources can improve an owner's understanding of the pet's needs and enable an owner to better meet those needs (Kidd et al. 1992; New et al., 2000; Patronek et al. 1996a; Patronek et al. 1996b). Knowing more about species-specific behavior may normalize the pet's behavior, which can reduce an owner's frustration.

Safety net programs also yield beneficial effects for the sheltering organization and the community at large. One obvious effect of reducing pet relinquishments is the potential to reduce shelter intakes. A reduction in shelter animal population better enables an organization to function within its capacity for care, improving the well-being of animals and personnel within the shelter, and potentially allowing care for animals that require more resources. In addition, reduced intakes may allow an organization to scale up or down or to shift focus, including expanding their community programs to support pet ownership. Such expansion may include strategic community partnerships that allow the organization to provide more comprehensive support through coordinated and targeted services. Greater engagement with the community improves knowledge of its pet ownership needs and challenges, facilitating more tailored programs and increasing their impact. Additionally, increased engagement with the community provides the organization multiple touchpoints, engendering positive perceptions and cementing the idea that an animal sheltering organization is a supportive resource for all pet owners.

5.3 Program Types

Programs vary in scope and achieve impact through a variety of strategies. All programs should be based on a foundation of cultural awareness and lack of judgment, where organizations believe that pet owners want to do the best thing possible for their pet(s). However, safety net programs do not replace legal or otherwise necessary action in situations of animal cruelty or neglect when the caregiver is unwilling or unable to accept assistance.

Safety net programs can be administered at the time of a potential relinquishment or proactively to address risk factors that may lead to relinquishment. They typically focus on three main areas: basic needs, accessible veterinary care, and accessible behavioral care. However, individual programs often blur the lines between these categorizations. For example, programs that focus on the provision of accessible veterinary care may present opportunities to provide support for concurrent behavioral needs (Weiss 2015). In addition, human health and social services may present an opportunity to identify at-risk pets and connect owners with beneficial safety net programs, using a One Health model that recognizes the interconnection of human, animal, and environmental health and well-being (https://www.avma.org/resources-tools/avma-policies/one-health). The following section provides an overview of many common safety net program types. These program types are summarized in Appendix 5.A.

5.3.1 Basic Needs

While nearly all safety net programs take basic pet and owner needs and well-being into consideration, the program types detailed in this section focus on those that provide resources such as food, shelter, and husbandry.

5.3.1.1 Food Bank Programs
Food bank programs provide pet food to companion animals at no cost to their owners. These programs can be set up as independent

pet food banks or in collaboration with human social services such as food pantries, soup kitchens, or homeless shelters. Limited published literature exists to document the impact of food bank programs, but one survey of staff members showed a high perceived client value of pet food banks (Rauktis et al. 2017). Further support for this perception was found in a recent study in which 60% of sheltering organizations surveyed offered a food bank program, and 60% of these organizations felt that it was their most used program (Russo et al. 2021).

The positive impact of a food bank program for the pet is clear: it addresses the pet's basic needs while also preventing relinquishment due to an owner's inability to provide adequate nutrition. Food-insecure pet owners may choose to feed their pet at the expense of their own nutrition (Rauktis et al. 2017); thus, pet food banks not only help the client via preservation of the human-animal bond but can also support that client's nutritional well-being.

Because pet food bank programs can be developed in conjunction with human food services, these programs can be an ideal opportunity for animal welfare organizations to begin or enhance collaboration with community partners. These community partnerships can then form a framework for other community outreach programs.

The resource commitment in establishing a pet food bank is generally quite reasonable, particularly when done in collaboration with community partners. Pet food banks are often established using donated pet food, which otherwise might be turned away or discarded by the shelter due to the health advantage of feeding shelter animals a consistent diet. Resources are necessary to ensure the physical space that is required to store food prior to distribution and to maintain the donated pet food inventory, including monitoring food expiration dates. Time must also be devoted to the actual distribution of the food. However, with some

variation based on the scope of the program, these resource investments are relatively small.

5.3.1.2 Pet-Friendly Housing Support

In addition to help with the basic need of nutrition, pet owners may need support in addressing the fundamental need of shelter, both for themselves and for their companion animals. This need is often particularly acute for clients living in rental housing. In one study, only 53% of rental accommodations were pet friendly, and of those only 11% allowed large-breed dogs. According to the same study, most landlords of pet-friendly housing required an additional pet deposit, and average rents for pet-friendly units were 20–30% higher per month than the overall average (Carlisle-Frank et al. 2005). In another study, 44% of renting pet owners reported having been declined as renters based on pet ownership, and 82% rated the process of finding their current residence as "difficult" (Power 2017).

Shelters can reduce relinquishments by providing pet-friendly housing support. This support can include accessible information on local renting laws to inform clients of their rights as tenants, both in private and public housing units (Huegel and MacMillan 2014). Support can also include a database of pet-friendly rental units and/or landlords. However, because not all pet-friendly units are advertised as such (Power 2017), developing a robust database requires the use of multiple research methods to identify landlords who allow companion animals and to clarify any restrictions on species and/or size. Such a database needs to be regularly updated.

Effective housing support programs reduce shelter relinquishment caused by housing restrictions while benefiting the pet and owner by maintaining the human-animal bond. They can also provide much-needed housing security for pet owners who choose not to relinquish their companion animal(s), despite restrictions. As with food bank programs, pet-friendly housing support presents another opportunity for collaboration with key stakeholders in the community, including attorneys, housing-assistance programs, and other social service programs. Such connections can serve as another avenue for shelters to build a framework of community collaboration and provide a comprehensive support network in the community.

The resources needed to implement housing support programs vary based on their scope. Simple programs may only provide access to information linked on the organization's website. Housing support that includes the development and maintenance of a pet-friendly housing database or advocacy for pet-friendly housing in the community requires a modest additional resource investment by the organization.

5.3.1.3 Rehoming Advice and Resources

If rehoming a pet is unavoidable, direct owner-to-owner rehoming services can prevent relinquishment and the need for sheltering. In one study exploring the rehoming of cats and dogs, 37% of respondents who had rehomed a pet within the last five years had given their pet to a friend or family member as compared to 36% who rehomed by taking their pet to a shelter (Weiss et al. 2015). Eleven percent of respondents rehomed their pet directly to a person not previously known. These findings suggest that owners may be willing, and even prefer, to directly rehome their pets, thus avoiding relinquishment to a shelter altogether.

The shelter's role in facilitating direct rehoming can include posting photos and information about available pets on an organization's website, offering tips for successful rehoming, or referring clients to credible organizations that focus on direct owner-to-owner rehoming. Shelters typically do not process directly rehomed animals as admissions or placements; thus, appropriate disclosure is necessary to ensure that adopters are aware that the shelter's normal evaluation processes have not taken place. However, direct rehoming allows the new adopter to receive information about

the pet right from the previous owner. This information is potentially even more valuable than information learned about an animal's behavior in the unfamiliar and stressful environment of the shelter.

A simplified process, with direct communication between a previous and future owner, is just one benefit of rehoming services. Additionally, the animal's welfare is enhanced by avoiding relinquishment to the shelter and, ideally, entering a well-counseled and well-prepared home. The organization avoids a shelter admission through a system that requires minimal resources to establish.

Of course, direct home-to-home transfer of ownership is not ideal for every circumstance. In a survey of sheltering organizations, while 55% of organizations offered rehoming advice and resources, only 36% of those organizations considered them highly used (Russo et al. 2021). However, given the low resource investment and potential benefits, direct rehoming services are still a valuable safety net program for appropriate scenarios.

5.3.1.4 Lost-and-Found Programs

In 2018, approximately 50% of all canine and feline admissions into sheltering organizations were animals identified as stray or at-large (Shelter Animals Count n.d.). Safety net programs that aim to prevent companion animals from becoming lost or facilitate reunification of stray pets with owners are vital to reducing shelter intakes and shelter length of stay.

Safety net programs targeting the stray pet population ideally include efforts to avoid the animal entering the shelter as a stray in the first place, including escape prevention initiatives. Some such programs aid in the construction of appropriate fencing for dogs. Others provide pet owners with information about how to secure gates and doors, how to train dogs to come when called, and how to recognize behavioral factors that may lead to escape attempts.

If a free-roaming companion animal is found, proper identification can facilitate reunification with their owner in the field by the finder or animal control officer, avoiding intake into the shelter. In one study of cats and dogs adopted with a free collar and identification, 94% of those pets were still wearing identification at follow-up approximately eight weeks later (Weiss et al. 2011). Reunification can be further facilitated by implanting microchips, which can increase reunification rates to twice those of unmicrochipped dogs and over 20 times those of unmicrochipped cats (Lord et al. 2009).

Shelters should maintain a thorough and up-to-date lost-and-found pet database and avoid unnecessary barriers to reunification such as heavy fees. An organization's website and social media outlets are ideal platforms to post photos and descriptions of found animals. Coordination and sharing of lost-and-found information with other community sheltering organizations is vital to ensure a robust reunification system.

Both preventive and reunification efforts are of clear benefit to pets and clients by helping to avoid the animal running at-large, impoundment, and the loss of the animal from the family. These efforts can also have a measurable effect within the community by reducing public safety and nuisance concerns related to free-roaming companion animals. In addition, stray pet safety net programs can provide the initial opportunity for connection with the client to encourage use of other services, such as accessible veterinary and behavioral care. In particular, owners reunited with a lost pet may want resources to address factors that led to the animal's loss, such as a reproductively intact status or an incomplete understanding of normal pet behavior.

Lost-and-found safety net programs are critical, and often required, operational components of organizations taking in stray animals. However, initiatives to prevent escape and facilitate reunification should also be considered by organizations not mandated to admit stray animals. Programs that go above and beyond the minimum lost-and-found standard of care, such as public microchipping clinics, can be an ideal opportunity for collaboration between private and municipal organizations in the community.

5.3.1.5 Temporary Sheltering

While safety net programs generally strive to keep animals in their homes, there are some circumstances in which temporary separation is necessary. Clients may be unable to care for their animals on a short-term basis for a variety of reasons, including disasters, health concerns, or domestic violence. The importance of care for the family pet in these times of crisis is emphasized by the inclusion of provisions for pet-directed response in the Robert T. Stafford Disaster Relief and Emergency Assistance Act (Bazan 2005) as well as by literature supporting the importance of companion animal safety in the decision-making of those affected by domestic violence (Ascione et al. 2007; Collins et al. 2018; Taylor et al. 2019). See Chapter 21 for more information on temporary sheltering as a component of disaster response.

Animal welfare organizations may voluntarily initiate or be called upon by governmental or human social services to aid in temporary sheltering of animals. Effective temporary sheltering programs avoid permanent relinquishment by facilitating reunification once clients' circumstances allow them to safely resume caring for their pet. Ideally, even this temporary separation would be avoided through co-sheltering of people and companion animals, but logistics and client circumstances often make co-sheltering impossible. As an alternative, the use of foster care for these animals is ideal to avoid the medical and behavioral detriments of sheltering as well as to avoid shelter crowding. Regardless of whether displaced animals are sheltered in foster homes or in a shelter's kennels, legally approved agreements and thorough guidelines should be set up for temporary sheltering programs to create clear expectations for all participants and to avoid ambiguity regarding the duration and extent of care.

Temporary sheltering programs require a fair investment of resources on the part of a sheltering organization to oversee the program and ensure adequate housing/caregiving without detrimental impact to the existing shelter population. However, their benefit to the client and animal has the potential to be significant. Times of crisis are likely to be periods in which maintenance of the human-animal bond is critical for the client's emotional health. Without these programs, clients may avoid seeking help for themselves due to fear about their pets' well-being (Ascione et al. 2007). Program oversight can be greatly aided by collaboration with governmental or non-profit human social services, allowing the animal welfare organization to focus primarily on animal care. Because of these connections, the benefits of a temporary sheltering program extend to the organization and community by strengthening a community framework of support for pet owners.

5.3.1.6 Humane Education

Humane education programs are a popular community outreach method for animal sheltering organizations. While often less directly applicable to relinquishment prevention, these programs still fall into the broad category of safety net programs by fostering a community that values and understands responsible pet ownership. Traditionally, these programs have focused on humane education for children. School- or camp-based humane education programs have a documented positive impact on children's knowledge of animal husbandry and emotional needs (Muldoon et al. 2016; Tardif-Williams and Bosacki 2015). In addition, there is evidence of the enhancement of prosocial behavior and empathy in children participating in these programs (Samuels et al. 2016). However, information is lacking regarding the impact of educational programs geared toward adults and the impact of these programs on pet retention.

The benefits of humane education programs for pets and clients vary widely with the scope of the program, and the impact is often less easily measured than for other safety net programs. However, there is value in the connection between the organization and community fostered by these programs and in their potential to enhance the visibility of the organization within the community. Humane education programs are also an excellent opportunity for collaboration between the sheltering organization and community groups such as schools, camps, childcare settings, and adult education programs. Depending on the community and the structure of these programs, these programs can also provide a revenue source for the animal welfare organization.

Like the benefits gained from the implementation of a humane education program, the resource investment required varies widely based on the scope of the program. Single visits by shelter staff to a classroom require minimal resources, while in-house educational programs such as after-school programs or camps can be resource intensive. Development of extensive humane education programs requires careful assessment of the available resources of the organization and existing community programs. However, as resources allow, humane education programs can be highly rewarding for shelter staff and volunteers and act as another building block in the connection between the shelter and the community.

5.3.2 Veterinary Care

Inability to access veterinary care has been documented as a common reason for companion animal relinquishment, with as many as 28% of surrenderers citing cost, in conjunction with medical issues, as the reasons for relinquishment in one study (Dolan et al. 2015). Safety net programs that address barriers to veterinary care have the potential to reduce relinquishment, thus facilitating behavioral well-being through stability in ownership and preservation of the human-animal bond.

5.3.2.1 Spay-Neuter Services

Surgical sterilization services for owned animals have become commonly established programs to reduce pet overpopulation by avoiding unwanted litters and preventing behavioral and medical concerns associated with an intact reproductive status. Effective spay-neuter programs can successfully increase the prevalence of altered animals in the community (Dolan et al. 2017; Frank and Carlisle-Frank 2007). A corresponding decrease in shelter relinquishment in communities with accessible spay-neuter programs has also been documented (Scarlett and Johnston 2012; White et al. 2010), though this reduction was only consistently identified for cats and not dogs. Research findings also support the reach of non-profit spay-neuter programs to animals that would not otherwise receive veterinary care (White et al. 2018) and show that client race and ethnicity are not barriers to program utilization (Decker Sparks et al. 2018; Poss and Bader 2008; Schurer et al. 2015).

Accessible spay-neuter services benefit the pet by enhancing animal health, avoiding unwanted litters, and preventing nuisance behaviors (American Veterinary Medical Association n.d.). When successful, these programs also positively impact the community through reduction of relinquishment, nuisance behaviors such as vocalization or urine marking, and, potentially, the incidence of serious dog bites, for which intact dogs are overrepresented (Patronek et al. 2013). Effective spay-neuter outreach also reduces pet overpopulation, a clear benefit for communities experiencing a significant homeless pet overpopulation. Even for communities with unmet adopter demand for puppies and kittens, effective spay-neuter outreach is an important population-level strategy to reduce disparity in the access to these services. Accessible spay-neuter services also allow for

thoughtful consideration of where new pets in the community are obtained, such as through animal transport (thus addressing pet overpopulation in other communities) or through responsible breeders. With careful program design and outreach, these programs can be an opportunity for collaboration with the local veterinary community. Practitioners can refer clients unable to afford full-cost sterilization or may participate in providing low-cost or free sterilization services.

While spay-neuter programs can have significant overall impact, they are resource intensive to establish and maintain. This is particularly true given that successful programs are accompanied by community outreach to build trust and interest in the program. Effective programs also address the issue that low-cost or even free spay-neuter programs may still include insurmountable barriers for clients who lack transportation or cannot take time off work to bring the pet for a surgical appointment. For these reasons, implementation of spay-neuter safety net programs should be carefully preceded by an analysis of the existing community landscape to assess the community need and to effectively target the desired population.

5.3.2.2 Access to Basic Veterinary Care

Spay-neuter programs typically include the provision of preventive care, such as vaccines and parasite treatment. Some may also administer basic treatment for minor conditions. However, medical concerns leading to relinquishment may not be fully addressed through these programs. There is growing interest in ensuring access to veterinary care that extends beyond wellness care to other medical concerns. Models for accessible veterinary care programs include academic programs at veterinary schools; programs run by animal welfare organizations; collaborative One Health programs with human health services; for-profit, low-cost veterinary services; and accessible services provided by private practitioners. The limited existing data support the efficacy of these programs at reaching the target demographic and providing accessible care (Ehnert et al. 2015; McCobb et al. 2018). Like spay-neuter programs, successful accessible veterinary care programs must carefully consider the community's needs and existing programs. While the impact and benefits of these programs mirror those of accessible spay-neuter services in potential significance, accessible veterinary care programs are resource intensive and may not be of strategic value for every organization and community. In addition, these programs may be perceived as a threat to the financial well-being of existing veterinary clinics. To mitigate this concern, successfully implemented accessible veterinary care programs include outreach to the local veterinary community in the early stages of planning and development (McCobb et al. 2018). Collaborative efforts such as vouchers for care at local clinics may be a less resource intensive and potentially better received alternative for many organizations.

5.3.2.3 Return-to-Field Programs

The behavioral health of free-roaming cats is often best served by avoiding sheltering and placement in a home, particularly for poorly socialized and feral cats. While more detail on these programs can be found in Chapter 7, their inclusion as a safety net program type is important to note.

5.3.3 Behavioral Care

All safety net programs address the emotional health of the animal by mitigating the risk of relinquishment and sheltering. However, an important subset of safety net programs specifically targets the behavioral health of the companion animal in the home. Behavioral reasons for rehoming have been reported in up to 40% of relinquished dogs and 28% of relinquished cats (Salman et al. 2000), though behavior concerns as the reason for relinquishment were reported by fewer than 20%

of respondents in a more recent study (Weiss et al. 2014). While behavior as a reason for relinquishment is complicated and multifactorial, behavioral interventions remain an important tool to prevent surrender. Behavioral safety net programs are broadly categorized in this section by type, but significant overlap can exist between these types based on program structure and individual circumstances.

5.3.3.1 Behavior Information Resources

One of the simplest strategies for behavioral support is to provide informational links or handouts on common behavior topics. In the aforementioned survey of sheltering organizations, while only 37% had safety net resources available on their website for pet owners, 80% of those organizations reported that the advice was focused on pet behavior (Russo et al. 2021). In addition to having freely accessible resources on its website, an organization can proactively share relevant information with adopters, with potential surrenderers, or at community outreach events. There are limited published data to support the impact of providing this information to prevent relinquishment, though given the wide availability of freely accessible material to use, the resource investment to collate this information for the organization's purpose is minimal.

One advantage to this provision of resources is that these resources can cover a broad range of concerns across species. Many behavioral interventions, such as training classes, focus on canine behavioral health, but resources can include information on feline behavior as well as on small mammal, avian, and large animal behavioral health. The benefit of providing such information is likely to be greatest if resources focus on common behavior problems that can be resolved by simple intervention strategies, making individualized counseling unnecessary. In one study, advice provided to puppy owners on puppy raising at a single veterinary visit had lasting impact in reducing undesirable behaviors (Gazzano et al. 2008). Effective advice provided on just one occasion may benefit the pet and client.

Sharing of information and advice through behavioral resources in an easily accessible format has the potential to reach a large number of people. However, its impact may be modest, particularly for challenging behavioral concerns, compared to more intensive intervention strategies. Impact is presumably enhanced by provision of resources in conjunction with an individualized discussion of behavior. An investment of staff or volunteer time is necessary to collate or create resources as well as to provide this individualized discussion when offered.

5.3.3.2 Training Classes

Another general behavioral support program provided by many animal welfare organizations is training classes. These programs vary in their quantity and scope as well as in their fee structure and target audience. There is limited information to assess their efficacy in preventing shelter relinquishment, and the information available is sometimes contradictory. In one study, puppies enrolled in learning and socialization classes were more likely to remain in their initial homes (Duxbury et al. 2003). However, other research has found that relinquished dogs were no more likely to have attended training classes than non-relinquished dogs (Kwan and Bain 2013) and that attendance at formal training classes did not significantly affect the total number of undesirable behaviors reported by pet owners (Blackwell et al. 2008).

Given these contradictory findings, the impact of these programs on preventing relinquishment is somewhat uncertain and is likely influenced by the individual program structure. There is intuitive benefit for the pet and client through the acquisition of training knowledge and socialization for the pet as well as through the shared bonding activity. However, whatever impact on pet retention there may be from training classes, it is limited

if only a small number of pet owners can access them. Many owners may experience barriers due to fees and lack of transportation to the class location. A strategy to mitigate these barriers is to provide fee-waived training classes directly in communities at high risk of animal relinquishment. This program structure facilitates the safety net benefit to clients and strengthens the relationship of the humane organization with the community. Virtual training classes are another strategy to enhance accessibility, though this format eliminates the socialization benefit and may reduce the learning and bonding experience.

When fees are incorporated into the program, the organization can benefit from the additional revenue. In addition, regardless of fee structure or location, classes can serve to introduce or further acquaint clients with the organization, potentially resulting in the recruitment of new volunteers or donors. Shelters that hold training classes may also choose to have staff or volunteers bring shelter dogs to participate, thus providing an additional benefit for animals awaiting placement.

Though these benefits are numerous, providing training classes can require a fair investment of resources to ensure that a qualified trainer is leading the classes and to manage the class schedule and enrollment. While this resource investment may be offset with class fee revenue, as mentioned, revenue must be balanced with achieving an underlying goal of preventing relinquishment. Creative solutions to achieve this balance can include the recruitment of volunteer trainers or partnership with reputable organizations or companies specializing in training services.

5.3.3.3 Behavior Helpline

Behavior helplines begin to delve into more individualized behavioral support. Helplines can often be staffed by trained volunteers, with questions escalated to the organization's behavioral staff if necessary. These services may be provided to adopters, potential surrenderers, or the general public and may overlap in structure and scope with the provision of behavior resources. Helplines can be run on-site or remotely, either electronically or via telephone, and they include an individualized discussion of the behavioral concerns for the pet. Efficient helplines can handle a high volume of contact. Similar services have long-standing use for human emotional health, and Shore et al. (2008) found a strong willingness to use such programs by pet owners if the services were free of charge.

Because there are limited data available to evaluate the efficacy of these programs, their impact on pet retention in the home is uncertain. However, as with the provision of general information, it is reasonable to assume some degree of benefit to the pet and client through the acquisition of knowledge about treatment strategies for behavior concerns. Similarly, it is likely that behavior helplines are more successful when addressing common concerns with relatively straightforward interventions. The benefit of these helplines is impacted by the quality of the advice and counseling. Therefore, while the resource investment in a helpline program can be modest, its benefit will presumably increase with a significant investment in time by behavior staff to train and provide ongoing support for helpline volunteers and staff.

5.3.3.4 Behavior Consultations

A more resource-intensive means of providing individualized behavior support is through behavior consultation services. These services are provided by a qualified behavior professional and may occur at the organization, in the client's home, or virtually. If the organization does not have qualified behavior personnel available for these services, partnerships can be developed with local trainers or training companies. While these services are most commonly provided to adopters to facilitate retention of the adopted pet in the home, their use can be extended to potential

surrenderers or the general public based on capacity and scope.

Data to evaluate the efficacy of individualized behavior consultations are lacking, but the potential benefit to the client and pet is presumably significant. Individualized and practical advice from a trained professional not only provides a treatment plan for the behavior problem(s), but it can also validate the client's concerns and help the client avoid feelings of isolation and permanence in dealing with the issue(s). The organization can experience the impact of avoiding relinquishment and the indirect benefit of positive word-of-mouth testimony of the client within their social network. In addition, if these services are provided through collaboration with professional trainers, clients may have the option, when accessible, of continuing long-term consultative services with the trainer. Finally, behavior consultation services can positively impact the entire community by reducing relinquishment and preventing companion animal public safety risks and nuisance behaviors.

To maximize these impacts and benefits, the behavior consultation program must be well implemented and accessible to those clients and pets in need of support. Pet owners have been found to be generally willing to pay for individualized counseling with an animal behaviorist, though, unsurprisingly, they are significantly more interested when behavior support services are offered for free (Shore et al. 2008). As with accessible veterinary care, any fee may be an insurmountable barrier to many clients. Similarly, the ability to travel to the animal welfare organization may be a significant barrier to receiving behavioral care. Providing services at a given location rather than in the home also limits the generalizability of these services to felines or other species. Virtual consultation improves accessibility but eliminates the ability to gain information through the consultant's interaction with the animal. Thus, while the benefits of behavior consultation services can be significant, careful planning and consideration should factor into the scope and structure of these programs for the organization.

5.4 How to Choose the Right Programs

Choosing which safety net programs to implement depends on a variety of factors that may differ by organization and community. Organizations should consider the needs of the community, existing services, the goal and potential impact of the program, and the resources needed to develop and run the program. A strategic approach that considers these factors will help identify high-priority programs for each individual organization. Picking the right mix of programs will maximize an organization's resources for optimal impact. That impact should be measurable in order to evaluate program success and guide ongoing program direction (see Figure 5.1).

5.4.1 Community Landscape– Assessing Pet Ownership Needs in the Community

Understanding the community in which pets and their owners live is critical when considering which safety net programs to implement. Trends in pet ownership, existing services that support pet ownership, and unmet needs combine to form the community's landscape of pet ownership. All pet owners need access to foundational services that support pet ownership, including provision of basic pet needs, veterinary care, and behavioral resources. However, strategies necessary to ensure access to these services will vary based on the community.

5.4.1.1 Pet Ownership Trends
Knowing pet ownership trends in the community, including ownership rates, general demographics of pets and owners, and community animal populations, is important for program development. National or local surveys about pet ownership are good sources with which to start (American Pet Products Association

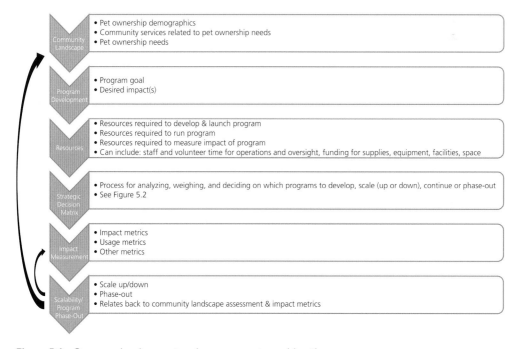

Figure 5.1 Program development and management considerations.

[APPA] 2017; American Veterinary Medical Association [AVMA] n.d.). Municipal licensing records, shelter intake data, veterinary patient data, pet food/supply store locations and sales, and grocery and convenience store sales of pet food and supplies, as well as other market research, are also useful sources of this information. New research assessing pet ownership trends may be necessary, so organizations should consider conducting their own surveys, polls, interviews, and focus groups. Ultimately, any organization planning to offer safety net programs will need an understanding of pet ownership trends in the communities they support. A model built on archival and direct research with community constituents will yield powerful insights an organization can use when planning safety net programs.

5.4.1.2   Services Supporting Pet Ownership

Because no animal sheltering organization exists in a vacuum, knowing which services already exist will help avoid unnecessary duplication and more effectively deploy limited resources. An inventory of services that support pet ownership can include both animal-oriented and people-oriented programs. Based on the information gleaned from a services inventory, an organization might decide that partnering with or supporting another organization on a new program may be the most efficient use of resources. Just as importantly, organizations need to know how the community uses existing services and what impact those services have. For example, self-administered animal food banks typically require minimal resources to implement and manage, but if a community already has well-used and impactful pet food banks offered by other organizations, even this minimal resource investment might not be needed.

5.4.1.3   Identifying Community Needs

Once an organization has identified pet ownership demographics and existing services, it is critical to then determine community needs.

Organizations can develop their own process or adapt an existing one, such as the Pets for Life community assessment (Humane Society of the United States n.d.). Identifying the goal and scope of the community needs assessment will help determine the direction to take; the assessment can be comprehensive or more targeted. Organizations should begin by mining their own intake data to assess trends in relinquishment reasons and intake types or locations. However, intake data can tell only part of the story; organizations will benefit from conducting their own surveys, interviews, and focus groups targeted to understanding the unmet needs of pet owners. These data-gathering efforts can be combined with efforts to identify pet ownership and demographic trends in the community for efficient data collection. Even informal conversations with relinquishing owners will yield a deeper understanding of ownership challenges than simple responses to questions in a form (DiGiacomo et al. 1998). Outreach should include not only pet owners but past owners as well as other agencies serving pets and owners. Information learned from these data-gathering efforts, both formal and informal, when collected in a systematic and accessible way, will provide a comprehensive understanding of the community's needs. Table 5.1 presents some options for information sources that can be used in program planning.

5.4.2   Program Goal and Potential Impact

After gathering data to understand pet ownership demographics, current services, and needs, an organization should be ready to determine which safety net programs would be valuable for the community. Successful safety net programs should have clear, concrete, and actionable goals that align with the organization's overall mission. Goals should reflect the identified needs, weighted in terms of desired impact (see Scarlett et al. 2017 for guidance on goal setting). A program may address issues that put a pet at high risk for surrender but that

Table 5.1 Sources of program-planning information.

Pet ownership demographics	Existing services		Community need
	Animal-oriented resources	People-oriented resources	
National surveys such as APPA, AVMA	Other animal shelters and rescues including municipal animal care and control agencies	Human health and welfare non-profit agencies such as: • Health clinics • Housing support services • Human shelter and homeless services • Human food banks	Animal shelter and rescue intake data (including municipal animal care and control): • Intake types and reasons • Intake locations
Regional/local surveys			
Municipal licensing data	Veterinarians and veterinary services	Similar resources as listed above run by governmental agencies	New research including surveys, interviews, and focus groups with pet owners, past owners, and agencies serving pets, owners, and other community members
Veterinary clinic patient data	Grooming services	Human-oriented programs run by other animal welfare organizations	
Pet food/supply store sales data	Pet food and supply stores		
Grocery/convenience store pet food and supplies sales data	Grocery/convenience stores that sell pet food and supplies		
Animal shelter and rescue intake data (including municipal animal care and control)	Pet food banks		
New research such as surveys, polls, interviews, focus groups	Dog-walking, daycare, and pet-boarding facilities		
	Animal-oriented resources run by human social services programs		

are less common, or it may address less risky but more common challenges or some combination. For example, problem behaviors put pets at risk for surrender (Dolan et al. 2015; Weiss et al. 2014), but those behaviors range from less serious but common problems like housetraining issues or high energy to more serious but less common problems like aggression or separation anxiety. More serious problems may best be served by a program that provides intensive behavioral consultations, while less serious concerns can be addressed through website information or helplines. Both types of programs are impactful but in different ways; that impact should support the desired goals. Organizations also need to examine potential impacts of any program outside of the desired goals, both positive and negative.

5.4.3 Resources Required

Program goals and their desired impacts must also align with available resources. Organizations must determine the necessary resources to develop and maintain planned safety net programs before moving forward. Even programs requiring few resources should be reviewed as part of this process, as numerous small programs can cumulatively drain an organization's resources. Non-strategic use of resources may

prevent an organization from offering a service to its community that might have a greater impact. Required resources may include staff and volunteer time for operations and oversight; funding for supplies, equipment, and facilities; and space. Organizations should have a realistic and comprehensive understanding of the resources needed to effectively develop and operate any program.

5.4.4 Strategic Decision-Making

At this stage, having determined the unmet needs of the pet-owning community, identified program goals and potential impacts, and made a realistic determination of the required resources to effectively develop and operate one or more safety net programs, organizations are ready to engage in a strategic decision-making process to determine the right program, or mix of programs, to maximize their investment for optimal impact. One way to do this would be to plot potential programs in a strategic decision matrix, weighing the needs and potential impacts against the resources required. The matrix may not yield a definitive conclusion, but developing it will clarify relevant factors that need to be considered. Figure 5.2 shows an example of a strategic decision-making matrix for one community.

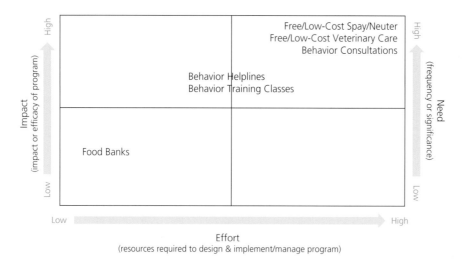

Figure 5.2 Example strategic decision-making matrix.

5.4.5 Measuring Impact and Program Evaluation

It is crucial that organizations design safety net programs for their communities in a way that allows for measurable impact. Program goals and the desired impact should be specified and quantified at the beginning of program development and modified as needed during program planning and after implementation. Organizations need to decide what metrics best measure program impact and how best to collect those data. Resources should be planned to support data collection, which should happen at multiple points in the program's lifetime. Data should be collected before the program is launched to determine a baseline, shortly after launch as a check-in to evaluate rollout and operations, and at regular intervals thereafter to calculate metrics and determine impact. Impact metrics measure the effects of the program in terms of the program's goals, but usage metrics are important to track as well. Usage metrics measure program use, such as number of clients (human and animal) served, number of calls to a behavior helpline, or amount of food used from a food pantry. Analyzing impact and usage metrics at regular intervals is critical to assessing success in meeting program goals and identifying issues.

It is also helpful to gather feedback from clients and personnel to understand their experiences and perceptions of the programs as well as suggestions for improvement. Surveys, interviews, and focus groups can be used, but more informal methods are valuable sources of information too. These include comment cards and forms (physical or virtual), emails or telephone calls, casual conversations, and even social media posts by clients, all of which may provide more immediate insight into program satisfaction. Feedback from clients and related personnel can help contextualize metrics as well as provide valuable insights into the client experience.

5.4.6 Scalability/Program Phase-out

When developing and managing safety net programs, organizations will want to consider the future of those programs. Scalability is the ability of a program to grow or contract depending on community needs and the organization's resources. Program scalability should be considered at the beginning of a program's life. It is unfortunate when a successful program cannot be scaled up to serve more clients due to an external restriction that was not thought of in the initial planning. On the other hand, not all programs need to grow; successful programs may serve their clients well and meet the program goals without expanding. It is important to revisit the community landscape assessment when determining scalability. Just like impact measurement, this assessment should be regularly updated to identify changes that may drive a desire for scaling a program up or down, such as a growth in pet ownership, a loss or addition of services at the organization or community, and so forth. Examining program impact and usage within the framework of the community assessment will help organizations determine how, or if, to scale their programs.

Finally, organizations need to consider the program's end-of-life. Is there a natural endpoint that would dictate the closure of the program? What resources are needed to sustain the program, and what happens if those resources are not there? Again, knowing the community landscape will help an organization with these decisions. Once the decision is made to end a program, a phase-out plan must be developed and should include how to communicate the closure to existing and past clients, how to transition those clients from the program to other services, if necessary, and how to best support those clients during the transition. Staff and volunteers, too, must be considered, as they may grapple with mixed feelings related to the program closure as well as worries about employment and volunteer opportunities. Thinking of these issues well in advance will help make the process for determining program closure clearer and ease the closure process for all involved.

5.5 Conclusions

Safety net programs are key to supporting pet retention and the behavioral health of pets at risk of shelter relinquishment. These programs benefit animals, pet owners, organizations, and communities. Given the multitude of program options, strategic program selection is critical, including consideration of goals, impact, and available resources. Programs must be thoughtfully planned, managed, and monitored to ensure that they meet pet ownership needs in the community and evolve as community needs change. With these considerations in mind, successful safety net programs are a critical tool in fostering an accessible and equitable support system for pet owners in the community.

References

American Pet Products Association. (2017). 2017–2018 APPA National Pet Owners Survey. Stamford, CT: American Pet Products Association. https://www.americanpetproducts.org/pubs_survey.asp (accessed 19 December 2019).

American Veterinary Medical Association. (n.d.). US Pet Ownership and Demographics Sourcebook. Schaumburg, Illinois: American Veterinary Medical Association. https://www.avma.org/resources/pet-owners/petcare/spaying-and-neutering (accessed 19 December 2019).

Ascione, F.R., Weber, C.V., Thompson, T.M. et al. (2007). Battered pets and domestic violence: Animal abuse reported by women experiencing intimate violence and by nonabused women. *Violence Against Women* 13 (4): 354–373.

Bazan, E.B. (2005, September). Robert T. Stafford Disaster Relief and Emergency Assistance Act: Legal requirements for federal and state roles in declarations of an emergency or a major disaster. Congressional Research Service, Library of Congress.

Blackwell, E.J., Twells, C., Seawright, A. et al. (2008). The relationship between training methods and the occurrence of behavior problems, as reported by owners, in a population of domestic dogs. *J. Vet. Behav.* 3 (5): 207–217.

Carlisle-Frank, P., Frank, J. M., and Nielsen, L. (2005). Companion animal renters and pet-friendly housing in the US. *Anthrozoös* 18 (1): 59–77.

Collins, E.A., Cody, A.M., McDonald, S.E., et al. (2018). A template analysis of intimate partner violence survivors' experiences of animal maltreatment: Implications for safety planning and intervention. *Violence Against Women.* https://doi.org/10.1177/1077801217697266.

Decker Sparks, J.L., Camacho, B., Tedeschi, P. et al. (2018). Race and ethnicity are not primary determinants in utilizing veterinary services in underserved communities in the United States. *J. Appl. Anim. Welf. Sci.* 21 (2): 120–129.

DiGiacomo, N., Arluke, A., and Patronek, G. (1998). Surrendering pets to shelters: The relinquisher's perspective. *Anthrozoös* 11 (1): 41–51.

Dolan, E.D., Scotto, J., Slater, M. et al. (2015). Risk factors for dog relinquishment to a Los Angeles municipal animal shelter. *Animals* 5 (4): 1311–1328.

Dolan, E.D., Weiss, E., and Slater, M.R. (2017). Welfare impacts of spay/neuter-focused outreach on companion animals in New York City public housing. *J. Appl. Anim. Welf. Sci.* 20 (3): 257–272.

Duxbury, M.M., Jackson, J.A., Line, S.W. et al. (2003). Evaluation of association between retention in the home and attendance at puppy socialization classes. *J. Am. Vet. Med. Assoc.* 223 (1): 61–66.

Ehnert, K., Lamielle, G., Scott, T. et al. (2015). The Healthy Pets Healthy Families initiative as an example of One Health in action. *J. Am. Vet. Med. Assoc.* 247 (2): 143–147.

Frank, J.M. and Carlisle-Frank, P.L. (2007). Analysis of programs to reduce overpopulation of companion animals: Do adoption and low-cost spay/neuter programs merely cause substitution of sources? *Ecol. Econom.* 62 (3–4): 740–746.

Gazzano, A., Mariti, C., Alvares, S. et al. (2008). The prevention of undesirable behaviors in dogs: Effectiveness of veterinary behaviorists' advice given to puppy owners. *J. Vet. Behav.* 3 (3): 125–133.

Hennessy, M.B. (2013). Using hypothalamic–pituitary–adrenal measures for assessing and reducing the stress of dogs in shelters: A review. *Appl. Anim. Behav. Sci.* 149 (1–4): 1–12.

Huegel, K. and MacMillan, I.B.N. (2014). No place like home. *Animal Sheltering*, 29–34.

Humane Society of the United States. (n.d.). Pets for Life Community Outreach Toolkit: Community Assessment. https://www. animalsheltering.org/sites/default/files/ documents/pfl-toolkit-community-assessment.pdf (accessed 19 December 2019).

Kidd, A.H., Kidd, R.M., and George, C.C. (1992). Successful and unsuccessful pet adoptions. *Psychol. Rep.* 70 (2): 547–561.

Kwan, J.Y. and Bain, M.J. (2013). Owner attachment and problem behaviors related to relinquishment and training techniques of dogs. *J. Appl. Anim. Welf. Sci.* 16 (2): 168–183.

Lord, L.K., Ingwersen, W., Gray, J.L. et al. (2009). Characterization of animals with microchips entering animal shelters. *J. Am. Vet. Med. Assoc.* 235 (2): 160–167.

McCobb, E., Rozanski, E.A., Malcolm, E.L. et al. (2018). A novel model for teaching primary care in a community practice setting: Tufts at Tech Community Veterinary Clinic. *J. Vet. Med. Educ.* 45 (1): 99–107.

McCune, S., Kruger, K.A., Griffin, J.A. et al. (2014). Evolution of research into the mutual benefits of human-animal interaction. *Anim. Front.* 4 (3): 49–58.

Muldoon, J.C., Williams, J.M., and Lawrence, A. (2016). Exploring children's perspectives on the welfare needs of pet animals. *Anthrozoös* 29 (3): 357–375.

New, J.C., Jr., Salman, M.D., King, M. et al. (2000). Characteristics of shelter-relinquished animals and their owners compared with animals and their owners in US pet-owning households. *J. Appl. Anim. Welf. Sci.* 3 (3): 179–201.

Patronek, G.J., Glickman, L.T., Beck, A.M. et al. (1996a). Risk factors for relinquishment of cats to an animal shelter. *J. Am. Vet. Med. Assoc.* 209 (3): 582–588.

Patronek, G.J., Glickman, L.T., Beck, A.M. et al. (1996b). Risk factors for relinquishment of dogs to an animal shelter. *J. Am. Vet. Med. Assoc.* 209 (3): 572–581.

Patronek, G.J., Sacks, J.J., Delise, K.M. et. al. (2013). Co-occurrence of potentially preventable factors in 256 dog bite-related fatalities in the United States (2000–2009). *J. Am. Vet. Med. Assoc.* 243 (12): 1726–1736.

Poss, J.E. and Bader, J.O. (2008). Results of a free spay/neuter program in a Hispanic *Colonia* on the Texas-Mexico border. *J. Appl. Anim. Welf. Sci.* 11 (4): 346–351.

Power, E.R. (2017). Renting with pets: A pathway to housing insecurity? *Hous. Stud.* 32 (3): 336–360.

Rauktis, M.E., Rose, L., Chen, Q. et al. (2017). "Their pets are loved members of their family": Animal ownership, food insecurity, and the value of having pet food available in food banks. *Anthrozoös* 30 (4): 581–593.

Russo, A., Dowling-Guyer, S., and McCobb, E. (2021) Community programming for companion dog retention: A survey of animal welfare organizations. *J. Appl. Anim. Welf. Sci.* https://doi.org/10.1080/10888705.2020. 1869551

Salman, M.D., Hutchison, J., Ruch-Gallie, R., et al. (2000). Behavioral reasons for relinquishment of dogs and cats to 12 shelters. *J. Appl. Anim. Welf. Sci.* https://doi. org/10.1207/S15327604JAWS0302_2.

Samuels, W.E., Meers, L.L., and Normando, S. (2016). Improving upper elementary students' humane attitudes and prosocial behaviors through an in-class humane education program. *Anthrozoös* 29 (4): 597–610.

Scarlett, J.M., Greenberg, M., and Hoshizaki, T. (2017). *Every Nose Counts: Using Metrics in Animal Shelters*. Middletown, DE: CreateSpace Independent Publishing Platform.

Scarlett, J. and Johnston, N. (2012). Impact of a subsidized spay neuter clinic on impounds and euthanasia in a community shelter and on service and complaint calls to animal control. *J. Appl. Anim. Welf. Sci.* 15 (1): 53–69.

Schurer, J.M., Phipps, K., Okemow, C. et al. (2015). Stabilizing dog populations and improving animal and public health through a participatory approach in indigenous communities. *Zoonoses Public Health* 62 (6): 445–455.

Shelter Animals Count. (n.d.) Dashboards. https://www.shelteranimalscount.org/ data-dashboards (accessed 2 December 2021).

Shore, E.R., Burdsal, C., and Douglas, D.K. (2008). Pet owners' views of pet behavior problems and willingness to consult experts for assistance. *J. Appl. Anim. Welf. Sci.* 11 (1): 63–73.

Tardif-Williams, C.Y. and Bosacki, S.L. (2015). Evaluating the impact of a humane education summer-camp program on school-aged children's relationships with companion animals. *Anthrozoös* 28 (4): 587–600.

Taylor, N., Riggs, D.W., Donovan, C. et al. (2019). People of diverse genders and/or sexualities caring for and protecting animal companions in the context of domestic violence. *Violence Against Women* 25 (9): 1096–1115.

Weiss, E. (2015). Safety nets and support for pets at risk of entering the sheltering system. In: *Animal Behavior for Shelter Veterinarians and Staff* (eds. E. Weiss, H. Mohan-Gibbons, and S. Zawistowski), 286–291. Hoboken, NJ: Wiley Blackwell.

Weiss, E., Gramann, S., Spain, C.V. et al. (2015). Goodbye to a good friend: An exploration of the re-homing of cats and dogs in the US. *Open J. Anim. Sci.* 5 (4): 435–456.

Weiss, E., Slater, M., Garrison, L. et al. (2014). Large dog relinquishment to two municipal facilities in New York City and Washington, DC: Identifying targets for intervention. *Animals* 4 (3): 409–433.

Weiss, E., Slater, M.R., and Lord, L.K. (2011). Retention of provided identification for dogs and cats seen in veterinary clinics and adopted from shelters in Oklahoma City, OK, USA. *Prev. Vet. Med.* 101 (3–4): 265–269.

Wells, D.L. (2019). The state of research on human–animal relations: Implications for human health. *Anthrozoös* 32 (2): 169–181.

White, S.C., Jefferson, E., and Levy, J.K. (2010). Impact of publicly sponsored neutering programs on animal population dynamics at animal shelters: The New Hampshire and Austin experiences. *J. Appl. Anim. Welf. Sci.* 13 (3): 191–212.

White, S.C., Scarlett, J.M., and Levy, J.K. (2018). Characteristics of clients and animals served by high-volume, stationary, nonprofit spay-neuter clinics. *J. Am. Vet. Med. Assoc.* 253 (6): 737–745.

Appendix 5.A Overview of Safety Net Program Types

		Benefits/Impact*			
Category	Program type	To the pet	To the owner	To the community	To the organization	Resources needed
Basic needs	Food banks	Address basic nutritional needs	Reduce food insecurity	Collaborative programs offer a One Health approach to meeting basic needs	Opportunity for collaboration with key community stakeholders	Minimal investment in time and resources, particularly if donated food is used
	Pet-friendly housing support	Addresses basic sheltering needs	Reduces housing insecurity	Collaborative programs create partnership with attorneys, human social services, and housing organizations	Opportunity for collaboration with key community stakeholders	Minimal resources to develop and maintain a database; more resources needed for advocacy
	Rehoming advice and resources	Avoid sheltering	Ideally ease the rehoming process and enhance communication with the new owner	Facilitate community member connections to address the need for rehoming	Place the onus for rehoming on the pet owner when feasible	Minimal
	Lost-and-found programs	Avoid the negative sequelae of roaming at-large	Reduce/prevent the emotional impact of losing a pet	Reduce the nuisance or dangerous behaviors related to stray pets	Often required for municipal organizations; touchpoint with the community to provide access to other services	Moderate to significant use of time but often within normal scope of responsibilities
	Temporary sheltering	Prevents permanent rehoming	Maintains the human-animal bond at a time of critical need	Removes a barrier for those in crisis to seek help for themselves	Opportunity for collaboration through programs that are often very well received by the organization's supporters	Moderate investment in time and resources to manage program and provide care
	Humane education	Potential for improved welfare	Increases knowledge regarding pet care and may improve children's emotional well-being	May enhance empathy and correlate with other positive behaviors in children	Strengthens ties to the community; provides potential for revenue through classes, parties, and camps	Variable based on the scope of the program
Veterinary care	Spay-neuter services	Health benefits of sterilization	Avoidance of unwanted litters and problematic pet behaviors associated with a sexually intact status	Reduced pet overpopulation and reduced free-roaming pets	Potential for outreach and collaboration with the local veterinary community	Significant financial and staffing resources typically necessary

(Continued)

Appendix 5.A   (Continued)

		Benefits/Impact*				
Category	Program type	To the pet	To the owner	To the community	To the organization	Resources needed
	Access to basic veterinary care	Health benefits of preventive health care and other primary veterinary care	Enhances the human-animal bond by preventing unmanaged medical concerns	Can be partnered with human health initiatives for a One Health community approach	Potential for strategic partnerships with human health agencies and/or private practitioners	Varies based on model but typically requires a moderate to significant resource investment as for spay-neuter services
	Return-to-field programs	Health benefits of sterilization and vaccination	If a caretaker is present, help to reduce colony size and improve colony health	Reduce the free-roaming cat population	Reduce euthanasia of healthy cats and foster collaboration with the community in trapping and caring for these cats	Require the resources to manage the program and provide sterilization services (but may be outweighed by reduced resources for sheltering and euthanasia)
Behavioral care	Behavior resources	Improved behavioral health	Increased knowledge regarding pet care	May reduce nuisance or dangerous pet behaviors	Enhance the knowledge base of clientele	Minimal resources to collate information and review the information with clients
	Training classes	Improved behavioral health	Increased training knowledge, an opportunity for socialization of the pet, and an opportunity for a relationship with a trainer and other pet owners	May reduce nuisance or dangerous pet behaviors	Strengthen organizational ties with adopters and potential for collaboration with local training services	Moderate to significant resource investment, particularly if combined with outreach
	Behavior hotlines	Improved behavioral health	Increased individualized knowledge regarding pet care	May reduce nuisance or dangerous pet behaviors	Strengthen organizational ties with adopters and the community	Minimal to modest resource investment dependent on program structure and expert support
	Behavior consultations	Improved behavioral health	Increased individualized knowledge and support in addressing pet behavior concerns	May reduce nuisance or dangerous pet behaviors	Strengthen organizational ties with adopters and potential for collaboration with local trainers	Significant resource investment dependent on program structure and scope

*The desired impact of all safety net programs is to prevent unnecessary companion animal relinquishment. Only benefits more specific to the individual programs are described.

6

Dog Behavior and Relinquishment to Shelters
Janis Bradley and Gary J. Patronek

6.1 Introduction

In order to critically assess the relative importance of pet owners' dissatisfaction with their dogs' behavior in relinquishment of dogs to shelters, it is first worth asking, "*How often are dogs relinquished overall? Are dogs being widely discarded by so-called irresponsible owners, or is the human-animal bond relatively stable?*" The short answer is, we don't know the answer to this question with any degree of precision, as there is no national shelter census or a single complete list from which a census could be conducted. Besides the lack of a reliable list, the definition of what constitutes an entity that might receive relinquished dogs is also hard to pin down, given the proliferation of small rescue organizations and groups lacking a physical structure that may accept relinquished dogs and keep them in temporary foster homes or otherwise act as intermediaries. Finally, the total size of the US owned dog population is also unknown, with estimates varying over time and by the source of the data. In 2016, the two largest-scale estimates ranged from 77.8 to 89.7 million dogs in the United States (Burns 2015; American Pet Products Association 2020). And, with the move to online survey platforms (as opposed to surveys by regular mail), the discrepancy seems to be widening (Downing and Lau 2014).

Nevertheless, it is still worth asking this question, with the understanding that the answer is at best an extrapolation that itself is based on estimates of unknown reliability, to try to put the problem in some perspective.

A 2019 study used a mark-capture method from different lists of shelters to try to enumerate the number of shelters in the United States, with the goal of making projections about the numbers of dogs received; they estimated 5.5 million dogs in the United States annually (Woodruff and Smith 2019). Depending on what figure from the estimates mentioned above is used for the total dog population, this would be between 6.1 and 7.1%. This is comparable to that reported by a modeling study in 1991, which estimated that about 7.6% of the US dog population entered shelters annually. The estimate of 7.1% is used here to be conservative (worst case) because it is based on the smaller of the two dog population estimates. Owner relinquishment accounts for an unknown proportion of dogs entering shelters, but some sources have put it around 28% of intakes, or about 1.1% of the total dog population (American Society for the Prevention of Cruelty to Animals [ASPCA] 2020; Zawistowski et al. 1998). If the reality is close to these estimates, people elect to end their relationships with their dogs at an annual rate roughly

Animal Behavior for Shelter Veterinarians and Staff, Second Edition. Edited by Brian A. DiGangi, Victoria A. Cussen, Pamela J. Reid, and Kristen A. Collins.
© 2022 John Wiley & Sons, Inc. Published 2022 by John Wiley & Sons, Inc.
Companion website: www.wiley.com/go/digangi/animal

similar to that of divorcing their spouses, the annual rate of which is about 2% (Amato 2010) (which we use here as more analogous than the commonly alluded to 50% lifetime divorce rate). We can reasonably assume that most of the human-human break-ups spring from behavioral incompatibilities. We don't know, however, what proportion of the sundered human-canine relationships are due not to incompatibility but rather to circumstances making it impractical for the person to continue to live with and care for a companion animal. Nevertheless, despite the overall stability of human-dog relationships, the consequences of those bonds that do break are encountered daily by those working in shelters. In this chapter, we will explore the state of the literature on canine behavior that pet owners report as having led to relinquishment and, to the extent possible, on interventions that have been suggested and attempted in an effort to prevent broken relationships and/or facilitate lasting rehoming.

6.2 A Brief History of Relinquishment Data

Understanding the impact of dog behavior on relinquishment can be informed by how shelters and researchers have approached the problem over the years. To the best of our knowledge, the issue of relinquished dogs and stray dogs and the subsequent euthanasia of healthy animals in shelters (so-called "pet overpopulation") was first discussed in the modern scientific literature in the early to mid 1970s—nearly half a century ago (Anonymous 1971; Schneider 1975). Growing concern about the problem led to two national conferences in 1974 and 1976, which brought numerous groups of stakeholders together for a discussion about causes and solutions (Anonymous 1974, 1976). The findings of those meetings indicated that a broad range of solutions needed to be explored, including research into methods of non-surgical

sterilization, more effective animal control policies, increased dog license fees to support the latter, sterilization of any intact dog before it was released from a shelter, and efforts to promote more responsible ownership.

A decade later, in 1985, the American Humane Association (AHA), a national advocacy group, began to systematically collect information from animal care and control agencies in the United States to attempt to quantify the problem nationwide; they eventually published a very influential report (Nassar et al. 1992). Those data, collected from more than 100 agencies, indicated that 42.2% of incoming dogs were relinquished (as opposed to being stray), and 62.8% of all dogs were euthanized. Data collected by ASPCA animal control services in New York City provided an even grimmer perspective. Although canine intake rates declined nearly fourfold between 1974 and 1994 (81,627 vs. 23,077 dogs, respectively), the proportion euthanized remained high and showed only a small decline over 20 years (82.7% vs. 74.0%, respectively) (Zawistowski et al. 1998). Nationally, a decade after the AHA study was published, a different convenience sample of 186 shelters suggested some improvement (52% of all dogs were euthanized), but regardless, 39% of dogs were considered unadoptable (Wenstrup and Dowidchuk 1999). The decisions about adoptability that occurred in tandem with such high euthanasia rates may appear almost unfathomable today, when an increasing number of communities in many parts of the United States report saving 85% or more of incoming dogs. But to some extent, those dark days continue to frame our present attitudes toward relinquishment.

In those early days, with the acknowledgment that data might help better characterize the problem of unwanted pets, some shelters also collected the reasons for relinquishment (along with other information about the dogs) at the time of surrender. For example, Rowan and Williams (1987) reported on a study by the Humane Society in Salem, Oregon, which surveyed 1,680 people relinquishing a dog to a shelter in that county. The leading reason was too many pets (27%), followed by other (22%), behavior (20%), old age (19%), and lifestyle changes (12%) (Rowan and Williams 1987). Arkow (1985) reported that in a 1981 survey conducted by the National Animal Control Association (NACA) of 918 relinquishers to 13 shelters distributed across 8 states, behavior was mentioned by 26.4%. Another study in the 1990s published in a major veterinary journal reported behavior as a major reason (30%) for relinquishment; however, it relied upon data from questionnaires distributed to relinquishing owners by shelter personnel and student interns only as time allowed (Miller et al. 1996). Given the non-random nature of the solicitations and low response rate (56 returned questionnaires from 1,406 dog relinquishers), those results were not generalizable, but they did serve to further educate readers (especially veterinarians) about important aspects of the relinquishment problem and reinforced the notion that behavior was an important contributor.

Despite the good intentions, enumerating reasons for relinquishment probably did little to reduce either intake or euthanasia. The list of stated reasons included all manner of owner lifestyle and dog behavioral factors (e.g., not being trained, illness, moving, receiving the pet as a gift, unwanted barking, housesoiling, allergies in the family, pulling on a leash, family member disliking the pet, new baby, having no time for the pet due to working, destructive behavior, being unable to afford veterinary care, incompatibility with other pets, and many others). In shelter lore, this grew to include more pejorative and fanciful things such as the pet "not matching the owner's furniture." The effect of these well-meaning efforts was largely counterproductive in that it led to shelter staff demonizing people relinquishing a pet, despite any mitigating personal circumstances. Given the high degree of emotional stress and guilt experienced by shelter workers, whose jobs entailed euthanizing large numbers of healthy

animals (Arkow 1985; Arluke 1991), it is not surprising that this mindset often carried over into the adoption process. Consequently, to try to ensure permanent homes for adopted pets, these reasons for relinquishment tended to be morphed into factors to be wary of when people were seeking to adopt a pet. This concern was reflected in ever-more-restrictive adoption policies, which made the very people shelters needed the most (i.e., those wanting to adopt a pet) the foil for the perceived shortcomings of those relinquishing dogs (Balcom and Arluke 2001).

Contemporaneously with the initial reports about pet overpopulation in the veterinary literature in the 1970s, and prior to the data-gathering efforts of the AHA in the mid-1980s, the Humane Society of the United States (HSUS), another national advocacy group, introduced and promoted their comprehensive "LES (Legislation, Education, Sterilization) is More" strategy to reduce the number of companion animals entering shelters (Rowan and Williams 1987). Although there were reports of shelter populations decreasing somewhat, it was clear to those in the shelter community that progress on euthanasia was insufficient.

The discussion about the importance of data for crafting potential solutions was reinvigorated in the late 1980s when Carol Moulton, an executive with the American Humane Association, approached veterinary theriogenologist Patricia Olson to discuss what was going on in US shelters. Coincidentally, in her teaching role, Dr. Olson encountered a veterinary student who challenged her to consider why the veterinary community overall had manifested such a tepid response to a situation that could legitimately be considered a crisis, as it represented the largest single cause of dog mortality in the United States.

Ultimately, those conversations led to two important developments, both spearheaded by Dr. Olson, veterinary epidemiologist M. D. Salman, and Ms. Moulton. One was a special edition of the *Journal of the American Veterinary Medical Association* (*JAVMA*) devoted for the first and only time to the topic of pet overpopulation (Vol. 198, No. 7, April 1, 1991; see Olson et al. 1991). This series of articles brought a detailed perspective on various aspects of pet overpopulation to the attention of the veterinary profession. The second development was a series of workshops (in June and November of 1992 and in August of 1993) also spearheaded by Dr. Olson, Dr. Salman, and Ms. Moulton, where scientists and other current or potential stakeholders gathered to further characterize the pet overpopulation problem and brainstorm future actions. One very important outcome of the workshops was the formation of the interdisciplinary National Council for Pet Population Study and Policy (NCPPSP), whose original members were the American Animal Hospital Association (AAHA), AHA, American Kennel Club (AKC), ASPCA, Association for Veterinary Epidemiology and Preventive Medicine, American Veterinary Medical Association (AVMA), Cat Fanciers Association (CFA), HSUS, Massachusetts Society for the Prevention of Cruelty to Animals (MSPCA), and NACA. The NCPPSP later designed and implemented an epidemiological study to better characterize the problem in the United States and to determine which of the oft-cited "reasons" for relinquishment was actually a risk factor and thus meriting caution and/or intervention (New et al. 2000). To draw any connections between the expression of particular behaviors in dogs and elevated relinquishment risk, we must first know the prevalence of the behavior of interest in the general pet dog population not surrendered or otherwise rehomed. This is of critical importance, because if the trait of interest (let's say unwanted barking) occurs as commonly in dogs living successfully in homes as in dogs being relinquished, there is no basis to conclude that it represents an elevated risk, even though it may well be a stated reason. As will be discussed later, determining the prevalence of various potential risk factors in the owned population is not easy,

and attempts to do this have met with only limited success.

Nevertheless, the practical implications and importance of distinguishing between a reason and a risk factor were highlighted by one finding in particular from the NCPPSP study—that receiving a pet as a gift, long believed to be particularly ill advised, was *not* a risk factor for relinquishment, as only 2.9% of relinquishers cited this reason compared with 4.5% of dog-owning households reporting having gotten a dog as a gift (New et al. 2000). This startled shelters, because based on that erroneous belief, some had gone so far as to close or place a moratorium on adoptions around the holiday season, thus denying many pets potential homes.

6.3 Lessons Learned from Risk Factor Studies

Three studies have formally assessed risk and ultimately evaluated some of the more common reasons for relinquishment (Patronek et al. 1996; New et al. 2000; Dolan et al. 2015). However, concerns remain. For example, Lambert et al. (2015) found methodological inconsistencies among studies reporting reasons for relinquishment, including the frequent lack of definition of a particular behavior itself and of behavior problems as a group, the inconsistency and frequent lack of reporting of the number of reasons relinquishers were instructed/allowed to report, and inconsistency in whether respondents were given a list to respond to or given open-ended questions. They note that when questioning owners, a prompt to provide "the reason" for relinquishment is likely to yield a very different response than one that asks the respondent to "check all that apply." For example, when "moving" is given as a reason, behavioral reasons are often also cited, leaving the relationship among these issues a matter of guesswork.

As indicated by the above, when given the opportunity, owners may cite more than one reason. Indeed, the NCPPSP provided a total of 71 different reasons for relinquishment for owners to select, with up to 5 reasons allowed per animal. Although behavioral issues were common (cited by up to 46.4% of owners), human health and personal issues, including moving, were cited even more frequently (cited by up to 69.1%) (Salman et al. 1998), reinforcing the fact that relinquishment is often complex (Salman et al. 1998; Scarlett et al. 1999; New et al. 2000). Another study also supported the role of behavior (48% of relinquishers indicated behavior was an important factor), but that study emphasized that owner attachment to the pet was also important (Kwan and Bain 2013). Using factor analysis, Shore et al. (2008) reported that objectionable behaviors clustered into groups they labeled destructiveness, unsociability, and timidity. There were moderate correlations between the factors, suggesting that multiple behavior issues in the same dog were not uncommon. Secondly, although some dogs may indeed be relinquished solely because of behavior problems, data suggest the role of behavior may also vary by geographic location and socioeconomic status. For example, a study at a single shelter in an underprivileged area of Los Angeles, California, reported that economic issues were the overriding factor, something that the authors recognized was potentially resolvable with assistance (Dolan et al. 2015). The relative importance of various reasons may also vary over time, reflecting other social changes, such as changing compliance with recommendations to sterilize a dog and/or the increasing cost of veterinary care.

Zeroing in on the role of behavior with surveys or more sophisticated epidemiological studies is further complicated because studies may lump all behaviors into a single category without distinguishing among different types of behavior, and/or they do not consistently capture the severity and/or frequency of the behavior under investigation, and even if they do, may not measure them in the same way. For example, New et al. (2000) asked owners to estimate whether a behavior occurred "always or almost always," "most of the time," "some of the time," or "rarely/never," whereas Patronek et al. (1996) asked owners to indicate whether a behavior occurred "daily, weekly," "≤2 times per month," or "never," making it difficult to compare the resulting findings with the NCPPSP study. Neither study captured information about perceived severity or impact of the behavior.

As discussed more fully later, even if the same label for behavior is used in a study, there may be inconsistency in how that behavior was actually defined, with aggression being one particularly problematic term. The choice of controls for comparison also differed among the three epidemiological studies. New et al. (2000) used a national mail sample from members of a consumer survey panel that included owners from across the United States (not just the communities where the participating shelters were located). By comparison, Patronek et al. (1996) interviewed local controls by telephone, whereas Dolan et al. (2015) conducted in-person interviews with owners bringing their pet to a low cost spay-neuter clinic for surgery.

6.4 The Importance of Definitions

As mentioned in Section 6.3, when trying to appreciate the role of a particular behavior in relinquishment, it is important that everyone have a reasonably shared understanding of what actions constitute the behavior in question. Thus, the problem with definitions goes beyond the issues with the scientifically imprecise term "behavior" itself, to the consistent lack of definitions of the various descriptors of specific problematic behaviors relinquishers are asked to report on. For example, it is commonly held that "aggression"—which can include, depending on the study, various warning and biting behaviors and/or simply the undefined label itself—is a leading behavioral reason for relinquishment. Unfortunately, there is nothing close to an accepted definition of "aggression," even on the part of behavior professionals, much less the owners being asked to describe their dog's behavior or the ultimate readers of the study. In common usage, the term is so pejorative as to be unlikely to elicit a description of an observable behavior (e.g., bite, snarl, snap, freeze, bark, etc.) from a pet owner but instead is more likely to prompt an inference about the dog's state of mind.

These issues with definitions may also explain inconsistency among and within studies. For example, in the study by Patronek et al. (1996), the odds ratios (OR) for relinquishment with "daily vs. never" aggression to people or toward other animals represented approximately a doubling or tripling in risk of relinquishment (OR = 2.14 and OR = 2.91, respectively), compared to a more than five-fold increase in risk with daily unwanted chewing (OR = 5.59) and a more than eight-fold increase in risk with daily inappropriate elimination (OR = 8.52), both of which are more easily defined than aggression. By comparison, in the NCPPSP study (New et al. 2000), when asked about frequency of "growling/hissing/snapping, or attempting to bite," compared to dogs who rarely or never did this, dogs who did it "Most of the time" were only at a somewhat increased risk of relinquishment (OR = 1.5, 95% confidence interval [CI] = 1.0–2.1), whereas paradoxically, dogs reported as doing this "Always/Most always" were not at increased risk (OR = 0.8, 95% CI = 0.4–1.5). In the same study, 246/2,020 (11.6%) of relinquished dogs had bitten a person versus 154/3,418 (4.5%) of owned dogs (OR = 2.9, 95% CI = 2.4–3.6). However, in a different sample recruited from owned dogs presented for veterinary care,

Guy et al. (2001) found that about 10% had bitten a familiar person.

No studies to our knowledge consistently used descriptions of specific and concrete behaviors in their questionnaires for people relinquishing dogs to a shelter. Segurson et al. (2005), for example, employed an abbreviated version of a widely used, but incompletely validated, pet owner questionnaire. That instrument uses some descriptions of specific and concrete behaviors (e.g., "bark," "growl," "snap") in their characterizations of "aggressive" behaviors but then resorts to asking respondents for subjective interpretations of the dog's emotional state (e.g., "no visible signs of fear or anxiety," "mild anxiety," "moderate fear/anxiety," etc.) in the section that attempts to diagnose fear responses. Other surveys of relinquishers rely either on owners' interpretations of the meaning of "yes/no" questions, which can imply limitations on appropriate answers even when open-ended prompts are also included. Open-ended responses (often prompted in interview-style surveys) require both accurate on-the-spot interpretation and later categorization that actually matches the interviewee's intent. Again, however, it is difficult to say how much the reported behaviors reflect subjective impressions rather than objectively definable behaviors. Even a novice behavior consultant will have learned that a seemingly concrete term like "bite" can mean anything from teething, puppy mouthing, an accidental nip during play with a toy, to a protracted hold. These still say nothing about the amount of pressure applied, which is a factor in determining whether an injury occurs as well as its severity, nor do they provide any information about context or possible motivation. For example, Guy et al. (2001), in a very large study of dogs being presented for veterinary care in facilities across Canada, found that 41% were reported by their owners to have expressed warning or biting behavior toward a familiar person, and 15.6% had actually bitten. Given that Guy et al. did not include warning and biting behavior toward *unfamiliar* people, and that findings exist suggesting that directing such behaviors toward familiars and unfamiliars does not typically co-occur in the same dog (Casey et al. 2014), we can hypothesize with some confidence that the percentage of owned dogs expressing these behaviors is considerably higher. Moreover, none of the dogs in Guy et al. (2001) had been relinquished to a shelter, so it is impossible to know the extent to which their behaviors were considered by the owners to be problematic at all. A more recent internet convenience sample in Finland found owners of pedigreed dogs reporting that 45% of dogs had expressed behaviors categorized as aggressive (barking, growling, snapping, biting) toward unfamiliar and familiar people, not including family members (Tiira et al. 2016). Actual bites to family members were reported at 8.2%. Again, these were not dogs being relinquished to shelters.

Dinwoodie et al. (2019) surveyed people from a self-selected internet sample and asked about biting specifically. They reported that 4.5% of dogs had bitten a person, and roughly two-thirds of those bites had broken skin. The survey did not ask about whether any medically treated injuries resulted. Such an injury might, of course, comprise a significant relinquishment risk. But even using our smaller dog population estimate mentioned in Section 6.1, fewer than one-half of one percent of dogs annually inflict a bite for which the victim seeks medical assessment. Of these, only 2.7% were severe enough to require hospitalization, a sample too small to be considered reliable (Centers for Disease Control and Prevention 2019). Nevertheless, no relinquishment study to our knowledge has examined the injury severity question.

All this renders the reason "aggression" (as well as many other descriptors that may or may not capture similar behaviors) nearly useless scientifically, absent the nuance that can only be acquired through detailed deconstruction of an event. This makes it less surprising that relinquishing owners' reports of their dog's behavior problems have been found to have poor predictive value with regard to subsequent guardians' accounts of the same dogs' behavior in their new homes (Stephen and Ledger 2007), leaving open the question of whether the difference is due to dogs not consistently expressing the behavior in varying environments and husbandry practices or to varying perceptions and definitions of behavior by owners.

6.5 The Challenge of Determining How and When Behaviors May Threaten Human-Canine Bonds

The issue of whether dog behaviors, even when designated as "problems," actually threaten human-canine relationships becomes even more critical when one considers that multiple studies have found high percentages of dog owners who have not relinquished their pets report living with behaviors they consider problematic. If dogs living successfully in homes are expressing similarly labeled behaviors to relinquished dogs, then it seems reasonable to look to the owner's perceptions and expectations as explanation for the threat to the relationship, rather than just to canine behavior itself. Indeed, as far back as the 1980s in the United States, behavior researchers found that as many as 40% of owners reported unwelcome behaviors without considering them to be relationship threatening (Voith et al. 1992). More recently, an internet survey of subscribers to a pet supply company in Japan found no less than 86% of respondents reporting at least one behavior their dogs expressed that they found troublesome, with barking and pica causing the most concern for owners (Yamada et al. 2019). Dinwoodie et al. (2019) surveyed an online, global convenience sample of 2,480 dog owners recruited using a variety of sources, including social media, TV, and radio, to assess a variety of behavior problem metrics. After excluding those respondents who said that their pet's behavior problems were their reason for completing the survey, the authors found that among responders completing the survey for another reason, most (85%) still reported their dogs had behavior problems. Fear and anxiety were the most common problems and showed significant overlap with aggression. At this point, it is unclear whether relationship-breaking behaviors in owned dogs occur at a different frequency or level of severity or whether relinquishing owners have a lower tolerance for or ability to manage them.

The issue of owners citing multiple reasons (when allowed) as described earlier suggests that relinquishment is often a complex decision, something more explicitly affirmed by qualitative studies (Balcom and Arluke 2001). The implication of this is that reasons examined in isolation are likely to be misleading, at least in terms of the strength of any association with relinquishment. Unless a multivariate analysis is performed to control for confounding variables and identify potential statistical interactions, looking at the unadjusted OR or relative risk may give a misleading view of the true role of behavior (or any other variable) in relinquishment. For example, one study at a single shelter in Indiana reported that in a multi-variate analysis, the OR for daily or weekly inappropriate elimination was reduced by about 50% when variables such as dog training, veterinary visits, sterilization, and expectations of work were simultaneously controlled for and other behavior variables (unwanted chewing, unwanted barking, hyperactivity, and aggression toward people or animals) were rendered not statistically significant (Patronek et al. 1996). The study in Los Angeles described in Section 6.3 also conducted a multivariate analysis to control for potential confounding factors (Dolan et al. 2015). In that population, only 7.4% of relinquishers mentioned behavior as a reason with or without mentioning cost, and when adjusted in a multivariate analysis, "behaving as expected" was not a risk factor.

When considering published studies, the choice of controls, the choice of reference categories, the definitions used, measurement methods (frequency and severity of the behavior), and identification of confounding factors and their degree of control using a multivariate analysis will all influence the interpretation of the OR as a measure of risk. Given that these features of design and analysis are so dissimilar among the three published studies, cross-study comparisons are not possible, and thus consistency of results cannot be assessed. Therefore, particularly given the frequency with which some behaviors are reported in the owned population, we are far from being able to conclude with any confidence from the published literature which, if any, behaviors (even if they were defined consistently) put the dog expressing them at elevated risk for relinquishment.

A final pitfall here is that even if an accurately described and quantified behavior was determined to have an elevated relative risk of relinquishment, if the behavior in question is relatively uncommon, then the absolute risk may be quite small. Thus, it is critical to appreciate the magnitude of the absolute risk when considering the appropriate amount of time and effort shelters should devote to behavioral screening and/or modification of specific behaviors for dogs in their care. However, an important caveat here is that despite the results of any observational study, common sense dictates that dogs deemed to be dangerous will rarely figure into rehoming strategies, as few shelters will accept the potential liability or ignore their responsibility with regard to their obligation to protect public safety that would arise in such rehoming.

6.6 Preventing Behavior-Related Relinquishment and Facilitating Adoptions: Compatible or Competing Priorities?

It may be worth asking what behaviors, if any, that dogs commonly express are likely to be "deal breakers" in their relationships with their human caretakers. Are some more difficult for people to live with than others, or do individual people respond so differently to the same behaviors as to make these questions unanswerable for practical purposes? Are risks related to the intensity and/or frequency of the expression of a behavior or to a cumulative effect of multiple problematic behaviors? What might be done to ameliorate these behavioral incompatibilities between dogs and their human caretakers? And how does any of this relate to the role of the caregiver's circumstances? Answers to these questions could be of concern to shelter behavior professionals, veterinarians, and staff for at least three reasons:

- They could help guide effective interventions to assist owners and/or recent adopters to prevent the need to surrender or return a dog.
- They could help guide rehoming and behavior modification decisions for dogs currently living in shelters to prevent returns.
- They could inform decisions regarding what proportion of shelter resources should be directed at behavior-related interventions to maximize prevention or repair of unsuccessful dog-human relationships.

Much of the literature would suggest that the first of these reasons might yield the most productive interventions—relinquishment prevention through support of behavior modification consultation with existing owners. However, this is also probably the least practical with regard to shelter resources and access to the target population of owners prior to relinquishment (i.e., the subgroup of people considering relinquishment for whom potentially modifiable dog behavior, and not human lifestyle issues, is the primary factor driving the decision).

With respect to behavior-driven relinquishment subsequent to adoption, one recent study suggests that it may be a mistake to conflate relinquishment with the return of adopted dogs or even to frame the latter as a failure (Patronek and Crowe 2018). In fact, the authors found that the small number of dogs returned after adoption (re-relinquished) from a large, open-admission shelter in the Southwest were re-adopted more quickly than the general shelter population. It is certainly possible that those dogs were more appealing to adopters in the first place. However, evidence is beginning to accumulate that time spent in a foster home has a stress-reducing effect on the dog (Gunter et al. 2019. If we assume that from a dog's point of view, re-relinquishment is no different from being returned from foster care, a time in a less stressful environment may have translated to behavior and even kennel presentation more attractive to potential adopters for some re-relinquished dogs. One study found that taking a fearful dog to a room fitted up to look like one in a home and interacting quietly with him for even 15 minutes a day for two or three days dramatically increased his likelihood of passing a behavior evaluation used to make adoptability versus euthanasia decisions, and it changed the dogs' behavior sufficiently to make staff comfortable placing them on the adoption floor (Willen et al. 2019). This supports the contention that context has a profound effect on such assessments but also suggests that the best environment for many dogs to practice appropriate behavior for an adoptive home is in a foster home. Aside from the dramatic marketing advantages of exposing the dog to a whole community of potential adopters in the hands of a foster person who knows him as an individual, it is a learning axiom that the best context for learning behaviors is the context in which those behaviors will actually be used. For domestic dogs, this is a human home.

6.7 How Have Relinquishment Prevention Measures Worked?

There are four points of potential opportunity for behavioral prevention measures to be applied: prior to bringing the dog to the shelter, at the point of intake, at the point of adoption from a shelter, and shortly after adoption.

With respect to the first, literature targeted to professional behaviorists might support the notion that shelters should provide behavior consultation resources for owners considering relinquishment, particularly since one study found owners to say that such support would allow them to keep their dog (Weiss et al. 2014). The authors are not aware of any empirical studies that have assessed the efficacy of interventions such as behavior counseling for owners in the community still at the contemplation stage. Such services, however, are beyond the resources of most shelter organizations. They require time-intensive interventions performed by highly trained practitioners. There is considerable literature going back decades documenting the efficacy of such interventions when help is initiated by the owner (Leuscher 2003; Line and Voith 1986; Takeuchi et al. 2000). However, all are based on case studies of owners who have already demonstrated a commitment to the relationship by seeking out consultation and following through on the instructions given. Behavior consultants, of course, routinely work with clients to help them avoid rehoming or euthanasia, but people who have taken this step probably represent a very small fraction of relinquishers. Also, from a practical perspective, it would be difficult to locate enough owners who would accept assistance in modifying their pet's behavior prior to

their appearance at the intake counter to make a substantial difference in overall relinquishment.

As far as the second potential opportunity, for most relinquishment, the shelter's first contact with a relinquishing owner is at the point of intake after the decision has likely already been made (DiGiacomo et al. 1998). Although there are anecdotal reports of intake personnel being able to prevent some intakes by offering help with veterinary care or temporary foster care during an emergency, that type of assistance is different from behavioral interventions that would require time and possibly expense by the owner. The in-depth interviews by DiGiacomo et al. (1998) were revealing in that most people had struggled with the decision to relinquish their pet for some time, with little room for behavioral intervention options by the time they appeared at the shelter.

The third opportunity occurs in the shelter prior to adoption. Some shelters use formal behavior evaluations consisting of a battery of tests, some of which are provocative by design. While such evaluations are primarily used to determine whether dogs can be made available for adoption at all, secondarily they may also be used to try to ensure a better match between dog and adopter. In some cases, behavioral tests may be used because of the belief they can accurately diagnose behavioral conditions that are stable as well as likely to be expressed in the future home, leaving the shelter the option of attempting behavioral modification while the dog is living in the shelter. See Chapter 9 for more information about assessing the behavior of shelter dogs.

The results of studies of behavior evaluations in shelters regarding the incidence of food aggression (i.e., expressing warning behaviors when approached and/or having their food manipulated by a plastic hand while eating) may shed some light on the value of this approach (Marder et al. 2013; Mohan-Gibbons et al. 2012). The primary findings were regarding the poor predictive validity of the test in the home; often dogs who froze, stared, growled, snarled, snapped, and bit the plastic hand in the test situation in the shelter did not express these behaviors, even when similarly provoked by real hands, in the home. Adopters were informed in each study that the dog they were adopting had expressed mild to moderate food aggression behaviors on a behavior evaluation (dogs diagnosed as expressing "severe" aggression were not made available for adoption[1]). Adopters were given instructions on situations to avoid in order to prevent triggering the behaviors and behavior modification techniques to employ (Marder et al. 2013; Mohan-Gibbons et al. 2012). Mohan-Gibbons et al. (2012) found that the rate of compliance with these instructions as reported by the adopters three months later was low.

Nevertheless, often a dog diagnosed as expressing these food-guarding behaviors in the shelter did not do so in the home. Moreover, adopters reported little concern about the behavior, whether it was actually present or hypothetical. Return rates were not affected, but since the prevalence of both adoption returns and food aggression is relatively low and the samples were not large, this remained inconclusive. Moreover, the adopters had been informed of the dogs' test results, so there may have been some self-selection for people who were not concerned about this behavior. One other study, however, looked at adoption return rates at nine shelters in seven states before and after suspending the use of food aggression testing from their behavior evaluations (Mohan-Gibbons et al. 2018). They found no statistically significant change in the overall 9% return rate among the shelters after suspending food-guarding testing.

Finally, also with respect to preventing re-relinquishment of adopted dogs, in an ideal

scenario, shelter behavior consultants would reach out periodically to all adopters to provide behavior modification or normalizing advice and coaching as soon as a conflict began to manifest and thus intervene before the relinquishment threshold was reached. However, results of admittedly limited attempts at preventing behavior-related relinquishment of adopted dogs have been mixed at best. In formal studies, pre-adoption counseling and instruction, for example, have not fared well so far. Interventions ranging from separation anxiety prevention instruction (Herron et al. 2014), attempts to motivate adopters to spend time walking their dogs in an effort to promote bonding (Gunter et al. 2017), and instruction on various potential behavior problems with an eye to early intervention (Weng et al. 2006) have all shown little difference between experimental and control groups, either in adopter behavior toward their dogs or the likelihood of relinquishment.

The role of adopters' decisions to take or not take their new pet to training classes has been somewhat more positive (Patronek et al. 1996; Salman et al. 1998). This raises the possibility that the commitment on the part of the adopter and/or the acknowledgment that a dog needs to be taught about human expectations may be the relevant variables, rather than the dog's personality or even his behavior. Many, if not most, pet owners are living with "problem behaviors" without ending their relationships, which suggests that the most efficacious time for intervention may be when the dog owner or new adopter begins to consider rehoming the dog. However, to our knowledge, no one has yet found a way to identify owners who are considering such a step.

Collectively, the authors believe that the data suggest we must at least consider the possibility that we cannot predict with any confidence what canine behaviors will be deal breakers for adopters as a group, even if we could reliably predict the occurrence of the behaviors themselves. Formal behavior evaluations based on a

---

1 While this is understandable from an ethical perspective, it compromises the validation aspect of the studies and leaves open questions regarding the role of the severity of a behavior in its influence on relinquishment.

series of provocative tests administered in shelter have been shown to be neither reliable nor predictively valid. As objective pass/fail tests, they simply cannot be depended upon to consistently predict behavior in subsequent homes, with many positive results (those suggesting problems) actually being false positives (Patronek and Bradley 2016; Patronek et al. 2019). Although imperfect, assessment of canine behavior (and matching dogs with suitable adopters) remains a subjective decision based on observed behavior in the shelter and history as well as the person's own limits and preferences.

6.8 Behavioral Interventions That May Promote Adoptions and Prevent Returns

Based on what we know about the cost-benefit of behavioral relinquishment prevention efforts, the most efficient use of shelter resources is likely to focus on encouraging behaviors that are attractive to adopters. The other potentially useful application of resources can be categorized as establishing good behavioral hygiene during a dog's stay in a shelter.

Shelters can create and maintain a physical environment and practice husbandry techniques that can help prevent the development or the strengthening of behaviors that have appeared in canine relinquishment studies. Such strategies are relevant to every dog in residence. Indeed, one underappreciated problem with the focus on reasons for (and risk of) relinquishment is that it diverts attention from what may be a much more important issue for shelters. Specifically, even though many people who have not relinquished their dogs report a wide variety of unwanted behaviors that they chose to live with, this choice presumably springs from their commitment to a dog they know and love. That does not mean that some of those behaviors, even if not risk factors for relinquishment, are equally irrelevant to choosing a dog for adoption or adoption success. Indeed, it is quite possible that these common behaviors that owners might well rate as merely an annoyance are in fact major impediments to adoption of a dog who brings those same behaviors into a new home. Therefore, we will focus our intervention recommendations on strategies directed at the dogs already in the shelter's care, with an eye to making those dogs more attractive behaviorally to potential adopters and, possibly, less likely to be returned, always bearing in mind that any proposed attempt to affect adoption/retention has not yet been demonstrated in field studies. For example, a study conducted at a Massachusetts shelter with a small population attributed an increase in adoption rate of dogs the shelter personnel had visually identified as "pit bull types"[2] to the implementation of a program to train volunteers in safe dog-walking practices, but the change could just as easily have been due to simply empowering volunteers to get the dogs out more and presenting them to the public in a positive light (Bright and Hadden 2017). Moreover, since the pre- and post-implementation periods were quite long (four and three years, respectively), it's difficult to say with confidence that all other factors remained unchanged and that the volunteer training program was the factor responsible. Another study attempted to gauge the effect of various enrichment interventions on length of stay but was unable to draw any conclusions since 80% of the dogs made available to the public were adopted in fewer than three days, much too short a period to reasonably observe differences in everyday behaviors among the study groups (Perry et al. 2020).

---

2 The common shelter practice of visually identifying breed(s) in a dog's ancestry has been soundly repudiated in the literature (Voith et al. 2009, 2013; Simpson et al. 2012)

6.8.1 Supporting Adoption-Promoting Behaviors

There is some correlation between length of stay and certain in-kennel behaviors. Examples include facing the back of the kennel and simply standing (Protopopova and Wynne 2014). However, training various alternative behaviors such as approaching the front of the kennel or making eye contact with visitors have been found to have little effect on potential adopter behavior (Protopopova and Wynne 2016) or length of stay (Protopopova et.al. 2012). Morphological preferences appear to be the major factors affecting choices of which dogs to interact with beyond a cursory glance into the kennel (Protopopova and Wynne 2016).

Fortunately, some behaviors do seem to encourage people to adopt a dog (albeit only after the person has already found the dog morphologically pleasing enough to take out of the kennel for a "get acquainted" session). Protopopova and Wynne (2014) observed 251 interactions between potential adopters and 150 dogs who were available for adoption in a large open-admission shelter in Florida. The only selection criterion applied to the dogs was that the potential adopter had expressed interest sufficient to request a "get acquainted" session with the dog outside his or her kennel. The authors found that maintaining proximity to the person and engaging in play (e.g., fetch or tug) when invited (Protopopova and Wynne 2014) increased the likelihood of adoption. These are behaviors that can be readily encouraged by adoption staff (Protopopova et al. 2016) and should be the priority behaviors elicited and reinforced by shelter staff across their canine population. In the 2016 study on active facilitation of the behaviors by shelter staff, the authors found that the adoption-enhancing effect of proximity occurred even when maintained by the dog being on leash (Protopopova et al. 2016). Both the samples studied and the ease of eliciting the desired behaviors suggest that these techniques are applicable to a general shelter population. There exist, of course, a very small minority of dogs expressing serious behavior issues, that is, considered by staff to be unsafe to interact with potential adopters in these ways. Such dogs may need major behavior modification before being made available for adoption. This kind of intervention requires the supervision of a qualified behaviorist, if attempted at all. For practical purposes, this would occur in a foster setting rather than within a conventional shelter. However, in some parts of the country, there are specialized facilities that can accept such dogs.

The simple behaviors described above can be applied to the general population of dogs and do not require sophisticated training skills. In fact, in the study intervention, the experimenters simply auditioned dogs for toy preferences, then supplied the preferred toy (e.g., ball, rope toy, stuffed toy, etc.) to the prospective adopter during the session, who was also given the leash to hold to maintain proximity (Protopopova et al. 2016). The voluntary likelihood of proximity to novel people can be increased, however, through a simple protocol of a series of novel people taking the dog to a "get acquainted" area and sitting passively, offering high-value treats whenever the dog approaches the person and continuing to deliver as long as the dog remains within a set distance. Once the dog forms a pleasant association with novel people, he often finds the social contact itself pleasant and is reinforced by it without the food reward.

Unless and until something equally effective is found, these two behaviors (responding to play solicitation and maintaining proximity to new people) should form the foundation for a shelter behavior program if the goal is to enhance potential adopters' inclination to form bonds with dogs who interest them. See Chapters 3 and 12 for more information on how animals learn and training and behavior modification for shelter dogs.

6.8.2 Supporting Behavioral Hygiene

It is critical for shelters to appreciate how various behaviors identified as problematic in studies of relinquishment are often inadvertently elicited and reinforced during routine housing and care in a shelter environment. These include indoor elimination, pulling on leash, barking and lunging at passing dogs, and jumping up on and mouthing people in greeting. Some dogs will have learned to use these behaviors to cope with their living situations in their previous homes, coming into the shelter with a reinforcement history already in place. However, for most dogs, the guidelines in Section 6.8.3 will work both for prevention and remediation. The dog who is new to the shelter, for example, may need only a few trials to learn that he must keep all four feet on the floor to entice the dog walker to come into his kennel with the leash. The dog who has already learned that jumping on the person to express his enthusiasm is always followed by the anticipated outing will require many more experiences of the walker leaving the kennel without him before he learns the desired behavior. The latter may require more repetition than is practical for staff and volunteers to support in some shelters. Dogs who have built up strong persistent undesirable behavior may be in most urgent need of foster placement where normal pet dog behavior interventions can be implemented with fewer time constraints. Section 6.8.3 will focus on supporting the presumably behaviorally mundane animals who make up most of the shelter population and doing this while they reside in the shelter.

6.8.3   The Kennel Environment: Context Can Train Undesirable Behaviors

The shelter environment in general presents challenges to behavioral hygiene not typically present in a home, which is one reason why fostering can be a beneficial housing option as the norm rather than just the exception when extra intervention is needed. The close confinement and elimination schedule needed for housetraining, for example, is made difficult by typical shelter kennel spaces and routines. Often the dog has no choice but to eliminate in his kennel, and he habituates, losing his natural aversion to urine and feces near his eating and sleeping space. This can erase any previous housetraining, and future housetraining efforts are rendered more difficult. The "gauntlet effect" of dogs needing to be taken past other dogs in close proximity every time they are taken out or having dogs paraded past them in their own kennels creates stress and frustration. The dog's only outlet, and thus relief for these emotions—an example of strengthening a behavior through negative reinforcement—is often barking and lunging at other dogs and sometimes at people. And this is exacerbated when combined with intraspecies social deprivation. In shelters, leashing dogs up for walks is often a quick and dirty business. When the walker approaches, the dog expresses his excitement with jumping and mouthing. Though the walker ignores these behaviors, the dog is rewarded for jumping and mouthing with the most pleasurable event in his day by being taken out of the kennel. The same pattern applies to learning to bark at approaching people. The dog barks as a release for excitement and frustration; the person continues to approach; the barking is reinforced.

While we cannot be certain these behaviors commonly cause re-relinquishment, we are fairly certain they are barriers to adoption, so shelters need to be mindful of the potential for eliciting and reinforcing them while dogs are in their care, develop strategies to prevent them, and simultaneously strengthen more desirable behaviors. The result is supporting behaviors that are more likely to be seen as positive by new adopters. The four examples in Sections 6.8.3.1–6.8.3.4 illustrate preventing indoor elimination, jumping up, and barking or lunging at passers-by, and learning to walk calmly on a leash. See Chapter 12 for more information on training and behavior modification for shelter dogs.

6.8.3.1   Example 1. Housetraining: Preventing Indoor Elimination
Preventing indoor elimination is largely a management procedure that exploits the dog's natural aversion to urine and feces near his eating and sleeping space. How much distance

he considers "enough" will be determined by how close to these areas he has been required to eliminate in the past. For many dogs, this can be accomplished by simply providing 24-hour access to safe, clean outdoor space free from frightening stimuli (e.g., things that bang unexpectedly, vehicles, power tools and machinery, nearby dogs barking or otherwise showing threatening behavior). Protecting the outdoor elimination space from such stimuli is important, as dogs are unlikely to voluntarily go to a scary place for the purpose of elimination even if the thing that frightened them there is not present at the moment.

Dogs also form strong associations with the kind of substrate available in their previous elimination area. This is much more salient than whether there is a roof overhead, so it is helpful if the outdoor space contains both dirt and concrete. At minimum, it needs to be obviously different from that in his indoor space. It is unacceptable to force a dog to eliminate in his sleeping and eating space. One simple way to avoid this scenario is to introduce a crate into the dog's housing space. This is the protocol of choice for a dog in foster care, where the first few days can involve crate confinement, with all elimination opportunities supervised and on leash. In a shelter with sufficient resources, future housetraining can be streamlined (or at least damage to past housetraining can be minimized) by keeping dogs on a schedule where they are taken out for brief walks several times a day when they are likely to need to eliminate (e.g., first thing in the morning, after meals, and last thing in the evening) and reinforced lavishly when they urinate or defecate during the walk.

6.8.3.2 Example 2. Keeping Feet on the Ground: Preventing Jumping Up

Jumping up on people is primarily an affiliative greeting behavior, expressing friendliness or anticipation or both, so the goal is to support the friendliness while teaching an alternative greeting behavior more acceptable to people. A shelter environment that includes walks or other outings for dogs presents an opportunity to achieve this within the daily routine. The objective is to teach the dog that his natural impulse to jump up will cause the person to go away and that the only way to get the person to attach his leash and take him out is to keep his feet off the person. It makes no difference to the efficacy of the procedure whether the primary motivation for the dog is proximity to a person or the outing itself. This means that if the dog puts feet on the person at any time during the procedure, the walker leaves the kennel and goes out of sight for 10–15 seconds. Typical points where a dog may give way to his enthusiasm and jump up are when the person appears at the kennel door, touches the gate/door latch, opens the door, enters the kennel, and reaches for the dog with the leash clasp or collar. The more intense the particular dog's expression of his enthusiasm, the more quickly he will learn this contingency, but only if it is consistently applied. Every time an exception is made, more trials will be required to regain the lost ground. In facilities that depend primarily on volunteers to walk the dogs, this protocol can be explained and practiced during volunteer orientation and training. Witnessing and practicing the dramatic effect of this technique in a single session will help alleviate skepticism about its effectiveness.

In shelters where dogs are co-housed—an effective and economical social enrichment strategy when done strategically—a way must be found for the walker to deal with only one dog at a time in order to implement this procedure. These include confining the non-target dog in another space (most commonly an attached outdoor elimination space) or scheduling co-housed dogs for walks at the same time, with a handler for each.

6.8.3.3 Example 3. Quiet: Preventing Barking and Lunging

Barking and lunging at passing dogs is very often an expression of frustration. The confined dog is constantly seeing dogs in tantalizing proximity but quickly learns that he can never actually access them. In these cases, the appearance of a dog ceases to predict social opportunities, that is, fun, and instead predicts extreme frustration. The more this is repeated, the more likely the dog is to develop an aversive response to dogs in general and feel the need to drive them away. This is an issue that is best addressed indirectly, through passive interventions. For the majority of dogs, who simply have a normal social attraction to other dogs, these interventions are twofold:

- *Prevent exposure that cannot lead to social interactions.* This usually means visual barriers between kenneled dogs and those dogs passing by the kennels. Without this facility modification, the stereotypical cacophonous kennel environment is almost inevitable. The authors are not aware of any formal studies that have examined the effect of full versus partial visual barriers in a shelter kennel. Until such studies are available, shelters are advised to determine which approach seems to work best in their environment or if different approaches may work better for individual dogs. At the very least, thought should be given to preventing dogs passing each other between kennels. Doing so creates a "gauntlet effect" for dogs being returned to kennels. Even the most amiable dog may be agitated by the dogs barking at him from either side and another dog approaching him directly head on, behaviors rarely exhibited in free social situations.
- *Provide opportunities for normal, positive, intraspecies social activity.* There are at least two practical ways to do this in a shelter environment.
  - *Playgroups* provide the maximum natural social stimulation for the smallest resource investment. Supervised off-leash play provides both mental and physical stimulation and for many dogs prevents the frustration-driven issues discussed above, even when the dog is on leash. It requires an enclosed play space, the size of which will determine the number of dogs in typical groups, and a playgroup leader who can train others to supervise groups. See Chapter 13 for more information on play and playgroups.
  - *Group dog walks* (pairs qualify in this case) should be the default dog-walking protocol

because, like playgroups, they provide intraspecies social stimulation and do this within the context of an activity already being provided. Environmentally fearful dogs often do better in the company of another dog. Social walks can benefit even dogs who are mildly fearful of other dogs or who are socially inappropriate with other dogs such that they consistently have conflicts in playgroups. For dogs in either category who are not ready to walk companionably with another dog, simply arranging for them to follow one another at a distance where both can remain calm provides reassurance that other dogs do not pose a threat. As with the other behaviors discussed here, for the dog who has already accumulated enough frightening or frustrating experience of other dogs to have learned to respond with strong barking and lunging at any dog at any distance, more elaborate interventions are indicated.

6.8.3.4 Example 4. Walking Calmly on Leash: Preventing Pulling

The leash is a form of restraint, albeit one that we understand as necessary for the safety of both the dog and the community when dogs are not confined. For the dog, pulling against this restraint is a very effective strategy if it results in moving toward whatever the dog's goal is in the environment. Dogs can be taught to maintain slack on a leash, but it is a difficult and counterintuitive skill for the dog, making training both technical and time-consuming. Fortunately, the dog who requires this kind of training is the exception because harnesses that attach the leash at the dog's chest are now available that manage this issue effectively and humanely for the majority of dogs (e.g., Easy Walk® harness [PetSafe®, Knoxville, TN], SENSE-ation® harness [National Webbing Products Company, Plainview, NY]). These devices work by transferring the forward pulling motion of the dog to the side and away from the goal and include simple directions for their use that can be incorporated into the routine of any regular outing. Combining the proper use of such harnesses with being mindful of the enrichment opportunities that are the underlying purpose of walks will result in most dogs walking without strong pulling. Thinking of these events as scent walks (rather than as an attempt to cover a given distance or exert physical energy) and allowing the dog to move from scent to scent to investigate will help deplete the motivation that initially drove him to pull on the leash.

6.9 Conclusions

To best direct limited resources to help dogs, it is important for shelters to have an accurate picture of why dogs enter shelters and how those dogs differ (if at all) from owned dogs. Although unwanted behavior figures prominently into reasons for relinquishment, it is important to appreciate two things: that most dogs being relinquished to shelters do not have adoption-preventing behavior problems and that many community-based studies have demonstrated that a large majority of owned dogs exhibit behaviors that their owners describe as problematic or undesirable. Three epidemiological studies have attempted to identify behavioral risk factors for relinquishment (i.e., behaviors reported more frequently in relinquished dogs than in owned dogs). However, it remains unknown if relinquished dogs display unwanted behaviors either more frequently or more intensely than owned dogs or if relinquishing owners simply have a lower tolerance for or ability to manage the same behaviors. Therefore, it is difficult to know which

behaviors may indeed be risk factors for relinquishment and how strong that risk may be. Both because of these unknowns and the logistical challenges in identifying dogs at risk of relinquishment before they arrive at the shelter, in most cases, preemptive intervention is not likely to be practical or cost-effective.

With respect to behavioral modification of preexisting behavior problems in the shelter, it is important to differentiate between measures of relative and absolute risk. A given behavior may be associated with a high relative risk of relinquishment compared to dogs not exhibiting that behavior in the home, but it may be uncommon among shelter dogs (have a low absolute risk). A careful cost-benefit analysis is warranted before devoting precious staff time to attempting to engage in modification of that behavior, as opposed to perhaps sending those few dogs to a skilled foster home where behavior modification can be attempted in a more typical environment.

Unwanted behaviors can be a product of the stressful environment of the shelter or be reinforced by the environment even if they pre-dated the dog's stay in the shelter. Such behaviors will not inevitably be expressed in a subsequent home, and steps can be taken to mitigate such risk in the shelter and thus enhance adoption prospects. These steps include modifying both the shelter environment and husbandry practices to improve the behavioral hygiene of all dogs in care. Once a potential adopter has identified a dog who interests them, the expression of simple behaviors that increase the likelihood of actual adoption can easily be elicited with simple training techniques.

References

Amato, P.R. (2010). Interpreting divorce rates, marriage rates, and data on the percentage of children with single parents. National Healthy Marriage Resource Center. Report.

American Pet Products Association. (2015). 2015–2016 APPA National Pet Owners Survey.

Stamford, CT: American Pet Products Association. Report.

American Society for the Prevention of Cruelty to Animals (ASPCA). (2020). Pet Statistics. https://www.aspca.org/animal-homelessness/shelter-intake-and-surrender/pet-statistics (accessed 2 April 2021).

Anonymous. (1971). Short fuse on the pet population bomb. *Mod. Vet. Pract.* 52 (3): 33–36.

Anonymous. (1974). *Proceedings of the National Conference on the Ecology of the Surplus Dog and Cat Problem.* (21–23 May 1974). American Humane Association.

Anonymous. (1976). *Proceedings of the National Conference on Dog and Cat Control*, Denver, CO (3–5 February 1976). American Humane Association.

Arkow, P. (1985). The Humane Society and the human-companion animal bond: Reflections on the broken bond. *Vet. Clin. N. Am. Small Anim. Pract.* 15 (2): 455–466.

Arluke, A. (1991). Coping with euthanasia: A case study of shelter culture. *J. Am. Vet. Med. Assoc.* 198 (7): 1176–1180.

Balcom, S. and Arluke, A. (2001). Animal adoption as negotiated order: A comparison of open versus traditional approaches. *Anthrozoös* 14 (3): 135–150.

Bright, T.M. and Hadden, L. (2017). Safewalk: Improving enrichment and adoption rates for shelter dogs by changing human behavior. *J. Appl. Anim. Welf. Sci.* 20 (1): 95–105.

Burns, K. (2019). Pet ownership stable, veterinary care variable. *J. Am. Vet. Med. Assoc.* 254 (2): 181–185.

Casey, R.A., Loftus, B., Bolster, C. et al. (2014). Human-directed aggression in domestic dogs (Canis familiaris): Occurrence in different contexts and risk factors. *Appl. Anim. Behav. Sci.* 152 (March): 52–63.

Centers for Disease Control and Prevention. (2019). Web-Based Injury Statistics Query and Reporting System (WISQARS). https:// webappa.cdc.gov/sasweb/ncipc/nfirates.html (accessed 2 April 2021).

DiGiacomo, N., Arluke, A., and Patronek, G.J. (1998). Surrendering pets to shelters: The relinquisher's perspective. *Anthrozoös* 11 (1): 41–51.

Dinwoodie, I.R., Dwyer, B., Zottola, V. et al. (2019). Demographics and comorbidity of behavior problems in dogs. *J. Vet. Behav.* 32 (July–August): 62–71.

Dolan, E.D., Scotto, J., Slater, M. et al. (2015). Risk factors for dog relinquishment to a Los Angeles municipal animal shelter. *Animals (Basel)* 5 (4): 1311–1328.

Downing, J. and Lau, E. (2014). Surveys yield conflicting trends in U.S. pet ownership. https://news.vin.com/VINNews. aspx?articleId=31369 (accessed 30 January 2020).

Gunter, L., Protopopova, A., Hooker, S.P. et al. (2017). Impacts of encouraging dog walking on returns of newly adopted dogs to a shelter. *J. Appl. Anim. Welf. Sci.* 20 (4): 357–371.

Gunter, L.M., Feuerbacher, E.N., Gilchrist, R.J., et al. (2019). Evaluating the effects of a temporary fostering program on shelter dog welfare. *Peer J.* https://doi.org/10.7717/ peerj.6620.

Guy, N.C., Luescher, U.A., Dohoo, S.E. et al. (2001). Demographic and aggressive characteristics of dogs in a general veterinary caseload. *Appl. Anim. Behav. Sci.* 74 (1): 15–28.

Herron, M.E., Lord, L.K., and Husseini, S.E., (2014). Effects of preadoption counseling on the prevention of separation anxiety in newly adopted shelter dogs. *J. Vet. Behav.* 9 (1): 13–21.

Kwan, J.Y. and Bain, M.J. (2013). Owner attachment and problem behaviors related to relinquishment and training techniques of dogs. *J. Appl. Anim. Welf. Sci.* 16 (2): 168–183.

Lambert, K., Coe, J., Niel, L. et al. (2015). A systematic review and meta-analysis of the proportion of dogs surrendered for dog-related and owner-related reasons. *Prev. Vet. Med.* 118 (1): 148–160.

Line, S. and Voith, V.L. (1986). Dominance aggression of dogs towards people: Behavior profile and response to treatment. *Appl. Anim. Behav. Sci.* 16 (1): 77–83.

Luescher, A.U. (2003). Diagnosis and management of compulsive disorders in dogs and cats. *Vet. Clin. N. Am. Small Anim. Pract.* 33 (2): 253–267.

Marder, A.R., Shabelansky, A., Patronek, G.J. et al. (2013). Food-related aggression in shelter dogs: A comparison of behavior identified by a behavior evaluation in the shelter and owner reports after adoption. *Appl. Anim. Behav. Sci.* 148 (1–2): 150–156.

Miller, D.D., Staats, S.R., Partlo, C. et al. (1996). Factors associated with the decision to surrender a pet to an animal shelter. *J. Am. Vet. Med. Assoc.* 209 (4): 738–742.

Mohan-Gibbons, H., Dolan, E., Reid, P. et al. (2018). The impact of excluding food guarding from a standardized behavioral canine assessment in animal shelters. *Animals (Basel).* https://doi:10.3390/ani8020027.

Mohan-Gibbons, H., Weiss, E., and Slater, M. (2012). Preliminary investigation of food guarding behavior in shelter dogs in the United States. *Animals (Basel)* 2 (3): 331–346.

Nassar, R., Talboy, J., and Moulton, C. (1992). Animal Shelter Reporting Study 1990. Englewood, NJ: American Humane Association. Report.

New, J.C., Jr., Salman, M.D., King, M. et al. (2000). Characteristics of shelter-relinquished animals and their owners compared with animals and their owners in U.S. pet-owning households. *J. Appl. Anim. Welf. Sci.* 3 (3): 179–201.

Olson, P.N., Moulton, C., Nett, T.M. et al. (1991). Pet overpopulation: A challenge for companion animal veterinarians in the 1990s. *J. Am. Vet. Med. Assoc.* 198 (7): 1151–1152.

Patronek, G.J. and Bradley, J. (2016). No better than flipping a coin: Reconsidering canine behavior evaluations in animal shelters. *J. Vet. Behav.* 15 (September–October): 66–67.

Patronek, G.J., Bradley, J., and Arps, E. (2019). What is the evidence for reliability and validity of behavior evaluations for shelter dogs? A prequel to "No better than flipping a coin." *J. Vet. Behav.* 31 (May–June): 43–58.

Patronek, G.J. and Crowe, A. (2018). Factors associated with high live release for dogs at a large, open-admission, municipal shelter. *Animals.* https://doi.org/10.3390/ani8040045.

Patronek, G.J., Glickman, L.T., Beck, A.M. et al. (1996). Risk factors for relinquishment of dogs to an animal shelter. *J. Am. Vet. Med. Assoc.* 209 (3): 572–581.

Perry, P.J., Scarlett, J.M., Houpt, K.A. et al. (2020). A comparison of four environmental enrichments on adoptability of shelter dogs. *J. Vet. Behav.* 35: 1–7.

Protopopova, A., Brandifino, M., and Wynne, C.D. (2016). Preference assessments and structured potential adopter-dog interactions increase adoptions. *Appl. Anim. Behav. Sci.* 176: 87–95.

Protopopova, A., Gilmour, A.J., Weiss, R.H. et al. (2012). The effects of social training and other factors on adoption success of shelter dogs. *Appl. Anim. Behav. Sci.* 142 (1–2): 61–68.

Protopopova, A. and Wynne, C.D.L. (2014). Adopter-dog interactions at the shelter: Behavioral and contextual predictors of adoption. *Appl. Anim. Behav. Sci.* 157: 109–116.

Protopopova, A. and Wynne, C.D. (2016). Judging a dog by its cover: Morphology but not training influences visitor behavior toward kenneled dogs at animal shelters. *Anthrozoös* 29 (3): 469–487.

Rowan, A.N. and Williams, J. (1987). The success of companion animal management programs: A review. *Anthrozoös* 1 (2): 110–122.

Salman, M.D., New, J.C., Scarlett, J.M. et al. (1998). Human and animal factors related to relinquishment of dogs and cats in 12 selected animal shelters in the United States. *J. Appl. Anim. Welf. Sci.* 1 (3): 207–222.

Scarlett, J.M., Salman, M.D., New, J.G. Jr., et al. (1999). Reasons for relinquishment of companion animals in U.S. animal shelters: Selected health and personal issues. *J. Appl. Anim. Welf. Sci.* 2 (1): 41–57.

Schneider, R. (1975). Observations on the overpopulation of dogs and cats. *J. Am. Vet. Med. Assoc.* 167 (4): 281–284.

Segurson, S.A., Serpell, J.A., and Hart, B.L. (2005). Evaluation of a behavioral assessment questionnaire for use in the characterization of behavioral problems of dogs relinquished to animal shelters. *J. Am. Vet. Med. Assoc.* 227 (11): 1755–1761.

Shore, E.R., Burdsal, C., and Douglas, D.K. (2008). Pet owners' views of pet behavior problems and willingness to consult experts for assistance. *J. Appl. Anim. Welf. Sci.* 11 (1): 63–73.

Simpson, R.J., Simpson, K.J., and VanKavage, L. (2012). Rethinking dog breed identification in veterinary practice. *J. Am. Vet. Med. Assoc.* 241 (9): 1163–1166.

Stephen, J. and Ledger, R. (2007). Relinquishing dog owners' ability to predict behavioural problems in shelter dogs post-adoption. *Appl. Anim. Behav. Sci.* 107 (1–2): 88–99.

Takeuchi, Y., Houpt, K.A., and Scarlett, J.M. (2000). Evaluation of treatments for separation anxiety in dogs. *J. Am. Vet. Med. Assoc.* 217 (3): 342–345.

Tiira, K., Sulkama, S., and Lohi, H. (2016). Prevalence, comorbidity, and behavioral variation in canine anxiety. *J. Vet. Behav.* 16: 36–44.

Voith, V.L., Ingram, E., Mitsouras, K., and Irizarry, K. (2009). Comparison of adoption agency breed identification and DNA breed identification of dogs. *J. Appl. Anim. Welf. Sci.* 12 (3): 253–262.

Voith, V.L., Trevejo, R., Dowling-Guyer, S. et al. (2013). Comparison of visual and DNA breed identification of dogs and inter-observer reliability. *Am. J. Sociol.* 3 (2): 17–29.

Voith, V.L., Wright, J.C., and Danneman, P.J. (1992). Is there a relationship between canine behavior problems and spoiling activities, anthropomorphism, and obedience training? *Appl. Anim. Behav. Sci.* 34 (3): 263–272.

Weiss, E., Slater, M., Garrison, L. et al. (2014). Large dog relinquishment to two municipal facilities in New York City and Washington, D.C.: Identifying targets for intervention. *Animals (Basel)* 4 (3): 409–433.

Weng, H.Y., Kass, P.H., Chomel, B.B. et al. (2006). Educational intervention on dog sterilization and retention in Taiwan. *Prev. Vet. Med.* 76 (3–4): 196–210.

Wenstrup, J. and Dowidchuk, A. (1999). Pet overpopulation: Data and measurement issues in shelters. *J. Appl. Anim. Welf. Sci.* 2 (4): 303–319.

Willen, R.M., Schiml, P.A., and Hennessy, M.B. (2019). Enrichment centered on human interaction moderates fear-induced aggression and increases positive expectancy in fearful shelter dogs. *Appl. Anim. Behav. Sci.* 217 (August): 57–62.

Woodruff, K. and Smith, D.R. (2019). An estimate of the number of dogs in US shelters in 2015 and the factors affecting their fate. *J. Appl. Anim. Welf. Sci.* https://doi:10.108 0/1088705.2019.1663735.

Yamada, R., Kuze-Arata, S., Kiyokawa, Y. et al. (2019). Prevalence of 25 canine behavioral problems and relevant factors of each behavior in Japan. *J. Vet. Sci* 81 (8): 1090–1096.

Zawistowski, S., Morris, J., Salman, M.D. et al. (1998). Population dynamics, overpopulation, and the welfare of companion animals: New insights on old and new data. *J. Appl. Anim. Welf. Sci.* 1 (3): 193–206.

7

Management of Community Cats

Margaret R. Slater

7.1 Introduction

Substantial change has occurred in many shelters around the United States and the world since the first edition of this book. One change is the increasing visibility of cats entering shelters. The Million Cat Challenge was certainly one reason for this (Million Cat Challenge 2015). Keeping cats out of the shelter, returning sheltered cats to their original locations (return to field [RTF]), ensuring adequate capacity to care for the animals in the shelter, and removing barriers to adoption are initiatives of the Challenge that many shelters adopted. This chapter will focus on ideas, options, and new data since the previous edition to help shelters address community cats more humanely, effectively, and safely. *Community cats* will be used to mean any outdoor, unconfined, unowned cat (Slater 2015). Community cats may or may not be fed by humans or be sterilized. They may be lost or abandoned (stray cats) or feral cats. Feral cats are too unaccustomed to humans to be placed as a typical pet. *Owned cats* are cats who have a person who states that this is their cat. A *caretaker* is someone who is providing food and spay-neuter for a cat or group of cats on a regular basis.

A *colony* of cats has been defined as a group of three or more sexually mature cats. However, the term "colony" has come to have negative connotations, leading to visions of dozens or hundreds of cats clustered together or of caretakers "making new colonies" of cats. The reality is that community cats typically exist in smaller groups of two or three cats (Spehar and Wolf 2018). For these reasons, "colony" will not be used in this chapter, rather the terms "individual" or "group of cats" will be used as appropriate. Trap-neuter-return (TNR) will also be used for all variations, including removal for adoption, vaccination, ear-tipping, documented or assumed monitoring by caretakers, and provision of shelter or water in addition to food. Cats will mean community cats unless otherwise specified.

One of the more subtle shifts in managing community cats is the separation between population-level and individual cat concerns. The former is clearly seen in the TNR literature, where there is a new emphasis as well as some upcoming tools to decrease the numbers of cats on the landscape and not "just" sterilize individual cats for their well-being. Focusing on decreasing the population of cats better addresses concerns about the cats' impact on the environment because fewer cats leads to less impact. Similarly, fewer community cats results in fewer cats whose welfare is of concern. Individual cats do, however, continue to need attention because there is still huge variability in cats' behavior, most notably in hunting interest and success.

Animal Behavior for Shelter Veterinarians and Staff, Second Edition. Edited by Brian A. DiGangi, Victoria A. Cussen, Pamela J. Reid, and Kristen A. Collins.
© 2022 John Wiley & Sons, Inc. Published 2022 by John Wiley & Sons, Inc.
Companion website: www.wiley.com/go/digangi/animal

7.2 Effective TNR

Veterinarians are uniquely positioned to help groups working with community cats make their efforts impactful as well as explain how modeling and real-world knowledge can inform TNR activities. TNR is not the sole solution. Rather it is one tool to address existing populations of cats.

7.2.1 Modeling TNR

To best apply TNR, simulation modeling of cat populations has continued to become more sophisticated. One study examined the number of "preventable cat deaths" based on various intensities and types of removal and TNR (Boone et al. 2019). Preventable deaths included removal for euthanasia as well as kittens born who ultimately died. Removal for euthanasia of 25% or 50% of all cats every six months as well as removal of 25% or 50% of cats in a six-month period followed by doing nothing until the population had rebounded (modeling the "culling" of cat populations) were four of the options. In these 10-year simulations of a 50-cat population, doing nothing led to the greatest number of preventable deaths, closely followed by removing 25% or 50% of cats for euthanasia in a six-month period then doing nothing until the population returned to capacity before removing cats again. Even more compelling was that doing TNR on 25% of the intact cats every six months resulted in more preventable deaths than removing 50% of all cats every six months for euthanasia. Overall, the number of preventable deaths was greatest for doing nothing (~1,000 cats/kittens), followed by both levels of removal for euthanasia and rebound, then removal for euthanasia at 25%, 25% TNR, 50% removal, and finally 75% TNR (32 cats/kittens).

Modeling suggests that effective TNR in the real world likely requires about 75% of intact cats be sterilized every six months to decrease the population over time and minimize the number of preventable deaths (Boone et al. 2019). This means that it is critical to define a cat population small enough to trap, sterilize, and return 75% of intact cats every six months. Performing intensive TNR up front results not only in faster and greater population declines but also fewer kittens born who then die.

Building on intensive TNR, Benka et al. (2021) examined the cost of various scenarios using price estimates from programs around the country. When TNR was done by trapping and sterilizing about 75% of intact cats every six months, the population decline in 10 years was comparable in cost to the 25% removal for euthanasia. TNR at this intensive level led to relatively small numbers of cats remaining intact to be trapped, with the actual number being dependent on the magnitude of immigration or abandonment. Fewer cats trapped means lower costs compared to removal for euthanasia, where 50% of ALL cats need to be removed every six months. Analysis of costs for TNR demonstrated that trapping costs were a small component of total cost—hiring someone to trap so that higher intensity, front-loaded TNR is not a cost barrier in the long term.

7.2.2 Counting Cats

If a goal is population decline, the relative numbers of cats across time and the density of cats in a community need to be known (Boone 2015). Then, intelligent management programs can be designed, success documented, and work adjusted as needed to track the impact of TNR. One major new initiative is the DC Cat Count, a collaboration of organizations working to create new knowledge about valid methods for the best ways to count cats (DC Cat Count 2018). This collaboration will develop tools to help animal shelter staff, volunteers, citizen scientists, and students determine just how many cats there are in a given geographic area.

The two main ways to count cats are using cameras and/or walking routes. The optimal placement of cameras to "trap" pictures of community cats has been studied and still needs refinement (Read et al. 2015; Carter et al. 2019; Nichols et al. 2019; Taggart et al. 2019). A Canadian study described how to create random walking paths (transects) in a city using primarily existing streets (Hand 2019). The author noted that this type of count could provide changes in cat population density over time when consistently repeated as well as identify specific locations with high cat populations, making targeting of interventions more feasible.

Geospatial mapping has been applied in New Zealand to predict locations of community cats. Individuals and groups of cats from TNR records were mapped. These locations were predicted by human population density, landscape characteristics, and socioeconomics in this region (Aguilar et al. 2015). Additional research is needed to determine if these variables are predictive in other geographical locations.

7.2.3 Recent Community Cat Management Research

A newly appropriated methodology in the study of cats is citizen science, a method of integrating outreach with data collection via the use of non-scientist volunteers (Cooper et al. 2007). It is cost-effective; however, its main value is that it permits coordinated, consistent data collection over time and larger geographies so trends can be studied. The use of trends makes the potential biases, such as lack of consistency by some observers, varied ability by observers to visualize cats, or a tendency to find cats in locations where there are more cats visible or active, less problematic. A study that used middle school and undergraduate students to collect data across a wide geography determined that cats and coyotes didn't share space except in small urban forest areas. Green spaces were found to have many coyotes and few cats (Kays et al. 2015). Instead, cats were found primarily in residential yards.

An urban Illinois resident developed a citizen science project and generated a rich TNR data set that led to important discoveries (Spehar and Wolf 2018). Between 2007 and 2016, 20 locations within a 1 km^2 area contained 195 cats who underwent TNR (92%) or were adopted. Of these cats, 30% were initially or eventually adopted, 34% disappeared, 7% died, 3% were euthanized due to serious injury or illness, 2% were returned to their owners, and 1% moved outside of the area. Peak group size within the area occurred within the first two years of starting management (from 1 to 35 cats). By 2016, only 44 total cats (23%) remained, with eight groups eliminated. The largest group decreased from 35 cats to 12 cats; all other groups ranged from 1 to 6 cats. These data illustrate the importance of ongoing efforts across longer periods to see population size impacts from TNR.

An indirect way to demonstrate the impact of TNR is surveys of caretakers. In Australia, where cats are particularly contentious, TNR is generally considered to be illegal, although the laws vary by state and local government (Rand et al. 2019). Adults involved in TNR in Australia were surveyed using an anonymous online tool (Tan et al. 2017). While this approach likely included only the most motivated and successful caretakers, the results demonstrate that a reduction in cat group size appears possible. For the 21 groups of cats with good data, the median initial group size was 11 (ranging from 3 to 40 cats) and declined over a two-year period to a median of 5 cats. There was variability in the trend for number of cats, with 17 groups becoming smaller, 4 groups staying the same, and 1 getting larger, as has been documented in other studies. Adoption was used in most but not all groups to decrease the population size; in some locations more than 50 cats and kittens had been removed. More than half of the groups had all adults sterilized, with the lowest sterilization at 47%. More respondents reported involvement in feeding and seeking resources for the cats than in trapping or transporting to the veterinarian, important findings when developing a program and identifying needs. A surprisingly high percentage of respondents indicated they provided treatments for fleas and intestinal parasites (69% and 73%, respectively) indicating that this could be a more common health service if the caretakers were made aware of its importance and provided with cost-effective products.

A more recent Australian survey of 30 residents involved in TNR reported that nearly all became involved out of a desire to effectively reduce cat populations over time and over concern for welfare and humane management (Rand et al. 2019). Seven respondents reported that they got involved because a friend or acquaintance asked them to, a potentially underused mechanism of engagement in TNR for other locations. Caretakers often received permission and sometimes support from police, housing representatives, or residents. Complaints were most commonly from neighbors, and attempts to resolve them were successful about half the time. These studies illustrate both the drive for people to help as well as the need for more options to manage cats.

Cat caretakers are key stakeholders whose trust can be difficult to gain when planning or implementing TNR. However, their wealth of information about the cats makes it worthwhile to make every effort to engage them, particularly those caretakers of larger groups of cats (Gunther et al. 2016). When working with caretakers, it is important to recognize that they often experience emotional stress and inability to afford treatment when caring for their cats (Young and Thompson 2019). TNR organizations can provide positive connections to other caretakers and organization members to help mitigate disillusionment, cynicism, and burnout.

The one element of managing cats with the least amount of research is stopping new cats from leaving the owned population and becoming community cats. Sterilizing owned cats as well as keeping owned cats in their homes are critical approaches (Miller et al. 2014). Substantive work in this area would be extremely valuable since immigration, including abandonment, continues to be a problem. In one example, a study in Canada identified 18 groups of cats around barns and stables with an average of 14 cats per group (Bissonnette et al. 2018). Ten groups of cats were intensively trapped for 48 hours and sterilized. The investigators were able to trap between 67% and 100% of cats in each group, with 90% median sterilization at 7 and 12 months of follow-up. In this short study, the original cats tended to leave and more new cats to enter the intact groups than the sterilized ones. In an urban example, cats in New York City also demonstrated very high turnover rates, from 78% to 98% (Kilgour et al. 2017).

Quite a few new articles on the impact of TNR on population size have been published. In Newburyport, Massachusetts, a 17-year program that included the creation of a limited-admission cats-only shelter, engagement of business owners, organized twice-daily feeding, and experienced cat trappers resulted in the elimination of approximately 300 cats (Spehar and Wolf 2017). TNR and the removal of socialized cats and kittens resulted in rapid population decline. These efforts, coupled with prompt, accurate identification of new cats, supported the eventual elimination of the population. This program is notable for how visible and comprehensive it was as well as how much the members of the group learned and problem solved. They used media coverage, tabling, and tours of the shelter to explain the work to the community—beginning in the early 1990s when little was known about TNR. Initially envisioned as solely TNR for unsocialized cats along the waterfront, it soon became evident that many of the cats were socialized. This led to two notable decisions: that adoption needed to be part of the solution and that these socialized cats were likely coming from residents who didn't feel they had a place to take cats they couldn't keep. They also learned that cats living in groups for years sometimes became adoptable (Spehar and Wolf 2017; Swarbrick and Rand 2018). Some could be rehomed with their caretakers. By 2009, the last cat died at the age of 16.

TNR success at population control was also studied at the community level. A long-term program's records from a gated community in Florida were used to estimate population size, change in population, cat outcomes, feline leukemia virus (FeLV), and feline immunodeficiency virus (FIV) prevalence across 23 years (Kreisler et al. 2019). This program began in 1995 and in 2006 added an adoption facility, sanctuary, and veterinary clinic. Again, it was clear that ongoing efforts were needed for a successful program managing more than 2,500 cats over the years. There were 1,111 cats returned and 1,419 were removed: 711 (50%) for adoption, 441 (31%) euthanized for FeLV- or FIV-positive tests, and 209 (15%) reported dead as part of the efforts to track cats; 58 (4%) died in care. Over 23 years, the number of cats estimated to be in the community declined from 661 cats to an estimated 83 cats in 2017. The average age of cats was about 7 years in 2006 with a decline to about 4 years in 2017. The prevalence of cats positive for FeLV or FIV also declined over time. This was a highly visible program within the gated community. The controlled access was believed to have decreased casual abandonment of cats, but there were many seasonal residents and staff who could have accounted for the continued arrival of new cats.

In Rome, data on cat sterilization was obtained across a 30-year period through 2018 (Natoli et al. 2019). Italy is a country where TNR has long been practiced, in some locations such as Rome, with government support. Groups of cats newly registered each year peaked in 2011 at about 160 after a city project to provide free sterilization for owned cats and have declined to about 80 in 2017. Of these groups of cats, 204/1,878 had stabilized their size and 89 gone extinct.

University campuses are different types of communities. In a 28-year follow-up of a university campus program in Florida, the original 204 cats declined to 10 (5%) and the 16 feeding locations to five (Spehar and Wolf 2019a). This was in the face of expanding student enrollment. The majority of new cats were seen in the first 10 years of the program. At first appearance, 43 socialized cats and 161 unsocialized cats were found. After 28 years, 45% of cats had been adopted, 24% disappeared, 11% were euthanized (for severe illness or injury or testing positive for FeLV or FIV in the early program years), 8% died, and 6% were known to have moved off campus. Cats who died or were euthanized had the longest median time on campus of 4 years, with one cat living 14 years. Factors that led to success were keeping a low profile for the program and having feeding stations in inconspicuous locations to discourage abandonment of cats as well as the university's "no pets" policy. The vigilance of caretakers in monitoring for new cats also contributed to sustained reductions long term. Clearly, this success required ongoing commitment, time, resources, and dedication but was possible!

A nine-year university program in Australia also was able to show substantial declines in cat population over time (Swarbrick and Rand 2018). This program began with a pest control company hired to trap and euthanize cats. In contrast to the program described in the previous paragraph, this was a very public activity. A key element for success was beginning as a one-year trial or pilot, having very explicit and population-oriented goals, holding regular meetings, and keeping good records. They also used feeding rosters, so the daily feedings were consistently done in inconspicuous feeding stations. During the program, 122 cats were handled, with 30% adopted or returned to their owners, 30% died or were euthanized, and 29% disappeared. Because the program actively encouraged reporting of any new, ill, injured, or deceased cats, the records were able to provide some additional details. Causes of death were accidents (5/14), serious diseases (4/14), one death during surgery, and four unknown. The most common reasons for euthanasia were cancer and renal disease (80% of euthanasia). An 8% per year mortality rate was calculated and was consistent with two other pet cat populations (New et al. 2004; O'Neill et al. 2015). The population on campus declined from a high of 69 at the beginning of the program to 15 adult, neutered cats in 2017, a 78% reduction in population size.

7.2.4 Community Cat Welfare

The question of welfare among community cats in light of deaths due to being hit by cars or "disappearances" continues to depend on one's values and beliefs. Recent discussions identified freedom from injury and disease, affective state (positive and negative feelings), and being able to behave naturally in the animals' environment as key considerations (Fraser 2008). TNR appears to support the first criterion. The last criterion is arguable: Is the lack of parenting and sexual behaviors a loss of "natural" behaviors? Of course, but so is less fighting and roaming leading to less injury and illness. And there are certainly short-term negative experiences from the TNR process (including trapping, transportation, injection of anesthetic, and overall stress) to weigh against better health. While these types of discussions are beginning, we are unlikely to come to consensus since we cannot ask the cats. Pragmatically, cats who could be adopted and removed from these risks presumably would have better welfare as pets. Remaining feral cat options are preemptive euthanasia, TNR, removal to a new environment with unfamiliar cats and people (a sanctuary), or doing nothing. Better knowledge of community cat welfare could help support which options might lead to the best welfare for a particular cat.

A newly developed cat welfare scale could be valuable for evidence-based best practices for cats. This promising tool used a simple visual scale for owned, managed (with a caretaker), and unmanaged (no caretaker) cats to assess their welfare (Zito et al. 2019). The visual scale included body condition score (9-point scale), coat condition, nose and/or eye discharge, ear crusting, and injuries (all a 4-point scale). The majority of cats in all three groups had ideal body condition, good coats, and no indicators of illness or injury. The authors suggested that this scale could be validated against hands-on examination and potentially blood work.

Another recent study in Austria added criteria to evaluate welfare including overall behavior, salivation, and general impaired health (Gilhofer et al. 2019). Five groups had from 12 to 30 cats; the remaining eight groups ranged from 1 to 9 cats; all had varying levels of sterilization. The presence of fewer clean feeding places was associated with more thin or apathetic cats (presumed ill) even when most cats were in good body condition and healthy. Cats approached caretakers who offered treats or diluted milk more closely (within 0.5 meters) than caretakers who did not. There was good to excellent agreement between the two observers, which meant that the criteria used may be reliably scored by different people.

In Israel, the welfare of cats in a city with TNR was evaluated by similar criteria (body condition score, visible illness or injury, and skin disease) (Gunther et al. 2018). Cat welfare was determined by walking transects through the city during a three-year period with 4,615 cat sightings. Among cats seen, 62% were sterilized and, within the 26 city neighborhoods, sterilization rates ranged from less than 20% to greater than 70%. In this city, kittens were significantly more likely to be emaciated and have severe injuries. Sterilized adult cats were more likely to be obese and less likely to have skin lesions than intact adults. These sterilized adult cats were more likely to have a permanent disability like missing an eye, tail, or leg; this was attributed in part to their potentially longer life span than intact adults. A new finding was that having a higher proportion of sterilized cats in the surrounding areas decreased the prevalence of emaciated or thin adult cats (intact or sterilized). The reasons for this weren't known but could have been related to decreased aggression and/or competition following sterilization.

7.2.5 Recent Shelter Intake and Community Cat Research

Intensive sterilization within small locations is generally considered to be necessary when decreasing shelter intake is a goal. The impact on shelter intake maybe be due to (i) the level of sterilization being high enough to decrease the cat populations, (ii) more owned cats being sterilized, and (iii) changing community awareness and philosophy about cats. In Chicago, TNR was performed in two zip codes from June 2011 to June 2013 with about 1,500 cats sterilized and 23% being removed for adoption (Spehar and Wolf 2018). There was a 30% to 40% reported reduction in intake from those zip codes attributed to this effort. The following two years, two more zip codes were added, about 2,000 cats sterilized, and similar results reported. These researchers attempted to account for other potential reasons for intake decline since intake data can be influenced by a variety of factors beyond TNR.

Another study targeted one large zip code (12 km^2) in Florida and aimed to trap at least 50% of the estimated population (based on survey findings) for return or adoption to decrease shelter intake (Levy et al. 2014). Over two years, 2,366 cats were trapped (a trapping rate of about 60 cats/year/1,000 residents), 52% returned, and the remainder adopted or transferred for adoption. Shelter intake from the targeted zip code decreased by 66%. By comparison, shelter intake outside that zip code had increased at the end of the study. Animal control officers also shifted from immediate impoundment to sharing information and connecting residents with other resources, a critical component.

Among six municipal shelters where TNR and RTF were implemented, four of these communities saw substantial decreases in cat intake after three years compared to the baseline year before the programs began (Spehar and Wolf 2019b). All reported a greater than 67% decline in feline euthanasia/1,000 residents and increases in live release rates for felines of 74% or higher. The median reduction of feline intake was 32%, with a median decline in euthanasia of 83%. The live release rate increased a median of 53%. Between 8% and 24% of cats in those programs were adopted or transferred for adoption. Only 0.3% to 1.1% of cats were ill enough to die or require euthanasia, supporting the overall good health of the cats.

The number of cats undergoing RTF was about 14,000 for all six of these communities (Spehar and Wolf 2019). That is a relatively small number compared to the aggregated intake of about 54,000 felines (about 26%) and not enough to be solely responsible for the 53% increase in live release rate. The number of households in the six communities was about 2.2 million based on US census data. Assuming 11% of households feed cats and multiplying by four for an estimate of numbers of cats, that equates to just under a million cats (Levy et al. 2014). Therefore, total surgeries of about 73,000 was 7% of all cats. That is a relatively small proportion and seems unlikely to have resulted in a reduction in the cat populations in those communities and subsequent reduction in intake numbers. Other factors are likely implicated in the reduction in euthanasia as well as intake.

7.3 Return to Field

RTF is also referred to as shelter, neuter, and return, which is distinct from shelters performing spay-neuter or other services with the initial caretaker's intention of return to the original location. RTF is for cats who enter the shelter, are sterilized and vaccinated, and then returned to their original location and counted as a live outcome. While this is often viewed as similar to TNR, it is actually quite a bit more controversial and less likely to be legal in many locations—in the era of pound seizures, many animal shelters specifically listed animal outcomes, and returning a cat to its location was not included. Additionally, shelters may be concerned that if they return cats to the community, they may be "abandoning" them, as they "owned" the cats in the shelter. A critical consideration is that some shelters have used this program to improve their live release rates without either improving their adoption programs or considering the welfare of the individual cats as deeply as they should. Determining whether an individual cat seems to be thriving, clearly identifying the specific location from which the cat came, and considering whether that cat might be better suited as a pet are all critical to doing RTF well. Because caretakers are often unknown in RTF programs, and because these programs, by themselves, don't influence the population size, this approach should be used thoughtfully and in combination with TNR.

The original RTF program was created by Jacksonville Animal Care and Protective Services in Florida (Kortis 2014). They also included targeted sterilization programs in key zip codes. The publicity for this program increased the nearly 500 cat surgeries in 2008 to nearly 11,000 surgeries in 2012. This combination of efforts partially supported a decline in shelter intake as well as in euthanasia of cats.

RTF has been proposed as a mechanism leading to feline shelter intake decline in a facility where stray cat intake predominated (Johnson and Cicirelli 2014). This shelter also was part of a large coalition and had been performing free or low-cost sterilization of owned and unowned cats for many years. Just over 10,000 cats were returned to their locations after being assessed as too fearful, fractious, or aggressive to consider for adoption. The feline intake in 2009 was 10.2/1,000 humans; by 2014 at the end of the reported study period, the intake had declined to 7/1,000 humans. The euthanasia rates declined even more

dramatically than intake. The shelter also reported that adult cat length of stay decreased, and the percentage of cats sterilized on intake increased to 60% (Edinboro et al. 2016). Decreasing length of stay decreased the risk of upper respiratory infection (URI) in this shelter. The shelter shifted their URI treatment protocols to a more cost-effective approach and increased the numbers of cats they were able to treat, further contributing to the decline in euthanasia. The shelter re-trapped 862 cats, with 90% of these cats trapped only a single time; when there were issues relating to cats in a location, mediation with the complainant was attempted by the shelter (Johnson and Cicirelli 2014). However, 47 cats (0.1% of all cats entering the shelter) during the RTF period were admitted as "nuisance" cats (Edinboro et al. 2016). Twenty of these cats were transferred to another organization for outcome. The number of cats found dead on the roads declined slightly over this time. In addition, only 150 of about 10,000 RTF cats were found dead (1%), providing a glimpse of welfare in this community.

7.4 Continuing Controversies around TNR

The controversies about TNR tend to center around a lack of nuance about what a "TNR" program includes—such as adoption—as well as the actual goals. This black-and-white approach only adds to the perceived polarization of the topic of managing cats without creating useful and potentially novel collaborations, such as the one between Portland Audubon Society and the Feral Cat Coalition of Oregon in the United States (Cats Safe at Home 2019).

A relatively small number of cats are the ones hunting wildlife based on research and highlights that learning about individual cat behavior may help to target cats who are most likely to impact wildlife populations and individuals (Moseby et al. 2015). This could lead to interventions to relocate those cats or move them into a working cat program. These more adept hunting cats could be the best rodent control cats in barns, warehouses, and other venues.

A recent paper discussing the ethical solution for stray cats in Australia stated that TNR supporters perceive TNR to "be the panacea for 'solving' issues of shelter overload" (quotes added) (Crawford et al. 2019). The referenced publications don't actually state that TNR is a panacea. Instead, many complementary approaches over long periods are the best options. In many locations, the approaches of "community education" and trapping cats for euthanasia have been ongoing for years without showing success at decreasing cat populations or shelter intake (Wolf et al. 2019). Instead, an honest, clearly articulated goal for a program, rigorous measurement of progress to that goal, an accounting of other potential influences on the goal, and adaptation when the goal is not being achieved are needed (Boone 2015).

Arguments are also made that TNR is too expensive (Crawford et al. 2019), yet the costs of removal and euthanasia are also high. These authors reference publications about cats who die or disappear and argue these outcomes make TNR inhumane. The authors go on to say that stray cats, including those that underwent TNR, are subject to stressors, injury, and disease, all of which is true for outdoor cats. Their only suggested solutions were prevention of abandonment and additional research into other methods of population control like contraception. They also propose additional legislation and campaigns to encourage more "responsible ownership" of cats and adoption of cats by non-cat owners, neither of which have yet shown to have the desired impacts. All are potentially viable options but without data and evaluation can't be the primary methods of preventing abandonment and don't address existing cat populations. Increasing sterilization of owned cats before they have litters and providing more funding to shelters are cornerstones for change, but making this happen is hard, and no new ideas to accomplish these were shared. By either doing nothing or proposing continued euthanasia of existing cats, the authors' welfare concerns are not addressed.

An often overlooked prerequisite when dealing with conflict around cats in the community is to develop and implement methods to measure the desired change (Doherty and Ritchie 2017). Demonstrating that the intervention will reduce predator damage to the species of interest and support the whole ecosystem needs to happen if that is the goal. Without this, poor decisions will be common and will waste time, money, and lives. Adding cost-benefit analyses will not only improve impact but also articulate and compare the actual options.

7.5 Communication

Community cats continue to exist and, in some cases, increase in numbers, due to the actions or inactions of humans, so human behavior change is critical (McLeod et al. 2019). Everyone who interacts with cats in a shelter or who interfaces with people outside of the shelter should begin by defining the words they are using to describe the cats. It is essential to recognize that sharing information (a much less judgmental and reciprocal phrase than "educating") has changed a lot over the past decade, and we now have some better information and resources.

One study specifically assessed the likely impact of existing messaging about managing cats, and the results were pretty dismal (McLeod et al. 2017). A few key findings are highlighted below. Most of the messaging focused on logic and facts; while those are important underpinnings, by themselves they don't generally lead to behavior change. When debunking myths, most messages started with the myth. However, that reinforces people's beliefs through a phenomenon called *backfire*.

Instead, keep the counter-message simple and don't state the myth. Research has shown that people are much more concerned about losing something they already have than about not gaining something new, so use this to frame the messaging: If you don't sterilize the cats you are feeding, others will step in and remove the cats. Local and immediate examples are more motivating and create better connections with people than distant and future focused ones. Sharing local social norms about doing as others are doing such as "90% of cat owners in your town have their cats altered" can be persuasive and are rarely used. These techniques create opportunities to really move the needle and make our messaging much more clear, impactful, and accessible.

A human behavior change framework was applied to get residents to report stray cats to support sustained TNR efforts (McDonald et al. 2018). The research clearly identified barriers for the residents, needs to accomplish the change, and location-specific interventions. Door knocking, posters, leaflets, social media, local news coverage, and TNR efforts were the methods of engagement. Two years later, active volunteers supported a local "Cat Watch," and 155 unowned cats had been trapped, neutered, and returned, 17 euthanized for health and 51 adopted, and 92 owned cats sterilized.

A survey in Australia found that there were complex drivers and barriers to getting owners to keep pet cats confined (McLeod et al. 2015). Both lowering barriers and increasing perceived benefits were deemed necessary. The first barrier was driven by cat owners' beliefs: roaming wasn't a problem, cats controlled the rodents, and roaming was important for the cats' well-being. The second barrier was a lack of interest or motivation about confining cats. There was reported variation in urban versus rural owners in how cats were confined, while age, gender, and education were not relevant. An intervention to share how to do outdoor containment and indoor enrichment to debunk the belief that full outdoor access was necessary was a suggested approach.

A recent article about the Danish public's perceptions and actions demonstrates some common inconsistencies (Sandøe et al. 2018). For example, 27% of respondents reported that outdoor roaming cats were a problem, yet respondents did not consistently report that cats should be kept indoors or consider them an issue for neighbors. Similar US data demonstrated that even within animal welfare or conservation groups, there were substantial disagreements in the respondents' beliefs about risks to people and wildlife (Wald et al. 2016).

Effective communication is crucial to keep cats in their community home when they are doing well. All stakeholders should be provided with options regarding cats based on the residents' concerns and problems. As public opinion has shifted to support the idea that cats are sentient and deserve non-lethal approaches to management like TNR (Wolf and Schaffner 2019), recent research has provided promising approaches to improve communication for achieving better welfare and outcomes for community cats.

7.6 Cat Impact in the Community

The impacts of cats on birds and wildlife continue to be topics of much debate and publication even among wildlife conservationists. Based on research and recommendations in the conservation field, integrated, nuanced, and thoughtful approaches are critical if we are to address the real issues of biodiversity (Lynn et al. 2019). There continues to be both policy and ethical issues about how humans, cats, and wildlife should and do coexist.

Over the decades, some conservationists have shifted their stance on cats. Recently, some have argued that those who express concern over the well-being of free-roaming cats are akin to science deniers (Lynn et al. 2019). There also are some difficult conversations about the intrinsic value of any animal that have begun within the conservation world, particularly within invasion biology, which will ultimately inform this work.

Drawing on outside disciplines such as philosophy can be helpful. An argument has been made that invasive or alien species are being "discriminated" against (Abbate and Fischer 2019). A compelling component was the idea that simply being an invasive species was enough to justify aggressive lethal management. The authors discuss that being "invasive" doesn't confirm harm to the environment or native species. Nor does being invasive mean that non-lethal options couldn't or shouldn't be considered as part of adaptive management approaches. By using these loaded terms, state or scientific organizations use their substantial influence and power to convey to citizens that these species are bad, and it is good to kill them, without having to provide rationale or data.

7.6.1 Predation Behavior

Our basic understanding of cat predation behavior hasn't changed: cats are still opportunistic and will hunt and/or eat what is available. In urban environments, cats commonly use the stalk-pounce-bite approach, but they can be creative in other settings and have been known to use a paw to fish (Fisher et al. 2015). There are still no data to indicate if cats prefer available carrion over hunting live prey.

New research has been published about the wide ranges in cat activity and interest in hunting as well as the seasonal or daily variability (Lepczyk et al. 2015). Some of this variability may be due to temperature as well as time of day. Recent work has also illustrated a general tendency for mammals to increase nocturnal activity where high human disturbance is found, across habitats, taxa, and types of human activities (Benítez-López 2018). The researchers hypothesized that humans were considered "super-predators" and therefore, were avoided by other species. This was supported by recent work on cats in the Philippines

as well (Bogdan et al. 2016). Cats would likely be variably influenced by human presence based on their comfort level with humans. One thing is clear, however: there are great differences among an individual cat's inclination toward and success in hunting as well as prey type.

Risks to prey species vary relative to space, time, and individual ability to detect predators. Risks have been studied in many species but only rarely for cats and their prey (Blanchard et al. 2018). One study found European starlings focused more intently on a stuffed cat than on other starlings (Butler and Fernández-Juric 2018). Even the same species of birds can show different levels and types of escape behaviors in rural versus urban environments, potentially due to different primary predators (Møller and Ibáñez-Álamo 2012). Two bird escape behaviors, biting and amount of wiggling, seem to have been clearly modified by exposure to cats within a 100-year period of urbanization. This is a fascinating research topic that could lead not only to a better understanding of predator-prey relationships but also to mechanisms to protect prey species.

Our efforts to study predation behavior can impact it. Recently some of the collar-mounted cameras used in cat studies were heavy enough to influence the movement and behavior of the cats (Coughlin and van Heezik 2014). Collars and devices should weigh less than 2% of the cats' weights or they could decrease distances traveled and home range size. Studies where a higher-weighted device was used could result in inaccurate range size, habitat use, or behaviors so results should be interpreted with caution.

One study highlighted the variability in hunting interest as well as potential impacts from heavier cameras (Hernandez et al. 2018). Twenty-nine cats that underwent TNR living in 11 locations around an island off the coast of the state of Georgia and fed daily were fitted with cameras. The 90-gm camera may have been heavy enough for smaller cats (under about 10 lbs.) to have impeded their movement, which was not known at the time of the study. Video averaged 22 hours per cat and revealed that only 83% of cats showed any hunting behavior. Of the 24 predatory cats, 18 (62% of total) killed prey with an average of about six kills per 24 hours. Three cats killed more than 12 animals in one day. The predatory cats' success at killing prey ranged from 0 to 100%, with an average of 44%. Cats were least successful at killing birds (only 17% of the time), which may have been related to carrying the camera. Cats nearer undeveloped habitats hunted more. Female cats and cats who hunted at night were more successful at killing prey. Seventy-three percent of hunting activity was between dusk and dawn. Some cats also had clearly preferred types of prey, including two who preferred arthropods and one who preferred amphibians.

Owned neutered cats in New Zealand showed slightly lower inclinations for hunting (62%) (Bruce et al. 2019) than the cats that underwent TNR on the island, which was still higher than owned neutered cats in the United States (45%) (Loyd et al. 2013). These differences could be related to the amount of time spent outside, variability among cats, a bias about which cats were volunteered to participate, size and age of the cats, or tolerance of the collars. This further supports the idea of identifying the key individual cats and considering managing them differently.

In Australia, 13 feral cats in several habitat types were fitted with cameras on collars—while these cameras weighed from 2% to 3.6% of the cats' weights, the cats had been wearing collar-mounted global positioning devices and were accustomed to this (McGregor et al. 2015). Some cats had quite a bit more video time in the 89 hours than others. Similar to the cats on the island, they were more successful at killing at night and killed about seven animals per 24 hours per cat. They also were much more likely to be successful in an open area (70% success) compared to a rocky or dense grass environment (17% success). Since the landscape type influenced cats' hunting ability, creating

landscapes that are less hospitable for cat success could change the cats' behavior. The cats spent about 60% of their time sleeping or resting, about 25% walking, about 8% grooming, and about 7% hunting.

A study in the Florida Keys demonstrated that among the 46 cats with hair analysis performed to determine dietary composition, the 38 cats near human settlements were found to have 88% of their diet from human sources (garbage, cat food) (Cove et al. 2018). The 5 cats farthest from humans had only 35% human food sources and 54% small mammals. Eight individual cats had wildlife as more than 50% of their diets.

7.6.2 New Understanding of Predator-Prey Behavior

The ways in which the behavior of predators and their prey influence predation is an area where cats are beginning to be studied (Banks et al. 2018). Learning more about how predator-prey interactions occur could provide new options for reintroducing native species such as exposing them to cats prior to reintroduction (Ross et al. 2019). This knowledge will also identify environments where cats are less likely to hunt or to hunt successfully. In one example, individually identifiable cats and rabbits were monitored on an Antarctic island in foraging areas with different levels of openness (ability to see for a distance) (Blanchard et al. 2018). Cats were the only predator in this location, simplifying interpretation. Cats were most active at night in less open areas, and rabbits were either less likely to spend time in those areas at night or were more vigilant if they did. The amount and direction of wind also influenced the behavior of the cats and rabbits. This study illustrates that the predator-prey dynamic is more complex than was previously described, even in a one predator–one prey species.

The presence of multiple predators is a more common situation. Even the scent of competitors like dogs and cats influenced the behavior of foxes (Banks et al. 2016). This illustrates that simple analysis of one predator-prey relationship could overlook potentially important behavior changes and impacts if the whole ecosystem isn't considered. Another study focused on reviewing some new approaches to understanding nest predation, a critical selective pressure for birds (Ibáñez-Álamo et al. 2015). The authors reported the need for more research on the interactions between predators, adult birds selecting nesting locations, and increased emphasis on what nestlings do to decrease predation. While cats are acknowledged by these authors as a predator of note, removal of cats had not consistently been shown to improve survival.

Interweaving the importance of the cat management goal with the complexity of ecosystems, one study was done on a ground-nesting bird in two habitats (Oppel et al. 2014). These authors reported that the type of environment (pasture vs. semi-desert) altered the impact of cat removal on bird survival as well as on rat, rabbit, and mouse activity. When this level of environmental variability is overlaid by prey not previously exposed to cats (Ross et al. 2019) as well as the variability in a cat's interest and ability to hunt, accurate broad generalizations are clearly difficult to make.

These intricacies make definitive and universal answers about what to do about cats impossible. Another entwined interaction is mesopredator release, where a higher-level (apex) predator is removed and lower-level predators (including cats) increase in number. The phenomenon seems to be dependent on additional factors including the specific habitat type and the extent of predator removal (Allen et al. 2013; McDonald et al. 2017). Furthermore, the removal of (introduced) cats may lead to a dramatic increase in prey species (Bergstrom et al. 2009). With multiple introduced species, removing one can lead to a variety of unintended consequences (Ballari et al. 2016). Reintroduction of mesopredators may also have implications: when the apex predators

Iberian lynx were successfully reintroduced in Spain, the few cat sightings in the area declined to nearly zero, and two feral cats were found apparently killed by the lynx (Jiménez et al. 2019).

There continues to be limited research on how the apparent fear of cats as indicated by behavior change may impact the reproductive success of birds. One model suggested this fear and subsequent behavior change on the part of urban songbirds could result in declining reproductive success of the birds through changes in foraging and use of different habitats (Beckerman et al. 2007). Even when few birds are predated by cats, this small change in reproductive success could have negative impacts on bird populations. This type of modeling has yet to be documented in the real world and may be too difficult to prove. It is likely a more serious concern when the bird species are under serious survival pressure by multiple factors. A different spin on fear of cats was suggested in a paper where the author argued that cats could decrease the presence of rodents, decreasing the need for rodenticides and their negative environmental impacts (Cuddington 2019).

These types of interwoven ecological interactions have led to a number of suggestions within the conservation field, one of which is to better use and understand existing tools such as population viability assessment and sensitivity (Ben-Ami et al. 2006). Given all of the contradictory and potentially incorrect statements as well as the real variability and interactions, an evidence-based approach is required. One article pointedly called into question the value of lethal control to reduce invasive predator impacts (Doherty and Ritchie 2017). The authors focused on introduced species in general and noted that lethal control is often assumed to benefit biodiversity in spite of practical, ecological, and ethical concerns. They recommend combinations of adaptive management (which evaluates impact and adjusts the effort accordingly), systematic use of expert information, and cost-benefit analyses to avoid unintended consequences such as mesopredator release. Expert elicitation is commonly done informally but should be done in a systematic and non-biased way (Martin et al. 2012).

Another unintended consequence is compensatory migration, where lethal or non-lethal removal may result in animals moving into that vacated area when resources are still available (Doherty and Ritchie 2017). Short-term, uncoordinated, or pulsed lethal control is likely ineffective; only long-term efforts have actually benefited native species. These authors conclude with the ethical considerations of lethal control. If prioritizing the conservation of native species over individual animals, especially non-native ones, is the justification for lethal removal, then it behooves the researchers to ensure that the desired impact will occur. If culling does more harm than good, limited resources and lives have been wasted. They do acknowledge that there may be inhumane lethal control methods; however, lethal control will remain a mainstay of predator management, making clear, evidence-based arguments for its use imperative.

The complexities of human society and our relationships with the species of concern also need to be considered. Some non-lethal and potentially more impactful options are to restore habitat complexity and provide additional shelter for prey species (Doherty and Ritchie 2017). Grazing, land clearing, and fire control all substantially impact more rural areas and the species that live there. Enclosing small areas where a critical part of the life cycle of the species of concern is carried out is another method. The opposite approach of enclosing the owned cats has been strongly suggested and has seen some success at keeping owned and feral cats safely confined (Cats Safe at Home 2019). Targeting the problem predators for removal or confinement, such as the cats who are most interested in and able to hunt, could be a viable option that needs more study.

7.7 Cat Behavior in the Community

The recognition that cats exhibit wide variability in their behavior is increasingly common. Since the last edition of this book, there have been updates on diseases in free-roaming cats and their interplay with behavior. One review discussed the importance of home range and longer distances traveled and how that leads to an increase in opportunities to acquire or transmit diseases (Lepczyk et al. 2015). For example, an unneutered male who is most likely to travel the longest distances may be the most important cat when it comes to controlling disease transmission. Because cat density is likely to be higher in urban areas, these are locations where disease transmission may happen most often. Note also that as prey species move or vectors of disease spread due to climate change, cats will also be impacted (Aguilar et al. 2015).

Preconceived ideas about how and where disease prevalence should be high may not be correct. One cross-sectional study of cats in Korea attempted to identify how supplemental feeding by humans, the population density of the cats, and the prevalence of eight pathogens were linked (Hwang et al. 2018). They found that the patterns of high prevalence of the diseases didn't always relate to the density or feeding variable and sometimes were only related to the sex of the cats.

Factors that influence the size and density of cat groups could expand beyond resources like food, shelter, and relatedness of the cats to the individual's behavior and personality influencing their abilities to live in social groups. This could be genetically influenced as well, making the study of cat sociability and behavior even more challenging. If TNR increases movement and recruitment (an open question), it could increase disease exposure (Lepczyk et al. 2015). These authors recommended placing cats in sanctuaries to help eliminate disease risk (at least of new exposures in small populations). However, sanctuaries are expensive and have finite capacity, making this recommendation useful only in very limited situations.

The impact of sterilization on behavior is still unclear. A small study in Rome of 17 cats did show some behavioral changes in the eight months post-sterilization compared to the nine months pre-sterilization (Cafazzo et al. 2019). There was some individual variation in that some of the more "dominant" cats (more aggression shown than received excluding hissing) were most likely to show less aggression and more affiliative behavior after sterilization; the hierarchy of cats was similar pre- and post-sterilization. Urine spraying was confirmed to stop or decrease dramatically in frequency.

The behavior of cats at a routine feeding time was studied in one group of 35 cats in a sanctuary (Damasceno et al. 2016). The authors reported that cats ate more when the person who brought food was present. Cats also stayed for a longer period of time when the person was present (four minutes on average) compared to when the person was not present (12 seconds on average). The cats also had a preferred spatial organization around the feeding locations. This suggests that having cats on a feeding schedule and staying at the location after bringing food may increase the likelihood of the cats eating promptly, decreasing the risk of attracting pest species to the feeding area.

Home range size of free-roaming cats has continued to be studied, primarily to improve management but also to better understand disease transmission possibilities. One study examined the assumption that the type of landscape including amount of vegetation and type of land use were important predictors of cat home range; they analyzed existing published research with cats in locations away from human settlements (Bengsen et al. 2015). They used estimates of the amount of vegetation and land use type as well as the average weights and sexes of cats from studies to develop models to predict range sizes. Female cats had smaller home ranges in landscapes with lots of vegetation when there was very little seasonal vegetation variation; their home range increased when seasonal variability increased. And the higher the seasonal variation in vegetation, the harder it was to predict home ranges. So, when we are working in locations with strong seasonal influences on plant growth, there will be higher variation in how far cats travel. Weight was only a weak predictor of range. Overall, males had parallel patterns but somewhat larger ranges than females. Results of studies like this can help with predicting home range size once the research is better developed to inform trap locations and cat density estimation.

In the Florida Keys, camera trapping and sophisticated mathematical modeling were used to document movement and activities of cats (Cove et al. 2018). Three populations were derived based on distances traveled, density of human housing, and time of day. This study demonstrated that, even within a fairly small area, cats showed different distances traveled and daily activity patterns. The smallest group of cats had the largest home ranges and were also more nocturnal and found farther away from human housing. Smaller home ranges and higher population densities were seen near houses; these cats were also crepuscular, and many were thought to be owned cats allowed outside during the day. Cats with moderately sized home ranges were hypothesized to be cats who were fed and/or underwent TNR.

7.8 Keeping Community Cats Out of the Shelter

Community cats who are thriving where they are, who are not in danger from unusual events like buildings being torn down, and who are not in habitats where their activities may have substantial impact on wildlife may not belong in an animal shelter. It will depend on the capacity of the shelter(s) or rescue(s) in that community whether socialized community cats and younger kittens could be adopted into homes. Healthy unsocialized cats often end up being euthanized, sometimes after being terrified by holding, and should not enter shelters. The challenge is that it is often difficult to know which cats are adoptable and which are not when they are living in the community. When that is the case, intertwined approaches to keeping cats out of shelters where they can lead good lives are needed including TNR, communication, and collaboration with other organizations.

A first consideration is a review of policies, ordinances, or laws impacting cats that make it difficult or illegal for animal shelters or residents to act. Some local or state laws are quite antiquated and need updating. Public opinion is often not in alignment with existing laws or policies. For example, a survey in Brisbane, Australia, found that once TNR was explained, 79% of respondents chose TNR as the preferred management strategy in juxtaposition to the current catching and culling cats for euthanasia (Rand et al. 2019). Only 18% of respondents supported the current lethal control program. Respondents who were male, older, did not own cats, and who believed euthanasia of stray cats was humane and that these cats spread diseases to humans were more likely to support lethal control. To appeal to this group of citizens, communications using a more practical approach focusing on cost and viability would be a better approach than a welfare appeal (Rand et al. 2019).

7.9 Community Cats in the Shelter

When community cats do enter the shelter, the cats will likely show a spectrum of socialization to humans from rarely seeing a human (feral) to very accustomed or socialized to humans. This heterogeneity creates challenges for shelter staff. Even well-socialized cats can be stressed or afraid when they arrive. Decreasing their stress as much as possible and using a

validated assessment like the Feline Spectrum Assessment (ASPCA 2018) is strongly recommended to accurately identify adult cats who are likely to be socialized. See Chapter 15 for more information on feline behavioral assessment.

Adult cats who appear frightened but assess as socialized could go to working cat programs, or if the shelter has the resources, receive intensive behavioral modification or fostering. Alternatively, these cats could be adopted as is using the "House Spirit Cat" program, particularly if this was an owned cat who was normal in the prior home; these cats are most likely to settle into a new home with time. (For details about how and when this program could be helpful, contact Dakin Humane Society [DHS], info@dakinhumane.org.) Offensively aggressive cats or those who need serious or ongoing medical care are not candidates for this program. Decreasing stress as much as possible, setting adopter expectations, and creative marketing of these cats is the key for adoption. In brief, these cats are housed in groups, or in offices, or in fosters to decrease stress. In a cage-free setup, include many hiding places consisting solely of carriers. The carriers make low-stress handling possible. A program where fosters can adopt straight from their homes will also help. Signage explaining the situation and what to expect, quiet interactions, petting with a toothbrush or backscratcher (see Figure 7.1), fun toys, and great treats are critical. Twice-weekly weighing and tracking food preferences will address the most common issue of not eating. A plan with the veterinary team is critical. Send home instructions on confining the cat to a room, providing hiding spaces, feeding guidelines and monitoring, and being patient.

DHS also developed a completely different adoption program for kittens between 2 and 3 lbs who were not obviously friendly and had arrived that day from the streets. This program is not instead of TNR; rather it is a supplement for organizations who have the capacity. The program should only be considered if (i) the shelter is readily adopting out friendly kittens

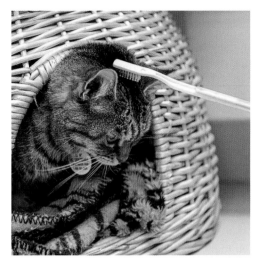

Figure 7.1 Using a toothbrush to interact safely and with less stress for a "House Spirit" cat in an office foster situation. *Source:* Courtesy of Dot Bernard, Dakin Humane Society.

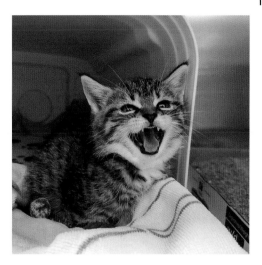

Figure 7.2 This is a candidate for the "Tiny Spirit" kitten program. *Source:* Courtesy of Meghan Delaney, Dakin Humane Society.

and there aren't lots of friendly kittens available at that time; (ii) it will not impact the shelter's ability to continue to do TNR since TNR can decrease population size more effectively than placing additional pets; (iii) staff can monitor kittens individually for their weights, health, and behavioral progress at the shelter; and (iv) the shelter has the capacity to care for the other animals in the facility.

DHS began this approach in 2015 after the organization explored the option of fostering slightly older kittens, just past that critical socialization period of about eight weeks, weighing at least 2 lbs (Bateson 2014). They found those kittens did well in foster, but they behaved in the same unsocialized way back in the shelter and weren't adoptable. To address this problem, they created the "Tiny Spirit" kitten program. They adopted these kittens "as is," still a bit hissy-spitty (see Figure 7.2), so they quickly got out of the shelter and into a home and didn't take up foster homes. About 85% of 91 kittens in this weight group could be successfully adopted; of the remaining 15%, some could be brought around with intensive efforts, but most could not and were sterilized and returned to their original locations. In

2016, DHS followed up on 87 adopted kittens. Adopters reported that 91% act like a "normal" cat, 98% still had the cat, and 88% confirmed that the information given to them was helpful. Seventy-six percent of adopters could touch the kitten within a week of adoption, 2% took longer than one month but all were able to touch them at the time of the survey. Of note was the fact that 28% of homes had kids in them, almost half with children under 10. Only 54% of homes were self-described as calm and quiet; the remainder ranged from some activity to "Grand Central Station" levels of activity.

Success with this program requires three components: (i) properly locating and housing the kittens for interaction while in the shelter, (ii) managing them for health and well-being, and (iii) the right marketing and setting adopter expectations. For most kittens, they should be individually housed in their own small kennel during the day (they can be returned to their littermates at night), preferably off the ground so they are at eye level and easy to interact with. Prepare an enclosure containing a hiding box 2 inches high to balance their stress with their exposure and accessibility. Add toys. Place these kennels in the busiest public part of the facility (DHS uses their front lobby). This makes these kittens easy for staff to access as well as visible to potential adopters. While this is very stressful for the kittens in the short term, it does help them to habituate more quickly and get out of the shelter and into a home. Kennel doors are locked except for cleaning (and kittens are burrito wrapped at that time) for the first 48 hours (see Figure 7.3). Staff will interact with the kitten using a toothbrush (which goes with the kitten) on a tongue depressor one minute at a time, 10 times each day. They also will burrito wrap the kittens, carry them around or to short meetings, and stroke their cheeks. After 48 hours, as many people as possible should interact using the toothbrush, talking to them, and petting and picking them up, in towels or not as the kitten indicates by behavior. Cues that are commonly seen as indicators of progress include a longer time until they jump around the kennel after a person arrives in front of the kennel, slow blinking, moving toward the front of the kennel (even if hissing), vocalizing, and a more relaxed body position. Great toys like peacock feathers and yummy food like human baby food (without garlic or onion) helps to counter-condition the kittens that a person (the scary thing) is paired with a positive thing (Bollen 2015). Positive reinforcement by leaving the kittens alone after they have relaxed is also an element of this approach (Halls 2018).

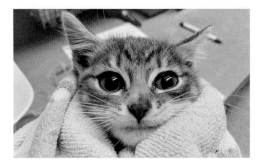

Figure 7.3 A "Tiny Spirit" kitten in a burrito wrap for safe handling, weighing, and while the kennel is being cleaned. *Source:* Courtesy of Meghan Delaney, Dakin Humane Society.

To ensure that the kittens are eating and staying healthy, they must be weighed daily and gain weight each day. Be very careful not to let them escape or hurt anyone in the first few days, and weigh kittens in a carrier or towel burrito, subtracting that weight. If they don't gain weight for two days in a row, they need an intervention.

Appropriate marketing and sharing of critical information to set expectations for new adopters is the final component. Potential adopters must work with an adoption counselor to interact with the kitten. If there aren't a lot of other kittens available, these kittens will sell themselves, hissing and all. Have the staff who have worked with the kittens talk to potential adopters. Tell adopters that this cat's first bond with a human will be with them. Post an information sheet on the kennel that explains the situation and starts with: "this kitten is not for everyone and here is why." Explain how they will likely behave with other cats (typically quite well) and what sort of investment by the adopter is needed. Send home instructions to contain the kitten in a small space and how to interact safely and effectively with these kittens, much as you might do for a foster situation.

Start this program small and get buy-in as success occurs. You may wish to call it a pilot program and have a preset time or number of kittens after which the program will be re-evaluated. Begin with easier kittens, those 2–2.5 lbs, healthy, and the colors that are popular in your community when kittens are in short supply. Work with your veterinary staff to have a plan for managing these kittens if they don't gain weight or become ill. Try it, track success (and failure), and adjust it to your needs. Success is (i) kittens are nearly all adopted within one week, (ii) very few humans are bitten or scratched, (iii) kittens are staying healthy and growing well, (iv) the shelter isn't accumulating more kittens than can be well cared for, and (v) adopter follow-ups show that the kittens are doing well in their homes and adopters are satisfied. If the kittens haven't made clear behavioral progress after the first 48 hours, re-evaluate them for the program. Kittens should be adopted within two weeks or sterilized and returned to their original location.

7.10 Conclusions

In the past few years, thinking has really become more nuanced about community cats, based in large part on recent publications and conversations. Sweeping, black-and-white statements about cats are increasingly recognized as inappropriate. Often, these statements won't be quite correct because cat behavior is very fluid and variable. Speaking this way polarizes the discussion in ways that are not helpful and can lead to pushback, simply over the words used rather than what is really meant, making common ground with others more difficult to find. Shifting the focus from providing an individual cat's spay or neuter surgery to how best to work with caretakers, trappers, and other groups involved with TNR to do effective, intensive TNR will be better for the cats in the long term. This will decrease the population of cats through attrition, lessening their impacts as the cats die or are euthanized from age-related diseases. Creative partnerships that are good for the community cats and shelters will involve compromise but may be life changing for the cats if we are open to this possibility. Clearly articulated goals for managing cats will need to have plans and measures that are adaptable rather than rigid or proscriptive. This will both allow us to better address the needs of communities and cats as well as help our staff make better decisions about individual cats in shelters and communities.

References

Abbate, C.E. and Fischer, B. (2019). Don't demean "invasives": Conservation and wrongful species discrimination. *Animals*. https://doi.org/10.3390/ani9110871.

Aguilar, G.D., Farnworth, M.J., and Winder, L. (2015). Mapping the stray domestic cat (*Felis catus*) population in New Zealand: Species distribution modelling with a climate change scenario and implications for protected areas. *Appl. Geogr.* https://doi.org/10.1016/j.apgeog.2015.06.019.

Allen, B.L., Allen, L.R, Engeman, R.M. et al. (2013). Intraguild relationships between sympatric predators exposed to lethal control: Predator manipulation experiments. *Front. Zoo.* https://doi.org/10.1186/1742-9994-10-39.

ASPCA (2018). Implement FSA at your shelter. https://www.aspcapro.org/research-feline-spectrum-assessment/implement-fsa-your-shelter (accessed 27 December 2019).

Ballari, S.A., Kuebbing, S.E., and Nuñez, M.A. (2016). Potential problems of removing one invasive species at a time: A meta-analysis of the interactions between invasive vertebrates and unexpected effects of removal programs. *Peer J.* https://doi.org/10.7717/peerj.2029.

Banks, P.B., Carthey, A.J.R., and Bytheway, J.P. (2018). Australian native mammals recognize and respond to alien predators: A meta-analysis. *Proc. R. Soc. Lond. [Biol]*. https://doi.org/10.1098/rspb.2018.0857.

Banks, P.B., Daly, A., and Bytheway, J.P. (2016). Predator odours attract other predators, creating an olfactory web of information. *Biol. Lett.* https://doi.org/10.1098/rsbl.2015.1053.

Bateson, P. (2014). Behavioural development in the cat. In: *The Domestic Cat: The Biology of Its Behaviour* (eds. D.C. Turner and P. Bateson), 3rd ed., 11–26. Cambridge, UK: Cambridge University Press.

Beckerman, A.P., Boots, M., and Gaston, K.J. (2007). Urban bird declines and the fear of cats. *Anim. Conserv.* https://doi.org/10.1111/j.1469-1795.2007.00115.x.

Ben-Ami, D., Ramp, D., and Croft, D.B. (2006). Population viability assessment and sensitivity analysis as a management tool for the peri-urban environment. *Urban Ecosyst.* https://doi.org/10.1007/s11252-006-9353-3.

Bengsen, A.J., Algar, D., Ballard, G. et al. (2015). Feral cat home-range size varies predictably with landscape productivity and population density. *J. Zoo.* https://doi.org/10.1111/jzo.12290.

Benítez-López, A. (2018). Animals feel safer from humans in the dark. *Science.* https://doi.org/10.1126/science.aau1311.

Benka, V.A., Boone, J.D., Miller, P.S. et al. (2021). Guidance for management of free-roaming community cats: A bioeconomic analysis. *J. Fel. Med. Surg.* https://doi.org/10.1177/1098612X211055685.

Bergstrom, D.M., Lucieer, A., Kiefer, K. et al. (2009). Indirect effects of invasive species removal devastate World Heritage Island. *J. Appl. Ecol.* https://doi.org/10.1111/j.1365-2664.2008.01601.x.

Bissonnette, V., Lussier, B., Doizé, B. et al. (2018). Impact of a trap-neuter-return event on the size of free-roaming cat colonies around barns and stables in Quebec: A randomized controlled trial. *Can. J. Vet. Res.* 82 (3): 192–197.

Blanchard, P., Lauzeral, C., Chamaillé-Jammes, S. et al. (2018). Coping with change in predation risk across space and time through complementary behavioral responses. *BMC Ecol.* https://doi.org/10.1186/s12898-018-0215-7.

Bogdan, V., Junek, T., and Vymyslicka, P.J. (2016). Temporal overlaps of feral cats with prey and competitors in primary and human-altered habitats on Bohol Island, Philippines. *Peer J.* https://doi.org/10.7717/peerj.2288.

Bollen, K.S. (2015). Training and behavior modification for shelter cats. In: *Animal Behavior for Shelter Veterinarians and Staff* (eds. E. Weiss, H. Mohan-Gibbons, and S. Zawistowski), 250–266. Hoboken, NJ: Wiley-Blackwell.

Boone, J.D. (2015). Better trap–neuter–return for free-roaming cats: Using models and monitoring to improve population management. *J. Fel. Med. Surg.* https://doi.org/10.1177/1098612X15594995.

Boone, J.D., Miller, P., Briggs, J. et al. (2019). A long-term lens: Cumulative impacts of free-roaming cat management strategy and intensity on preventable cat mortalities. **Front**. *Vet. Sci.* https://doi.org/10.3389/fvets.2019.00238.

Bruce, S.J., Zito, S., Gates, M. et al. (2019). Predation and risk behaviors of free-roaming owned cats in Auckland, New Zealand via the use of animal-borne cameras. *Front. Vet. Sci.* https://doi.org/10.3389/fvets.2019.00205.

Butler, S.R. and Fernández-Juricic, E. (2018). European starlings use their acute vision to check on feline predators but not on conspecifics. *PLOS ONE.* https://doi.org/10.1371/journal.pone.0188857.

Cafazzo, S., Bonanni, R., and Natoli, E. (2019). Neutering effects on social behaviour of urban unowned free-roaming domestic cats. *Animals.* https://doi.org/10.3390/ani9121105.

Carter, A., Potts, J.M., and Roshier, D.A. (2019). Toward reliable population density estimates of partially marked populations using spatially explicit mark–resight methods. Ecol. *Evol.* https://doi.org/10.1002/ece3.4907.

Cats Safe at Home. (2019). http://www.feralcats.com/csah (accessed 26 December 2019).

Cooper, C.B., Dickinson, J., Phillips, T. et al. (2007). Citizen science as a tool for conservation in residential ecosystems. *Ecol. Soc.* https://doi.org/10.5751/ES-02197-120211.

Coughlin, C.E. and van Heezik, Y. (2014). Weighed down by science: Do collar-mounted devices affect domestic cat behaviour and movement? *Wildl. Res.* https://doi.org/10.1071/wr14160.

Cove, M.V., Gardner, B., Simons, T. et al. (2017). Free-ranging domestic cats (*Felis catus*) on public lands: Estimating density, activity, and diet in the Florida Keys. *Biol. Invasions.* https://doi.org/10.1007/s10530-017-1534-x.

Crawford, H.M., Calver, M.C., and Fleming, P.A. (2019). A case of letting the cat out of the bag—why trap-neuter-return is not an ethical solution for stray cat (*Felis catus*) management. *Animals.* https://doi.org/10.3390/ani9040171.

Cuddington, K. (2019). Would a reduction in the number of owned cats outdoors in Canada and the US increase animal welfare? https://www.rethinkpriorities.org/blog/2019/10/28/would-a-reduction-in-the-number-of-owned-cats-outdoors-in-canada-and-the-us-increase-animal-welfare (accessed 27 December 2019).

Damasceno, J., Genaro, G., Terçariol, C. et al. (2016). Effect of the presence of a person known to the cats on the feeding behavior and placement of feeders of a domestic cat colony. *J. Vet. Behav.* https://doi.org/10.1016/j.jveb.2015.11.002.

DC Cat Count (2018). hub.dccatcount.org (accessed 26 December 2019).

Doherty, T.S. and Ritchie, E.G. (2017). Stop jumping the gun: A call for evidence-based invasive predator management. *Conserv. Lett.* https://doi.org/10.1111/conl.12251.

Edinboro, C.H., Watson, H.N., and Fairbrother, A. (2016). Association between a shelter-neuter-return program and cat health at a large municipal animal shelter. *J. Am. Vet. Med. Assoc.* https://doi.org/10.2460/javma.248.3.298.

Fisher, P., Algar, D., Murphy, E. et al. (2015). How does cat behaviour influence the development and implementation of monitoring techniques and lethal control methods for feral cats? *Appl. Anim. Behav. Sci.* https://doi.org/10.1016/j.applanim.2014.09.010.

Fraser, D. (2008). Understanding animal welfare. In: *Abstracts of the 21st Symposium of the Nordic Committee for Veterinary Scientific Cooperation (NKVet).* Vaerløse, Denmark: Acta veterinaria Scandinavica. https://doi.org/10.1186/1751-0147-50-S1-S1.

Gilhofer, E.M., Windschnurer, I., Troxler, J. et al. (2019). Welfare of feral cats and potential influencing factors. *J. Vet. Behav.* https://doi.org/10.1016/j.jveb.2018.12.012.

Gunther, I., Raz, T., and Klement, E. (2018). Association of neutering with health and welfare of urban free-roaming cat population in Israel, during 2012–2014. *Prev. Vet. Med.* https://doi.org/10.1016/j.prevetmed.2018.05.018.

Gunther, I., Raz, T., Zor, Y.E. et al. (2016). Feeders of free-roaming cats: Personal characteristics, feeding practices, and data on cat health and welfare in an urban setting of Israel. *Front. Vet. Sci.* https://doi.org/10.3389/fvets.2016.00021.

Halls, V. (2018). Tools for managing feline problem behaviours: Environmental and behavioural modification. *J. Fel. Med. Surg.* https://doi.org/10.1177/1098612X18806757.

Hand, A. (2019). Estimating feral cat densities using distance sampling in an urban environment. *Ecol. Evol.* https://doi.org/doi:10.1002/ece3.4938.

Hernandez, S.M., Loyd, K.T., Newton, A.N. et al. (2018). The use of point-of-view cameras (Kittycams) to quantify predation by colony cats (*Felis catus*) on wildlife. *Wildl. Res.* https://doi.org/10.1071/WR17155.

Hwang, J., Gottdenker, N.L., Oh, D. et al. (2018). Disentangling the link between supplemental feeding, population density, and the prevalence of pathogens in urban stray cats. *Peer J.* https://doi.org/10.7717/peerj.4988.

Ibáñez-Álamo, J.D., Magrath, R.D., Oteyza, J.C. et al. (2015). Nest predation research: Recent findings and future perspectives. *J. Ornithol.* https://doi.org/10.1007/s10336-015-1207-4.

Jiménez, J., Nuñez-Arjona, J., Mougeot, F. et al. (2019). Restoring apex predators can reduce mesopredator abundances. *Biol. Conserv.* https://doi.org/10.1016/j.biocon.2019.108234.

Johnson, K.L. and Cicirelli, J. (2014). Study of the effect on shelter cat intakes and euthanasia from a shelter neuter return project of 10,080 cats from March 2010 to June 2014. *Peer J.* https://doi.org/10.7717/peerj.646.

Kays, R., Costello, R., Forrester, T. et al. (2015). Cats are rare where coyotes roam. *J. Mammal.* https://doi.org/10.1093/jmammal/gyv100.

Kilgour, R.J., Magle, S.B., Slater, M.R. et al. (2017). Estimating free-roaming cat populations and the effects of one year trap-neuter-return management effort in a highly urban area. *Urban Ecosyst.* https://doi.org/10.1007/s11252-016-0583-8.

Kortis, B. (2014). Community TNR: Tactics and Tools. Phoenix, AZ: Petsmart Charities.

Kreisler, R.E., Cornell, H.N., and Levy, J.K. (2019). Decrease in population and increase in welfare of community cats in a twenty-three year trap-neuter-return program in Key Largo, FL: The ORCAT program. *Front. Vet. Sci.* https://doi.org/10.3389/fvets.2019.00007.

Lepczyk, C.A., Lohr, C.A., and Duffy, D.C. (2015). A review of cat behavior in relation to disease risk and management options. *Appl. Anim. Behav. Sci.* https://doi.org/10.1016/j.applanim.2015.07.002.

Levy, J.K., Isaza, N.M., and Scott, K.C. (2014). Effect of high-impact targeted trap-neuter-return and adoption of community cats on cat intake to a shelter. *Vet. J.* 201 (3): 269–274. https://doi.org/10.1016/j.tvjl.2014.05.001

Loyd, K.T., Hernandez, S.M., Carrol, J.P. et al. (2013). Quantifying free-roaming domestic cat predation using animal-borne video cameras. *Biol. Conserv.* https://doi.org/10.1016/j.biocon.2013.01.008.

Lynn, W.S., Santiago-Ávila, F., Lindenmayer, J. et al. (2019). A moral panic over cats. *Conserv. Biol.* https://doi.org/10.1111/cobi.13346.

Martin, T.G., Burgman, M.A., Fidler, F. et al. (2012). Eliciting expert knowledge in conservation science. *Conserv. Biol.* https://doi.org/10.1111/j.1523-1739.2011.01806.x.

McDonald, J.L., Farnworth, M.J., and Clements, J. (2018). Integrating trap-neuter-return campaigns into a social framework: Developing long-term positive behavior change toward unowned cats in urban areas. *Front. Vet. Sci.* https://doi.org/10.3389/fvets.2018.00258.

McDonald, P.J., Nano, C.E.M., Ward, S.J. et al. (2017). Habitat as a mediator of mesopredator-driven mammal extinction. *Conserv. Biol.* 31 (5): 1183–1191.

McGregor, H., Legge, S., Jones., M.E. et al. (2015). Feral cats are better killers in open habitats, revealed by animal-borne video. *PLOS ONE.* https://doi.org/10.1371/journal.pone.0133915.

McLeod, L.J., Driver, A.B., Bengsen, A.J. et al. (2017). Refining online communication strategies for domestic cat management. *Anthrozoös.* https://doi.org/10.1080/08927936.2017.1370237.

McLeod, L.J., Hine, D.W., and Bengsen, A.J. (2015). Born to roam? Surveying cat owners in Tasmania, Australia, to identify the drivers and barriers to cat containment. *Prev. Vet. Med.* https://doi.org/10.1016/j.prevetmed.2015.11.007.

McLeod, L.J., Hine, D.W., and Driver, A.B. (2019). Change the humans first: Principles for improving the management of free-roaming cats. *Animals.* https://doi.org/10.3390/ani9080555.

Miller, P.S., Boone, J.D., Briggs, J.R. et al. (2014). Simulating free-roaming cat population management options in open demographic environments. *PLOS ONE.* https://doi.org/10.1371/journal.pone.0113553.

Million Cat Challenge (2015). www.millioncatchallenge.org (accessed 26 December 2019).

Møller, A.P. and Ibáñez-Álamo, J.D. (2012). Escape behaviour of birds provides evidence of predation being involved in urbanization. *Anim. Behav.* https://doi.org/http://dx.doi.org/10.1016/j.anbehav.2012.04.030.

Moseby, K.E., Peacock, D.E., and Read, J.L. (2015). Catastrophic cat predation: A call for predator profiling in wildlife protection programs. *Biol. Conserv.* https://doi.org/10.1016/j.biocon.2015.07.026.

Natoli, E., Malandrucco, L., Minati, L. et al. (2019). Evaluation of unowned domestic cat management in the urban environment of Rome after 30 years of implementation of the no-kill policy (national and regional laws). Front. *Vet. Sci.* https://doi.org/10.3389/fvets.2019.00031.

New, J.C., Kelch, W.J., Hutchison, J.M. et al. (2004). Birth and death rate estimates of cats and dogs in U.S. households and related factors. *J. Appl. Anim. Welf. Sci.* https://doi.org/10.1207/s15327604jaws0704_1.

Nichols, M., Ross, J., and Glen, A.S. (2019). An evaluation of systematic versus strategically-placed camera traps for monitoring feral cats in New Zealand. *Animals.* https://doi.org/10.3390/ani9090687.

O'Neill, D.G., Church, D.B., McGreevy, P.D. et al. (2015). Longevity and mortality of cats attending primary care veterinary practices in England. *J. Fel. Med. Surg.* https://doi.org/10.1177/1098612X14536176.

Oppel, S., Burns, F., Vickery, J. et al. (2014). Habitat-specific effectiveness of feral cat control for the conservation of an endemic ground-nesting bird species. *J. Appl. Ecol.* https://doi.org/10.1111/1365-2664.12292.

Rand, J., Fisher, G., Lamb, K. et al. (2019). Public opinions on strategies for managing stray cats and predictors of opposition to trap-neuter and return in Brisbane, Australia. *Front. Vet. Sci.* https://doi.org/10.3389/fvets.2018.00290.

Rand, J., Hayward, A., and Tan, K. (2019). Cat colony caretakers' perceptions of support and opposition to TNR. *Front. Vet. Sci.* https://doi.org/10.3389/fvets.2019.00057.

Read, J.L., Bengsen, A.J., Meek, P.D. et al. (2015). How to snap your cat: Optimum lures and their placement for attracting mammalian predators in arid Australia. *Wildl. Res.* https://doi.org/10.1071/wr14193.

Ross, A.K., Letnic, M., Blumstein, D.T. et al. (2019). Reversing the effects of evolutionary prey naiveté through controlled predator exposure. *J. Appl. Ecol.* https://doi.org/10.1111/1365-2664.13406.

Sandøe, P., Nørspang, A.P., Kondrup, S.V. et al. (2018). Roaming companion cats as potential causes of conflict and controversy: A representative questionnaire study of the Danish public. *Anthrozoös.* https://doi.org/10.1080/08927936.2018.1483870.

Slater, M.R. (2015). Behavioral ecology of free-roaming/community cats. In: *Animal Behavior for Shelter Veterinarians and Staff* (eds. E. Weiss, H. Mohan-Gibbons, and S. Zawistowski), 102–128. Hoboken, NJ: Wiley-Blackwell.

Spehar, D.D. and Wolf, P.J. (2017). An examination of an iconic trap-neuter-return program: The Newburyport, Massachusetts case study. *Animals.* https://doi.org/10.3390/ani7110081.

Spehar, D.D. and Wolf, P.J. (2018). A case study in citizen science: The effectiveness of a trap-neuter-return program in a Chicago neighborhood. *Animals.* https://doi.org/10.3390/ani8010014.

Spehar, D.D. and Wolf, P.J. (2019a). Back to school : An updated evaluation of the effectiveness of a long-term trap-neuter-return program on a university's free-roaming cat population. *Animals* 9 (10): 768–782.

Spehar, D.D. and Wolf, P.J. (2019b). Integrated return-to-field and targeted trap-neuter-vaccinate-return programs result in reductions of feline intake and euthanasia at six municipal animal shelters. *Front. Vet. Sci.* https://doi.org/10.3389/fvets.2019.00077.

Swarbrick, H. and Rand, J. (2018). Application of a protocol based on trap-neuter-return (TNR) to manage unowned urban cats on an Australian university campus. *Animals.* https://doi.org/10.3390/ani8050077.

Taggart, P.L., Peacock, D.E., and Fancourt, B.E. (2019). Camera trap flash-type does not influence the behaviour of feral cats (*Felis catus*). *Aust. Mammal.* https://doi.org/10.1071/am18056.

Tan, K., Rand, J., and Morton, J. (2017). Trap-neuter-return activities in urban stray cat colonies in Australia. *Animals.* https://doi.org/10.3390/ani7060046 10.3390/ani7060046.

Wald, D.M., Lohr, C.A., Lepczyk, C.A. et al. (2016). A comparison of cat-related risk perceptions and tolerance for outdoor cats in

Florida and Hawaii. *Conserv. Biol.* https://doi.org/10.1111/cobi.12671 10.1111/cobi.12671.

Wolf, P.J., Rand, J., Swarbrick, H. et al. (2019). Reply to Crawford et al.: Why trap-neuter-return (TNR) cat management is an ethical solution for stray cat management. *Animals.* https://doi.org/10.3390/ani9090689.

Wolf, P.J. and Schaffner, J.E. (2019). The road to TNR: Examining trap-neuter-return through the lens of our evolving ethics. *Front. Vet. Sci.* https://doi.org/10.3389/fvets.2018.00341.

Young, R.L. and Thompson, C.Y. (2019). Exploring empathy, compassion fatigue, and burnout among feral cat caregivers. *Soc. Anim.* https://doi.org/10.1163/15685306-00001704.

Zito, S., Walker, J., Gates, M.C. et al. (2019). A preliminary description of companion cat, managed stray cat, and unmanaged stray cat welfare in Auckland, New Zealand using a 5-component assessment scale. *Front. Vet. Sci.* https://doi.org/10.3389/fvets.2019.00040.

Part III

Dogs in the Shelter

8

Handling Shelter Dogs
Trish McMillan and Kristina Spaulding

8.1 Introduction

Being in a shelter exposes dogs to stress in myriad ways. Shelter dogs are plucked out of their environment and transported to a new and unfamiliar place. For some dogs, this may be an improvement over conditions of cruelty or neglect. For others, it may be a loss of space, freedom, social interaction, and/or the creature comforts of the previous home. For all dogs, it's a major change. When they arrive at the shelter, they are placed in a kennel, often surrounded by other frightened or stressed animals. They are handled by unfamiliar people in unpredictable ways. Often they are moved from intake and led through a gauntlet of barking dogs to be put in another kennel. Periodically, people may come to walk them outside. Other times, they may be taken out and subjected to bathing or other procedures. They never know what's going to happen from one time to the next—it might be a pleasant event or it might be an unpleasant one. Imagine how you would feel if you went through this experience!

The shelter experience can be very stressful for dogs. This raises potential welfare concerns, and many shelters are understandably interested in reducing stress in dogs. In addition, shelters often house dogs that are scared, aggressive, or otherwise difficult to manage. This causes stress and safety concerns for staff and volunteers.

There are many things shelter staff can do to make the shelter experience less stressful for dogs. This chapter will discuss how to reduce stress while handling shelter dogs, including how to handle potentially dangerous dogs safely and defensively. It will also cover ways to make euthanasia as stress-free as possible. There are many other steps that shelters can take to reduce stress including facility design and management, enrichment, and training. See Chapters 10, 11, and 12 for more information on those topics.

8.2 What Is Stress?

Before discussing handling techniques, a closer look at the concept of "stress" is warranted. Stress occurs when an animal faces a challenge (McEwen 2017). This challenge triggers a stress response that activates two systems—the sympathetic-adrenal-medullary (SAM) and hypothalamic-pituitary-adrenal (HPA) systems (Sapolsky et al. 2000; Lupien et al. 2009). Immediately upon exposure to a stressor, the SAM system is activated. The adrenal glands release epinephrine and norepinephrine, which cause a number of physiological responses,

Animal Behavior for Shelter Veterinarians and Staff, Second Edition. Edited by Brian A. DiGangi, Victoria A. Cussen, Pamela J. Reid, and Kristen A. Collins.
© 2022 John Wiley & Sons, Inc. Published 2022 by John Wiley & Sons, Inc.
Companion website: www.wiley.com/go/digangi/animal

such as pupil dilation and increased heart rate and respiration.

In addition, the HPA axis responds by releasing stress hormones. Corticotropin-releasing hormone (CRH) and arginine vasopressin (AVP) are released by the hypothalamus. They signal the pituitary gland to release adrenocorticotropic hormone (ACTH). ACTH signals the release of glucocorticoids (aka stress hormones) from the adrenal cortex (Lupien et al. 2009). In dogs, the primary stress hormone is cortisol. The HPA axis takes a little longer (several minutes) to respond than the SAM system. The exact timing of the stress response varies widely. However, in many cases it takes 20–30 minutes for cortisol levels to peak, and they can remain elevated for 90 minutes or more (Beerda et al. 1996; Dickerson and Kemeny 2004).

The triggering event that causes the challenge to baseline is called a stressor. Examples of a challenge to baseline include being hit by a car, going for a run, or catching a virus. These are all physical stressors. There are also psychosocial stressors. Psychosocial stressors are stressors that involve psychological or social factors but no actual physical perturbation. Examples of psychosocial stressors include meeting a new person or dog, being attacked without being physically injured, lack of control over the environment, or social isolation.

The activation of the SAM and HPA axes causes a number of physiological responses that prepare the animal for fight or flight (Lupien et al. 2009). Blood pressure, heart rate, and respiration increase, and stored energy is converted into glucose. Pupils dilate, sensory perception increases, and pain perception decreases. At the same time, systems that are not immediately necessary—such as immune function, growth, digestion, and reproduction—are shut down. All of these changes prepare the body for survival in the moment.

Low to moderate levels of acute stress are generally considered beneficial and adaptive, as they help the animal cope with the immediate situation. However, extreme levels of acute stress or stress that is chronic can have serious and long-lasting impacts on the physical and emotional health of the animal (Seeman et al. 1997; Beerda et al. 1999; Sánchez et al. 2001; Yamamoto et al. 2009; van der Kooij et al. 2014).

Stress researcher Bruce McEwen (2017) groups stress into three categories: good, tolerable, and toxic. Good stress (or eustress) occurs when the animal experiences a challenge and is able to successfully cope with that challenge such that they experience a positive outcome. Tolerable stress happens when an animal experiences a challenge that is *distressing* at the time, but they are able to cope with that stress and do not suffer any negative long-term consequences. The type of stress depends on the animal's response to the stressor. Consider going to college. For many, this would be considered good stress. In this case, the college experience is challenging but is still very enjoyable for the individual and is beneficial in the long run. For others, college may be difficult and distressing. Despite this, they manage to pull through and earn their degree without any long-term negative consequences. Experiences just about anyone would find distressing—such as the death of a family member—also fall into the category of tolerable stress as long as the individual is able to cope without showing a persistent deterioration in mental, emotional, or physical health.

The type of stress that this chapter is focused on is toxic stress. Toxic stress is distressing and exceeds an animal's ability to cope. As a result, they often suffer long-term consequences to their emotional and physical health. This can include changes to the brain that will also make it more difficult for them to cope with future stressors. For the remainder of the chapter, references to "stress" will be referring to toxic stress.

There is ample evidence that stress can increase the likelihood of maladaptive behavior down the road, so it's very important that shelters implement strategies aimed at minimizing stress. Social and spatial restriction in dogs—as often occurs in shelters—have been associated with increased displays of aggression (Beerda et al. 1999). Chronic stress is widely accepted to cause a number of negative impacts on mental and physical health. In general, chronic stress has been linked to increased aggression, anxiety, and depression-like behaviors in a variety of species (Sánchez et al. 2001; Wood et al. 2003; Zoladz et al. 2008; van der Kooij et al. 2014; Ménard et al. 2016). It has also been shown to impair social behavior, memory, and cognition (Schwabe et al. 2012; Nazeri et al. 2015; Sandi and Haller 2015) and enhance fear (Rau et al. 2005). Physical health can also be dramatically impacted in a number of ways including increased susceptibility to disease, slower healing, and shortened lifespan (Glaser and Kiecolt-Glaser 2005; Dreschel 2010; Juster et al. 2010). This means that reducing stress will likely increase the emotional, mental, and physical well-being of dogs in shelter care.

Once a dog has an aversive experience in a particular context, that encounter influences their future behavior in that same context, even if the current experience is not itself unpleasant (Döring et al. 2009). This is called *context learning*. Another issue is that animals often show a more intense response to stress when they experience multiple triggers at once, or in quick succession. Trigger stacking occurs when stress accumulates due to the introduction of so many stressors in a short period of time that there is no opportunity for the animal to return to baseline (Edwards et al. 2019). Context learning and trigger stacking indicate that it is especially important to prevent or minimize stressful experiences in the first place, as they can have a cumulative effect.

Because stressed animals may be more likely to react aggressively (Sandi and Haller 2015), using low-stress techniques and defensive handling also increases safety for staff, volunteers, and shelter visitors.

8.3 Stress in Shelter Dogs

The shelter experience has the potential to be very stressful for dogs. They are placed in a crowded and unfamiliar environment with limited access to social interaction and restricted movement and freedom. Shelter dogs also require regular handling and medical care; even outside of a shelter or veterinary environment, these interactions and their associated contexts can be sources of fear, anxiety, and stress (Grandin 1998; Edwards et al. 2019).

What does the research tell us about stress in shelter dogs? A number of studies have demonstrated that cortisol levels are elevated when dogs first enter the shelter (Protopopova 2016; Hennessy et al. 2020). However, after the first several days to a week, cortisol levels tend to gradually decrease until they return to baseline (Protopopova 2016). Does this mean dogs are no longer stressed? Not necessarily—interpretation of these results is complex.

First, it is important to understand that cortisol alone cannot tell us about the well-being of an animal. Cortisol levels are influenced by several factors in addition to stress. These factors include time of day, spay-neuter status, age, and sampling method (Chmelíková et al. 2020). Furthermore, cortisol levels only indicate the activation of the stress response without providing any information on the animal's emotional state. It seems clear that entering a shelter environment is stressful. However, cortisol levels do not indicate what *type* of stress (good, tolerable, or toxic) an animal is experiencing. Therefore, it's not possible to make inferences about their emotional state or their welfare based solely on changes in cortisol. Because of this, it's important that assessments of shelter dog welfare are not limited to measurements of cortisol levels.

It is not yet clear why cortisol levels are returning to baseline. Under conditions of chronic stress, biological systems eventually become dysregulated (McEwen and Stellar 1993; Juster et al. 2010). One possible explanation is that the decrease in cortisol levels is an indication of a malfunctioning stress response system. It's also possible that cortisol levels return to baseline because dogs are becoming habituated to the shelter environment and are no longer experiencing stress. Indeed, several studies have shown that cortisol levels in kenneled dogs remain responsive to acute triggers (e.g., restraint, venipuncture) and interventions (e.g., petting) (Tuber et al. 1996; Beerda et al. 1998; Coppola et al. 2006; Shiverdecker et al. 2013). This suggests that the stress response system is still responding normally.

In addition, stress impacts individuals differently. Averaging cortisol levels together eliminates individual variation. Therefore, even if dogs *on average* are becoming less stressed, that doesn't mean that *none* of the dogs are experiencing stress. Anyone with shelter experience knows that certain individual dogs can suffer greatly in a shelter environment. Other dogs may cope well with a shelter environment. There is also evidence from research that different dogs respond differently to an extended stay at a shelter (Hiby et al. 2006; Stephen and Ledger 2006). Aggressive and fearful dogs are often eliminated from study samples, and these may be the very individuals that are most susceptible to stress. The age and source of dogs are other factors that may impact an individual's reaction to stress. In particular, dogs that are still undergoing development (puppies and adolescent dogs) and seniors are most susceptible to the effects of stress. In addition, there is evidence that the ability to cope with stress is influenced by an animal's personality (Koolhaas 1999; Corsetti et al. 2018; Protopopova et al. 2019). Finally, dogs coming from particularly difficult environments, such as cruelty and neglect, may experience an increase in their quality of life after arriving at—and adjusting to—the animal shelter.

In summary, much more research is needed to understand what is driving the decrease in cortisol levels after the first several days to a week at the shelter. There are three key points that can be taken from these data. First, the first week in the shelter appears to be particularly difficult for the population as a whole, so it's important to target that week in an attempt to reduce stress levels. Second,

certain individuals suffer more from the impacts of stress. Being able to identify these individuals will enable staff to target them for stress intervention programs. Shelters with limited staff and financial resources may not be able to administer comprehensive enrichment or training programs to every dog. If especially vulnerable individuals can be singled out, these individuals can receive the resources that are available. Finally, our understanding of how stress impacts dogs—and the individual characteristics that matter—is still incomplete, and additional research in this area is needed.

8.4 Body Language

One of the most important ways to keep ourselves, our coworkers, our adopters, and our animals safe is to become experts at reading canine body language. Early recognition of signs of arousal, fear, or aggression will allow for quicker intervention, a change in handling technique, and a reduction in the chances of a fearful or aggressive response. See Chapter 1 for more information on reading canine body language.

8.5 Responding to the Dog's Emotional State

Once a stressed dog is identified, how should a handler respond? The first step is to stop and reassess. What is causing the stress? What options are there for alleviating that stress? Is the procedure or activity absolutely necessary at this time? Responding to the dog's emotional state means assessing needs versus wants. If the activity falls into the "want" rather than "need" category, perhaps it could be eliminated completely.

In cases where potentially stressful experiences cannot be avoided, there are a number of tactics that can help to reduce stress in the dog. Is it something that needs to be done immediately? Or, if the dog will be undergoing an anesthetic event in the near future, could the procedure be done at that time? Is there something that could be changed—a different approach—that would reduce the dog's stress?

The following sections outline several different options for changing tactics to reduce or minimize stress in dogs. Shelters have varying levels of resources in terms of time, space, staff, volunteers, and money. Some of the following recommendations will be difficult or impossible for certain shelters to implement. Follow the recommendations that make the most sense for your shelter—even small changes can make a big difference!

8.5.1 Timing

Being in a shelter often bombards dogs with several different stressors in quick succession, at least until they can adjust to their new environment. They are likely to be stressed even before reaching the shelter. Research on wild animals has shown that translocation creates stress in four primary ways: capture, captivity, transport, and release (Dickens et al. 2010). This is even more true for animal shelters where some percentage of the dogs were stray before entering the shelter environment. Even dogs that are surrendered by their owners experience some degree of capture by being placed in a crate, carried in, or having a leash attached.

As described in Section 8.3, evidence suggests that stress levels are highest during the first week of the shelter stay. For this reason, whenever possible, defer any potentially unpleasant experiences until after the first week. This limits the impact of trigger stacking and gives dogs some time to adjust to change before experiencing additional stress. It also gives shelter workers a chance to develop a relationship with the dog and start training plans designed to prevent or mitigate stressful experiences.

8.6 Low-Stress Handling

Low-stress handling includes any process or procedure that reduces stress in the animal being handled. In addition to improving welfare and increasing safety, it will decrease the likelihood of developing (or accelerating) negative handling-related associations and help keep shelter workers safe from dog bites and other injuries. The first step is being able to correctly recognize and interpret body language signals in dogs so that workers can accurately assess their emotional state and adjust as needed. Staff and volunteers should be taught how to approach a dog in a non-threatening manner. Most dogs do not respond well to being approached directly, reached for, or leaned over. This is especially true if they are confined (such as in a kennel), restrained, or already fearful for another reason.

8.6.1 Entering and Exiting Kennels

There are a number of strategies that can be used to get a dog safely in and out of a kennel. In some cases, dogs need to be moved immediately, without having time to condition them to going in the kennel or walking past other dogs. There are long-term training interventions that can help with this for shelters that have the resources, but this chapter will focus on techniques that workers can use to handle dogs in the moment. For dogs that have already been taught to sit on cue, asking for a sit before opening the kennel door and leashing the dog up can help teach more manageable behavior.

8.6.1.1 Getting Difficult Dogs Out of Kennels

If a dog is difficult to get out of the kennel or is exhibiting fearful or aggressive behavior, the staff member can show her the leash and speak kindly and happily to her, using a potentially familiar phrase such as "wanna go for a walk?" They can crack the front of the kennel open, bracing it with a foot so the dog can't burst out. Some dogs quickly change how they feel about the person at the front of the kennel when they recognize the person is going to take them for a walk. A handler can place their hand and the leash just inside the door and, with a treat, lure the dog's head through the leash opening. Another handy trick is to slide a long sausage treat through the door from the outside in order to let the dog put her head into the loop of the slip lead, rather than going in and attempting to throw the lead over her head.

If the dog remains fearful at the back of the kennel, or is lunging and barking at the front, it's time to break out the *really* good treats, which every staff member should carry in their treat pouch. If staff members toss the dog a small piece of chicken, cheese, hot dog, or other high-value treat every time they walk by, the dog should start feeling better about their presence. Extremely fearful or reactive dogs might take longer to learn this association, but this is a wise protocol to begin with any dog who arrives with poor kennel presentation. A treat bucket on the outside of the kennel makes it easy for volunteers and potential adopters to also toss the dogs treats, thereby generalizing these positive feelings to volunteers and adopters.

Some handlers worry that feeding a barking dog reinforces undesirable behavior. If the behavior decreases, by definition, it is not being reinforced. Watch the dog's body language and demeanor—most dogs can't help but start to like the "cookie people." Pavlovian conditioning is a powerful tool.

Very fearful or feral-type dogs may not respond quickly to this protocol, or they may have a harder time generalizing affiliative behavior toward new people. If a fearful dog is dog-social, co-kenneling her with a more outgoing companion can help her start feeling better about humans, too. If her companion is at the front of the kennel wagging, social facilitation (as well as the enrichment of having a social companion) can make a big difference in the fearful

dog's willingness to come forward for treats, attention, and, eventually, leashing. The opportunity to go to an exercise area together may also be a chance for positive human interaction. Staff should be coached in treating two dogs with hands far apart so they won't compete for treats, and dogs should be separated at mealtimes and if either of them is likely to guard food from the other.

If co-kenneling is not possible, scheduled daily play sessions with social dogs can be helpful for teaching a positive association between leashing in the kennel and getting out to do something fun. It may be wise to kennel a fearful dog near the play areas, so the dog can easily move to the play yard, especially if she's not good at walking on lead. Fitting a fearful dog with a harness and light drag leash can enable catching her once the play session is over.

In general, when handling unknown or difficult dogs, it's easiest to use a slip lead, so that the handler doesn't have to go all the way into the kennel with the dog in order to leash her up. With dogs who may direct aggression toward the handler, a raised bed or plastic crate pan can be used to protect the handler's legs as they open the kennel, keeping the barrier between them and the dog as they get a slip lead on to get her out. Sometimes using two people and two slip leads is safer. With one handler on each side of the dog, holding the leashes in opposition to one another, the handlers can work together to keep one another safe from potential bites. Alternatively, a control pole and a slip lead with a second handler can be used when handling of dangerous dogs cannot be avoided (see Figure 8.1). The dog should be guided with the leash as much as possible, with the control pole only used as a backup for safety, to avoid the dog panicking and flailing at the end of the pole. If the dog is unused to being on leash, or if walking through the shelter is too stressful, a rolling

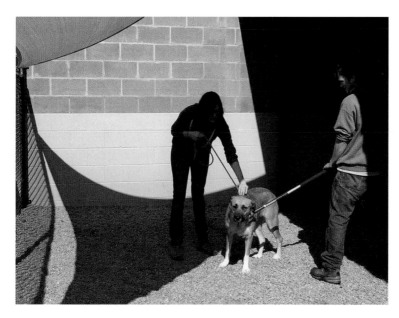

Figure 8.1   Simultaneous use of control pole and slip lead for handling of a dangerous dog.

crate can be used to move the dog around the shelter and minimize control pole use.

8.6.1.2   Returning Dogs to Kennels

When returning the dog to a single-housed kennel, toss treats in the back corner. This will help her associate returning with something pleasant. If resources allow, you can even give the dog an interactive food-stuffed toy. Note that food—even high-value food—will not be enough to counter some dogs' desire to avoid the kennel or stay with people. However, this method should be helpful for some percentage of kenneled dogs, particularly if employed from the very beginning *before* a dog develops an aversion to the kennel.

When handling a dog that tends to lunge as the kennel door is closed after putting her back, or a fearful dog who will bolt away as the door is opened, it may be helpful to fashion a quick-release by attaching a lightweight clip lead to the O-ring of the neck loop. The clip lead can be attached to the O-ring just moments before the dog is returned to her kennel to avoid loosening the neck loop while walking the dog. Once the dog is secure inside her kennel, the handler can remove

the leash by gently tugging on the leash where it connects to the O-ring, making the procedure hands-free. This way, the leash can be removed with the kennel door closed and braced with a foot (see Figure 8.2).

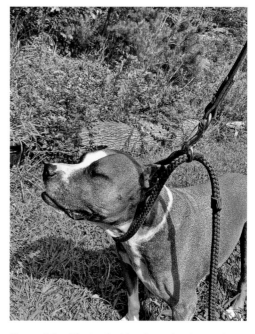

Figure 8.2   Slip lead with release leash attached.

8.6.2 Moving Dogs Around the Shelter

Once the dog is out of the kennel, it's best to avoid passing other dogs if possible. Some shelters will put all of the dogs on one side of the kennel runs with the guillotine door shut, just before walking time. When each individual dog is ready for their walk (or needs to be transported for some other reason), the door for that dog's kennel can be opened, and the dog can be leashed and taken out of the kennel on the empty side of the run. If there are dogs across the aisle, they should be put on the opposite side as well. This means that any dog walking down the center aisle will not be exposed to other dogs in kennels. If there are dogs only on one side, the handlers should position themselves on the side farthest from the kenneled dogs, to avoid the potential for a redirected bite to the handler. If having dogs on both sides of the aisle is unavoidable, the handler should try to keep the dog in the center of the aisle to maintain greatest distance.

When moving about the facility, avoid allowing dogs to come face-to-face or pass each other in close quarters, as this could result in a fight between dogs or cause a dog to redirect onto the handler (Overall 2013; Herron and Shreyer 2014). Even in cases not involving aggression, this is very stressful for many dogs and can lead to the development of aggressive behaviors. To prevent such interaction, have a designated entry and exit door if at all possible, as well as "one-way" traffic areas in kennel runs. If this is not an option, choose a path that passes by as few other dogs as possible. If kenneled dogs are on the handler's right side, the handler should be on the left side of the dog they're moving, so the human's body won't be directly between the dog they're moving and other dogs that dog might want to bite. It is important to keep enough distance between the dogs that they can't bite one another, and the handler should try not to bump the dog with their leg as they're walking as this can also cause a redirected bite. When moving through an area where another person, dog, or animal may be encountered, look around corners and calmly announce your approach, so that other workers have warning and can move out of the way or ask you to wait if necessary. Mirrors can be helpful on blind corners.

Handlers should also be aware of other sights, sounds, or smells that may be stressful for the dog. Loud noises, strong smells, and high traffic areas can be distressing for many dogs and should be avoided when possible (Overall 2013; Herron and Shreyer 2014; Edwards et al. 2019). Rooms can be wiped down with a veterinary deodorizer after an animal leaves to minimize lingering scents that may be distressing (Herron 2015).

Consider alternative strategies for dogs that are particularly fearful or have difficulty moving through the shelter for some other reason, such as physical limitations. Rolling cages can be used to transport dogs from one area of the shelter to another. A blanket or towel draped over the cage can provide further protection from stimulation and help the dog stay calm. Smaller dogs that tolerate handling may be able to be carried. In some cases, wrapping a dog with a blanket or towel and covering their face may help them relax. Each dog will need to be assessed individually to decide on their individual handling plan. Remember to observe body language closely and to stop and re-evaluate if the dog appears to be extremely stressed, is struggling, or is showing increasing levels of distress. Keep notes on each dog so that other staff and volunteers know which strategies work best for a particular dog. These notes can also be used to make adjustments to the plan for that particular dog.

8.6.3 Getting a Dog Comfortable with a New Handler

Some dogs may need some additional work in order to be comfortable with basic handling. For those dogs, it is very helpful to go through the process outlined in this section *before* a dog needs to be handled or removed from its kennel. That will allow them to have several positive experiences before asking them to tolerate touch or move from one place to another.

Whenever possible, handlers should give the dog the opportunity to approach them, rather than the handler approaching the dog. It is important to take this slow and to proceed at the dog's pace. Lack of control is a major factor influencing how stressful a particular experience is (Seligman and Maier 1967; Lucas et al. 2014). Giving the dog more control (such as approaching you when they are ready) will help reduce their stress. Taking a few extra minutes to let the dog get to know the handler before they take a dog out of their kennel can go a long way to making a fearful or anxious dog easier to handle down the road. When doing in-kennel socialization work, handlers should limit contact to 10–15 minutes at first, so that the dog does not become overwhelmed. Some dogs may need even shorter sessions or "drive-by treats" to start. Ideally, the dog should become more affiliative and easier to handle after every contact with a volunteer or staff member. If this is not the case, the training plan needs to be changed.

If taking a fearful dog out for a walk or other procedure, approach with non-threatening body language. Turn sideways and, if safe to do so, crouch down. Gently toss high-value treats toward them. Avoid making sudden or dramatic moves when tossing treats, as this can be scary. Instead, try to throw treats using a subtle flick of the wrist, rather than moving the entire forearm or arm. Avoid making direct eye contact. Talk quietly and calmly, using a welcoming tone of voice. Some dogs react better to silence, but some dogs seem to be spooked by this and will become more afraid if someone is completely quiet and still.

As the dog gains confidence, gradually toss treats closer to the handler. If the dog approaches, let them sniff without reaching for them or speaking suddenly or loudly. Many dogs need plenty of time to sniff (or sniff and

retreat) before they are ready for more direct interaction. Continue to ignore the dog until she solicits contact. Most dogs will do this by leaning against or pawing the handler, or pushing their nose or head under the handler's hand. If petting a shy or unknown dog, avoid reaching over their head or back. Instead, pet them gently on the side of the shoulder or neck. Many dogs dislike being touched on the head or hugged. Many dogs are also sensitive around their feet, belly, and rear end. Avoid sudden, fast movements, reaching toward or leaning over the dog, and sudden, loud noises.

Feeding high-value treats can help the dog to warm up more quickly, but be mindful that this can also make them approach more closely than they otherwise would. This makes it particularly important to avoid sudden movement and sound. If you do need to shift positions or stand up, toss food away so the dog is not right next to you when you stand. Watch them carefully for the signs of fear and stress discussed above. It can be helpful to teach fearful dogs to place their heads through a wide-open slip lead, luring with food at first.

8.6.4 Handling for Procedures

Additional steps can be taken for more invasive handling, such as grooming and medical procedures. The goal is to reduce the animal's stress as much as possible. Keeping dogs as calm as possible will also reduce the risk of injury to staff as well as the amount of time needed for procedures. The least amount of restraint necessary should be used. If an animal is struggling, stop and reassess. The general rule of thumb is three seconds for dogs and no more than three tries (Edwards et al. 2019). Animals should be restrained in a way that makes them as comfortable as possible. This includes giving them a non-slip surface and holding limbs in natural and comfortable positions (Overall 2013; Hammerle et al. 2015). Towels and blankets can also be a good option, particularly for smaller dogs (Overall 2013). When possible, also let the dog choose the location of the exam that they are most comfortable with—such as the table or the floor. Many animals are more comfortable on the floor than on the table (Döring et al. 2009).

Fear Free® (Fear Free, LLC, Denver, CO) training programs advocate for the use of a touch gradient. This involves touching the animal lightly first and continuing the exam with gradually escalating intensity of touch. For example, pet, tap, pinch, inject. During this process, the handler should maintain constant contact with at least one hand on the dog. This will help avoid a startle effect that can occur when the hands are removed and touch is initiated again. Again, dogs should be approached from the side, rather than from behind or head on. Many dogs are most comfortable being touched on the shoulder or side, so this is a good starting point. Avoid beginning the process by handling areas that are painful or frequently sensitive, such as the head, ears, feet, or tail.

During an exam or grooming procedure, food can be used as a distraction. This is most beneficial when circumstances or staff resources do not allow for gradually acclimating a dog to a procedure. This will probably be the case in most shelter environments. Food should be highly palatable. Examples include peanut butter, canned tuna, canned dog food, baby food, squeeze cheese, and freeze-dried real meat. Food can be placed in small disposable cups for the dogs to lick to avoid additional sanitization and cleanup time. Offer food even to dogs that are calm. This will help maintain their positive emotional state and reduce the likelihood of becoming fearful of handling, grooming, or veterinary procedures down the line.

8.6.5 Developing Positive Associations

The strategies described in Sections 8.6.1–8.6.4 are best for minimizing stress in the moment. However, they are not necessarily effective at preventing stress in the long run because the dog may start to associate the presence of food

(for example) with unpleasant experiences. In a shelter environment that has a training and/or behavior department, there are additional steps that can be taken to aid in handling. These processes can also be passed on to any new adopters for them to continue at home and during vet clinic visits.

8.6.5.1 Muzzle Training

Muzzle training is very beneficial for a number of reasons. Staff or volunteers can train dogs to wear a muzzle so that if they do need to be muzzled at some point, it doesn't add to their stress during a procedure. The Muzzle Up! Project is a great resource for information on muzzle training a dog (www.muzzleupproject.com).

8.6.5.2 Developing a Positive Emotional Response to Specific Locations

It can also be very helpful to establish a conditioned emotional response to the rooms where dogs are likely to be handled (such as grooming areas and clinic areas). If they have had multiple positive experiences in a room prior to having a potentially aversive experience, they may be more resilient. This will also minimize trigger stacking because the animal will not be stressed simply by being in an unfamiliar room.

The first step involves bringing the dog into the new space and letting them investigate at their own pace. High-value treats can be scattered on the ground or offered by hand. Scattering on the ground has the additional benefit of encouraging the dog to explore and associating multiple areas of the room (not just the area where the human is) with good things. However, it is also beneficial to teach the dog that good things come from the people in the room. It's important during this process to make sure inappropriate behavior is not being reinforced. For example, staff and volunteers should turn their back or stand up if the dog is barking, jumping, or pawing for attention or food and should not feed the dog during or immediately after any of these behaviors.

Once the dog is comfortable in the room and indicates they are ready for interaction, start to interact with the dog through training, quiet play, or gentle petting. If the dog does not approach, sit on a chair, sideways to the dog, and use the procedure detailed in Section 8.6.3 to increase comfort with the handler.

Taking measures to help the dog feel comfortable can extend beyond the veterinary and grooming areas to other appropriate areas of the shelter such as the room where potential adopters get acquainted with dogs. This can help maintain already positive feelings or reduce feelings of fear or stress associated with these contexts. It has the added benefit of starting to teach the dog that new areas *in general* are good, and they are more likely to show their best behavior to adopters when they are comfortable with the location.

8.6.6 Reducing Stress through Handling

Several studies have shown that petting and personal interaction reduce stress in shelter dogs. McGowan et al. (2018) found that 15 minutes of petting resulted in decreased signs of stress. This was the case even though the volunteer was unfamiliar to the dog. There is some evidence that petting may have a particularly strong impact on social dogs (Shin and Shin 2017). It even appears to help mitigate the impacts of an aversive experience, such as a blood draw (Hennessy et al. 1998). It's possible that petting per se is not the key factor—Shiverdecker and colleagues (2013) found that play and the passive (non-interactive) presence of a human also decreased cortisol—and there was no significant difference between dogs in those conditions and dogs that received petting. Therefore, shelters do not need to focus solely on petting as a possible source of stress reduction. Time spent together interacting in other ways, such as play or walking together, is likely to be beneficial as well.

8.7 Defensive Handling

What is defensive handling? It is a set of skills and techniques that keep the handler safe, starting with reading the dog's body language accurately, then learning to use a leash and the tools at hand to stay safe, and, finally, handling gently and calmly to minimize fear and reduce the risk of aggressive behavior.

8.7.1 Why Do We Need These Skills?

Learning how to safely handle dogs includes learning how to lengthen and shorten the leash to keep the dog away from triggers, as well as how to use body weight and center of balance to convince the dogs that the handler is strong and not easily budged by a hard pull. Defensive handling also includes some basic techniques to stay safe if a dog tries to bite a person or another dog.

Gentle, reward-based training and low-stress handling methods take a lot of the risk out of working with difficult dogs, but any time handlers work with animals that have teeth, they're at risk of a bite. We need to respect dogs' speed and strength in order to keep ourselves and other shelter animals safe.

One of the best investments a shelter can make is in training their staff and volunteers in safe, humane handling. Increasing the skills of the employees who work with the dogs every day is a win/win, as the dogs will behave better every time they're handled, and the employees will gain valuable skills to make them safer. Shelter workers and volunteers who haven't been properly trained in how to handle and work with dogs with behavior issues will have trouble staying safe around dogs who become stressed, fearful, or aggressive. This may result in injuries and perhaps fear of working with these types of animals in the future. As sheltering professionals, it is our responsibility to keep ourselves, our volunteers, our adopters, and the community as safe as possible.

8.7.2 Have a Plan

When working with dogs, it's important to be aware of your environment and to always be prepared for worst-case scenarios. If an off-leash dog charges a handler and their dog during a walk, what tools are available? Which way should they go? If a person comes around the corner while a handler is working with a reactive or fearful dog, should they cross the street? Get behind a car? Do a U-turn? If a dog-fight breaks out during shelter dog playgroups, what tools should be used, and in what order?

8.7.3 Equipment

8.7.3.1 Leashes

Many shelters choose to use slip leads for daily dog handling. If you have a short length of stay and dogs get adequate in- and out-of-kennel enrichment, the slip lead can be an effective tool. The other advantage to slip leads is that they can be tossed or gently dropped onto a dog without needing to fumble around their head or neck area to fit equipment or attach a leash. A correctly fitted slip lead can be safer than using a collar or harness with a clip leash, especially for the handler working with fearful or potentially aggressive dogs (see Figure 8.3). The downside to using slip leads is that, in the absence of actively teaching the dogs to walk on a loose leash, dogs can damage their tracheas or even choke themselves when they pull hard, out of excitement or fear. It is advised that at least the long-stay shelter dogs be taught to walk politely without pulling.

When using a slip lead to take a dog for a walk, it's important to fit the lead correctly for the side on which the handler will stand. Conventionally, dogs are handled on the handler's left, but shelter dogs generally don't have any formal training; whichever side feels strongest or safest to the handler is fine. The slip lead is properly positioned by making the lead into the letter "P," and then dropping it onto the dog at the left side of the handler. In this way, it will tighten across the top of the

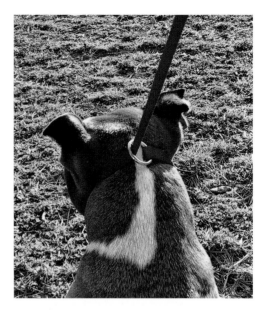

Figure 8.3 Correctly fitted slip lead.

dog's neck and release easily when the tension is relieved (see Figure 8.4).

When handling an excited shelter dog, it's important not to leave a lot of slack leash in

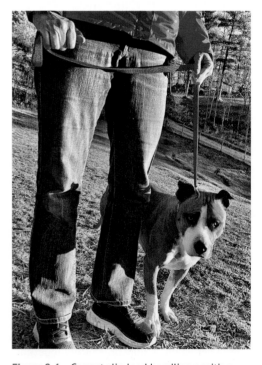

Figure 8.4 Correct slip lead handling position.

front of her face—this will easily start a game of tug-of-war and cause a loss of leash control. Ideally, the slip lead will be fitted high up on the dog's neck, right behind the ears, with the lead going straight up behind the dog's head, so it's not so easy for the dog to grab.

Leash width is also important. Rather than fitting the leash to the size of the dog, it's safest to use a leash that fits the handler's hand such that they can maintain a firm grip and easily use the techniques in this section. The leash should be able to lengthen and shorten easily, "lock" in the hand to keep it from slipping, and be of sufficient width so as not to cut into the hand if the dog pulls hard.

An average person's hand tends to fit a 5/8-inch leash well. A person with larger hands might choose a 3/4-inch leash. Leashes made of BioThane® (BioThane Coated Webbing Corp., North Ridgeville, OH) or leather are easy to grip and don't slip unless they're wet but can be expensive. Cotton or nylon leashes are strong but can slide through fingers. Handlers should use a leash that they can easily close their fingers around and that is easy to lengthen and shorten. Many shelters use rope leashes; these are fine for most people's hands, though they are inappropriate for shortening with the finger lock technique, as this spreads your fingers and reduces grip strength. Rope leads can be more easily shortened with a thumb lock (see Section 8.7.4.3).

The length of the leash should be adjusted for the work to be done with the dog and the environment. A 6-ft. leash is adequate for most situations, as it can be lengthened or shortened as needed, even with dogs who have behavioral issues. The shorter, thinner, 3- or 4-ft. nylon leads that many shelters buy are hard on people's hands and dogs' necks and are too short for most of the leash work described in this chapter. If this is all that is available, two of these can be attached together to give the handler and the dog more options.

8.7.3.2 Walking Equipment

If you are using 5- to 6-ft. shelter slip leads, these can be made into harnesses to take the

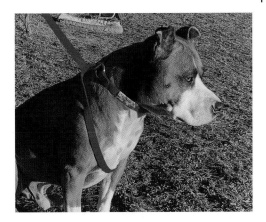

Figure 8.5 A slip lead positioned for use as a leash harness.

pressure off the dogs' throats. This can be a solution for hard pullers as well; just displacing the pressure to a different part of the body can help them stop pulling so hard. There are a few ways to do this, depending on the type of slip lead. If there is a large enough O-ring on the slip, pass the leash behind the dog's legs and back through the ring (see Figure 8.5). The Harness Lead (Beach Haven, NJ) and The Walkie™ (W Squared, Inc.) use similar mechanisms. For puppies, dogs who are unused to a collar, toy-breed dogs, and brachycephalic breeds, a vest style, H-back, or step-in harness with a clip on the back are all safe and gentle.

Front-attach harnesses are very popular and can work well to keep dogs from pulling hard. However, some brands can be difficult to get on squirmy dogs, and this design puts the leash right in front of the dog's mouth, where it's fun for them to grab. Some dogs get defensive about being harnessed if they ever get the skin behind their elbows pinched while clipping the harness. Staff and volunteers should be taught to be careful about this. Putting a hand between the plastic clip and the dog will ensure that if anyone gets pinched, it will be the human. Walking harnesses are often fitted incorrectly, which can create an escape risk and can also be painful for the dogs or chafe behind the front legs. Staff and volunteer training in low-stress equipment handling is vital, as is a good understanding of how the manufacturers intended their equipment to be fitted. Using treats while putting on head halters, martingale collars, or harnesses can help desensitize dogs to the equipment every time you take them out or put them back. A smear of peanut butter on the wall or lick mat or a scattering of treats on the ground can also distract the dog while they're getting "dressed," and these simple counterconditioning techniques should be part of staff and volunteer training if this equipment is used.

One other equipment tip: if using coats to walk dogs during frigid winter weather, use only coats with VELCRO® (Velcro IP Holdings, LLC, Manchester, NH) closures. Many a dog has been upset and many a shelter worker has been bitten trying to squeeze a dog's head or legs into a sweater.

8.7.3.3 Collars

For most shelter dog handling, if not using slip leads alone, a martingale collar is safe and, when adjusted properly, hard for the dog to slip out of. If the metal pieces are able to touch one another when the collar is pulled tight, the collar needs to be shortened up a bit, so there's at least a couple of fingers' width between the rings. The loop should not hang so loosely that a leg or jaw can get stuck. A martingale collar with a clip attachment is easier to put on nervous dogs than those that have to be pushed over their heads, but the plastic clip may be a weak point.

A well-fitted flat buckle collar can be a good tool for dogs who aren't good at slipping out of them and for dogs who don't pull hard. They may not safely fit dogs with thick necks and smaller heads.

8.7.3.4 Head Halters

There are several types of head halters. These can be great tools for controlling extremely large dogs or dogs who have a tendency to redirect aggression onto their handler. This equipment does need to be fitted correctly,

and some dogs, even with careful desensitization, will always protest wearing them. A frequent mistake with the commonly used Gentle Leader® (Radio Systems Corporation, Knoxville, TN) is the neck strap fitting too loosely. Follow the manufacturer's instructions and ensure that only one finger fits under the neck strap. The muzzle strap should be loose enough to allow panting. Gentle leash handling is particularly important with this powerful tool; the leash should be loose unless you are giving direct information to the dog about slowing down, moving forward, or turning. It can also be helpful to use a more lightweight leash clip so there isn't as much weight on the dog's nose.

8.7.4 Leash Handling

Using low-stress, reward-based methods will make dogs less likely to become offensively or defensively aggressive toward their handlers. Even so, handlers occasionally meet dogs who will try to bite or who will redirect aggression on them when frustrated by something out of reach. It is important to know how to defend oneself if this sort of thing happens.

8.7.4.1 How to Hold a Leash

Dogs' jaws are very fast and well coordinated. When working with shelter dogs, the leash is the handler's primary tool. Holding a leash correctly and firmly can save milliseconds in the event of a bite attempt. Hold the leash sloppily, and one can end up with a bite wound or a broken hand. It is safest to hold the leash with the hand closest to the dog, in order to keep it short while walking through tight spaces in the shelter.

8.7.4.2 Hand Holds

When handling a potentially aggressive dog, arm strength is best used by ensuring the "dog end" of the leash always comes out of the pinkie finger side of the hand. If the leash comes out of the index finger side of the hand while holding a snapping dog at arm's length, the handler will have far less strength, the hand and arm may twist, and there may be the risk of a bite or other injury. While handling a strong or difficult dog, it's important to keep the leash in the hand closest to the dog and to never put one's body between the dog and the kennels, if possible.

8.7.4.3 Leash Locks

It is important to ensure the leash cannot slip through the hands. If the leash accidentally slips out and lengthens, a fearful or aggressive dog may have room to bite a dog or human who is passing by. Here's where the leash lock comes in. While shortening the leash, the piece that is shortened will go over the finger (see Figure 8.6) or thumb (see Figure 8.7). When the hand is closed again *around the whole leash*, it will be far less likely to slip through the

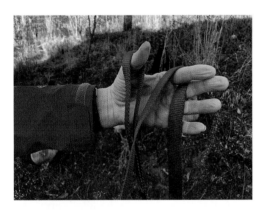

Figure 8.6   Finger lock.

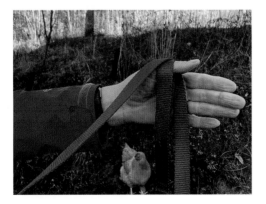

Figure 8.7   Thumb lock.

hand, at least if the handler's grip strength is good. If round rope leashes are used, the thumb lock is preferable to the finger lock. Many people prefer to wrap the leash around their wrist or the palm of their hands, but these grips are not as easy to let go of if a handler needs to back tie the dog or get away from her. Under no circumstance should a leash be wrapped around a hand or a wrist multiple times, as this can seriously injure a handler (Forrester 2020), and it will be much more difficult to get away from a dog who becomes aggressive. Handlers should use the leash grip that is most comfortable AND safe.

8.7.4.4 Accordion

There may be times that handlers want to shorten the leash without using the leash lock—perhaps they find themselves lengthening and shortening the leash many times while walking through the shelter, or perhaps they're working a dog on a long line and need to gather a number of loops into one hand.

In these cases, the "accordion" leash-shortening method might be most appropriate: starting the hold, as always, with the leash handle over just a thumb, and then folding it into "bunny ears" in the hand (see Figure 8.8). This hold is easy to lengthen, as the handler just needs to open and close the hand once, and the dog has the full 6 ft. again. This will allow handlers to more easily increase distance from an aggressive or over-aroused dog and shut the leash in a door, or to wrap the leash around a pole or handle, in order to back tie the dog (see Section 8.7.6.3).

8.7.5   Balance and Body Awareness

When working with dogs, especially dogs who may panic or aggress, it is important to stay balanced and ready to counteract any of the dog's movements to avoid being pulled off one's feet or lose control of the dog. It is best to wear safe, practical clothing when handling dogs—closed-toe shoes or boots with good grip

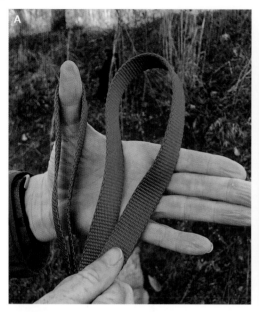 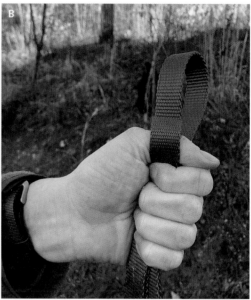

Figure 8.8 An accordion leash hold can be formed by folding the leash into "bunny ears" (A) and then closing the hand (B). Opening the hand instantly allows the dog to have the full leash length.

for the surface underfoot. If the dog being handled has a tendency to redirect aggression onto the handler, sturdy jeans or work pants will offer leg protection, and for some dogs, Kevlar® (DuPont de Nemours, Inc.) handling gloves may be advised. There will be less dexterity with gloves, but when it is necessary to work in closer contact with dogs who may bite, the trade-off may be worth it.

In general, when working with more difficult or unknown dogs, it's best to stay standing up. If appearing smaller might gain a dog's trust, the handler might squat or go down on one knee rather than sitting or kneeling all the way down. That way if the dog's behavior changes, it is easy for the person to stand up and get out of the way. When standing still with a dog, it is best to keep feet roughly shoulder width apart. If the dog is pulling in one direction, the handler's weight can be positioned over the opposite foot, to counterbalance the dog's weight. Most people's center of balance is around belly button height, so keeping hands low and close to the body will increase safety and strength. This will also more easily allow leash shortening for better defensive handling, if needed.

When walking with a dog, hands should be low and weight should be solidly over the feet so that the handler can't easily be pulled off balance. If a dog needs to be restrained or walked in the opposite direction as a distraction passes, the handler can smoothly slide a hand down the leash to a short hold that doesn't leave the dog room to reach another dog or person if she decides to lunge or bite. The exact distance will depend on the size of the dog, the length of the handler's arm, and the equipment being used. It is important to give the dog slack on the leash as soon as the distraction passes. If the dog is trying to jump up on someone in a friendly way, try dropping treats on the ground or putting a foot on the leash to keep the dog from being reinforced by the person's attention.

8.7.6 Handling Scenarios

8.7.6.1 Redirected Aggression
A lot of redirected bites can be avoided by good leash handling and body positioning, as well as by avoiding blind corners and maintaining an appropriate distance from potential triggers. Handlers should try to avoid coming between

the dog they're walking and a row of kennels. If a dog is actively trying to bite, they should straighten the leash arm (consider a two-handed leash hold for stronger dogs) and hold the dog away. It may be wise to walk a known redirector on either a head halter, a muzzle, or both so that control of her mouth is maintained.

8.7.6.2 Highly Aroused Dogs

Maintaining dogs in social isolation can cause behavioral deterioration, especially in shelters with longer lengths of stay and in the absence of effective in-kennel and out-of-kennel enrichment programs. Shelters should aspire to stay within their capacity for care in part by reducing length of stay. Institutional living can be stressful for social animals, so it is important to move them into adoptive homes without unnecessary delay (Newbury et al. 2010).

Giving dogs social time with humans and dogs outside of their kennels and giving them lots of feeding and chewing enrichment in their kennels will also help avoid over-arousal and leash climbing. Co-kenneling can also help, especially with dog-social, mouthy adolescents. Consider sending behaviorally deteriorating dogs to foster care—even for one night or a weekend. Positive traits that may enhance adoptability may be discovered once the dog is in a home environment.

A common behavior issue while walking shelter dogs is leash-grabbing, which can escalate to biting at the clothing, arms, or legs of the handler. This should be considered a cry for help from the dog, and steps should be taken to get them out of the shelter environment completely and help them cope with shelter life until that time.

Some techniques to discourage leash-grabbing in the short term include:

- Making the leash taste terrible (vinegar or bitter-flavored spray)
- Using a chain leash, making the part of the leash closest to the dog out of a sturdy choke chain, or covering the dog side of the leash with a piece of PVC pipe
- Offering the dog a stuffed toy, chewy, or rope toy they would rather carry or play tug with

during the walk (the handler may need to keep holding the other end of a rope toy to keep it interesting)
- Ensuring that the slip lead is fitted high up, behind the dog's ears, and then goes straight up behind her head to the handler
- Straightening the arms and holding the dog away from the handler with the leash if the dog is grabbing at the sleeves or body.

8.7.6.3 Back Ties

There should be places in each area of the shelter where the leash can be run through a hook, handle, rail, or carabiner to pull the dog away from the handler or against the wall. These back ties are a safe way to maintain control while waiting for the dog to calm down, for a second handler and second leash, or for a control pole to get the dog back to their kennel. If an aggressive dog needs to be held away from a handler on a walk, running the leash around a tree or fence post can serve a similar function.

8.7.6.4 Control Pole Use and Storage

A control pole (sometimes referred to as a "catch" pole) is an infrequently used emergency measure to move a dog who can't be secured by any other means. It should never be used on a small dog or cat, as severe injury or death may result. Alternatives to a control pole must always be considered, such as a rolling crate, a towel, a Snappy Snare, a squeeze cage, or sedation. Many dogs are reactive when confined in a kennel. Prior to using a control pole on such dogs, and if movement of the dog is not urgent, try housing the dog in a guillotine kennel and spending a few days winning her over with food or walks. Most dogs who have once been pets can be walked using a simple leash once they adjust to shelter life.

Every ward should have a control pole near the fight kit (see Section 8.7.7)—it is wise to put an appropriate length pole in each area, for the job it is likely to have to do. Shorter poles may be easier to manage, especially in a smaller kennel run or for certain types of veterinary handling, but they will also put the dog closer to the handler, which can be more dangerous.

Never store a control pole by hanging it by the wire noose or by propping the noose end on the ground. These practices will kink the line, making it harder to tighten and loosen, and may present a safety hazard to both the handler and the dog. Control poles should be hung via attachments to the pole handle and should be regularly checked for wear and to ensure they still work properly.

A control pole needs to be positioned correctly, with the pole at the top of the dog's neck, to avoid having the wire twist. Handlers should practice tightening and loosening the noose on a stuffed dog or other suitable-sized object, even a coworker's wrist, before attempting to use it on a live dog. Adrenaline can often cause people to pull the neck loop too tight, easily hurting or choking a dog with this powerful tool. Application of the techniques described in this chapter will help minimize the need for using a control pole.

The control pole needs to be used like a rigid leash; it is important to avoid pushing on it or putting excessive pressure on the dog's neck. Ask the dog to move gently, beside the handler, and give her a clear path forward. Never use the pole to drag a dog behind the handler or to lift the dog onto an elevated surface. Circle with her if necessary. Again, a rolling crate or chemical restraint may be safer and more humane options if moving a fearful or potentially aggressive dog a considerable distance. Using a second handler and leash and doing most of the guiding with the leash rather than the pole may be less stressful for the dog.

8.7.6.5 Off-Leash Dogs

If an off-leash dog is trying to bite, first try to defuse the situation by using non-confrontational body language. Slow movements, avoiding direct eye contact, and backing away slowly are often safer options than physically confronting a potentially aggressive dog.

If the dog continues to threaten, handlers should use whatever tools are at hand. All workers should have training on the location of fight kits and the use of the tools in them (see Section 8.7.7). Doors or escape routes should be noted. Handlers who are threatened by an unleashed, potentially aggressive dog might put themselves in a kennel run or climb on or over a table, fence, or vehicle.

Handlers should be taught to scan the environment for objects to put between them and the dog, like a chair or a trash can, and to look for something they might "feed" to the dog, such as an item of clothing, a toy, or a leash. They might direct the dog's attention onto this inanimate object by wiggling it in front of them. It is really important to remain on one's feet. Handlers might grab something with one hand to avoid falling down, turn their body sideways, and use their feet to keep the dog away from more vital body parts. As a last resort, positioning one's back against a wall or in a corner means the dog can't easily pull a handler down.

If the dog has a grip on clothing or a body part and is shaking her head, the handler should grab the collar, scruff, or sides of her head to minimize that head movement. Handlers might try standing over the dog and gripping her waist between their knees in "control position" if she's biting someone else (see Figure 8.9). If there is a break stick in the nearest fight kit, this can be an effective way to get a dog to release their grip. Handlers can also try "feeding the bite" (i.e., pushing the biting dog forward into the victim, causing the dog to recoil and release) or using a noise interrupter to get the dog to release and back off. The goal is to get the dog on a leash and behind a door, preferably in a kennel. Closing the door on the leash can keep the dog from biting others on the other side, if it is not a kennel door. See Section 8.7.7 for further discussion of these techniques.

As a last resort, and if there is not a break stick or other tool handy, getting water into a dog's nose and mouth may get her to release her grip. It is important that someone has the dog in control position when the grip is released, so that the dog cannot then redirect

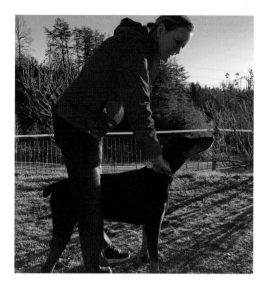

Figure 8.9 "Control position" for restraining a dog that is attempting to bite.

her aggression on the handler. Dogs can be harder to handle when wet and slippery, so using a break stick or other dogfight tools may be preferable.

If a dangerous dog does manage to pull a handler down, it may be safest to curl up into a ball and play dead, using the hands to cover the neck. If veterinary staff are available, a gripping dog can be sedated intramuscularly in order to get them to release a grip on a human or another dog. Another option is to use a slip lead, collar, or belt and lift up on the dog's neck until the dog lets go in order to get a breath of air. A taser may be another option to get a dog to back off or let go—sometimes just the crackling sound is enough to accomplish this.

8.7.7 Breaking Up a Dogfight

Although it's important to try to avoid dogfights, they will happen from time to time, when attention slips, when a dog escapes, or when someone makes a miscalculation about behavior. The defensive maneuvers that come naturally to us as humans are often quite dangerous when applied to a dogfight. Grabbing collars, punching, kicking, trying to pry mouths apart with our fingers—these are all potentially very risky moves.

When faced with a dogfight, first take a breath and think. Where are the tools? Who else is around? And most importantly, which dog is the aggressor? That is the one who will need to be removed from the situation first. The goal, in order to keep people and dogs safe, is to get this dog behind a door, through a gate, or into a kennel. Sometimes there is more than one dog actively aggressing and, in these cases, there should be a second handler to deal with that dog or to remove one and then attempt to contain the second. Alternatively, one dog can be tied to something secure, and then the second dog can be broken away and removed from the area. A loud alarm, such as an air horn or walkie-talkie button, can function as a call for help if a handler is alone when a dogfight breaks out in a ward or play yard. There should be one in each fight kit, and/or a "panic button" in each ward, so shelter workers can easily summon help.

If a fight breaks out in a playgroup and someone is actively breaking up the fight, other helpers should quickly and efficiently remove each of the non-combatant dogs and take them to a safe place or attach them to the fence with a carabiner. Ideally, dogs who are interacting in a play or adoption area will be wearing drag leashes so that their leashes can simply be picked up. If not, use (or make) a slip lead to get the other dogs out of the area safely, one at a time. Slip leads can be fashioned out of clip leads by running the clip through the handle, creating a circle at one end for the dog's head.

Next, concentrate on the aggressor. Fight kits should be available in each play yard and in areas of the facility that people can easily access during an emergency (see Box 8.1).

Fight kits should be inventoried at least every two months. Make sure the spray devices are checked as would be done for a fire extinguisher, to ensure they're still pressurized and full, and check the condition and function of control poles at the same time.

Box 8.1 Fight Kit Contents
● Extra slip leads ● Squirt bottle with water ● Citronella spray ● Compressed air ● Air horn ● Break sticks

It is also important to realize that most dog-fights are just spit and noise and often sound a lot worse than they actually are. Even dogs who are trained and conditioned to fight can fight for many minutes, even hours—so in most cases there is time to get the tools and help needed to break up the fight without injury to humans. Exceptions to this, which often require an urgent response, include:

● Large dog versus small dog
● Blocked airway
● Blocked blood flow (tight neck grip and victim dog losing consciousness).

Even in many of these cases, it may still be preferable to take time to get the proper tools than to wade in without anything other than one's own body to break up the fight.

It is important that staff be trained in canine body language and play behavior, so that they can tell the difference between normal dog play and actual aggression that needs to be interrupted. There are two general types of dogfights: "slash and dash," where the dogs are biting or snapping and releasing, and "gripping" fights, where one or both dogs are holding on tightly and may be shaking their heads from side to side. Some tools and techniques to break up a dogfight are more appropriate for "slash and dash" fights and some work better for "gripping" fights; while a variety of tools and techniques can be used, these should generally proceed from least to most invasive for each given scenario.

The least invasive way to break up a fight is by picking up each dog's drag leash and walking in opposite directions. Please note, this will not work on a "gripping" fight; indeed, pulling dogs apart who are gripping can increase damage. The next least invasive way to break up a dogfight involves using a squirt bottle. Many dogs will back down from an altercation or release their grip if they get even slightly wet. In a more severe, gripping fight, a hose or water bottle can be used to put water into the dog's nose or mouth. Other objects you might have at hand are a bowl or bottle of water, or a pressurized water fire extinguisher.

A loud voice or noise maker can also be an effective method of breaking up a fight. Anything that makes a loud noise can startle dogs into backing off from a fight, providing time to leash or corral the aggressor and get them out of the situation. The noise should be emitted fairly close to the dog's head, but not so close that they can easily redirect their bite onto the handler or the noisemaker itself. It is also important to use these tools judiciously; noisemakers may frighten other dogs in the area who are not involved in the fight. Box 8.2 lists common noisemakers to include in a fight kit.

Hands-on techniques may also be used to break up a dogfight. These techniques carry increased risk of bites to the handlers, so the hands-off techniques should be tried first. These include placing something between fighting dogs, throwing something over the dogs, the "wheelbarrow," "feeding the bite," and using a break stick.

Anything in the environment can be used to split two dogs up: a trash can, a folding table or chair, a pig board. Bring the object in between the two dogs, and then remove the aggressor once they are split apart. This may not be the best option if one dog is gripping the other, as you may cause skin and flesh to tear. Throwing something over the dogs will briefly make their world "go dark"; dogs may then stop fighting long enough for one of them to be removed. A blanket, towel, or jacket can be tossed over the dogs' heads. Throwing a thick towel or blanket over smaller dogs can also make it safer to pick them up once they split up.

Box 8.2   Common Fight Kit Noisemakers

Shake can

Fill a can or bottle with pebbles or pennies and shake near the dog's head.

Large shake bottle

Fill a half-gallon or gallon size jug with some pennies or pebbles; shake near the dog's head and, if large enough to do so safely, insert between fighting dogs before shaking.

Bowls

Clang two metal bowls together near the dog's head.

Compressed air

Activate the device near the dog's head to emit a loud hissing noise (do not point this at the dog's skin or face).

Air horn

Use as a last resort to disrupt a fight and/or as an emergency call for help.

Citronella spray

Spray directly into the dog's nose or mouth to get her to back off or release a grip. Take the can outside and practice releasing the safety catch and hitting rocks or other inanimate objects prior to use. Scent also acts as a disruptor.

If the dogs are not gripping one another, the "wheelbarrow" can be a fairly safe, hands-on way to separate them. This can be done with one handler "wheelbarrowing" each dog, or if alone, the handler should concentrate on the aggressor. Grasp the dog by the top of the thighs, where they meet the abdomen. Lift the dog's hind end in the air, and back up in order to walk or swing her away. Ideally the handler will circle to break the aggressor's eye contact with the other dog. If the aggressor is a larger dog, lift her back end and walk backward, circling to keep the dog from being able to come around and bite. The goal is to back the dog into another area and get her away from the dog she is biting long enough to get leashed, into control position, or to remove the other dog.

If the dogs are gripping and a fight kit is not available, "feeding the bite" is another way to get a dog to release. When using this technique, it is very important to first get the dog into control position—stabilizing the dog by stepping over her with your legs between her ribcage and hip bones (see Figure 8.9). Hold the dog who is gripping by the collar or the scruff, and then push her head into the body part she's gripping. This technique will work better if she's gripping a solid body part like a shoulder, rather than a moveable part like an ear or a tail. This move can part the aggressor's jaws enough to pull the dogs apart.

Also known as a "parting stick" or incorrectly as a "bite stick," a break stick is a piece of equipment, usually made of wood or hard plastic, specially made to pry open a dog's jaws during a gripping fight. Starting with the gripping dog in control position and grabbing the collar right at the base of the skull are essential so that the dog can't redirect and bite the handler once they release. If the dog is not wearing a collar, a leash may be wrapped around her neck or the dog may be grasped by the scruff. Holding the break stick parallel to the jaw, work it into the dog's mouth, right behind the canine teeth so that approximately 1 inch of the stick is in the dog's mouth. Caution and discretion should be used as this may result in fractured teeth, but this technique can also minimize damage to the victim dog. Twist the handle, rotating the stick until the grip is broken, and then get the aggressor out of the situation; onto a back tie or through a gate or door. If both dogs are gripping, one person will need to release each dog's grip. If working with a particularly large or strong dog, two people may be needed, with a break stick inserted on either side of the dog's mouth. If the handler is alone, one dog should be secured by a leash to something sturdy before attempting to get the other dog to release.

Any time two dogs with teeth are together, deliberately or accidentally, there is the possibility of a fight that can lead to serious injury. Shelter handlers should have the equipment and training to break altercations up quickly and safely.

8.8 Handling Dogs during the Process of Euthanasia

Euthanasia is an unfortunate reality in animal shelters. Some animals are euthanized in order to end suffering brought on by illness or injury. Others need to be euthanized for behavior or space reasons. Regardless of the circumstances, it is our obligation to make sure that shelter dogs experience a "good death" (euthanasia means "good death" in Greek). A complete discussion of handling dogs during the euthanasia process is beyond the scope of this chapter, and the reader is referred to the Association of Shelter Veterinarians' *Guidelines for Standards of Care in Animal Shelters* (Newbury et al. 2010), the 2nd edition of *Shelter Medicine for Veterinarians and Staff* (Smith-Blackmore 2012), and the American Veterinary Medical Association's *Guidelines for the Euthanasia of Animals* (Leary et al. 2020) for more details. This chapter will focus on environmental management, euthanasia techniques, and animal handling most pertinent for behavioral euthanasia of dogs (e.g., for reasons of aggression, severe anxiety or undersocialization, fear). There are several steps that can help make this a less stressful experience for both the dog and the shelter personnel.

8.8.1 Environment

If possible, spend some time prior to euthanasia doing something the dog enjoys such as playing, petting, or taking a walk. Offer them delectable food. Euthanasia should be done in a quiet, comfortable room away from highly trafficked areas. A white noise machine may help mask additional sounds. It should have comfortable bedding; the use of dog-appeasing pheromone (DAP) may also help reduce anxiety in the shelter environment (Tod et al. 2005). Some shelters have an area that is furnished similar to a room in a home that can be used as a location for euthanasia. Many shelters have the resources to teach a dog to develop a positive conditioned emotional response to various locations in the shelter; this is a great room to add to the list. That way, if a dog needs to be euthanized, she will be familiar with and comfortable in the room.

Measures should be taken to ensure that good sanitation procedures are followed between each euthanasia procedure. We know that dogs are highly sensitive to chemical signals and social animals release alarm pheromones when distressed (Verheggen et al. 2010) so, while this has not been studied in dogs, it's reasonable to expect that dogs could become distressed simply by being in a room where dogs have recently died. Similarly, potentially aversive or disruptive auditory stimuli should be silenced (e.g., two-way radios, telephones, public address systems). Animals should not be permitted to observe or hear the euthanasia of other animals or permitted to view the bodies of dead animals (with the possible exception of euthanasia of multiple neonatal littermates or closely bonded animals for whom separation may be more distressing). When euthanasia is in progress, a clearly visible sign should be placed on each entry point to the room prohibiting entry.

Although a designated euthanasia room is often desirable from a logistical and shelter management standpoint, it is crucial to recognize that many animals will be stressed by novel environments. Extremely undersocialized, fearful dogs will be traumatized simply by moving the dog to a euthanasia room. For this reason, electing to perform euthanasia in the kennel or ward where the animal resides should be considered and may be the most humane option. In these cases, exposure for adjacent animals can be minimized by temporarily relocating them or by using curtains to obscure the view and mask any vocalizations. Additional planning, precautions, and communication with all shelter personnel may be necessary to ensure the same level of environmental control over the kennel or ward can be maintained as if the euthanasia were taking place in a designated room.

Once the dog is present in the space where euthanasia will take place, ensure she has time to acclimate to the area (if novel) and get comfortable. If possible and safe, have at least one person present with whom the dog is familiar and comfortable; however, the total number of personnel present should be limited to those directly involved in the euthanasia process. The low-stress handling and restraint methods outlined throughout this chapter should be employed during the euthanasia process, remembering to always use the minimum amount of restraint. Use high-value food as a distraction to keep the dog calm and happy.

8.8.2 Euthanasia Techniques and Handling Methods

Humane euthanasia should be achieved through the administration of a sodium pentobarbital solution (often called "euthanasia solution"). For dogs, intravenous (IV) administration is the only acceptable route in the majority of circumstances. The intraperitoneal route may be used for puppies less than 10 lbs (Smith-Blackmore 2012). For dogs that are unconscious or anesthetized prior to injection, intracardiac is also acceptable (Newbury et al. 2010). Each of these routes of administration has advantages and disadvantages, including variations in time to effect, which must be considered for each animal. In all instances, using a new needle of the smallest gauge possible will serve to reduce pain and discomfort during administration.

If the dog is dangerous, difficult to manage, or very anxious, the use of antianxiety medications and/or sedatives to reduce the dog's stress and keep everyone safe should be considered. The choice of sedative, dose, and route should be discussed with and prescribed by the shelter veterinarian. This discussion should occur before the euthanasia process has begun, even in cases where the use of antianxiety medications or sedatives may not be needed.

Humane handling during administration of pre-euthanasia sedatives is critical; dogs must be kept as calm as possible through the point of loss of consciousness. In the cases of dogs that are overtly aggressive, severely undersocialized, or exhibiting extreme fear, creative restraint techniques may be needed to minimize stress and ensure staff safety. Least invasive may be chemical restraint through the administration of oral sedatives (including unconstituted sodium pentobarbital powder) mixed in a high-value food item (e.g., raw ground meat). (Note that if unconsciousness is achieved through oral administration of sodium pentobarbital powder, IV injection of sodium pentobarbital solution is still required to induce death.) Trans-mucosal administration of anesthetics (e.g., ketamine, dexmedetomidine) may be possible without direct handling by squirting the anesthetic solution directly into the dog's mouth. A third option that does not require direct animal handling is the delivery of tranquilizing agents through a blow dart; this method requires specialized equipment and is not recommended in the absence of formal training and a skilled, experienced darter.

When physical handling is required, a variety of tools and techniques can be employed to minimize handling and reduce associated stress. For dogs housed in cages or small kennels and that are unlikely to lunge toward the cage front, a pole syringe can be passed through cage or kennel bars to deliver an intramuscular (IM) sedative. For dogs that can be handled on a leash, use of a restraint gate (a single panel gate, usually chain link, mounted to the middle of a solid wall) may be effective. The dog can be walked up to the open gate (facing the hinge) and gently compressed between the wall and the gate. While the handler holds the leash taut, another trained staff member can safely administer an IM sedative in the hind end. An existing door that abuts a wall, pig board, or other large solid item can also be used in this manner in the absence of a restraint gate. Finally, a squeeze cage (also called a transfer or restraint cage) may also be an option when less invasive options are not feasible. A squeeze cage contains a built-in mechanism that allows for one side wall of the cage to be pulled toward the other, with the dog compressed and immobilized in between, for administration of IM sedatives. It may be possible to train dogs to enter the squeeze cage prior to use to facilitate this process. Once the dog is sedated or unconscious, they can be systematically scanned for a microchip, and euthanasia by IV injection can safely proceed as planned.

8.9 Conclusions

Great handling can make all the difference in keeping shelter staff safe, increasing the well-being of shelter dogs, and increasing adoptions. Training on low-stress handling, starting with learning to read body language, is one of the most important trainings shelter staff and volunteers can receive. With proper techniques, each animal should become more comfortable, not less comfortable, each time they're handled. Animal handlers must also be trained in basic safety measures including what to do if a dog tries to bite and how to break up a dogfight. When euthanasia is necessary, careful planning and consideration of the environment and route of euthanasia along with practicing low-stress animal handling techniques can ensure the process is humane.

Please visit the companion website for video clips and downloadable resources associated with this chapter.

References

Beerda, B., Schilder, M., Janssen, N. et al. (1996). The use of saliva cortisol, urinary cortisol and catecholamine measurements for noninvasive assessment of stress responses in dogs. *Horm. Behav.* 30: 272–279.

Beerda, B., Schilder, M.B.H., van Hooff, J.A.R.A.M. et al. (1998). Behavioural, saliva cortisol and heart rate responses to different types of stimuli in dogs. *App. Anim. Behav. Sci.* 58: 365–381.

Beerda, B., Schilder, M., van Hooff, J.A.R.A.M. et al. (1999). Chronic stress in dogs subjected to social and spatial restriction. *I. Behavioral responses. Physiol. Behav.* 66 (2): 233–242.

Chmelíková, E., Bolechová, P., Chaloupková, H. et al. (2020). Salivary cortisol as a marker of acute stress in dogs: A review. *Domest. Anim. Endocrinol.* 72: 106428.

Coppola, C.L., Grandin, T.R., and Enns, M.R. (2006). Human interaction and cortisol: Can human contact reduce stress for shelter dogs? *Physiol. Behav.* 87: 537–541.

Corsetti, S., Borruso, S., Di Traglia, M. et. al. (2018). Bold personality makes domestic dogs entering a shelter less vulnerable to disease. *PLOS ONE.* https://doi.org/10.1371/journal.pone.0193794.

Dickens, M.J., Delehanty, D.J., and Romero, L.M. 2010. Stress: An inevitable component of animal translocation. *Biol. Conserv.* 143: 1329–1341.

Dickerson, S.S. and Kemeny, M.E. (2004). Acute stressors and cortisol responses: A theoretical integration and synthesis of laboratory research. *Psychol. Bull.* 130 (3): 355–391.

Döring, D., Roscher, A., Scheipl, F. et al. (2009). Fear-related behavior of dogs in veterinary practice. *Vet. J.* 182: 38–43.

Dreschel, N.A. (2010). The effects of fear and anxiety on health and lifespan in pet dogs. *Appl. Anim. Behav. Sci.* 125 (3): 157–162.

Edwards, P.T., Smith, B.P., McArthur, M.L. et al. (2019). Fearful Fido: Investigating dog experience in the veterinary context in an effort to reduce distress. *Appl. Anim. Behav. Sci.* 213: 14–25.

Forrester, M. (2020). Dog leash-related injuries treated at emergency departments. *Am. J. Emerg. Med.* 38 (9): 1782–1786.

Glaser, R. and Kiecolt-Glaser, J.K. (2005). Stress-induced immune dysfunction: Implications for health. *Nat. Rev. Immunol.* 5: 243–251.

Grandin, T. (1998). Review: Reducing handling stress improves both productivity and welfare. *Prof. Anim. Sci.* 14: 1–10.

Hammerle, M., Horst, C., Levine, E. et al. (2015). 2015 AAHA canine and feline behavior management guidelines. *J. Am. Anim. Hosp. Assoc.* 51: 205–221.

Hennessy, M.B., Morris, A., and Linden, F. (2006). Evaluation of the effects of a socialization program in a prison on behavior and pituitary-adrenal hormone levels of shelter dogs. *Appl. Anim. Behav. Sci.* 99 (1): 157–171.

Hennessy, M.B., Williams, M.T., Miller. D.D. et al. (1998). Influence of male and female petters on plasma cortisol and behaviour: Can human interaction reduce the stress of dogs in a public animal shelter? *Appl. Anim. Behav. Sci.* 61: 63–77.

Hennessy, M.B., Willen, R.M., and Schiml, P.A. (2020). Psychological stress, its reduction, and long-term consequences: What studies with laboratory animals might teach us about life in the dog shelter. *Animals* 10 (11): 2061.

Herron, M.E. (2015). Low-stress handling in veterinary practice—The new norm or still a novel concept? *Adv. Small Anim. Med. Surg.* 28 (9): 1–2.

Herron, M.E. and Shreyer, T. (2014). The pet-friendly veterinary practice: A guide for practitioners. *Vet. Clin. North Am. Small Anim. Pract.* 44: 451–481.

Hiby, E.F., Rooney, N.J., and Bradshaw, J.W.S. (2006). Behavioural and physiological responses of dogs entering re-homing kennels. *Physiol. Behav.* 89: 385–391.

Juster, R., McEwen, B.S., and Lupien, S.J. (2010). Allostatic load biomarkers of chronic stress and impact on health and cognition. *Neurosci. Biobehav. Rev.* 35: 2–16.

Koolhaas, J.M., Korte, S.M., De Boer, S.F. et al. (1999). Coping styles in animals: Current status in behavior and stress-physiology. *Neurosci. Biobehav. Rev.* 23 (7): 925–935.

Leary, S., Underwood, W., Anthony R. et al. (2020). AVMA Guidelines for the Euthanasia of Animals: 2020 Edition. Schaumburg, IL: American Veterinary Medical Association.

Lucas, M., Ilin, Y., Anunu, R. et al. (2014). Long-term effects of controllability or the lack of it on coping abilities and stress resilience in the rat. *Stress* 17 (5): 423–430.

Lupien, S.J., McEwen, B.S., Gunnar, M.R. et al. (2009). Effects of stress throughout the lifespan on the brain, behaviour and cognition. *Nat. Rev. Neurosci.* 10: 434–445.

McEwen, B.S. (2017). Neurobiological and systemic effects of chronic stress. *Chronic Stress* 1: 2470547017692328.

McEwen, B.S. and Stellar, E. (1993). Stress and the individual: Mechanisms leading to disease. *Arch. Intern. Med.* 153: 2093–2101.

McGowan, R.T.S., Bolte, C., Barnett, H.R. et al. (2018). Can you spare 15 min? The measurable positive impact of a 15-min petting session on shelter dog well-being. *Appl. Anim. Behav. Sci.* 203: 42–54.

Ménard, C., Hodes, G.E., and Russo, S.J. (2016). Pathogenesis of depression: Insights from human and rodent studies. *Neuroscience* 321: 138–162.

Nazeri, M., Shabani, M., Ravandi, S.G. et al. (2015). Psychological or physical prenatal stress differentially affects cognition behaviors. *Physiol. Behav.* 142: 155–160.

Newbury, S., Blinn, M.K., Bushby, P.A. et al. (2010). *Guidelines for Standards of Care in*

Animal Shelters. Apex, NC: Association of Shelter Veterinarians.

Overall, K. 2013. *Manual of Clinical Behavioral Medicine for Dogs and Cats*. St. Louis, MO: Elsevier.

Protopopova, A. (2016). Effects of sheltering on physiology, immune function, behavior, and the welfare of dogs. *Physiol. Behav.* 159: 95–103.

Protopopova, A., Hall, N.J., Brown, K.M. et al. (2019). Behavioral predictors of subsequent respiratory illness signs in dogs admitted to an animal shelter. *PLOS ONE*. https://doi.org/10.1371/journal.pone.0224252.

Rau, V., DeCola, J.P., and Fanselow, M.S. (2005). Stress-induced enhancement of fear learning: An animal model of posttraumatic stress disorder. *Neurosci. Biobehav. Rev.* 29 (8): 1207–1223.

Sánchez, M.M., Ladd, C.O., and Plotsky, P.M. (2001). Early adverse experience as a developmental risk factor for later psychopathology: Evidence from rodent and primate models. *Dev. Psychopathol.* 13: 419–449.

Sandi, C. and Haller, J. (2015). Stress and the social brain: Behavioural effects and neurobiological mechanisms. *Nat. Rev. Neurosci.* 16: 290–304.

Sapolsky, R.M., Romero, M., and Munck, A.U. (2000). How do glucocorticoids influence stress responses? Integrating permissive, suppressive, stimulatory, and preparative actions. *Endocr. Rev.* 21 (1): 55–89.

Schwabe, L., Joëls, M., Roozendaal, B. et al. (2012). Stress effects on memory: An update and integration. *Neurosci. Biobehav. Rev.* 36 (7): 1740–1749.

Seeman, T.E., Singer, B.H., Rowe, J.W. et al. (1997). Price of adaptation—Allostatic load and its health consequences: MacArthur Studies on Successful Aging. *Arch. Intern Med.* 157: 2259–2268.

Seligman, M.E. and Maier, S.F. (1967). Failure to escape traumatic shock. *J. Exp. Psychol.* 74 (1): 1–9.

Shin, Y. and Shin, N. (2017). Relationship between sociability toward humans and physiological stress in dogs. *J. Vet. Med. Sci.*, 79 (7): 1278–1283.

Shiverdecker, M.D., Schiml, P.A., and Hennessy, M.B. (2013). Human interaction moderates plasma cortisol and behavioral responses of dogs to shelter housing. *Physiol. Behav.* 109: 75–79.

Smith-Blackmore, M. (2012). Euthanasia. In: *Shelter Medicine for Veterinarians and Staff*, 2nd ed. (eds. L. Miller and S. Zawistowski), 469–494. Hoboken, NJ: Wiley-Blackwell.

Stephen, J.M. and Ledger, R.A. (2006). A longitudinal evaluation of urinary cortisol in kennelled dogs, *Canis familiaris*, *Physiol. Behav.* 87 (5): 911–916.

Tod, E., Brander, D., and Waran, N. (2005). Efficacy of dog appeasing pheromone in reducing stress and fear related behaviour in shelter dogs. *Appl. Anim. Behav Sci.* 93 (3–4): 295–308.

Tuber, D.S., Hennessy, M.B., Sanders, S. et al. (1996). Behavioral and glucocorticoid response of adult domestic dogs (*Canis familiaris*) to companionship and social separation. *J. Comp. Psychol.* 110 (1): 103.

van der Kooij, M.A., Fantin, M., Kraev, I. et al. (2014). Impaired hippocampal neuroligin-2 function by chronic stress or synthetic peptide treatment is linked to social deficits and increased aggression. *NPP* 39: 1148–1158.

Verheggen, F.J., Haubruge, E., and Mescher, M.C. (2010). Alarm pheromones: Chemical signaling in response to danger. *Vitam. Horm.* https://doi.org/10.1016/S0083-6729(10)83009-2.

Wood, G.E., Young, L.T., Reagan, L.P. et al. (2003). Acute and chronic restrain stress alter the incidence of social conflict in male rats. *Horm. Behav.* 42: 205–213.

Yamamoto, S., Morinobu, S., Takei, S. et al. (2009). Single prolonged stress: Toward an animal model of posttraumatic stress disorder. *Depress. Anxiety* 26: 1110–1117.

Zoladz, P.R., Conrad, C.D., Fleshner, M. et al. (2008). Acute episodes of predator exposure in conjunction with chronic social instability as an animal model of post-traumatic stress disorder. *Stress* 11 (4): 259–281.

9

Assessing the Behavior of Shelter Dogs
Pamela J. Reid

9.1   Introduction

When a dog appears at the doors of an animal shelter, he is a behavioral puzzle. He may have come in as a stray or been brought in by a Good Samaritan. He may be accompanied by an owner who can no longer keep the dog. He may have been seized as a cruelty victim or a dangerous dog. The task of shelter personnel is to discover who this dog is—to assemble the puzzle pieces and create a behavioral picture of the dog.

To do this, every shelter should have a structured system for continually assessing the behavior of the dog throughout the time the dog is in the shelter. The assessment process can be a high-stakes endeavor. In some cases, the information gathered may determine if the dog lives or dies. Is this dog appropriate for adoption, or is he unsuitable for sheltering or placement because of safety concerns or unacceptable welfare? Information about a dog's behavior also guides good matching with potential adopters. For shelters with a behavior program, further goals include identifying dogs who need behavior modification or help coping with the stressors of the shelter environment—as well as tracking the efficacy of interventions for these dogs. Finally, in dangerous dog or cruelty cases, gathering data

about a dog's behavior may also serve as forensic evidence (Reid 2013; see Chapter 21).

While the behavior assessment process should be especially intensive early in a dog's stay, when the dog is still an enigma, it is also important to continue monitoring his behavior. Not only does this result in the accumulation of additional data to build a more accurate profile, it also ensures that changes in behavior are detected quickly. Behavior changes could signal a shift in the animal's quality of life (see Chapter 19) or the emergence of an underlying medical condition. For instance, maybe the dog would benefit from a change in housing, increased enrichment, or a move to a foster home. For dogs that are undergoing behavioral rehabilitation, there is a need for routine monitoring to gauge the impact of treatment. Perhaps the dog has improved to the point that he can be made available for adoption, maybe the dog is not making reasonable progress and the treatment plan needs to be adjusted, or maybe the dog's behavior has worsened and a decision needs to be made about whether to continue with treatment.

Learning about the dog for the purpose of making good dog-adopter matches is important because we know that some adopted dogs are returned for behavioral reasons (see Chapter 6). In some cases, the reason for a return wouldn't

Animal Behavior for Shelter Veterinarians and Staff, Second Edition. Edited by Brian A. DiGangi, Victoria A. Cussen, Pamela J. Reid, and Kristen A. Collins.
© 2022 John Wiley & Sons, Inc. Published 2022 by John Wiley & Sons, Inc.
Companion website: www.wiley.com/go/digangi/animal

have been a concern for a different adopter, such as incompatibility with resident pets (Mondelli et al. 2004; Shore 2005). The more that is known by shelter personnel about the dog—his personality, energy level, compatibility with children or animals—the better informed adopters will be when selecting the right dog for them.

What shelters want is a way to efficiently capture information about a dog's personality or temperament (these terms tend to be used interchangeably, but they are distinct; see Raymment et al. [2015] for an extensive discussion of dog temperament and personality) by observing the dog's behavior. Indeed, it would be ideal if exposing a dog to a set of structured experiences in the form of a standardized behavior evaluation, or "temperament test," could reveal how they will behave in a variety of future contexts (Sternberg 2002; Weiss 2007). However, the reality is that behavior is dynamic. That is not to say that behavior is random or unpredictable, but behavior at any time is influenced by numerous factors, including genetics, experience, motivation, learning, and the current environment (Clay et al. 2020b; Ley and Bennett 2007). Further complicating matters, some individuals' behavior is more plastic than others (Goold and Newberry 2017b), resulting in increased variability. Moreover, shelters are novel, stressful, and socially isolating—all of which further impact behavior. Thus, behavior observed in any one specific context may not be predictive of behavior in other situations or even in the same situation in the future. To differentiate between behavioral tendencies due to personality traits and behaviors that are specific to their context, it is imperative to control for situational and motivational factors by having multiple people observe the dog in many different situations (Raymment et al. 2015). What this means is that the only way we can hope to predict how a dog will behave outside the shelter world with any degree of confidence is to observe his behavior in a wide variety of circumstances.

9.1.1 Decision-Making

It's not surprising that the quality of a decision about an animal is assumed to be directly related to the amount of information gathered about that animal, especially when it comes to complex challenges like predicting future behavior. The more puzzle pieces gathered, the more complete the picture. For example, staff in Australian shelters felt that they could make better decisions if they were given more time to get to know the dogs in their care (Mornement et al. 2010). Goold and Newberry (2017b) suggest that shelters should wait as long as possible before deciding on the fate of an animal. Not only does that allow for increased behavior observations of the dog in various scenarios; there is also evidence that a dog's behavior is particularly unstable during the first few days or weeks in the shelter environment (Goold and Newberry 2017a, 2017b; Kis et al. 2014). For instance, Goold and Newberry (2017b) found that shelter dogs increased their friendly behavior toward humans over the first two weeks in the shelter, with the most sizable change happening in the early days after arrival. The magnitude of the change varied across individuals; dogs who were the most social on the first day in the shelter were not necessarily the most social on day 15. They note that individual differences in the day-to-day variation of shelter dog behavior have been largely unstudied.

However, there is a substantial cost to gathering information. It takes time and resources. The quest for information should not come at the cost of holding dogs in the shelter for longer than necessary. Lengthening a dog's stay is not only likely to have a detrimental effect on that dog, it also prevents housing, supplies, and personnel from being directed toward other dogs in need. A shelter's overarching goal should be to identify adoption candidates as quickly as possible and move them into adoptive or foster homes or into a relocation program. Likewise, dogs who are *not* adoption candidates should be identified and swiftly moved along a path to outcome; dogs with treatable behavior problems that make them immediately unadoptable can be placed in a behavior modification program, and dogs with untreatable behavior problems or unacceptably poor welfare should be humanely euthanized.

Striking an optimal balance between speed and accuracy when making decisions is no easy feat. Effective decision-making involves collecting information in an efficient manner and gauging when enough information has been accumulated to be confident in the decision (Drugowitsch et al. 2015). How much evidence is required depends in part on the consequences of inaccurate decisions. In the case of decisions about shelter dogs, the consequences are considerable. As mentioned above, mistaken judgments about a dog can result in his needless death. Errors in the opposite direction can result in a dangerous dog being placed in the community. Both types of miscalculations are likely to weigh heavily on shelter personnel, possibly leading to compassion fatigue (Hill et al. 2020; Scotney et al. 2015).

Not all decisions are necessarily fraught with uncertainty, though. Dogs that are brought to the shelter with credible reports of severe aggression toward people or other dogs should be euthanized as quickly as legally possible. There is no benefit to holding these dogs in a stressful shelter, during which time staff may become attached to them. Dogs that come in with trustworthy reports from a surrendering owner and dogs that are highly social with people and dogs, seemingly unfazed by the stresses of the shelter, can be fast-tracked for adoption. Be aware, though, that quick decisions based on only a few observations ("thin-slicing") are most likely to be accurate when made by behavior experts; thin-slicing by non-experts is notoriously prone to error (Croskerry 2006). Dogs who fall in between these two extremes—the ambiguous ones—are the dogs for whom decisions should be based on an adequate accumulation of behavioral observations.

9.1.2 The Observational Assessment Model

Traditionally, many shelters have placed their faith almost exclusively in standardized behavior evaluations to reveal information critical to pathway planning. But, as discussed in Section 9.2.9, behavior evaluations have not proven highly accurate nor precise when used to predict behavior, particularly aggression, after adoption. It has been suggested that standardized evaluations, in part because of their provocativeness, result in a significant number of dogs exhibiting aggression who ultimately would not do so in a home (Patronek and Bradley 2016). Thus, rather than relying on a single "snapshot" of behavior, a more rational approach is to implement what has been called a "mixed assessment model" (Rayment et al. 2015) or a "longitudinal observational assessment model" (Goold and Newberry 2017b) (hereafter referred to as the observational assessment model). Such an approach relies on collecting behavioral data from all of the players who are likely to know or learn something about a dog in a variety of contexts, in addition to conducting a standardized evaluation. Shelter personnel, volunteers, adoption counselors, and even members of the public may interact with the dog and, without a formalized process for collecting their observations, those data are lost. Moreover, observing the dog in naturally occurring situations, such as walking by a children's playground or meeting a potential adoptive family, can uncover information that wouldn't be revealed in a standardized evaluation. This approach, by definition, involves multiple sources weighing in on the dog's behavior in numerous contexts, which is expected to reveal behavioral consistencies and, thus, is more likely to capture the dog's personality. A drawback, however, is that most of the people observing the animal and generating these data are not trained experts in canine behavior. Currently, there are very few studies addressing the integrity of such information. Including a standardized behavior evaluation in the assessment process is advisable, as this ensures that behavior staff also interact with the dog.

A distinct advantage of the observational assessment model is that if concerning behavior is exhibited in one context, it can be further explored in other situations. This is especially important for behaviors that might warrant euthanasia. Shelters should only make euthanasia decisions based on a single incident of aggression if the aggression is truly egregious, such as a severe attack on a person or other dog. Otherwise, problematic behavior should be safely confirmed in other situations to guard against potential errors. As more research accumulates, it may prove feasible for shelters to also substantiate behavioral observations with correlated physiological measures, such as heart rate and heart rate variability via heart rate monitors (Bergamasco et al. 2010; Rayment et al. 2013; Vincent and Leahy 1997), activity levels via accelerometers (Hoffman et al. 2019; Jones et al. 2014), and arousal via leash tension meters (Shih et al. 2020).

Dowling-Guyer et al. (2011) express the legitimate concern that this model may be difficult to implement in shelters because of the limited situations and stimuli to which shelter dogs are exposed. However, many shelters already rely on behavior information collected from more than one source, including surrendering owners, daily care staff observations, and a brief medical/behavior intake exam (Marder 2015). Even staff at high-intake shelters are likely to be able to observe dogs with ambiguous behavior in at least six to nine situations; Goold and Newberry (2017a, 2017b) felt this was an adequate number of observations of shelter dogs' interactions with people and other dogs to provide an accurate indication of future behavior. More potentially worrisome is the concern that busy shelter staff do not have the time to record their observations or that behavior staff do not have the time to compile and assimilate the data. The good news is that

with new technologies emerging, such as mobile apps that feed directly into a shelter's database, staff can quickly and efficiently enter behavior data. Records can be autofilled with the dog's previous data so that only significant changes in behavior are flagged for the behavior team.

9.2 Sources of Behavior Information

Shelters need to consider their individual circumstances and resources when deciding on a behavior assessment process, using their best judgment to determine how they can expediently gather as much information as is needed for each animal. To aid shelters in making educated decisions about where to focus their information-gathering efforts and how to weigh and assimilate the data they receive, presented in Sections 9.2.1–9.2.9 are the benefits and limitations of the various sources of information typically available in the shelter environment.

9.2.1 Information from Relinquishing Owners

It is a commonly held belief among shelter professionals that owners won't be honest about the behavior of the dog they are surrendering (Duffy et al. 2014; Stephen and Ledger 2007). The reasons for this distrust are many. One perspective is that owners may exaggerate their dog's behavior problems because they feel the need to justify why they are giving up the dog. Alternatively, owners might downplay behavior problems to improve their dog's chances for rehoming. Yet another possibility is that once owners have made the decision to surrender their pet, they are uninterested in providing information and will respond to questions carelessly. In addition, relinquishing owners have been shown to have weaker attachment to their pets, leading Kwan and Bain (2013) to speculate that perhaps relinquishing owners are less observant and, therefore, less knowledgeable about their dog's behavior. However, DiGiacomo et al. (1998) found that many owners struggle with the decision to surrender, often resorting to the shelter after expending considerable effort to keep or rehome the animal, which suggests that some owners do at least have a strong sense of responsibility toward the pet and probably a reasonably accurate perspective on their behavior.

Contrary to those concerns, research indicates that owners often do disclose information that is valuable for making outcome and placement decisions. Segurson et al. (2005) asked people surrendering their dogs to complete the 103-item Canine Behavioral Assessment and Research Questionnaire (C-BARQ). Half of the people were told that their responses were confidential and would not be shared with shelter personnel; the other half were told that their responses would be used by the shelter to match their dog to a new owner. The researchers found that when owners believed the information would be kept confidential, they were more likely to disclose that their dog exhibited aggression toward family members or fear of strangers. There was no difference between the groups in their willingness to report that their dogs showed aggression to strangers, aggression toward or fear of dogs, non-social fear, separation-related behaviors, or attachment/attention-seeking behaviors. Both groups reported higher incidences of problem behavior than a control group of owners surveyed when bringing their dogs to a medical referral clinic.

In contrast, a subsequent study that used a shorter 42-item version of the questionnaire, called C-BARQ^(S), found no difference between the responses of owners who were told that their information would be kept confidential, owners who were told that their information would be shared with the shelter, and owners who weren't told anything about how their information would be used (Duffy et al. 2014).

The most apparent difference between the studies, other than the length of the questionnaire, was that Segurson et al. (2005) approached owners face-to-face, explaining the questionnaire and asking them to complete it, whereas the questionnaires were simply made available and self-administered in the Duffy et al. (2014) study. In general, face-to-face interactions are more susceptible to social desirability biases; people feel pressured to give answers that they believe the other person wants to hear (Durmaz et al. 2020; Lelkes et al. 2012; Richman et al. 1999). Thus, it's possible that self-administered questionnaires are more likely to result in accurate disclosures of problem behavior, but more research is needed to fully understand the best way to gather such information from owners.

As a tool to predict how a dog is likely to behave in an adoptive home, owner reports do not appear to be terribly useful on their own. Stephen and Ledger (2007) followed up with adopters at two- and six-weeks post-adoption and found only a few consistencies with what owners had reported about their dogs at surrender. At two weeks, fear, anxiety, or aggression toward veterinarians, aggression to unfamiliar dogs or unfamiliar people, stealing food, chewing furniture, mounting, and anxiety when left alone were the behaviors correlated with surrendering owner reports. By six weeks there were fewer correlations. Duffy et al. (2014) found that adopter reports only corresponded to surrendering owner reports for aggression toward unfamiliar people, urination when left alone, and destructive chewing. McGuire et al. (2020) specifically asked surrendering owners about their dogs' tendency to guard food, toys, or chew items and found no positive relationship with resource guarding reported in the adoptive home. They did confirm, though, that dogs who were reported by their owners to *not* guard resources were similarly unlikely to guard in the new home.

If a Good Samaritan brings a stray dog to the shelter, it is worth collecting whatever behavioral information the finder might know about the dog. They presumably captured and handled the dog, at least minimally, or they may have even kept the dog at their home for a time while they tried to find the owner themselves. Those interpreting this information should take into consideration the amount of time the person spent with the dog, the circumstances under which the information was gathered, and the nature of the information reported. Likewise, with increasing numbers of dogs being relocated from one shelter to another, the author advises that the receiving shelter request any behavioral records from the originating shelter, bearing in mind that the value of those records is a function of the shelter's behavior assessment process and the time the dog spent there.

9.2.2 Medical Staff Observations

Every dog coming into a shelter typically undergoes, at the very least, a medical intake exam, so medical personnel can be an economical and valuable source of information about the dog's reaction to unfamiliar people, physical handling, restraint, and potentially unpleasant experiences. However, it is important to keep in mind that how a dog behaves during a medical exam may be influenced by his discomfort with the procedures being performed during the exam and his history with medical care. Some dogs who are tolerant of or even friendly toward people in every other situation may become defensively aggressive or extremely fearful when handled by medical personnel, especially if they are in pain, because of previous unpleasant experiences in medical contexts (Mills et al. 2020).

There is reason to suspect that an animal's behavior during a veterinary exam may not be reflective of behavior in other circumstances. Research substantiates that veterinary exams are stressful for most dogs (Riemer et al. 2021; Travain et al. 2015). Döring et al. (2009) found that close to 80% of owned dogs exhibited

fearful behavior during a standardized veterinary exam. Dogs unaccompanied by their owners experience significantly more stress (Csoltova et al. 2017; Stellato et al. 2020), especially when physically manipulated (Stellato et al. 2019). Owner-surrendered dogs admitted to a shelter are essentially in a comparable situation, with a stranger rather than the owner taking them for their exam. Furthermore, intake exams typically occur shortly after admission to the shelter, when dogs' stress levels are found to be highest, as indicated by elevations in cortisol (Coppola et al. 2006; Hennessy et al. 1997; Hiby et al. 2006).

While there is no published research specifically examining the value of behavioral information gleaned during a standard veterinary exam in the shelter environment, Lind et al. (2017) found no correlation between veterinarians' assessments of stress and a behavior evaluation of owned dogs at a veterinary clinic. However, there is at least some indication that dogs who are frightened during a veterinary exam are likely to also show fear in other circumstances. Edwards et al. (2019) found that dogs reported by their owners to exhibit fear when examined by a veterinarian (55%) are also likely to exhibit fear in new situations (68%) and suffer from pain/touch sensitivity (35%) and non-social fear (37%).

Behavior observations during a medical intake exam may be primarily useful for learning how the dog responds to stressful events, developing a handling plan for the dog during future medical procedures, and creating a behavior modification plan to reduce sensitivity to handling or restraint if necessary. Behavior information from medical personnel should be considered in light of the circumstances of the interaction and in conjunction with other observations in different contexts. Box 9.1 contains sample questions that medical staff can answer to collect critical data on the nature of the interaction and Box 9.2 contains a word bank to consistently characterize responses.

Box 9.1 Example Medical Observation Form

Your Name:
Your Title:
Animal Name/ID:
Date and Time of Interaction:
Facility:

Are you (Familiar is more than 3 interactions):
- Familiar
- Unfamiliar

What type of medical procedure was required?
- Visual (e.g., hands-off, no restraint required)
- Tactile (e.g., palpating, looking in ears/mouth, restraint necessary)
- Invasive (e.g., temperature, injections, blood draw)

If medical staff was unable to complete a full exam, please describe why:

Where did the exam/procedure take place (in kennel, medical office, on ground, on exam table, etc.)?

Did the dog receive any pre-exam anxiolytics or require sedation to be handled?
- Yes
- No

If yes, why?

Did you restrain the dog?
- Yes
- No

If yes, please record ALL behaviors you saw during restraint (see word bank).

Did you muzzle the dog?
- Yes
- No

Did the dog require a designated handler/defensive handling? Please describe what type of handling occurred.

How did the dog behave when you stood in front of their kennel? Please record all behaviors observed (see word bank).

How did the dog respond socially to you? Please record all behaviors observed (see word bank).

Did you physically move (pick up, gently push body, move by collar) the dog? If yes, please select all behaviors observed (see word bank).

Did you attempt to walk the dog? If yes, please record ALL behaviors you saw when attempting to walk the dog (see word bank).

How would you characterize the dog's overall emotional response throughout your interaction?
- Happy
- Sad

- Angry
- Nervous
- Excited
- Scared
- Neutral

Box 9.2   Survey Response Word Bank

Stayed close and/or followed you (Affiliative Behavior)
Took treats/toys from you (Affiliative Behavior)
Licked you socially (Affiliative Behavior)
Sought contact with you (Affiliative Behavior)
Pawed at you (Affiliative Behavior)
Bounced/wiggly toward you (Affiliative Behavior)
Play bowed (Affiliative Behavior)
Flipped upside down (Affiliative Behavior)
Jumped on you in greeting (Affiliative Behavior)
Moved away from you (Fear/Anxiety)
Repeatedly approached and moved away (Fear/Anxiety)
Moved slowly and/or hesitantly (Fear/Anxiety)
Paced (Fear/Anxiety)
Yelped/shrieked (Fear/Anxiety)
Excessively drooled (Fear/Anxiety)
Startled—did not recover (Fear/Anxiety)
Trembled (Fear/Anxiety)
Crawled and/or barked (Fear/Anxiety)
Cowered (Fear/Anxiety)
Hid (Fear/Anxiety)
Urinated/defecated while exhibiting fear (Fear/Anxiety)
Fled/attempted to escape (Fear/Anxiety)
Catatonic/shut down (Fear/Anxiety)
Bit at leash (Fear/Anxiety)
Flailed or rolled on leash (Fear/Anxiety)
Hard stared and/or whale eye (Aggression)
Raised hackles/fur stood on end (Aggression)
Froze (Aggression)
Growled (Aggression)
Muzzle punched/hard jab with closed mouth (Aggression)
Lunged toward a person/dog (Aggression)
Bared teeth (Aggression)
Attempted to bite (Aggression)
Bit (Aggression)
Mouthed—light pressure (Arousal)
Jumped on you—difficult to interrupt (Arousal)

Grabbed clothes/limbs/leash (released) (Arousal)
Mounted/humped (Arousal)
Grabbed leash and tugged (Arousal)
Grabbed clothing and tugged (Arousal)
Body slammed (Arousal)
Mouthed — not painful (Arousal)
Mouthed — painful (Arousal)
Paced, repetitive, abnormally patterned movement (Arousal)
Barked

9.2.3 Daily Care Staff and Volunteer Observations

Daily care staff and volunteers often have more direct contact with a dog than anyone else in the shelter system. They typically interact with the dog during routine cleaning, watering, and feeding. In some shelters, daily care personnel and volunteers are also responsible for providing in-kennel enrichment (beds, toys, chew items, etc.), transferring the dog to and from outdoor exercise areas or play yards, supervising playgroups, and walking and socializing with the dog.

However, behavior observations collected by daily care staff who haven't received targeted training on that task may not be very accurate. In one study, dogs underwent a standardized behavioral evaluation and, simultaneously, shelter staff completed a questionnaire about each dog's behavior toward adults, children, dogs, and cats; their reaction to being handled; how well they walked on leash; and so forth (van der Borg et al. 1991). Staff correctly predicted only one-third of the behavior problems ultimately reported by adopters one to two months after adoption, whereas the behavioral tests predicted almost 75% of the problems.

One understandable explanation for the poor accuracy of daily care staff observations is that people may be reluctant to disclose negative information about a dog because they don't want to jeopardize the dog's chances for adoption. Therefore, daily care staff and volunteers may be biased toward providing positive feedback, as was the case in the van der Borg et al. (1991) study, in which staff predicted that

dogs would not exhibit problem behaviors in the adoptive home when, in fact, they did. Goold and Newberry (2017a) found that close to half of the shelter staff they studied mistook aggressive behavior for excitement and frustration, but rarely did they mistakenly classify non-aggressive behaviors as aggression. The staff ratings, therefore, indicated a tendency to judge dogs' behavior positively.

In addition to an optimistic judgment bias, staff and volunteers who are untrained in animal behavior may misinterpret behaviors or be unable to recognize more subtle variations in behavior. Research on the validity of inexpert judgments of dog behavior provides mixed support for this. For instance, in comparisons of dog professionals, dog owners, and non-dog owners rating behavior from video footage, familiarity with dogs wasn't necessary for the accurate identification of friendly or happy dogs, but fearful dogs were better recognized by the professionals (Wan et al. 2012). Tami and Gallagher (2009), however, found that both experts and non-experts were equally capable of identifying fear in dogs. When it came to identifying other types of behavior, being an expert didn't seem to help that much. Tami and Gallagher (2009) found that both experts and non-experts were equally poor at differentiating play from aggression. Wan et al. (2012) found that even highly proficient experts had trouble agreeing on when dogs were exhibiting behavior suggestive of "sadness" and "anger."

It is particularly fascinating that as people gain more familiarity with dogs, they pay more attention to the whole dog. Experts reported that they were more likely to rely on multiple features of the dog when making their judgments than non-experts (Wan et al. 2012). An eye-tracking study showed that non-experts focused more on dogs' heads while dog trainers paid more attention to dogs' bodies (Kujala et al. 2012). This attention to the whole dog may enable experts to more readily interpret dogs' overall affective state. Expert dog trainers in the Tami and Gallagher (2009) study provided more information about the dogs' motivations and emotions than the non-experts. Similarly, in the Kujala et al. (2012) study, experts were more likely than non-experts to make inferences about the dogs' mental states, such as "the dog was reserved" or "the dog was friendly and playful."

Fortunately, when non-experts are provided with training, their proficiency improves. Flint et al. (2018) showed that providing people with written descriptions, pictures, and video examples of mild-to-moderate and high-to-extreme levels of fear significantly increased their ability to accurately identify levels of fear in new videotaped examples. Likewise, non-experts who were provided with a one-hour training session on reading and interpreting dog behavior were almost as adept at assessing dogs for their aptitude as military working dogs as professionals with 9–22 years of assessment experience (Fratkin et al. 2015).

Clearly, if we wish to collect accurate behavioral information from shelter staff and volunteers, targeted training is required. Training programs should emphasize the importance of attending to each of the relevant component features as well as the whole picture of the dog, enabling people to differentiate aggression from play and frustration and to detect subtle variations in emotional states, including fear, sadness, and anger. The ideal instructional format for learning to perceive and interpret dog behavior has not been investigated, so it is probably best to combine written descriptions with still images and video examples. There is evidence to suggest that incorporating all three

media capitalizes on each of their strengths. Simplifying the task with photographs and written text may enhance initial acquisition of knowledge, whereas providing more complex video examples improves the learner's ultimate performance (Arguel and Jamet 2009; Ganier and de Vries 2016; Höffler and Leutner 2007; van Hooijdonk and Krahmer 2008).

9.2.4 Walks and Field Trips

Shelters often incorporate walks by staff or volunteers into the routines of their dogs. Walks are believed to improve the health and mental well-being of the dogs and reduce stress associated with being in their kennels (Coppola et al. 2006; Perry et al. 2020). In a study that specifically looked at the relationship between the impressions of volunteer dog walkers about certain dogs and the same dogs' behavior during a standardized behavior evaluation, Shih et al. (2020) found that dogs who pulled less on the leash during walks were rated as more social during the evaluation. Other than that, the researchers found little correlation between volunteer reports and the evaluation results, although that may be because the judgments asked of the volunteers were quite zoomed out, such as "I don't think this dog is suitable for a non-experienced adopter." The researchers felt that the volunteers might have been more tolerant of the dogs' behavior than the evaluators and that they may have been reluctant to disclose behavior that would be perceived as negative.

Notwithstanding the findings of the Shih et al. (2020) study, a walk can reveal much about a dog's behavior: his enthusiasm for getting out of his kennel, his comfort with having his collar held and a leash applied, how he reacts to other dogs as he walks through the shelter, his interest in interacting with the handler versus checking out the environment, his confidence in novel and outdoor locations, his inclination to pull on the leash, and his willingness to return to the kennel. Walks that take place off shelter property are even more

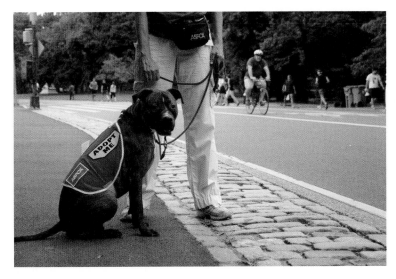

Figure 9.1 Walking on city streets exposes the shelter dog to a variety of everyday experiences.

informative. How does the dog react to passersby, children, joggers, cyclists, skateboarders, and/or other potentially provoking or frightening stimuli (see Figure 9.1)? Providing these details, along with strategies for managing any problematic behavior observed on walks, may promote regular dog walking post-adoption. While encouraging adopters to walk their dogs doesn't necessarily reduce return rates (Gunter et al. 2017), owners who walk their dogs report a greater sense of obligation toward their pets (Gunter et al. 2017; Hoerster et al. 2011), so educating them about dog-specific walking strategies based on information from shelter walks could promote the human-animal bond post-adoption.

9.2.5 Socialization Sessions

We know that one-on-one interactions with people can be highly beneficial for reducing stress in shelter dogs (Coppola et al. 2006; Dudley et al. 2015; Hennessy et al. 1998; Shiverdecker et al. 2013; Willen et al. 2017). In addition to being important for stress reduction, socialization sessions can provide useful information about how a dog interacts with people. When gathering information, ask

questions of the socializer that will inform good adoption matches and provide helpful information for new adopters. Is the dog motivated to interact with people? Does the dog enjoy petting? Is the dog comfortable playing with people? Is he content to stay in proximity? Does he respond to common verbal instructions, such as "Sit," "Down," and "Come?" Is the dog eager to perform behaviors to earn treats? What kind of treats most motivate him? Like reports provided by daily care staff and volunteers, information garnered from socialization sessions may be impacted by people's level of behavioral expertise and by their desire to paint the dog in a positive light.

Another source of socialization information that should not be overlooked is adoption counselors, sometimes known as "matchmakers." During meet-and-greet sessions with potential adopters, matchmakers are privy to observations that may not be attainable in other situations. How did the dog react to meeting an entire family? Did he gravitate to the adults or the children? Did he show a preference for males or females? How did he handle children's loud voices and erratic movements? Was he comfortable being handled by an "average" adopter? Did he exhibit behaviors that have been shown to be particularly appealing to adopters, such as playing with a toy and lying down in proximity to people (Protopopova and Wynne 2014)? If the adopters rejected the dog, was it because of his behavior? The answers to these questions are extremely helpful not only to the behavior team but also to the match-makers to prepare for future meet-and-greet opportunities.

9.2.6 In-Kennel Behavior

The behavior of dogs in their kennels is typically monitored to detect potential welfare concerns but is not usually considered useful in predicting behavior outside of the kennel environment. In fact, a prevailing belief is that even friendly dogs may exhibit aggression when confined to a kennel. Goold and Newberry (2017a) found support for this. When dogs (at least those under six years of age) were in their kennels, the probability of displaying aggression toward people was highest compared to a variety of other situations. Curiously, they also found that when dogs were in their kennels, aggression toward other dogs was lowest. Anecdotally, this has not been the experience of many shelter professionals.

Clay et al. (2019) claim that monitoring in-kennel behavior allows for early detection of potential problems ultimately revealed during a standardized behavior evaluation. They found that observing dogs in their kennels for one hour a day for the first five days in the shelter predicted the dogs' behavior in an evaluation performed on the sixth day. Dogs who exhibited behaviors associated with fear, anxiety, and arousal (whining, panting, tenseness, lowered body, standing by the wall, etc.) in their kennels were likely to show the same behaviors during the evaluation. Aggression was rare both in kennel and in the evaluation. Over the course of the five days, fearful behavior declined for most dogs, and the dogs spent more time at the front of their kennels or resting in their beds, suggesting that they were acclimating to the environment. Dogs who were eventually euthanized were less relaxed and jumped up more in their kennels than dogs who were adopted. While monitoring in-kennel behavior for an hour each day is not feasible for most shelters, the same information may be gathered through daily care observations and routine quality of life monitoring, possibly combined with accelerometer data, as accelerometers become more affordable and sophisticated (see Chapter 19).

9.2.7 Playgroups

Increasingly, shelters are offering playgroups for their dogs (see Chapter 13). Not only is participation in playgroups an excellent form of enrichment and physical exercise for dog-friendly dogs, there is limited evidence that it also results in fewer stress-related behaviors once the dogs return to their kennels (Belpedio et al. 2010; Johnson et al. 2013). Participation in playgroups has also been shown to influence how dogs respond to other dogs during a standardized behavior evaluation. Dogs who joined a playgroup session prior to undergoing an evaluation reacted more positively to a stimulus dog than control dogs who were evaluated without a playgroup session, although the two groups of dogs were studied at different times, so other factors could have accounted for the disparity (Flower 2016). Gfrerer et al. (2018) also found that regular interactions between adult dogs reduced the likelihood of aggression toward dogs in a standardized behavior evaluation. Over the course of eight weeks, adult military working dogs, housed in much the same way as shelter dogs, were provided with three hours of interaction with other dogs weekly. Most interaction occurred in a playgroup context, but some dogs could only safely interact leashed or behind a fence. These dogs subsequently exhibited less aggression toward a model dog and a live stimulus dog than control dogs who had not been exposed to other dogs (Gfrerer et al. 2018). Lacking long-term follow-up on these specific dogs, it is impossible to know whether the playgroup

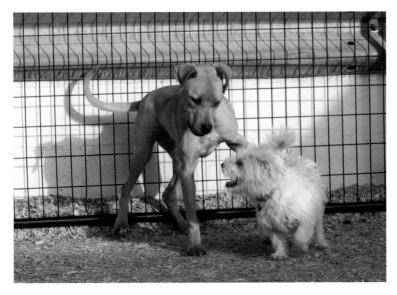

Figure 9.2 A large dog learning to play with a small dog during playgroup. *Source:* Courtesy of Barb Davis.

experience produced only a short-term reduction in conspecific aggression, perhaps due to habituation, or a lasting change resulting from learning how to interact non-aggressively with dogs.

In addition to the benefits of shelter playgroups for the participating dogs, playgroups can provide worthwhile information for matching a dog to an appropriate adopter. How does the dog react to being off leash in an enclosed area? Is the dog more interested in interacting with people or dogs, or does he prefer to explore the environment? How playful or energetic is he? Does he get along well with all dogs or only certain individuals (see Figure 9.2)?

The dog's behavior toward other dogs while in a playgroup can be particularly enlightening because dogs may react differently toward other dogs when uninfluenced by a leash and handler (McConnell and London 2009). How does the dog respond to corrections from other dogs, and how appropriately does the dog deliver corrections to other dogs? Depending on the situation, the dog may also reveal how he responds to people intervening in his interactions with other dogs (verbal corrections, physical restraint, etc.) and to aversive stimuli

(water spray, startling noise, compressed air, citronella spray, etc.) should their use be necessary to interrupt inappropriate behavior or a dogfight. On the other hand, a limitation of playgroup observations is that a dog's motivation to play with other dogs may completely overwhelm his desire to interact with people. Also, some dogs simply don't enjoy playgroups, and their anxiety in playgroup situations may inhibit their behavior in general or cause defensive behavior not provoked in other contexts. Thus, it is important to assess dogs' behavior toward people and dogs outside of the playgroup context as well. An on-leash assessment is particularly important, as this is how most dogs encounter other dogs and people in their everyday lives.

9.2.8 Foster Stay and Adopter Returns

Observations of a dog's behavior as he transitions from the shelter to a home environment are extremely helpful in matching the dog to a new adopter. A stay in a foster home is presumed to be the most accurate reflection of how the dog will behave in an adoptive home, at least during the time just after adoption. For the purposes of information gathering, an adoption return may also fall into this category.

Many shelters have volunteer foster programs that provide a temporary stay for dogs who need medical or behavioral rehabilitation before being returned to the shelter for adoption. A stay with an experienced foster volunteer can be invaluable for determining if a behaviorally challenged dog is safe to place or can experience a good quality of life in a home. In a review of the records of a large, open-admission municipal shelter in the United States, Patronek and Crowe (2018) discovered that adult dogs returning from a foster stay were 20 times more likely to be adopted (or transferred to another shelter or rescue group, which implies that the dog met some sort of criteria for adoption suitability) than dogs who had remained in the shelter. Similarly, 85% of adopted dogs who were returned within 30 days were quickly and successfully readopted. While it could be that dogs are better behaved as a result of their experience when they return to the shelter (Hennessy et al. 2006), Patronek and Crowe (2018) surmise that the shelter obtains valuable information about the dogs' time out of the shelter to facilitate good matching with adopters. Regrettably, they didn't delve into the process by which the shelter gathers and documents that information.

Foster programs are considered beneficial for promoting adoption, either through increased visibility to potential adopters or by so-called "foster fails," when the fosterer ends up adopting the dog. Mohan-Gibbons et al. (2014) examined a program called Adoption Ambassadors in which the foster volunteer is responsible not only for caring for the dog but also for identifying an adopter and facilitating the transfer. Significantly fewer fostered dogs were subsequently returned by their adopters than dogs who had been adopted directly from the shelter. However, it took longer for dogs in the foster program to be adopted than dogs in the shelter. This could be because fosterers are pickier when it comes to selecting adopters or because dogs in foster homes are not exposed

to as many potential adopters as they would be in the shelter. It's also possible that the longer the dog spends in foster, the better prepared he is for a successful adoption. Without a full understanding of the factors at play, placement in a foster home should be considered carefully. Dogs who are likely to fit into anyone's home may be best served staying at the shelter, where they will be adopted quickly, whereas dogs who may need more careful matching for a successful adoption could be prioritized for foster homes.

Adoption of dogs who have been fostered may be more successful because of the higher quality of information provided by fosterers. Potential adopters also have the chance to observe the dog in more realistic situations than staff do in the shelter. Nearly one-quarter of the adopters of foster dogs in the Adoption Ambassadors program said they based their decision to adopt in part on information imparted by the fosterer, compared with only 3% of adopters who said they relied on information from shelter personnel (Mohan-Gibbons et al. 2014). Gilchrist (2019) examined the agreement between fosterers' and adopters' impressions of their dogs and found that fosterers' responses about their dogs on the C-BARQ matched much more closely with the subsequent adopters' responses, even six months post-adoption, than with those provided by shelter staff.

Coordinating a sustainable foster program is resource- and time-intensive, and not all shelter professionals are convinced that transitioning a dog from the shelter to a foster home and potentially back to the shelter is good for the dog's well-being. However, research reveals that getting the dog out of the shelter, even for one to two nights, reduces stress and improves quality of life by promoting uninterrupted rest during the time away from the shelter (Fehringer and Dreschel 2014; Gunter et al. 2019). While the benefits do not continue after the dog returns to the shelter, cortisol levels were no different than they were before the dog left (Gunter et al. 2019), suggesting that the transition back to the shelter is not unduly distressing. Unfortunately, a "sleepover" is unlikely to reveal much useful information about a dog's behavior, simply because most dogs spend that time catching up on their sleep.

Many shelters transferred their animals into foster homes during the COVID-19 pandemic and, with all the potential benefits, the hope is that robust foster and sleepover programs will become a sustainable component of care for homeless dogs (Morgan et al. 2021). Dogs experiencing high levels of distress or displaying undesirable behavior in the kennel or those suffering from long lengths of stay may benefit the most from time out of the shelter to reduce their stress and enable them to reveal how they would behave in a home environment. See Box 9.3 for an example survey for collecting behavior information from fosterers (and associated word bank in Box 9.2).

9.2.9 Standardized Behavior Evaluations

As mentioned previously, shelters have long relied on regimented behavior evaluations (sometimes erroneously referred to as "temperament tests" or "personality tests") as a consistent, practical way to gather information about a dog in a short period of time (Marder 2015; Reid et al. 2004). In an evaluation, the dog is exposed to a battery of tests designed to simulate experiences commonly encountered by a pet dog (Mornement et al. 2009). Some of the experiences are potentially provocative, such as unpleasant handling, and possibly scary, such as being approached by a threatening stranger. Most evaluations try to capture information about the dog's sociability with people and with dogs, his tolerance of handling, his activity level and playfulness, his propensity for aggression, his reaction to novelty, and his ability to recover from a frightening event. A list of standardized behavior evaluations that have received scientific attention appears in Table 9.1.

Despite their widespread acceptance (Mohan-Gibbons et al. 2012), there is little scientific evidence to support the use of behavior evaluations as predictive sources of information. A good behavior evaluation ought to fare well on three important criteria: (i) feasibility, (ii) reliability, and (iii) validity (Taylor and Mills 2006). A discussion of each of these criteria follows. For a comprehensive review of the relevant published literature on behavior evaluations, see Patronek et al. (2019).

9.2.9.1 Feasibility

Many of the standardized behavior evaluations documented in the literature are impractical for a shelter because they require too much time (Dowling-Guyer et al. 2011; Ledger and Baxter 1997; van der Borg et al. 1991) or too much specialized training to conduct (Netto and Planta 1997). Time is a particular concern in busy shelters because animals can end up waiting for their evaluation before being cleared for outcome. The ASPCA's short SAFER® (ASPCA, New York, NY) test was developed in part to address the concern with evaluation bottleneck (E. Weiss, personal communication). Shelters frequently report that they have modified an existing behavior evaluation or have designed their own to suit their needs (D'Arpino et al. 2012). Most of these were probably created without input from a psychometrician or an applied animal behaviorist (Taylor and Mills 2006) and lack scientific investigation (Mornement et al. 2009). Balancing the desire to collect behavioral information with the need to move animals through the system quickly, the author feels that a practical shelter behavior evaluation should take no longer than 30 minutes, require no more than two handlers and a stimulus dog, be well documented in a step-by-step protocol, and be accompanied by a scoring system that is easy to use and interpret.

9.2.9.2 Reliability

Measures of test reliability include intra-rater reliability, inter-rater reliability, test-retest

Box 9.3   Example Foster Dog Survey

Thank you for fostering one of our dogs! We will ask you to fill out this survey periodically while the dog is with you. Please fill it out each time you receive a request from us. Any information you share will help us learn more about the dog.

Foster Dog:
Date:
Your Name:
Animal Name:

Does the dog/puppy reliably use an appropriate potty area? Select all that apply.
- Yes—Outside
- Yes—Pee Pads
- Yes—Other
- No—Regularly eliminates in inappropriate areas

How many hours a day is the dog/puppy used to being alone?

Where do you leave the dog/puppy when no one is home? Select all that apply.
- Loose in home
- Crated
- Baby gate or exercise pen
- Dog is never alone

How does the dog behave when left alone?

Does the dog show interest in food/treats?
- Yes
- No

How does the dog respond when a familiar adult of the household approaches? Record all behaviors observed (see word bank).

Are there children in the household?
- Yes
- No

If yes, how does the dog respond when a familiar child of the household approaches? Record all behaviors observed (see word bank).

How does the dog respond when approached by a familiar person while eating? Record all behaviors observed (see word bank).

How does the dog respond when approached by a familiar person while playing with a toy? Record all behaviors observed (see word bank).

How does the dog respond when approached by a familiar person while chewing on a highly valued treat/bone? Record all behaviors observed (see word bank).

How does the dog respond when unfamiliar people visit the home? Record all behaviors observed (see word bank) or write "N/A" if this hasn't happened.

Are there other pets in the home?
- Yes
- No

If yes, what behaviors does the dog display toward other pets in the home? Record all behaviors observed (see word bank).

Does the dog display any signs of fear, stress, or aggression when touched on particular parts of his or her body (such as the feet, ears, or tail)?
- Yes
- No

If yes, list all of the behaviors/body parts.

How frequently does the dog go on leash walks?

How frequently is the dog off-leash in a fenced area?

Have you encountered other dogs on walks?
- Yes
- No

If yes, what behaviors have you observed? Record all behaviors observed (see word bank).

Have you been approached by familiar people on walks?
- Yes
- No

If yes, what behaviors have you observed? Record all behaviors observed (see word bank)

Have you been approached by unfamiliar people on walks?
- Yes
- No

If yes, what behaviors have you observed? Record all behaviors observed (see word bank).

Have you encountered joggers/runners on walks?
- Yes
- No

If yes, what behaviors have you observed? Record all behaviors observed (see word bank).

Have you encountered bicycles/scooters/wheeled carts on walks?
- Yes
- No

If yes, what behaviors have you observed? Record all behaviors observed (see word bank).

Have you encountered loud traffic (i.e., honking horns, air brakes, garbage trucks) on walks?
- Yes
- No

If yes, what behaviors have you observed? Record all behaviors observed (see word bank).

If present, what is the dog's reaction to climbing/descending stairs? Riding on an elevator? Record all behaviors observed (see word bank).

How does the dog behave in the car? Record all behaviors observed (see word bank).

Any other behaviors that you think we should know about?

Table 9.1 Behavior evaluations in the published literature.

Standardized behavior evaluation	Reference
Behavioural Assessment for Re-homing K9s (B.A.R.K.)	Mornement et al. 2014
	Mornement et al. 2015
Dutch Socially Acceptable Behavior (SAB) test	Van der Borg et al. 2010
Match-Up	Dowling-Guyer et al. 2011
Modified Assess-a-Pet	Bennett et al. 2012
	Bollen and Horowitz 2008
	Christensen et al. 2007
	McGuire et al. 2020
Royal Society for the Prevention of Cruelty to Animals Canine Behavioural Assessment, Queensland, Australia	Clay et al. 2020
	Poulsen et al. 2010
	Shih et al. 2020
Safety Assessment for Evaluating Rehoming (SAFER)	Bennett et al. 2012
Unnamed shelter dog test developed by Dog's Trust, UK	Diesel et al. 2008
Unnamed test for human-directed aggression	Klausz et al. 2014
Unnamed test for human- and dog-directed aggression	Netto and Planta 1997
Unnamed shelter dog test developed by authors	Valsecchi et al. 2011
Unnamed shelter dog test developed by authors	Van der Borg et al. 1991

reliability, and internal consistency (which examines different subtests that are intended to measure the same behavior) (Diederich and Giffroy 2006). For shelters that have more than one evaluator, inter-rater reliability (IRR) is the most relevant measure because it refers to consistency across evaluators. Naturally, if a test has good IRR, it will invariably have good intra-rater reliability as well (Patronek et al. 2019). A few studies, using different behavior evaluations, looked at agreement on ratings across evaluators and found good IRR (Klausz et al. 2014; Mornement et al. 2014; van der Borg et al. 2010), whereas others found acceptable IRR on some subtests and less than acceptable IRR on others (Diesel et al. 2008; Kroll et al. 2004; Valsecchi et al. 2011). In the Diesel et al. (2008) study, evaluators with extensive experience or those who had received formal training in dog behavior were more likely to agree on ratings of at least highly prevalent behaviors. Unfortunately, in a survey of Australian shelters, Mornement et al. (2010) found that only two-thirds of evaluators received any training at all, and at least half of those received informal, on-the-job training.

Wickens et al. (1995) found poor IRR between male and female evaluators, but the researchers believe that the differences were not solely because males and females scored behavior differently but also possibly because they may have administered the tests inconsistently and/or they elicited different reactions from the dogs (Hennessy et al. 1998; Wells and Hepper 1999). However, in a different study, Valsecchi et al. (2011) found that the gender of evaluators had no effect on dogs' responses in their behavior evaluation.

In an examination of internal consistency, Brown et al. (2020) found that even apparently minor modifications in procedure resulted in substantially different ratings of sociability toward humans. Published behavior evaluations vary in how tests of sociability are performed. The evaluator may either stand, kneel, or sit in a chair. The dog may be leashed or free to move about an enclosed area. In some evaluations, the person ignores the dog; in others, the person actively calls the dog and may pet him if he approaches. Not surprisingly, Brown et al. (2020) found that dogs displayed more social behavior when evaluators knelt or sat in a chair than when they stood and when the dog was leashed rather than loose. Dogs were also more social when the evaluator interacted with them than when they were ignored. However, there were substantial individual differences, rendering no specific procedure as more predictive of social behavior in other contexts.

9.2.9.3 Validity

There are several types of validity that make for an overall good test. Patronek et al. (2019) provide a comprehensive explanation of the differences between content or construct validity, convergent validity, criterion validity, face validity, and predictive validity. While all of these forms of validity are relevant to establishing that a behavior evaluation is a useful tool, the ability of the evaluation to predict future behavior is most germane to shelters.

To assess the predictive validity of a behavior evaluation, a "gold standard" against which to compare the results of the evaluation is needed. Not surprisingly, given that the goal is to predict future behavior, most studies compare shelter dogs' scores on the evaluation with their subsequent behavior in the adoptive home. However, for ethical and legal reasons, this approach limits the study population to only dogs who "passed" the evaluation and were adopted. Dogs identified as having significant behavior problems that render them unsuitable for adoption, such as aggression, are not included. Other studies have avoided this complication by using reports from relinquishing owners as the true indication of problematic behavior in the sample of dogs being tested and have looked to see if their evaluation is able to accurately identify those dogs described as problematic. A third approach is to exclude shelter dogs altogether and focus on the evaluation's ability to detect problem behavior in owned dogs. Owned dogs are run through the behavior evaluation, and the results are compared with reports of the dogs' behavior by their owners.

The next step is to determine how accurate the evaluation is at identifying dogs who have been reported as exhibiting the specific problem behavior and dogs who have not. Sensitivity is the proportion of dogs who the test detects as exhibiting the behavior of interest who truly do (true positives or "hits"). For instance, a test with a sensitivity of 80% will correctly catch 80 out of every 100 problematic dogs but will miss 20% of dogs who exhibit the problem behavior but test negative (false negatives or "misses"). Specificity is the proportion of dogs who the test detects as not exhibiting the behavior of interest who truly do not (true negatives or correct rejections). A test with a specificity of 60% will only catch 60 out of every 100 dogs who are problem-free but will misidentify 40% of the problem-free dogs as exhibiting the problem behavior (false positives or "false alarms"). Typically, as sensitivity increases, specificity decreases and vice versa.

While sensitivity and specificity provide an indication of the evaluation's ability to correctly identify dogs with and without the behavior of concern, to fully understand the usefulness of the evaluation, it is necessary to also address the question, "How likely is it that a dog who has tested positive truly has the problem behavior of interest?" That is the positive predictive validity of the evaluation, which is the proportion of true positives in the population of dogs tested who exhibited the behavior of interest. For example, if an evaluation has a positive predictive value of 90%, that means that 9 out of 10 dogs who test positive are true positives. Likewise, the negative predictive value is the proportion of true negatives in the set of dogs who tested as not exhibiting the behavior of interest. A negative predictive value of 70% means that 7 out of 10 dogs who test negative are true negatives. The predictive value is determined by the sensitivity and the specificity of the evaluation AND the prevalence of the behavior of concern in the population of animals being tested. If prevalence is low, most errors will necessarily be false positives, while if prevalence is high, errors will be false negatives.

While ideally, the overall error rate for a test will be low, some number of errors is unavoidable, and the choice of a good behavior test requires an informed decision about an acceptable balance of false positives and false negatives. For certain problem behaviors, such as aggression, it might be appropriate to use a test that has a higher negative predictive value because the cost of missing an aggressive dog and adopting him out is unacceptably high. For problems such as mild fear of being handled or mouthiness, it might be best to use a test that better balances positive and negative predictive value—while knowing this information could avoid a possible mismatch with an adopter, the cost of missing such behaviors is likely to be low.

In conclusion, to fully assess the usefulness of a behavior evaluation as a component of the assessment process, the predictive value should be considered along with an acceptable balance of erroneous results. The prevalence of a particular behavior, such as aggression, in the population of dogs in your shelter has a direct impact on the likelihood that a dog who has tested as aggressive truly is aggressive. Sensitivity and specificity are characteristics of the behavior evaluation, prevalence is a characteristic of the population you are testing, and the predictive value of the evaluation for any specific population is a function of sensitivity, specificity, and prevalence. Unfortunately, as revealed in the review below, few researchers have approached validation testing in the same way, so only a handful of published studies report sensitivity, specificity, and predictive value. The following review is categorized by the gold standard used.

9.2.9.3.1 Shelter Dogs: Behavior Evaluation Results and Behavior in the New Home

Studies that compare evaluation results with behavior in the adoptive home rely largely on reports of behavior after the dog has been in the home for some period of time, anywhere from 1–13 months post-adoption. Van der Borg et al. (1991) found that their evaluation predicted 75% of all of the problem behaviors described by owners 1–2 months after adoption. Looking specifically at aggression, the evaluation accurately identified 82% of the dogs who exhibited human-directed aggression post-adoption, with a positive predictive value of 59%, and 86% of dogs who exhibited conspecific aggression post-adoption, with a positive predictive value of 52%. Specificity rates were correspondingly lower, and negative predictive values were higher. Their evaluation errs on the side of caution when it comes to assessing for aggression.

Bollen and Horowitz (2008) determined that dogs who were classified as unsocial toward people during a modified version of the Assess-a-Pet (mAAP) evaluation were more likely to be reported by their adopters to exhibit non-aggressive behavior problems (e.g., barking, destructive behavior, separation anxiety, fearful behavior) at a six-month follow-up check. They also found that dogs who were rated as mildly aggressive on one or two subtests of the evaluation were more likely to be returned for aggression by their adopters. In contrast, Christensen et al. (2007) found that the mAAP evaluation did a relatively poor job of detecting aggression, with 41% of dogs who had "passed" the evaluation reported by their adopters as showing behaviors consistent with aggression (lunging, growling, snapping, biting). Similarly, a comparison of behavior ratings from the Behavioural Assessment for Rehoming K9s (B.A.R.K.) evaluation with adopter reports revealed only moderate correlations for fear and friendliness/aggression and no relationship for ratings of anxiety, compliance, or activity level (Mornement et al. 2014). A further analysis of the predictive validity of B.A.R.K. (Mornement et al. 2015) found that the test missed 25% of the 73 dogs who exhibited aggression post-adoption.

A few studies have looked specifically at predicting dogs' guarding of coveted items, such as food, bones, and toys. For instance, Marder et al. (2013) followed up with adopters of dogs who had exhibited food aggression on the Match-Up II behavior evaluation and found that only 55% of those dogs showed aggression over food in the new home. However, the ability to predict the absence of food guarding was better—78% of the dogs who did not show food aggression in the evaluation also did not in the home—thus, the test is useful for identifying non-guarders. McGuire et al. (2020) too found that roughly half of the dogs who showed guarding of a variety of resources during the behavior evaluation did not show the same behavior in the adoptive home. Like Marder et al. (2013), they found that the behavior evaluation, in this case the mAAP, more reliably identified non-guarders (specificity of 92%; negative predictive value of 89%), Mohan-Gibbons et al. (2012) also found that the presence of food aggression in the SAFER behavior evaluation was not predictive of the same behavior in the home.

The decision of whether to test for aggression over resources should be based on the individual shelter's comfort with adopting out dogs that might show this behavior. While Marder et al. (2013) found that few adopters cared if their dogs guarded food, McGuire (2019) reported that dogs exhibiting severe resource guarding were returned to the shelter at a higher rate than the general population. In a different study, though, Mohan-Gibbons et al. (2018) found that severe food guarders were at no greater risk of return than mild or moderate guarders. They did, however, see a higher rate of bites to adopters from food-guarding dogs than non-guarders, although the percentage of bites did not increase when shelters ceased formal testing for the behavior.

A primary drawback of these studies is the reliance on adopter reports of behavior. When there is disagreement between evaluation results and post-adoption behavior reports, there is no way to determine if the evaluation is flawed, the adopter reports are inaccurate, or both are at fault. A different approach to comparing the behavior of the dog in the shelter and in the adoptive home is to first evaluate the dog in the shelter and then conduct the same evaluation after the dog has been adopted. Valsecchi et al. (2011) re-tested dogs in their new homes approximately four months after adoption and reported moderate correlations with the dogs' in-shelter evaluation responses. In contrast, Poulsen et al.'s (2010) findings were mixed. Eighty days after adoption, dogs' tendency to guard resources and their reactions to noise, movement, toys, and play were consistent across evaluations, but their interactions with the unfamiliar evaluator were not consistent.

9.2.9.3.2 *Shelter Dogs: Behavior in the Former Home and Behavior Evaluation Results*

Bearing in mind the adage that "the best predictor of future behavior is past behavior," a few studies have examined agreement between reports from the relinquishing owner and subsequent evaluation test results. Duffy et al. (2014) looked at the correlation between aggression reported on the C-BARQ[(S)] by the surrendering owner and aggression during a behavior evaluation conducted after the dogs were in the shelter. Dogs who showed aggression during the evaluation were more likely to have been rated as aggressive by their former owners. Dogs euthanized at the shelter were more likely to have been reported by their owners as having behaved aggressively toward strangers. These results are consistent with an earlier finding by Bollen and Horowitz (2008) that 90% of surrendered dogs reported by their owners to have exhibited aggressive behavior failed one or more subtests of the mAAP evaluation. However, evaluators knew in advance the dogs who had been relinquished for aggression, which could have led to conscious or unconscious biases in the interpretation of their behavior during the evaluation. In the Valsecchi et al. (2011) study, 10 long-term shelter dogs with established histories of human-directed aggression were included in their sample. All 10 dogs exhibited such severe aggression during the evaluation that handling was unsafe to perform. Like the previous study, the evaluator in this case was also not blind to the status of the dogs being evaluated, and so this could have led to biases in interpretation.

9.2.9.3.3 *Owned Dogs: Behavior Evaluation Results and Owner Reports*

A significant limitation of validation studies performed on shelter dogs is that shelters cannot responsibly adopt out dogs who exhibit serious aggression during the evaluation, and, as a result, it is impossible to ever know the true rate of false positives on the test. A solution to this shortcoming is to conduct the behavior evaluation on owned dogs. It is well established that problem behavior, including aggression toward family members, strangers, and other dogs, is present in the owned dog population (Casey et al. 2014; Duffy et al. 2008; Martínez et al. 2011).

Bennett et al. (2012) recruited owned dogs coming into a veterinary teaching hospital and put the dogs through two standardized behavior evaluations: the mAAP and SAFER. At the same time, owners completed the C-BARQ to reveal the dogs' aggression histories. For SAFER, sensitivity was 60% and specificity was 50%. For mAAP, sensitivity was 73% and specificity was 59%. When the researchers categorized the severity of the aggression as none/mild, moderate, or severe, the mAAP results correlated significantly with owner reports. In contrast, the SAFER test was able to differentiate between dogs with none/mild or severe aggression but missed identifying dogs with moderate levels of aggression. However, both tests were still prone to substantial error rates, and the authors recommend relying on additional sources of information to best obtain a picture of a dog's aggressive behavior.

In their study of owner reports and performance on a behavior evaluation, Clay et al. (2020a) employed the unique approach of bringing owned dogs into an animal shelter to be evaluated while owners waited in a separate room. The owners had previously completed the C-BARQ questionnaire for their dogs. The researchers reported positive correlations for fear, arousal, friendliness, and anxiousness. In addition, aggression toward humans on the evaluation was correlated with owner reports; however, the incidence of aggression during the evaluation was exceedingly low. Similarly, few dogs exhibited aggression toward other dogs in the evaluation, despite a relatively high number of owners (60%) reporting conspecific aggression in their dogs.

Evaluations that are designed specifically to detect aggressive behavior have produced mixed results. For example, Netto and Planta's (1997) battery of 43 tests for aggression, some of which are highly provocative, distinguished between dogs with and without a bite history with an overall accuracy rate of 57%. The prevalence of aggression in the population was unusually high (60%) because they actively recruited owners of aggressive dogs to participate. As a result, their false positive rate was low (7%), and their false negative rate was quite high (36%). Van der Borg et al. (2010) found that the Dutch Socially Acceptable Behavior test identified dogs with a history of human-directed aggression with an overall accuracy rate of 62% or 67%, depending upon whether the test was conducted inside or outside. Combining the results for dogs tested indoors and outdoors, the positive predictive value was 47%, and the negative predictive value was 68.5%. Using a different evaluation, Klausz et al. (2014) reported good agreement between aggression exhibited by owned dogs during the test and owner reports of aggression toward strangers but not toward familiar people.

9.2.9.3.4 *The Use of Simulations*

Standardized behavior evaluations often incorporate the use of simulations to increase safety. For instance, a fake hand on a stick is frequently used to touch the dog while he is eating or chewing. A doll is used to assess how the dog might be expected to react toward children. Kroll et al. (2004) tested owned dogs, some with a history of aggression toward children, and found that the aggressive dogs were prone to aggress not only toward the doll but also toward the fake hand. Unfortunately, false positive and false negative errors were highly prevalent. Another study found that reactions to a doll and a model dog partially correlated with dogs' histories of aggression, as measured by the owners' responses on the C-BARQ (Barnard et al. 2012). In a study that compared shelter dogs' reactions to a model dog and a real dog, Shabelansky et al. (2015) found good agreement for friendliness, moderate agreement for fearfulness, and poor agreement for aggressiveness. Clearly, this is dissatisfying, as the primary reason for using a replica of a dog is to reduce the risk of aggression toward a real dog. Given these results, the author cautions against relying solely on these mockups for predicting future aggressive behavior in shelter dogs. Mockups may be useful as an initial screen to flag individual dogs for further assessment.

9.2.9.3.5 *The Champagne and the Cork?*

The published research clearly calls into question the merit of information gleaned from a standardized behavior evaluation conducted in a shelter environment. The disappointing reliability and validity evidence is further substantiated by Patronek and Bradley's (2016) contention that behavior evaluations designed to detect aggressive dogs are likely to result in a high number of false positives. They argue that aggression toward people is a relatively rare phenomenon; probably present in no more than 16% of the general dog population, based on dog bite statistics. Guessing that behavior evaluations might share roughly the same sensitivity (92%) and specificity (36%) as diagnostic tests for aggressive or delinquent behavior in people (such as those designed to predict future violent offending), Patronek and Bradley ran simulations to reveal that as many as 78% of dogs identified as aggressive in an evaluation are likely false positives. Even under the best-case scenario of improbably high sensitivity (85%) and specificity (85%), the false positive rate was still 48%, hence the title of their paper "No Better than Flipping a Coin." They conclude that no subtest or full test battery has been demonstrated to be reliable and valid and the tests are likely to produce high false positive rates; therefore, they recommend that

shelters discontinue the use of standardized behavior evaluations.

Wynne (2016), however, argues in a *Psychology Today* blog that just because our current behavior evaluations are not very good, we shouldn't throw up our hands in defeat. Instead, Wynne suggests that, much like what happened with psychological tests for humans, we should be inspired to develop more accurate tests. Wynne also points out that Patronek and Bradley's (2016) analysis only takes the risk to the dog into consideration, not the risk to humans. It's true that if a shelter's primary concern is public safety, it may be worth accepting a high rate of false positives to ensure that truly dangerous dogs are identified and kept from re-entering the community. In the Patronek and Bradley analysis, a shelter using their fictitious evaluation would only adopt out three false negatives—dogs who didn't exhibit aggressive behavior during the evaluation but would do so in the home—for every 100 dogs adopted. However, that is at the cost of euthanizing 174 false positive dogs. That's a heavy price for dogs to pay. Granted, it's a price that may be justified. Each shelter must decide where they lie in terms of risk aversion.

Neither Patronek and Bradley (2016) nor Wynne (2016) paint a complete picture of reality. First, both of their analyses assume that all aggressive behavior is equally dangerous and that shelters would euthanize a dog exhibiting any level of aggression. That is untrue. Some shelters successfully deal with dogs exhibiting certain types of mild to moderate aggressive behavior, either by modifying the behavior prior to adoption or supporting the adopter once the dog is in the home (see Chapter 12). Second, as Patronek and Bradley (2016) point out, some unknown number of truly dangerous dogs would be detected in the shelter outside of the behavior evaluation and filtered from the pool of adoption candidates. Finally, accepting that a reasonable segment of the shelter dog population may exhibit aggression purely because they are stressed by their circumstances further cements the argument that safely corroborating aggression in additional contexts is an indispensable process for balancing the risks to both shelter dogs and the public.

Furthermore, as discussed above, the predictive validity of any test relates not only to the quality of the test but also to the prevalence of the behavior being tested. If the true prevalence of aggression in dogs is lower than the 16% estimate used in the Patronek and Bradley (2016) simulations, then false positives are even more likely. If, on the other hand, the true prevalence is higher than 16%—as may increasingly be the case in some shelters as populations shift toward more problematic dogs—then false positives are less likely, thus increasing the likelihood of false negatives.

The decision of whether to reject standardized behavior evaluations in their entirety—essentially throwing out the champagne along with the cork—is not a straightforward one. There are more empirical data on the worth of behavior evaluations than on any of the other sources of information recommended in this chapter. And there is no question that individual dogs behave differently in response to the stimuli presented during an evaluation. Some dogs find the experience terrifying, some find it threatening, and some behave as though it's a fun and enriching activity. The significance of these differences in terms of how well, or even if, they relate to future behavior remains unknown.

Ultimately, it is up to individual shelters to decide if they wish to include an evaluation as a source of behavioral data. In the grand scheme of a mixed assessment model, a standardized behavior evaluation may be the only opportunity for behavior staff to interact directly with the dog. It's also an efficient way to gather information about the dog's behavior in a range of consistent scenarios. Furthermore, observing a dog during a behavior evaluation allows staff to assess his behavior relative to other dogs in the shelter, thereby maintaining a behavioral yardstick on the overall population. If a shelter chooses to incorporate an evaluative procedure, the author recommends that they select one of the test batteries published in the scientific

literature, as these have at least received some empirical attention. Detailed written protocols, with clear limits on the extent to which provocation is permitted, are a must. In addition, the evaluation should be performed in the recommended order. How a dog responds on a particular subtest can't help but influence his responses, and the evaluator's, on subsequent subtests, so it is important to keep the order consistent. Evaluators should be trained on how to administer the evaluation and on how to record and interpret dogs' responses. Routine audits ought to be performed to ensure accuracy and consistency. Filming evaluations is useful not only to allow for review of dogs exhibiting concerning behavior but also for auditing and instructing. Evaluations should be performed no earlier than the fourth day after arrival in the shelter to allow for some lowering of stress (Hennessy et al. 1997).

If a shelter opts to use a standardized behavior evaluation, the test should, like all of the other sources of information outlined in this chapter, comprise part of a series of assessments that together inform pathway planning as well as treatment and outcome decisions for an individual dog (Bennett et al. 2012; Patronek et al. 2019). Whenever safe and feasible, observations of problematic behavior should be corroborated in other circumstances outside of the testing environment, by additional observers, before considering it truly reflective of the dog's future behavior (Rayment et al. 2015). An exception to this should be made only if truly egregious aggression is exhibited during the evaluation. In such a case, the shelter should be prepared to accept that it might be deeming a false positive dog as unsuitable for adoption rather than risk placing a dangerous dog into the community.

9.3 Behavior Information and Pathway Planning

When a dog enters the shelter system, the process of collecting behavior information begins and should persist until the dog is either adopted, transferred to another organization, or humanely euthanized. Some dogs can be fast-tracked—suitable for placement with very few behavior observations. Even with such a designation, a fast-tracked dog's status could change at any time prior to adoption, so it's necessary to continue to collect behavior observations with some regularity. Other dogs will be identified as candidates for humane euthanasia right away because of a credible history of severe aggression or an instance of egregious aggression in the shelter. All others fall into the category of needing further behavior information to determine if they meet the organization's adoptability guidelines or treatment inclusion criteria. If a dog is a candidate for behavior treatment, the behavior assessment process continues until the dog improves to the extent that he meets adoptability guidelines or fails to make progress. At any time during a dog's stay, it may be determined that the dog suffers from a behavior condition that is considered untreatable by the organization or is suffering from an unacceptable quality of life. At that point, unless there are alternatives

for treatment or improved quality of life elsewhere, humane euthanasia is appropriate. A visual depiction of one possible behavior assessment process appears in Figure 9.3.

Of course, behavior is rarely, if ever, the sole determinant of a shelter dog's ultimate outcome; medical conditions, operational considerations, and placement opportunities all contribute to pathway planning. Data gathered through the assessment process should be compiled, reviewed, and interpreted by the behavior team, bearing in mind the limitations inherent within each source of information and the lack of supportive reliability and validity evidence, to assemble a picture of the individual dog's behavior. This picture, however complete or incomplete, is then brought forth by the behavior team for a holistic discussion about the most suitable pathway for the dog.

9.4 Conclusions

Shelters are responsible for distinguishing between dogs who are appropriate for

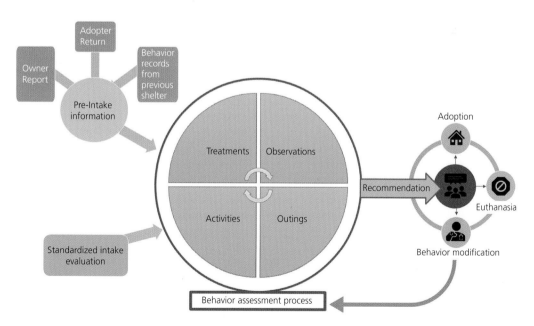

Figure 9.3 A visualization of how the various sources of behavioral information come together to inform a behavior team's outcome recommendation for a particular dog.

adoption, dogs who need rehabilitation, and dogs who are unsuitable for placement either because of safety concerns or unacceptable welfare. Toward that end, shelters need processes for gathering accurate behavior information that enables them to gauge the dog's current state and, to the best of their ability, predict future behavior. Ideally, once compiled, these processes will provide not just snapshots of behavior but rather a glimpse into the dog's personality, which is believed to reflect more reliable information about behavior outside of the shelter environment. Personality is formed by a complex interplay between a dog's genetic predispositions, developmental circumstances, and life experiences. However, a dog's behavior at any given time is also heavily influenced by his emotional and motivational states, stress level, and the specific environment. Thus, any single observation of behavior should be considered but a piece of a larger puzzle. The more pieces you have, in different contexts and by different observers, the more complete the puzzle picture. Shelters face the challenge of collecting just the right amount of information—too little and not enough of the puzzle is filled in; too much and the puzzle is more complete, but the dog's stay has been lengthened, perhaps unnecessarily. By striking the right balance, sufficient information is gathered in an optimal amount of time to make the best and most expedient outcome decision for each animal in the shelter.

Acknowledgments

The author would like to acknowledge Maya Gupta for her willingness to discuss and review various drafts of this chapter.

References

Arguel, A. and Jamet, E. (2009). Using video and statis pictures to improve learning of procedural contents. *Comput. Hum. Behav.* 25:354–359.

Barnard, S., Siracusa, C., Reisner, I. et al. (2012). Validity of model devices used to assess canine temperament in behavioral tests. *Appl. Anim. Behav. Sci.* 138: 79–87.

Belpedio, C., Buffington, L., Clusman, S. et al. (2010). Effect of multidog play groups on cortisol levels and behavior of dogs (*Canis lupus familiaris*) housed in a humane society. *J. Appl. Compan. Anim. Behav.* 4: 15–27.

Bennett, S.L., Litster, A., Weng, H-Y. et al. (2012). Investigating behavior assessment instruments to predict aggression in dogs. *Appl. Anim. Behav. Sci.* 141: 139–148.

Bergamasco, L., Osella, M.C., Savarino, P. et al. (2010). Heart rate variability and saliva cortisol assessment in shelter dog: Human-animal interaction effects. *Appl. Anim. Behav. Sci.* 125: 56–68.

Bollen, K.S. and Horowitz, J. (2008). Behavioral evaluation and demographic information in the assessment of aggressiveness in shelter dogs. *Appl. Anim. Behav. Sci.* 112: 120–135.

Brown, K.M., Feuerbacher, E.N., Hall, N.J. et al. (2020). Minor procedural variations affect canine behavior during sociability assessments. *Behav.* https://doi.org/10.1016/j.beproc.2020.104145.

Casey, R.A., Loftus, B., Bolster, C. et al. (2014). Human directed aggression in domestic dogs (*Canis familiaris*): Occurrence in different contexts and risk factors. *Appl. Anim. Behav. Sci.* 152: 52–63.

Christensen, E., Scarlett, J., Campagna, M. et al. (2007). Aggressive behavior in adopted dogs that passed a temperament test. *Appl. Anim. Behav. Sci.* 106: 85–95.

Clay, L., Paterson, M.B.A., Bennett, P. et al. (2019). Early recognition of behaviour problems in shelter dogs by monitoring them in their kennels after admission to a shelter. *Animals.* https://doi.org/10.3390/ani9110875.

Clay, L., Paterson, M.B.A., Bennett, P. et al. (2020a). *Comparison of canine behaviour scored using a shelter behaviour assessment and an owner completed questionnaire, C-BARQ*. *Animals*. https://doi.org/10.3390/ani10101797.

Clay, L., Paterson, M.B.A., Bennett, P. et al. (2020b). In defense of canine behavioral assessments in shelters: Outlining their positive applications. *J. Vet. Behav.* 38: 74–81.

Coppola, C.L., Grandin, T., and Enns, R.M. (2006). Human interaction and cortisol: Can human contact reduce stress for shelter dogs? *Physiol. Behav.* 87: 537–541.

Croskerry, P. (2006). Critical thinking and decisionmaking: Avoiding the perils of thin-slicing. *Ann. Emerg. Med.* 48: 720–722.

Csoltova, E., Martineau, M., Boissy, A. et al. (2017). Behavioral and physiological reactions in dogs to a veterinary examination: Owner-dog interactions improve canine well-being. *Physiol. Behav.* 177: 270–281.

D'Arpino, S., Dowling-Guyer, S., Shabelansky, A. et al. (2012). The use and perception of canine behavioral assessments in sheltering organizations. *Proceedings of the American College of Veterinary Behaviorists/American Veterinary Society of Animal Behavior Veterinary Behavior Symposium*, San Diego, CA.

Diederich, C. and Giffroy, J.-M. (2006). Behavioural testing in dogs: A review of methodology in search for standardization. *Appl. Anim. Behav. Sci.* 97: 51–72.

Diesel, G., Brodbelt, D., and Pfeiffer, D.U. (2008). Reliability of assessment of dogs' behavioural responses by staff working at a welfare charity in the UK. *Appl. Anim. Behav. Sci.* 115: 171–181.

DiGiacomo, N., Arluke, A., and Patronek, G. (1998). Surrendering pets to shelters: The relinquisher's perspective. *Anthrozoös* 11: 41–45.

Döring, D., Roscher, A., Scheipl, F. et al. (2009). Fear-related behavior of dogs in veterinary practice. *Vet. J.* 182: 38–43.

Dowling-Guyer, S., Marder, A., and D'Arpino, S. (2011). Behavioral traits detected in shelter dogs by a behavior evaluation. *Appl. Anim. Behav. Sci.* 130: 107–114.

Drugowitsch, J., DeAngelis, G.C., Angelaki, D.E. (2015). Tuning the speed-accuracy trade-off to maximize reward rate in multisensory decision-making. *eLife* 4: e06678.

Dudley, E.S., Schiml, P.A., and Hennessy, M.B. (2015). Effects of repeated petting sessions on leukocyte counts, intestinal parasite prevalence, and plasma cortisol concentration of dogs housed in a county animal shelter. *J. Am. Vet. Med. Assoc.* 247: 1289–1298.

Duffy, D.L., Hsu, Y., and Serpell, J.A. (2008). Breed differences in canine aggression. *Appl. Anim. Behav. Sci.* 114: 441–460.

Duffy, D.L., Kruger, K.A., and Serpell, J.A. (2014). Evaluation of a behavioral assessment tool for dogs relinquished to shelters. *Prev. Vet. Med.* 117: 601–609.

Durmaz, A., Dursun, İ., and Kabadayi, E.T. (2020). Mitigating the effects of social desirability bias in self-report surveys: Classical and new techniques. In: *Applied Social Science Approaches to Mixed Methods Research* (eds. M.L. Baran and J.E. Jones), 146–185. Hershey, PA: IGI Global.

Edwards, P.T., Hazel, S.J., Browne, M. et al. (2019). Investigating risk factors that predict a dog's fear during veterinary consultations. *PLOS ONE* 14: e0215416.

Fehringer, A. and Dreschel, N.A. (2014). Stress in shelter dogs and the use of foster care to improve animal welfare. *J. Vet. Behav.* 9: e1–19.

Flint, H.E., Coe, J.B., Pearl, D.L. et al. (2018). Effect of training for dog fear identification on dog owner ratings of fear in familiar and unfamiliar dogs. *Appl. Anim. Behav. Sci.* 208: 66–74.

Flower, S. (2016). The effect of play group on the behavior of shelter dogs. *CUNY Academic Works*. https://academicworks.cuny.edu/cgi/viewcontent.cgi?article=1122&context=hc_sas_etds (accessed 5 September 2021).

Fratkin, J.L., Sinn, D.L., Thomas, S. et al. (2015). Do you see what I see? Can non-experts with minimal training reproduce expert ratings in behavioral assessment of working dogs? *Behav.* 110: 105–116.

Ganier, F. and de Vries, P. (2016). Are instructions in video format always better than photographs when learning manual techniques? The case of learning how to do sutures. *Learn. Instr* 44: 87–96.

Gfrerer, N., Taborsky, M., and Würbel, H. (2018). Benefits of intraspecific social exposure in adult Swiss military dogs. *Appl. Anim. Behav. Sci.* 201: 54–60.

Gilchrist, R.J. (2019). Using the C-BARQ to predict in-home behaviors of adopted dogs. Speech presented at the Canine Science Conference in Phoenix, AZ (18–20 October 2019).

Goold, C. and Newberry, R.C. (2017a). Aggressiveness as a latent personality trait of domestic dogs: Testing local independence and measurement invariance. *PLOS One* 12 (8): e0183595.

Goold, C. and Newberry, R.C. (2017b). Modelling personality, plasticity and predictability in shelter dogs. *R. Soc. Open Sci.* 4: e170618.

Gunter, L.M., Feuerbacher, E.N., Gilchrist, R. et al. (2019). Evaluating the effects of a temporary fostering program on shelter dog welfare. *Peer J.* 7: e6620.

Gunter, L., Protopopova, A., Hooker, S.P. et al. (2017). Impacts of encouraging dog walking on returns of newly adopted dogs to a shelter. *J. Appl. Anim. Welf. Sci.* https://doi.org/10.108 0/10888705.2017.1341318.

Hennessy, M.B., Davis, H.N., Williams, M.T. et al. (1997). Plasma cortisol levels of dogs at a county animal shelter. *Physiol. Behav.* 62: 485–490.

Hennessy, M.B., Morris, A., and Linden, F. (2006). Evaluation of the effects of a socialization program in a prison on behavior and pituitary-adrenal hormone levels of shelter dogs. *Appl. Anim. Behav. Sci.* 99: 157–171.

Hennessy, M.B., Williams, M.T., Miller, D.D. et al. (1998). Influence of male and female petters on plasma cortisol and behaviour: Can human interaction reduce the stress of dogs in a public animal shelter? *Appl. Anim. Behav. Sci.* 61: 63–77.

Hiby, E.F., Rooney, N.J., and Bradshaw, J.W.S. (2006). Behavioural and physiological responses of dogs entering rehoming kennels. *Physiol. Behav.* 89: 385–391.

Hill, E.M., LaLonde, C.M., and Reese, L.A. (2020). Compassion fatigue in animal care workers. *Traumatology* 26: 96–108.

Hoerster, K.D., Mayer, J.A., Sallis, J.F. et al. (2011). Dog walking: Its association with physical activity guideline adherence and its correlates. *Prev. Med.* 52: 33–38.

Höffler, T.N. and Leutner, D. (2007). Instructional animation versus static pictures: A meta-analysis. *Learn. Instr.* 17: 722–738.

Hoffman, C.L., Ladha, C., and Wilcox, S. (2019). An actigraphy-based comparison of shelter dog and owned dog activity patterns. *J. Vet. Behav.* 34: 30–36.

Johnson, A., Dougherty, H., Sunday, P. et al. (2013). *Independent study 490A: Do play groups for shelter dogs reduce in-kennel arousal and excitability levels?* Iowa State University Animal Industry Report.

Jones, S., Houpt, K.A., Dowling-Guyer, S. et al. (2014). Use of accelerometers to measure stress levels in shelter dogs. *J. Appl. Anim. Welf. Sci.* 17: 18–28.

Kis, A., Klausz, B., Persa, E. et al. (2014). Timing and presence of an attachment person affect sensitivity of aggression tests in shelter dogs. *Vet. Rec.* https://doi.org/10.1136/vr.101955.

Klausz, B., Kis, A., Persa, E. et al. (2014). A quick assessment tool for human-directed aggression in pet dogs. *Aggressive Behav.* 40 (2): 178–188.

Kroll, T.L., Houpt, K.A., and Erb, H.N. (2004). The use of novel stimuli as indicators of aggressive behavior in dogs. *J. Am. Anim. Hosp. Assoc.* 40: 13–19.

Kujala, M.V., Kujala J., Carlson, S. et al. (2012). Dog experts' brains distinguish socially relevant body postures similarly in dogs and humans. *PLOS One* 7: e39145.

Kwan, J.Y. and Bain, M.J. (2013). Owner attachment and problem behaviors related to relinquishment and training techniques of dogs. *J. Appl. Anim. Welf. Sci.* https://doi.org/10.1080/10888705.2013.768923.

Ledger, R.A. and Baxter, M.R. (1997). The development of a validated test to assess the temperament of dogs in a rescue shelter. *Proceedings of the First International Conference on Veterinary Behavioral Medicine* (eds. D.S. Mills, S.E. Heath, and L.J. Harrington). Birmingham: UK Universities Federation for Animal Welfare.

Lelkes, Y., Krosnick, J.A., Marx, D.M. et al. (2012). Complete anonymity compromises the accuracy of self-reports. *J. Exp. Soc. Psychol.* 48: 1291–1299.

Ley, J.M. and Bennett, P.C. (2007). Understanding personality by understanding companion dogs. *Anthrozoös* 20: 113–124.

Lind, A.-K., Hydbring-Sandberg, E., Forkman, B. et al. (2017). Assessing stress in dogs during a visit to the veterinary clinic: Correlations between dog behavior in standardized tests and assessments by veterinary staff and owners. *J. Vet. Behav.* 17: 24–31.

Marder, A.R. (2015). Intake and assessment. In: *Animal Behavior for Shelter Veterinarians and Staff* (eds. E. Weiss, H. Mohan-Gibbons, and S. Zawistowski), 131–144. Hoboken, NJ: Wiley-Blackwell.

Marder, A.R., Shabelansky, A., Patronek, G.J. et al. (2013). Food-related aggression in shelter dogs: A comparison of behavior identified by a behavior evaluation in the shelter and owner reports after adoption. *Appl. Anim. Behav. Sci.* 148: 150–156.

Martínez, Á.G., Pernas, G.S., Casalta, F.J.D. et al. (2011). Risk factors associated with behavioral problems in dogs. *J. Vet. Behav.* 6: 225–231.

McConnell, P.B. and London, K.B. (2009). *Feisty Fido: Help for the Leash-Reactive Dog*, 2nd ed. Black Earth, WI: McConnell Publishing.

McGuire, B. (2019). Characteristics and adoption success of shelter dogs assessed as resource guarders. *Animals.* https://doi.org/10.3390/ani9110982.

McGuire, B., Orantes, D., Xue, S. et al. (2020). Abilities of canine shelter behavioral evaluations and owner surrender profiles to predict resource guarding in adoptive homes. *Animals.* https://doi.org/10.3390/ani10091702.

Mills, D.S., Demontigny-Bédard, I., Gruen, M. et al. (2020). Pain and problem behavior in cats and dogs. *Animals.* https://doi.org/10.3390/ani10020318.

Mohan-Gibbons, H., Dolan, D.E., Reid, P. et al. (2018). The impact of excluding food guarding from a standardized behavioral canine assessment in animal shelters. *Animals* 8: 27.

Mohan-Gibbons, H., Weiss, E., Garrison, L. et al. (2014). Evaluation of a novel dog adoption program in two US communities. *PLOS ONE* 9: e91959.

Mohan-Gibbons, H., Weiss, E., and Slater, M. (2012). Preliminary investigation of food guarding in shelter dogs in the United States. *Animals* 2: 331–346.

Mondelli, F, Prato-Previde, E., Verga, M. et al. (2004). The bond that never developed: Adoption and relinquishment of dogs in a rescue shelter. *J. Appl. Anim. Welf. Sci.* 7: 253–266.

Morgan, L., Protopopova, A., Birkler, R.I.D. et al. (2021). Human-dog relationships during the COVID-19 pandemic: Booming dog adoption during social isolation. *Humanit. Soc. Sci. Commun.* https://doi.org/10.1057/s41599-020-00649-x.

Mornement, K.M., Coleman, G.J., Toukhsati, S. et al. (2010). A review of behavioral assessment protocols used by Australian animal shelters to determine the adoption suitability of dogs. *J. Appl. Anim. Welf. Sci.* 13: 314–329.

Mornement, K.M., Coleman, G.J., Toukhsati, S. et al. (2014). Development of the Behavioral Assessment for Re-homing K9s's (B.A.R.K.) protocol. *Appl. Anim. Behav. Sci.* 151: 75–83.

Mornement, K.M., Coleman, G.J., Toukhsati, S.R. et al. (2015). Evaluation of the predictive validity of the Behavioral Assessment for Re-homing K9s's (B.A.R.K.) protocol and owner satisfaction with adopted dogs. *Appl. Anim. Behav. Sci.* 167: 35–42.

Mornement, K., Toukhsati, S., Coleman, G. et al. (2009). Reliability, validity and feasibility of existing tests of canine behaviour. In: *AIAM Annual Conference on Urban Animal Management*, Geelong, Australia. Australian Institute of Animal Management.

Netto, W.J. and Planta, D.J.U. (1997). Behavioural testing for aggression in the domestic dog. *Appl. Anim. Behav. Sci.* 52: 243–263.

Patronek, G.J. and Bradley, J. (2016). No better than flipping a coin: Reconsidering canine behavior evaluations in animal shelters. *J. Vet. Behav.* 15: 66–77.

Patronek, G.J., Bradley, J., and Arps, E. (2019). What is the evidence for reliability and validity of behavior evaluations for shelter dogs? A prequel to "No better than flipping a coin," *J. Vet. Behav.* 31: 43–58.

Patronek, G.J. and Crowe, A. (2018). Factors associated with high live release for dogs at a large, open-admission, municipal shelter. *Animals.* https://doi.org/10.3390/ani8040045.

Perry, P.J., Scarlett, J.M., Houpt, K.A. et al. (2020). A comparison of four environmental enrichments on adoptability of shelter dogs. *J. Vet. Behav.* 35: 1–7.

Poulsen, A., Lisle, A., and Phillips, C.J.C. (2010). An evaluation of a behavior assessment to determine the suitability of shelter dogs for rehoming. *Vet. Med. Int.* 1: 1–9.

Protopopova, A. and Wynne, C.D.L. (2014). Adopter-dog interactions at the shelter: Behavioral and contextual predictors of adoption. *Appl. Anim. Behav. Sci.* 157: 109–116.

Rayment, D.J., De Groef, B., Peters, R.A. et al. (2013). The use of real-time heart rate monitors to assess arousal levels during canine behavioural test batteries. *Australian Institute of Animal Management Proceedings*, Alice Springs, Australia (16 October 2013). Victoria, Australia: AIAM.

Rayment, D.J., De Groef, B., Peters, R.A. et al. (2015). Applied personality assessment in domestic dogs: Limitations and caveats. *Appl. Anim. Behav. Sci.* 163: 1–18.

Reid, P.J. (2013). Animal behavior forensics: Evaluation of dangerous dogs and cruelty victims. In: *Shelter Medicine for Veterinarians and Staff*, 2nd ed. (eds. L. Miller and S. Zawistowski), 559–567. Hoboken, NJ: Wiley-Blackwell.

Reid, P., Goldman, J., and Zawistowski, S. (2004). Animal shelter behavior programs. In: *Shelter Medicine for Veterinarians and Staff* (eds. L. Miller and S. Zawistowski), 317–331. Ames, IA: Blackwell.

Richman, W.L., Kiesler, S., Weisband, S. et al. (1999). A meta-analytic study of social desirability distortion in computer-administered questionnaires, traditional questionnaires, and interviews. *J. Appl. Psychol.* 84: 754–775.

Riemer, S., Heritier, C., Windschnurer, I. et al. (2021). A review on mitigating fear and aggression in dogs and cats in a veterinary setting. *Animals.* https://doi.org/10.3390/ani11010158.

Scotney, R.L., McLaughlin, D., and Keates, H.L. (2015). A systematic review of the effects of euthanasia and occupational stress in personnel working with animals in animal shelters, veterinary clinics, and biomedical research facilities. *J. Am. Vet. Med. Assoc.* 247: 1121–1130.

Segurson, S.A., Serpell, J.A., and Hart, B.L. (2005). Evaluation of a behavioral assessment questionnaire for use in the characterization of behavioral problems of dogs relinquished to animal shelters. *J. Am. Vet. Med. Assoc.* 227: 1755–1761.

Shabelansky, A., Dowling-Guyer, S., Quist, H. et al. (2015). Consistency of shelter dogs' behavior toward a fake versus real stimulus dog during a behavior evaluation. *Appl. Anim. Behav. Sci.* 163: 158–166.

Shih, H-Y., Paterson, M.B.A., Georgiou, F. et al. (2020). Do canine behavioural assessments and characteristics predict the human-dog interaction when walking on a leash in a shelter setting? *Animals* 11 (1): 26. https://doi.org/10.3390/ani11010026.

Shiverdecker, M.D., Schiml, P.A., and Hennessy, M.B. (2013). Human interaction moderates plasma cortisol and behavioral responses of dogs to shelter housing. *Physiol. Behav.* 109: 75–79.

Shore, E.R. (2005). Returning a recently adopted companion animal: Adopters' reasons for and reactions to the failed adoption experience. *J. Appl. Anim. Welf. Sci.* 8: 187–198.

Stellato, A.C., Dewey, C.E., Widowski, T.M. et al. (2020). Evaluation of associations between owner presence and indicators of fear in dogs during routine veterinary examinations. *J. Am. Vet. Med. Assoc.* 257: 1031–1040.

Stellato, A.C., Hoffman, H., Gowland, S. et al. (2019). Effect of high levels of background noise on dog responses to a routine physical examination in a veterinary setting. *Appl. Anim. Behav. Sci.* 214: 64–71.

Stephen, J. and Ledger, R. (2007). Relinquishing dog owners' ability to predict behavioural problems in shelter dogs post adoption. *Appl. Anim. Behav. Sci.* 107: 88–99.

Sternberg, S. (2002). *Great Dog Adoptions: A Guide for Shelters*. Alameda, CA: Latham Foundation.

Tami, G. and Gallagher, A. (2009). Description of the behaviour of domestic dog (*Canis familiaris*) by experience and inexperienced people. *Appl. Anim. Behav. Sci.* 120: 159–169.

Taylor, K.D. and Mills, D.S. (2006). The development and assessment of temperament tests for adult companion dogs. *J. Vet. Behav.* 1: 94–108.

Travain, T., Colombo, E.S., Heinzl, E. et al. (2015). Hot dogs: Thermography in the assessment of stress in dogs (*Canis familiaris*)—A pilot study. *J. Vet. Behav.* 10: 17–23.

Valsecchi, P., Barnard, S., Stefanini, C. et al. (2011). Temperament test for re-homed dogs validated through direct behavioral observation in shelter and home environment. *J. Vet. Behav.* 6: 161–177.

Van der Borg, J.A.M., Beerda, B., Ooms, M. et al. (2010). Evaluation of behaviour testing for human directed aggression in dogs. *Appl. Anim. Behav. Sci.* 128: 78–90.

Van der Borg, J.A.M., Netto, W., and Planta, J.U. (1991). Behavioural testing of dogs in animal shelters to predict problem behaviour. *Appl. Anim. Behav. Sci.* 32: 237–251.

Van Hooijdonk, C. and Krahmer, E. (2008). Information modalities for procedural instructions: The influence of text, pictures, and film clips on learning and executing RSI exercises. *IEEE T. Prof. Commun.* 51: 50–62.

Vincent, I.C. and Leahy, R.A. (1997). Real-time non-invasive measurement of heart rate in working dogs: A technique with potential applications in the objective assessment of welfare problems. *Vet. J.* 153: 179–183.

Wan, M., Bolger, N., and Champagne, F.A. (2012). Human perception of fear in dogs varies according to experience with dogs. *PLOS One* 7: e51775.

Weiss, E. (2007). Meet Your Match SAFER™ Manual and Training Guide. https://www.aspcapro.org/research/meet-your-match-0 (accessed 6 August 2021).

Wells, D.L. and Hepper, P.G. (1999). Male and female dogs respond differently to men and women. *Appl. Anim. Behav. Sci.* 61: 341–349.

Wickens, S.M., Astell-Billings, I., McPherson, J.A. et al. (1995). The behavioural assessment of dogs in animal shelters: Interobserver reliability and data redundancy. *Proceedings of the 29th International Congress of the International Society for Applied Ethology*, Potters Bar, UK. Universities Federation for Animal Welfare.

Willen, R.M., Mutwill, A., MacDonald, L.J. et al. (2017). Factors determining the effects of human interaction on the cortisol levels of shelter dogs. *Appl. Anim. Behav. Sci.* 186: 41–48.

Wynne, C.D.L. (2006). Should shelters bother assessing their dogs? *Psychol. Today.* August 19. https://www.psychologytoday.com/us/blog/dogs-and-their-people/201608/should-shelters-bother-assessing-their-dogs.

10

Canine Housing and Husbandry for Behavioral Well-Being
Stephanie Janeczko, Lila Miller, and Stephen Zawistowski

10.1 Introduction

It is generally believed that dogs living in animal shelters are subject to a range of conditions and stimuli that are not conducive to good physical and behavioral health. Environmental design and facility management practices impact the quality of life of sheltered dogs (Kiddie and Collins 2015), and there is a growing body of data and anecdotal information showing that appropriate housing and husbandry can mitigate the negative impact of many detrimental features commonly attributed to shelters.

An evaluation of how dogs in animal shelters are cared for must begin with the initial observation that almost all dogs were removed from where they were living previously, unless they were born in the shelter. This may be the only aspect of their life history that most shelter dogs have in common. Some dogs may have lived in homes where they received excellent care for both their physical and behavioral needs, whereas others may have been subjected to neglect and abusive treatment. Still others may have been strays scratching out a living by scavenging for food and sleeping wherever they could. Between these extremes are a range of conditions that ensure that each dog brings her own unique life experience to the shelter. This individual variation in prior experiences, as well as the substantial genetic variations, are increasingly recognized as relevant considerations in providing appropriate housing and husbandry to dogs. This in turn presents a challenge to shelters in how they design their physical structures and implement animal care practices beneficial for individual animals and the population as a whole. A uniform approach will not provide each dog with the environment they require to attain the best possible welfare while in the shelter's care. Ongoing observation and assessment of each animal's behavior must begin at the point of intake and continue throughout their time in the shelter's care, with this information used to tailor animal care to meet the needs of the individual. Alternate housing, including in foster care, as well as placement options should be urgently considered for animals exhibiting significant fear, anxiety, stress, or frustration in the shelter.

Breed, sex, and age play a role in the onset and prevalence of poor welfare in kenneled dogs (Stephen and Ledger 2005). For example, younger dogs were found to be more likely to chew their bedding, breeds differed in their tendency to bark, and females engaged in tail chasing sooner than males, though this was a rare behavior. Fear-related behaviors (hiding, escape attempts, and lack of appetite) were observed earlier in the shelter stay than

Animal Behavior for Shelter Veterinarians and Staff, Second Edition. Edited by Brian A. DiGangi, Victoria A. Cussen, Pamela J. Reid, and Kristen A. Collins.
© 2022 John Wiley & Sons, Inc. Published 2022 by John Wiley & Sons, Inc.
Companion website: www.wiley.com/go/digangi/animal

wall bouncing, pacing, and circling. The frequency of the behaviors observed changed over several weeks, with substantial variation among dogs. It is therefore important to continuously evaluate each dog as an individual, so care and husbandry can be adapted in a way that meets their needs, provides the best possible quality of life while in the shelter, and helps prepare that dog for a successful life in a new home (Coppinger and Zuccotti 1999; Tuber et al. 1999).

10.2 Admission to the Animal Shelter

Within the animal welfare field, there is increasing recognition that intake by a sheltering organization is not always necessary nor in the best interest of a particular animal, the larger population of animals cared for by that organization, or the larger community. Instead, robust programs that provide resources, such as accessible veterinary care, behavioral counseling and training, or temporary boarding, support the human-animal bond and help keep pets and people together. As a result, intake can be reduced and prioritized, allowing organizations to provide a higher level of individualized care for the animals that truly need traditional sheltering services (e.g., animals in need of significant veterinary and/or behavioral care, victims of cruelty) and do so in a more efficient manner. When rehoming is necessary, assisting the owner in doing so themselves or caring for and placing the animal directly via foster care is often an appropriate and preferable alternative to shelter intake and housing. Critical evaluation of whether each dog needs to be admitted by the shelter, and, if so, whether housing on-site is the best option should be the first consideration when evaluating housing options in a shelter.

When intake is the appropriate option, it is important to recognize that entry into an animal shelter environment is extremely stressful for most dogs (Hiby et al. 2006). Regardless of their living arrangements prior to intake,

virtually all dogs entering the shelter will be without their human and/or animal attachment figures, and they will face an environment that is inherently more restrictive and lacking in choice than they had previously experienced. Dogs will be confronted with novel experiences, including contact with different humans and animals, changes to their movements and routines, and new surfaces, odors, sounds, and diets, among other changes.

In each case, dogs experience psychological stressors that are known to activate stress-related physiological responses through stimulation of the sympathetic branch of the autonomic nervous system and the hypothalamic-pituitary-adrenal axis (Tuber et al. 1999). Physical and behavioral ailments may develop as a result of stress, which can further diminish animal health and welfare and may confuse the diagnosis of a variety of medical conditions. Stressed animals may act in unexpected or unpredictable ways. To further complicate matters, the same stressor or stressors will impact individual animals differently. For example, there is evidence that salivary cortisol levels are higher in intact dogs compared with those who were spayed or neutered and in small compared to large and giant dogs housed in an animal shelter (Sandri et al. 2015). Similarly, the severity and manifestation of the stress response is likely to vary across individuals. Some dogs may express their distress by becoming more active, while other dogs may become inactive (Hiby et al. 2006). Several studies have shown that dogs entering shelters will show an elevated plasma cortisol level (Hennessy et al. 1997, 1998), which is one physiological indicator of stress. This research indicates that the elevated cortisol levels will persist for several days but that brief 15- to 30-minute sessions of positive interaction with a person can have a beneficial effect (Shiverdecker et al. 2013; McGowan et al. 2018; Willen et al. 2019).

Starting at the time of intake, it is critical that concerted efforts are made to reduce stress-inducing stimuli (e.g., excessive noise, random placement with other animals, rough handling) and proactively provide comfort and gentle handling to every dog. Staff involved in the intake process must take the dog's behavior and demeanor, as well as his or her physical condition, into account, and they should use low-stress handling techniques to minimize fear, anxiety, and stress (see Chapter 8).

Psychopharmaceuticals should be considered during the peri-intake period to alleviate stress and facilitate acclimation to the shelter environment. There is limited evidence from one study that administration of low doses of trazodone for up to 48 hours around the time of intake was associated with lower rates of infectious respiratory disease, shorter lengths of stay, and greater likelihood of adoption (Abrams et al. 2020). However, it is important to remember that association does not imply causation, and there are numerous effective interventions to control infectious disease, reduce time in shelter, and increase live outcomes. Further research is necessary to better understand what role psychopharmaceuticals may have in alleviating the stress of intake and housing in a shelter setting including which medications may be effective, when, at what dose, and for what time and duration. All medications should be prescribed judiciously and as part of a comprehensive plan to address the specific concern(s) for which a drug is prescribed; such use should not be considered a replacement for other interventions.

The history, physical exam findings, and behavior of a dog will inform staff as to which initial housing options are most appropriate for that individual. Housing should be separated based on the dog's species, age, health, behavior, and reproductive status (Newbury et al. 2010). Animals with evidence of contagious disease must be isolated from the general population to reduce the risk of disease transmission. Animals who are shy, fearful, or anxious should be provided with a consistent and structured environment that minimizes reassignment of enclosures and provides the same assigned caregivers on a regular basis.

10.3 General Housing Considerations

Over the years, dog husbandry and housing in shelters has moved away from what was largely a "one size fits all" strategy, instead adopting an approach focused on meeting the needs of the individual animal. In veterinary medicine, this is reflected in how vaccination protocols are now designed to fit an animal's age, immune status, lifestyle, and risk of exposure to disease. Similarly, optimum feeding protocols now require matching nutrition to the life stage and health condition of the animal. In animal shelters, the change is reflected in how animals are increasingly housed and fed according to their individual needs, with attention paid to both their physical and behavioral health and welfare. Hubrecht (1993) asserted that a good housing system for dogs should allow them to exercise choice, to manipulate and chew safe objects, and to socialize with people and other dogs.

The Association of Shelter Veterinarians' (ASV) Guidelines for Standards of Care in Animal Shelters are based on the Five Freedoms, originally developed in 1965 for farm animals in intensive husbandry settings in the United Kingdom but considered appropriate for shelter animals as well (Newbury et al. 2010). While all of the Freedoms are important, the second and fourth are particularly relevant to housing shelter animals. The second Freedom states that animals must be "free from discomfort by providing an appropriate environment, including shelter and a comfortable resting area," and the fourth Freedom states that animals must be free to "express normal behaviors by providing sufficient space, proper facilities and company of the animal's own kind." Specifically, the ASV Guidelines state the following:

> Primary enclosures must provide sufficient space to allow each animal, regardless of species, to make normal postural adjustments, for example, to turn freely

and to easily stand, sit, stretch, move their head without touching the top of the enclosure, lie in a comfortable position with limbs extended, move about and assume a comfortable posture for feeding, drinking, urinating and defecating. In addition, cats and dogs should be able to hold their tails erect when in a normal standing position. Primary enclosures should allow animals to see out but should also provide at least some opportunity to avoid visual contact with other animals.

(Newbury et al. 2010, p. 7)

The British Veterinary Association (Animal Welfare Fund), the Fund for the Replacement of Animals in Medical Experiments, the Royal Society for the Prevention of Cruelty to Animals, and the Universities Federation for Animal Welfare (BVAAWF/FRAME/RSPCA/UFAW) Joint Working Group on Refinement recommended "providing an enriched environment for dogs which permits them to express a wide range of normal behaviour and to exercise a degree of choice. . .combining this with a socialization, habituation and training programme" (Prescott et al. 2004).

Both of these guidelines represent a departure from many previous recommendations for appropriate dog housing that focused on space designations only. Although it has been theorized for years that poor housing can lead to behavior problems in dogs, many facilities continue to house them in small, unenriched cages that do not take into account the importance of enrichment and do not permit the dog to make normal postural adjustments or exhibit normal behavior. Single, small, unenriched cages typically reflect a regulatory or engineering approach to caring for dogs that uses minimal space recommendations based on the dog's size, rather than a results-oriented welfare approach that considers the importance of providing for behavioral needs.

10.3.1 Size, Layout, and Construction of Enclosures

The minimum and ideal space requirements per dog are unknown and could be expected to vary based on individual factors such as age, size, breed, physical health, behavioral health and well-being, and prior experiences. Shelter medicine texts have previously recommended providing 35–64 ft^2 of space per dog, best configured for an individual dog's welfare as 8 ft. × 8 ft. rather than the traditional long and narrow 4 ft. × 16 ft. layout typical of runs in older facilities (Schlaffer and Bonacci 2013). While several studies (e.g., Hubrecht et al. 1992; Jongman et al. 2018) of sheltered or kenneled dogs have failed to find significant increases in activity with increasing cage size, the changes in the sizes studied may have still been too small to result in any measurable behavioral differences. However, when significant variation in enclosure size was investigated, dogs in larger pens were found to be more active and spent less time engaged in stereotypy (Hetts et al. 1992). More recently, Normando et al. (2014) found that shelter-housed dogs given 9 m^2 (approximately 100 ft^2) of space showed increased general activity levels and visual exploration of the environment compared to dogs housed in enclosures half that size. Housing in larger enclosures also increased the probability of behaviors likely to increase chances of adoption, such as positive interactions with toys, co-housed dogs, and people. In another study, dogs were found to spend more time in the front of their enclosure when housed in large kennels (10 m^2 floor space) than in smaller kennels (3 m^2 floor space) (Jongman et al. 2018). Dogs at the front of their enclosures were more likely to view other dogs and people, which may have a direct positive effect on welfare as well as an indirect effect by improving chances of adoption. Studies have shown adopter preference for dogs positioned at the front as opposed to the back of their enclosures (Wells and Hepper 1992) and that dogs selected for adoption were most likely to approach or greet the adopter when first met (Weiss et al. 2012).

All portions of the primary enclosure, regardless if it is a pen, cage, run, kennel, condo unit, or double-sided compartment, should be made from durable nonporous materials that are easily disinfected, safe, and sturdy, with no jagged or sharp edges that can injure the inhabitant. Wood should be avoided in primary enclosures and animal areas, as it cannot be effectively disinfected and can be damaged by chewing. If the enclosure contains a drain, it should be covered to prevent nails, paws, or even limbs from getting trapped in its holes. Flooring must be safe and comfortable for the dog when standing, walking, lying down, or eliminating. Floors should be solid, preferably with a non-slip finish. Wire floors are not recommended (Prescott et al. 2004; Newbury et al. 2010) and should be avoided to prevent foot injuries and general discomfort.

At least a portion of the enclosure that is accessible to the dog should always be dry, ventilated, fully shaded, and provide protection from temperature extremes. A strong preference to eliminate away from the area where they eat, drink, and sleep has been shown in shelter-housed dogs (Wagner et al. 2014), and access to an area where the dog can urinate and defecate away from the "living areas" should be provided. The primary enclosure should be large enough to provide the dog with bedding or a bed, a platform (bedding may be placed on the platform if the dog indicates a preference to sleep there), toys, and the ability to hide or at least a partial visual barrier. The movement of dogs throughout the shelter should be minimized as much as possible so the dog can become familiar with her immediate scents and environment. In fact, unless there is a compelling reason to move dogs, they should remain in the same enclosure whenever possible for the duration of their stay.

Shelters will ideally have some variety in the styles and sizes of primary enclosures available for housing dogs, arranged in a way that allows for appropriate separation.

Housing must be available to sufficiently isolate dogs with contagious illnesses away from the general population. Similarly, separate areas must be available to safely house and care for dogs that may pose a safety risk to people or other animals. Housing areas must be served by heating, ventilation, and air-conditioning systems that are adequate to maintain a comfortable environment, with suitable temperature, humidity, and air quality conducive to maintaining the dogs' health and welfare. Separate ventilation for areas used to house dogs in isolation is necessary because canine respiratory pathogens may be spread through aerosolization.

10.3.2 Social Interactions and Environmental Enrichment

Regardless of the size, configuration, and location of the primary enclosure, providing social contact and environmental enrichment is critical for animals' well-being. One could reasonably expect dogs to benefit from larger enclosures up to a certain point, particularly when increasing their space also includes the provision of outdoor space. At the same time, the cost of housing dogs in significantly larger enclosures—either in a new building or when retrofitting an existing facility—is likely to be substantial and may not be the best use of limited resources. There is no compelling evidence that simply enlarging a dog's living space without providing enrichment and social engagement will result in better welfare (Taylor and Mills 2007). One study of dogs housed long-term in Italian shelters found the most important variable that improved the dogs' welfare was the opportunity to regularly get out of the cage for a walk, while size of the enclosure had no effect (Cafazzo et al. 2014). Shelters are encouraged to direct their efforts and resources toward increasing the quality of the environment, interaction with people and conspecifics, and, perhaps most importantly, time out of the enclosure to have the greatest impact on the health and well-being of dogs in their care. Additional information about enrichment and playgroups can be found in Chapters 11 and 13, respectively.

10.3.3 Daily Rounds and Pathway Planning

There is increasing recognition that minimizing an animal's length of stay is one of the most important things shelters can do to improve the health and welfare of individual animals as well as the population as a whole. This requires actively tracking and guiding each animal's stay, starting at the time of intake and extending throughout her stay until the animal leaves—a process known as "pathway planning." It involves making an initial assessment of the animal's likely outcome(s), identifying all of the steps necessary to get the animal to that outcome, and ensuring that everything that needs to happen is scheduled and completed in a timely manner.

The daily rounds process serves as the foundation for the active planning and daily evaluation necessary to efficiently and effectively care for animals. It involves a physical walkthrough and discussion of all animals in the facility by representatives from key teams (i.e., medical, behavior, operations). The purpose of this exercise is to identify the physical and behavioral needs of each animal and determine or confirm the animal's pathway (see Chapter 19). Adjustments can be made to the pathway if necessary, and delays addressed promptly. Immediate actions should be taken to address each animal's needs, with more robust response plans updated and enacted as necessary.

Daily rounds and pathway planning together form a critical framework that ensures accountability across teams for humane and efficient individualized care. This approach emphasizes consideration of the whole animal, with continuous adjustments and adaptations to maximize the animal's quality of life. All shelters have a finite capacity for care, which they cannot exceed if they are to meet the medical and

behavioral needs of their animals to provide them with good welfare. This requires careful and continuous evaluation of the facility, housing, staffing, and available resources alongside the unique needs of the animals in the shelter's care.

10.3.4 Foster Care

Consideration should be given to placing dogs in foster care whenever appropriate and possible, rather than housing on-site at the shelter. This is particularly important for dogs that have been in the facility for prolonged periods of time or are expected to have long lengths of stay, that are particularly vulnerable to infectious diseases, or that require a greater level of individual attention, care, and treatment than is possible in the shelter setting. While foster care is especially important for the unique needs of animals just described, its value in better meeting the physical and behavioral needs of all individual animals should not be overlooked. The observations reported by foster caregivers are likely to provide a more accurate picture of a dog's health and behavior than what could be obtained in the shelter, and this additional information may lead to a more informed, complete assessment that will help the shelter to better plan for appropriate care and placement options. Foster caregivers are often able to provide a greater level of individual animal attention and treatment than is possible in a busy shelter, increasing the feasibility and success of assessing, treating, and managing a variety of medical and behavioral conditions. Placement in foster care can be particularly helpful in evaluating a dog's behavior, reducing stress, and providing treatment for known or subsequently identified behavioral concerns, often with support from shelter behavior and veterinary staff.

10.3.5 Sanitation Considerations

Cleaning and disinfecting, collectively referred to as sanitation, comprise a critical part of daily shelter operations. The impact of sanitation protocols on dog behavior will be discussed here, and the reader is referred to several other readily available sources for further information on the subject (Newbury et al. 2010; Karsten 2021).

Removing dogs from their enclosures for daily cleaning and disinfecting can be very stressful. It can be challenging for staff to take a shy, fearful, anxious, or aggressive dog from his or her cage every day without further exacerbating that dog's negative emotional state and potentially putting themselves at risk. Housing dogs in double-sided compartments so they can freely move from one side to the other without being handled is often the best husbandry and welfare option, especially for these dogs. Importantly, it also increases the efficiency of sanitation procedures, leaving more time for staff and volunteers to provide the dogs with enrichment, positive social contact, exercise, and training or behavior modification. Even if this option is available, it is important for all staff and volunteers who handle animals to receive training in animal behavior and low-stress handling techniques so that the least amount of handling and restraint necessary can be used whenever possible. Routine husbandry practices should be as predictable as possible to further minimize stress (Rooney et al. 2009). It is important to establish a schedule for cleaning that ensures the same procedures are performed at the same time each day and by the same caregivers to the greatest extent possible. These procedures should be performed as quietly and efficiently as possible. If a dog must be removed from the enclosure for sanitation procedures but is resistant, it may be better to delay the activity until a later time, to use a different technique such as coaxing the dog into a crate that can then be gently moved, or to designate a different person who can better handle that particular dog. Staff and volunteers must understand that stress is a major contributing factor to disease transmission, reduced

welfare, and the development of abnormal behaviors and that it should be avoided when possible.

Removal of dogs from their enclosures for complete cleaning and disinfection is not only potentially detrimental but is also not always necessary. Spot cleaning is often preferable for dogs five months of age and older remaining in their primary enclosure. This process allows a dog to stay within his or her enclosure while feces, visible dirt, and debris are removed; food and water receptacles are cleaned and replenished; and the space is tidied up. Daily cleaning in this manner is necessary to maintain a comfortable and sanitary environment, while disinfection necessitating the removal of the dog should take place only when a new occupant is introduced into the enclosure or for disease-control purposes. Spot cleaning can also help reduce animal stress by preserving the dog's scent within the environment and minimizing movement in and out of the enclosure.

If full cleaning and disinfection is necessary, dogs should be removed from the portion of the cage, kennel, or room by placing them on the other side of a partition, confining them to a solid-sided or covered crate within the enclosure, or taking them out of the enclosure completely. Ideally, sanitation activities will be scheduled to occur at the same time dogs are walked or placed in playgroups (as appropriate to their physical and behavioral health conditions). When this is not feasible, dogs should be secured on the side of the kennel opposite to that being cleaned via a guillotine door or similar divider, placed in an outdoor exercise yard (weather permitting) or an indoor training/play area, or temporarily placed in a different, sanitized enclosure. The "move one down" method should be avoided whenever possible because it can be stressful for the dogs and because the need to thoroughly disinfect each enclosure sequentially and between dogs is labor intensive. Dogs should not be tethered during cleaning, as this may contribute to disease spread, lead to negative interactions between dogs, and pose a safety risk for personnel. Similarly, the practice of allowing a dog to run free in a room while his or her cage is being fully cleaned and disinfected should also be discouraged because of the challenges that poses to adequately and safely sanitizing the room afterward.

Enclosures must never be hosed down while the dog is still inside that portion of the housing unit, as this is highly distressing and increases physical discomfort and disease susceptibility. For the same reasons, housing units should be fully dried before the dog is returned to the area. Disinfectants and cleansers that do not have strong or noxious odors should be chosen, remembering that a dog's sense of smell is highly sensitive. All chemicals and products should be approved for use around dogs, effective against pathogens of concern in the given environmental conditions, and prepared according to the manufacturer's instructions. Rinsing enclosures to remove chemical residues may be a necessary step for safety reasons. Even when not required, rinsing should be considered to further reduce odors that could be unpleasant to dogs, as long as rinsing is not contradicted by the manufacturer's instructions for efficacy or safety reasons. Increasing the concentration of chemicals or indiscriminate mixing is likely to increase the risk of human and animal discomfort, toxicity, and safety concerns. Products that have shorter contact times and are environmentally friendly should be selected whenever possible.

10.4 Behavior and Sensory Factors to Consider for Dog Housing

10.4.1 Smell

Dogs have a highly developed sense of smell, which is key to communication, exploration, foraging, and hunting. They are very sensitive to trace odors that may not be noticed by or even seem pleasant to humans.

Olfactory stimulation as a form of sensory enrichment has been documented in a variety of species with a variety of scents, but only limited studies have investigated the impact on kenneled or shelter-housed dogs. A small number of studies suggest that essential oils and other scents may also provide beneficial effects for dogs in shelters. Coconut and ginger were found to decrease vocalizations and movement and to increase sleeping in shelter-housed dogs (Binks et al. 2018). In another study, lavender and chamomile seemed to increase behaviors associated with relaxation in shelter dogs—more resting, less movement, and less vocalization—while rosemary and peppermint stimulated more standing, movement, and vocalization (Graham et al. 2005). These behaviors are likely to be attractive to potential adopters and the scents may also appeal to visitors, enhancing their perception of the shelter. Some essential oils that are beneficial (or harmless) to humans may be toxic to dogs, and a veterinarian should be consulted before instituting their use as part of a shelter enrichment program or for treatment of individual dogs. Although these oils may be intended for aromatherapy use only, an accident or careless handling could result in some of these oils being spilled or coming into inadvertent contact with the dog's skin and then being licked off and ingested. Similarly, oils and other scents should not be applied to bedding due to the risk of irritation, absorption, or ingestion and because such use may result in the lack of a comfortable sleeping space if a dog finds the scent aversive.

Dog-appeasing pheromone (DAP) has been used with mixed results to calm dogs and relieve anxiety. Much of the literature surrounding the use of DAP has focused on pet dogs in typical home settings, and there is a lack of consensus regarding its benefit and value in alleviating stress and anxiety in shelter-housed dogs. A study by Tod et al. (2005) suggested that DAP continuously administered over a seven-day period may help reduce some behavioral indicators of stress, such as barking, and increase resting and sniffing behavior in kenneled dogs. However, in other studies the use of DAP spray failed to reduce the frequency of barking or stress-related behaviors in shelter dogs (Hermiston et al. 2018), and a DAP diffuser was not shown to have an effect on the behavior of beagles separated from their owners in a laboratory environment (Taylor et al. 2020). The presence of other natural pheromones may mute the impact of DAP. It is important to keep in mind that if a shelter has a high-efficiency ventilation system that generates 10–15 air exchanges per hour in the kennel area, circulating DAP may be quickly removed from the environment, so the use of a DAP collar or spraying a suitable object in the enclosure may be more efficacious, but there is little data to support this. Pheromone products are likely to be most beneficial when used in conjunction with other techniques as part of a comprehensive plan to reduce stress and provide an enriched environment. Most shelters, particularly those with limited resources, would be better served by focusing on opportunities to increase dogs' interactions with people and other dogs and to reduce the time spent in their enclosures, as well as through efforts to efficiently move dogs to foster care or successful placement.

10.4.2 Hearing

Staff should be made aware that excessive noise, including barking, is harmful to both human and dog hearing and can cause stress that is detrimental to welfare. It must be remembered that dog hearing is substantially more sensitive than human hearing, and dogs confined in shelter settings may be exposed to noise for prolonged periods of time. The non-absorbent surfaces that facilitate good sanitation also tend to reflect rather than absorb sound, and poor shelter design can contribute to loud noise levels. Some acoustical vibrations in the 20–40 kHz range, which are not detectable by humans, will still be heard by dogs given

the differences in the species' auditory ranges, and efforts must be made to identify and control these sources of excess noise as well.

It can be challenging to provide an acoustical environment that supports animal health and welfare in an animal shelter. Staff should be trained to work as quietly as possible to keep noise levels at a minimum. Practices such as slamming cage and kennel doors should be avoided, especially during cleaning and when dogs are inside their enclosures. Quieter, plastic latches that prevent the slamming of cage doors are preferred over metal latches. Auditory input from animal and non-animal sources (fans, phones, overhead speakers, high-pressure hosing units, etc.) should be minimized to the extent possible. Loud machinery and equipment should be located at a distance away from all animal enclosures. Exposure to noises such as firecrackers, car alarms, and sirens as well as prolonged construction and building maintenance noise can all compromise an animal's welfare (Patterson-Kane and Farnworth 2006). All efforts should be made to ensure that animals are protected from loud noise to the extent possible and are provided with opportunities to hide when avoidance is impractical.

One of the most common sources of noise in an animal shelter is likely to be the dogs themselves. Studies have shown that sound levels in a shelter can exceed 100 dB on a regular basis (Sales et al. 1997; Coppola et al. 2006). The Occupational Safety and Health Administration (OSHA) recommends that humans wear protective gear when exposure to noise exceeding 100 dB occurs for two hours per day (OSHA 2014), yet dogs with more sensitive hearing than humans may be exposed to these and higher levels for much longer periods of time. Regular or continuous exposure to sound at these levels is stressful and can have a profound negative impact on the physical and psychological health of animals. Long-term exposure to noise levels in this range (over six months) has been shown to cause measurable harm to dogs' hearing (Scheifele et al. 2012).

Dogs bark for a variety of reasons, including over- or understimulation, and barking is a socially facilitated behavior. While sound levels naturally increase with the number of dogs barking, the excitement level of the dogs has been found to be a more significant factor impacting noise levels than the specific number of dogs present (Myer and Conlon 2012). Efficient and consistently scheduled daily care activities can help reduce barking. Dogs should not be deprived of human contact to reduce barking, but thoughtful adjustments to daily routines may help reduce stimulation, especially when it is unpredictable. In one shelter-based study, the general kennel noise levels were found to be significantly lower when visitor access was restricted in dog housing areas (Hewison et al. 2014). While consistently or excessively restricting the public's access to shelter dogs could have negative impacts by increasing their length of stay and/or reducing chances of adoption, dedicated time each day without any humans in the kennel areas can prove beneficial. For example, one to two hours can be set aside each afternoon for a predictable break from stimulation. During this time, dogs are provided with additional enrichment in their enclosures, the lights are dimmed, soft music is played, and staff, volunteers, and members of the public do not enter the area.

Dogs are more likely to bark when staff, other animals, and visitors pass by their kennels. When retrofitting an existing shelter facility or designing a new building, careful attention should be given to housing configurations to reduce this type of stimulation. When possible, kennel designs that require dogs to walk down a long row or aisle of enclosures to enter or exit an area should be avoided; smaller rooms and/or multiple entry/exit doors to housing spaces should be chosen instead. Housing in small rooms or self-contained enclosures compared to traditional kennels may also reduce the level of noise from barking dogs for humans and other animals in

the shelter. In facilities where this isn't possible, staff can use other strategies to decrease the likelihood of barking. For example, more reactive dogs should be housed away from doors and heavily trafficked areas. Partial barriers can also help prevent visual access to activity, and their use also gives dogs some choice in how they engage with the environment. Care should be taken, however, not to fully restrict visual access as that can lead to increased barking in some dogs. Group housing dogs sometimes seems to reduce barking (Hetts et al. 1992; Mertens and Unshelm 1996; Coppola et al. 2006; Grigg et al. 2017). Dog enclosures should be located at a sufficient distance away from feline housing to minimize or avoid the negative impact barking has on cats.

Because a single dog barking can quickly result in all dogs in a kennel barking, efforts targeted to dogs observed to repeatedly initiate this behavior or to bark excessively are likely to be beneficial. Determining whether the dog is under- or overstimulated will help refine interventions, which may include additional enrichment in the enclosure; increased time out of the kennel to exercise, socialize with people, and relax in a quiet area; co-housing with one or more other dogs; inclusion in playgroups if appropriate; and/or moving the dog to a kennel in a different area.

Sound-dampening and absorbent materials and acoustic panels should be used to reduce noise levels whenever possible, and especially if operational adjustments have been insufficient in reducing excessive noise. Sound-absorbing baffles may also be hung from the ceiling (Garvey et al. 2016).

Although the reduction of unnecessary noise is an important focus in shelters, auditory enrichment may also prove beneficial. Some studies suggest that soft classical music may have a soothing effect on dogs (Wells et al. 2002; Kogan et al. 2012; Bowman et al. 2017). Non-musical, white noise has been found to reduce the amount and intensity of barking in laboratory-housed dogs (Kilcullen-Steiner and Mitchell 2001).

Kenneled dogs exposed to audiobooks have been shown to display increasing resting behaviors, even more so than dogs exposed to classical music or psychoacoustically designed dog music (Brayley and Montrose 2016). However, in some cases, music may actually act as a stressor for dogs; heavy metal music was found to increase body shaking in one study (Kogan et al. 2012). Music, white noise, or audiobooks should never be on continuously or played when dogs are sleeping. See Chapter 11 for additional information on the use of auditory enrichment.

10.4.3 Vision

To facilitate husbandry procedures, the kennel area should be well lit with natural light and/or artificial light that closely approximates natural light in both duration and intensity (Newbury et al. 2010). Lighting systems should be in good working condition. The flicker of a poorly functioning fluorescent light or the buzz of a defective lighting ballast is generally considered aversive by people and would also likely be aversive for dogs. Lighting should be provided on a diurnal cycle to allow for both light and dark periods for dogs, who will develop corresponding activity cycles as a result. Although there is some evidence that shelter dogs will adjust to overnight exposure to artificial light and sleep relatively undisturbed (Houpt et al. 2019), this has not been studied in large numbers of animals, in varying populations, or with a variety of lighting systems. The physiologic and long-term impacts remain undetermined in dogs, but there is ample evidence of deleterious health effects in people exposed to artificial light at night (Cho et al. 2015). Thus, shelters should aim for consistent schedules approximating 12 hours of light and 12 hours of darkness, with staff taking care to turn the lights off for the evening before leaving.

Although natural light is considered preferable in animal housing areas, data on the differences between natural versus artificial light is limited. Similarly, little research has been done to investigate specific concerns regarding the type of artificial light that might be used, including incandescent, fluorescent, compact fluorescent bulbs, or light-emitting diode. There is some evidence that dogs with indoor/outdoor housing options and dogs that are exposed to natural sunlight will more strongly synchronize their activity cycle to light/dark periods. It is thought that this may be due to the brighter sunlight and the more gradual transition from light to dark that occurs outdoors when compared with the instantaneous transition that results from using artificial lighting indoors (Siwak et al. 2003). Despite the potential benefits of natural light, it is important to keep track of the sun's path throughout the day to ensure that individual housing areas or enclosures are not subjected to excessive sun and possible overheating via windows or skylights. Dogs must be moved or able to access shade at will when adverse conditions occur. The sun's path will vary with the season, so this will need to be checked on a regular basis throughout the year.

Dogs should be able to see out of enclosures to satisfy their natural curiosity. Wells and Hepper (1998) indicate that dogs allowed to see other dogs will take advantage of the opportunity and position themselves in their kennel to facilitate the observation of other dogs. This frequently results in dogs who are at the front of their enclosure, a position that may improve the dogs' chances of being adopted (Weiss et al. 2012). If visual stimuli cause excessive barking in a dog, a partial visual barrier or partition that does not totally obscure the dog's ability to see out of the enclosure may be necessary. If the stimuli are predictable, the use of a full barrier at limited, specific times of the day may also be an appropriate option. As mentioned above, if an enclosure is near a door or other highly trafficked area that stimulates excessive activity or barking, it may be necessary to move the dog to another enclosure.

10.5 Types of Primary Enclosures

10.5.1 Small Unenriched Cages

Small cages designed to house one dog, or single, crate-like cages, as illustrated in Figure 10.1, are commonly found in shelters. The potential advantages of placing dogs in small, single cages include allowing the staff to closely monitor individual health, including eating, drinking, bowel movements, and other bodily functions. These enclosures also are advantageous for dogs that are injured, severely diseased, or debilitated and need restricted movement on a temporary basis. However, there are many more disadvantages to this type of housing, and its routine use in shelters is not recommended.

It is often mistakenly believed that use of small single enclosures will reduce disease transmission by eliminating direct contact between animals. However, the most common method of disease spread is via fomites or inanimate objects, so simply housing dogs individually in any sized enclosure will not eliminate disease spread. Single cages are actually more likely to facilitate disease susceptibility and spread because the additional animal handling required during sanitation procedures creates more occasions for fomite spread and because dogs housed in this way are generally stressed due to the inadequate environment. Cages are often made of stainless steel, fiberglass, or other non-porous materials that permit ease of cleaning and disinfection but do not provide for comfort or noise reduction. They are often too small to provide sufficient space to separate resting, sleeping, and feeding areas from elimination areas or to include enrichment essentials such as a bed, platform, or hiding place. They also do not allow for choice or control over the environment and preclude the expression of most normal behaviors. Singly housed dogs who are socially isolated and housed in unenriched environments have been found to have low overall activity, are

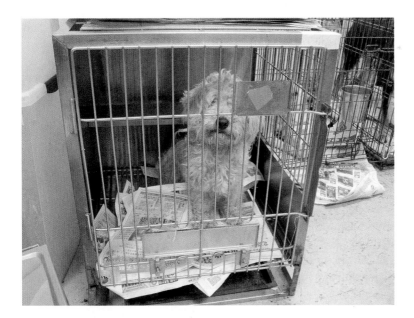

Figure 10.1 Example of single unenriched cage where there is insufficient space to separate the food and resting area from excrement and introduce any enrichment articles, and the dog has no choices and cannot perform normal behaviors or postural adjustments. This type of housing fails to meet basic requirements outlined in the ASV Guidelines for Standards of Care in Animal Shelters and numerous other guidelines and requirements for kenneled dogs. *Source:* Reproduced with permission from L. Miller.

more passive, are more likely to become bored or frustrated, and have a tendency to exhibit stereotypical circling and increased behavioral abnormalities (Hubrecht 2002; Prescott et al. 2004).

Shelters routinely using small, single cages are strongly encouraged to phase them out for use in all but the few limited circumstances noted above. Particular emphasis should be placed on prioritizing housing changes for dogs experiencing social isolation and replacing enclosures that are too small to allow for adequate environmental enrichment or the expression of normal behavior. Small cages may be temporarily used for seriously ill animals with infectious disease or for those receiving intensive medical care where movement and social contact with conspecifics should be restricted. However, these dogs may be better served by receiving care in a veterinary hospital or other venue that can better meet their individual needs without endangering the health and well-being of the rest of the shelter population.

When single cages must be used for healthy dogs, the largest available enclosures should be used. Every effort should be made to restrict their use to very short-term stays, perhaps only at initial admittance for very small dogs who may have enough space for postural and behavioral adjustments. It is vital to provide some distance between elimination and resting/eating areas and to provide soft bedding and a hiding place (or at least a partial visual barrier). It is essential that dogs in single cages receive walks at least twice a day for exercise and to eliminate, and they should spend as much time out of the enclosure as possible. At a minimum, dogs housed in these enclosures should receive at least one opportunity for social interaction with humans and/or conspecifics per day (as appropriate to their individual needs, preferences, heath, and behavior). It is important to note that the need for exercise and positive social interaction is not met by simply handling the dog for essential husbandry chores, such as cleaning and feeding. These dogs should be prioritized for evaluation to determine if they are candidates for foster care and/or for placement in playgroups with other dogs during the day if they must remain in the shelter.

10.5.2 Single Enriched Enclosures

Single enriched enclosures are single cages, "condos," pens, runs, or even small rooms that are large enough to allow a dog enough space to perform the postural movements described in the ASV Guidelines and to allow for some separation between elimination, resting, and eating/drinking areas. These enclosures also have enough space to include enrichment, such as toys, a bed, a hiding space, and a platform or elevated perch (see Figure 10.2). They should meet or exceed the specific size dimensions recommended in Section 10.3. Some condo units may be large enough to house a pair of compatible dogs.

This type of housing can be appropriate for most dogs when the enclosure is adequately sized relative to the dog and if staff provides sufficient time out of the enclosure, as well as positive social interactions with people and other dogs, if appropriate. It is important to note that regardless of the amount of space and environmental enrichment, social opportunities and walks must be provided for dogs housed in any kind of enclosure. Single enriched enclosures may be especially useful as housing for dog-aggressive dogs who cannot be housed with other dogs, dogs who simply do not prefer the company of other dogs, and dogs who require individual monitoring for behavioral and health reasons. One of the main disadvantages to this model is that, like the small, unenriched cage, it limits the dog's choices. Another disadvantage is that dogs housed in these enclosures generally require more handling for daily care activities. This can increase the risk of disease transmission, increase the risk to staff handling dogs that show aggression toward people, and may increase fear, anxiety, or stress in some dogs. A single enclosure is a poor housing choice for dogs that respond fearfully or aggressively

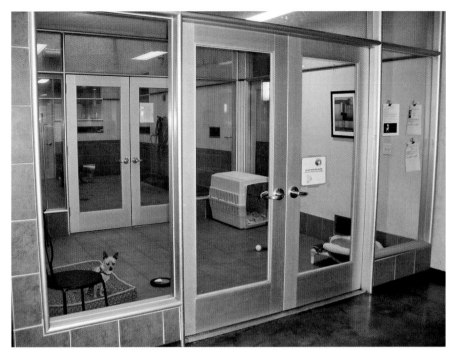

Figure 10.2 Example of single enriched dog housing. This space would be suitable for two small compatible dogs. Note the bed, toys, and kennel suitable for hiding, perching, or resting. *Source:* Reproduced with permission from S. Janeczko.

when handled. Despite the challenges that these enclosures present with respect to daily care activities, they may provide a greater level of biosecurity and be preferable for housing vulnerable puppies (pending placement in foster care) if the alternative is housing in unsealed and/or damaged runs.

10.5.3 Double-Sided Enclosures

Double-sided enclosures (including cages, runs, and kennels) allow dogs access to and movement from one side of the enclosure to the other when a partition that separates the two areas is opened (see Figure 10.3). The most common variation of a double-sided enclosure is a long run divided by a guillotine door that can be raised and lowered, often providing indoor/outdoor access. These enclosures may also be arranged so that the compartments are side by side, and some use different styles of partitions, such as saloon doors. For very small

dogs or puppies, housing in a double-sided cage that has a portal between the two sections, as is often seen in retrofitted feline housing units, may be an option.

Typically, double-sided enclosures are the most flexible and desirable configuration for housing dogs and puppies in shelters. They provide enough space for environmental enrichment to be added, for dogs to have more choice and control over their environment compared to most single-sided enclosures, and to perform all postural adjustments and movements. Normal behavior patterns can be observed and welfare can be increased by placing a bed, elevated platform, hiding place, and food on one side of the partition, while the other side functions as the dog's elimination area. This contributes to the dog's ability to engage in normal behaviors, as shelter-housed dogs have been found to display a strong preference to eliminate away from areas where they eat and rest (Wagner et al. 2014). This may

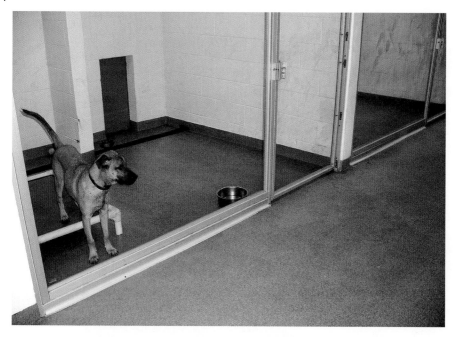

Figure 10.3 Example of one compartment of a double-sided enclosure. Note the guillotine door in the back of the unit and the resting platform. *Source:* Reproduced with permission from S. Janeczko.

also enhance adoptability because it may be easier for a house-trained dog to maintain her housetraining. A common variation of double-sided enclosures includes both indoor and outdoor access, sometimes referred to as indoor/outdoor runs (see Figure 10.4). They have the same advantages as double-sided indoor compartments with the added benefit of allowing dogs free choice to access fresh air and sunshine. Double-sided enclosures are also considered the most versatile model because they can be used for almost all circumstances: housing puppies or adult dogs; single animals, pairs, or small groups (if large enough for the size and number of dogs); newly admitted or short- or long-term residents; and animals with a range of medical and behavioral conditions. These units facilitate animal care without removal from the enclosure, which is of particular benefit for animals who may pose a safety concern; who exhibit significant fear, anxiety, or stress related to daily care activities; and who are particularly vulnerable to infectious disease. While one side is being cleaned,

dogs can be moved to the other side, reducing stress to the dogs, minimizing the risk of disease transmission via fomites, and increasing staff safety. Importantly, these enclosures also allow for more efficient completion of basic husbandry tasks, thereby increasing the amount of staff and volunteer time available for assessment, treatment, playgroups, or other activities.

There are, however, drawbacks to this design. Double-sided enclosures require a greater amount of square footage per dog and can be expensive to build. While not inherent to the design itself, traditional layouts usually have a long and narrow configuration that does not provide for optimal use of space. For example, larger dogs often hit their noses and tails on the walls when they turn around, which has been reported to be stressful to some dogs (Schlaffer and Bonacci 2013). Wear and tear that occurs with general usage or damage done by an individual dog can create safety concerns with double-sided enclosures. It is essential that periodic inspections be

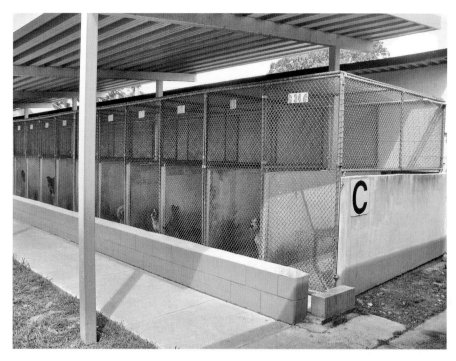

Figure 10.4 Example of a traditional double-sided enclosure providing indoor and outdoor access. Note the overhead roof to protect dogs from excessive sun and inclement weather. *Source:* Reproduced with permission from S. Janeczko.

performed to check for the absence of frayed cords and rust, ease of opening and closing of the guillotine door, and so forth. Enclosures that provide both indoor and outdoor areas will waste energy if the partition door is not sealed properly to prevent the escape of air-conditioning during hot weather and heat during cold weather. The doors may freeze in cold climates or allow too much humidity in the building in hot weather, contributing to moist conditions that facilitate pathogen survival and can lead to the development of mold. Both the indoor and outdoor portions must be physically secure and offer dogs protection from direct sunlight, inclement weather conditions, predators, and vandalism.

Shelters should not keep the dividing door closed in order to use a double-sided enclosure to separately house two (or more) dogs. Shelters doing so are typically trying to increase their capacity, but this is a misplaced effort. Doubling up of animals eliminates the

advantages of double-sided compartments, which were created specifically to provide dogs with additional space, enrichment, and choice. This practice is likely to negatively impact the dogs' health, behavior, and well-being, and it also increases the amount of staff time necessary to provide basic animal care. The result is that a greater number of animals are housed in the facility, and it takes more time per dog to provide an adequate level of animal care. Most organizations struggle with having adequate staffing capacity as much or more so than they struggle with having adequate housing capacity. Using both sides of the enclosure further exacerbates that imbalance and leads the organization to operate even further outside its capacity for care. Challenges are further compounded when an organization uses this practice to house dogs in unequally partitioned double-sided enclosures (i.e., one side is much larger than the other) or in indoor/outdoor runs, leading to a situation where some or all dogs are subjected to inadequate, uncomfortable, and, in some cases, unsafe housing.

10.6 Co-housing in Pairs or Small Groups

Paired or group housing can provide dogs with opportunities for enrichment that alleviate loneliness and boredom, allow for the expression of normal behaviors and social interactions such as sniffing and play, and create a more interesting environment that helps reduce stress and promotes mental well-being. Group-housed dogs have been observed not only to interact socially but also to spend more time investigating the floor of their enclosures, presumably because of the increased olfactory stimuli from other dogs (Hubrecht et al. 1992). Conversely, increases in active behaviors and stereotypies indicative of stress and reductions in play behavior have been reported in shelter dogs following separation from conspecifics (Walker et al. 2014). Because co-housing provides ongoing social contact with conspecifics and may promote an interest in the environment, it can offer a distinct welfare advantage over individual housing for dogs who enjoy social interaction and can safely and appropriately be housed with other dogs.

Careful planning is necessary to ensure that the benefits of co-housing can be achieved without increasing disease transmission and stress, conflict, or overt fighting. It is important to treat dogs as individuals; though beneficial for many, co-housing is not beneficial for all. Thorough consideration must be given to appropriately pairing dogs or matching them with a group. Dogs who are uncomfortable with other dogs may find pair or group housing more stressful than being housed individually. Not surprisingly, variability has been reported in affiliative behavior between pairs, which may suggest that some pair-housed dogs enjoy each other's company, while others merely tolerate the presence of their partner (Walker et al. 2014). In one study where kenneled dogs were housed in pairs, only a minority of pairings showed significant declines in multiple stress-related behaviors, but cortisol levels deposited in hair were lower in samples collected after paired housing was initiated. The overall level of barking in the facility, among both paired and individually housed dogs, was also reduced, suggesting positive impacts of this housing strategy for at least some dogs (Grigg et al. 2017). Importantly, published research on pair and group housing generally indicates few negative impacts, with agonistic behavior rarely reported (Mertens and Unshelm 1996; Petak 2013; Walker et al. 2014; Grigg et al. 2017).

Equal consideration should be given to meeting the dog's behavioral needs while appropriately managing the risk of infectious disease transmission and other detriments to physical health. The physical facility, individual dog and population-level needs, and available resources will influence the suitability of co-housing as an appropriate option. Only compatible animals should be co-housed, and thoughtful selection and pairing is necessary to ensure a beneficial experience for all dogs involved. Paired or group housing is not appropriate for all dogs. Dogs must each be carefully observed and evaluated for their health, behavior, and compatibility with the other dog(s) in the group before they can be safely placed together and left alone. Because of the amount of time it can take to adequately assess the dog, to find one or more suitable companions, and for the dogs to become adequately adjusted to one another, group housing dogs who arrived at the shelter separately from one another is generally not recommended if they are likely to have a relatively short length of stay (i.e., less than two weeks). When longer lengths of stay are expected, co-housing dogs is an important welfare option to consider, especially when foster care is not appropriate or available.

There have not been enough studies performed to determine a specific number for maximum group size or definitive amount of space per dog housed in a group in a shelter. As noted previously, the minimum and ideal space requirements per dog are unknown and could be expected to vary based on individual factors such as age, size, breed, physical health, behavioral health and well-being, and prior experiences. When dogs are communally housed, it is often in pairs or threes only (see Figure 10.5), although exceptions can be made for housing larger, carefully screened and monitored groups together when adequate space is available. In general, groups should not exceed four to six dogs. Requirements for the physical enclosure where the dogs will reside apply equally if one, two, or several dogs will be housed therein, and most US shelters have little or no housing suitable for groups of dogs. Regardless of the exact group size and arrangements, all co-housed dogs must have enough space between eating, resting, and elimination areas, access to sufficient and appropriately spaced resources, and the ability to distance themselves from other dogs. Each

dog should have his or her own bed, platform, or soft resting place and, ideally, a place to hide or retreat from other dogs. Water should be provided in a way that provides sufficient and ready access to all dogs. However, multiple food bowls are generally not necessary or desirable because co-housed dogs should generally be separated at feeding times. The space may have partial visual barriers but should allow for dogs to see out of the enclosure without jumping off the ground, sniff the area, explore the space, and exercise control over their movements within the space. Staff should be able to see and have easy access to all of the dogs (Prescott et al. 2004). When two or more dogs are housed together, the enclosure should also provide sufficient space for the dogs to comfortably interact with one another should they choose to do so. There should also be enough room to accommodate people entering the enclosure to perform basic tasks, such as leashing the dog(s) prior to removal. The likelihood of social conflict and infectious disease

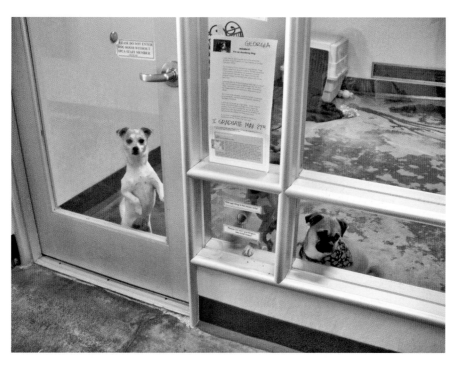

Figure 10.5 Example of single enriched dog housing with three small dogs. Note the portable kennel suitable for hiding. *Source:* Reproduced with permission from S. Janeczko.

transmission is generally proportional to the number of dogs and will be further increased if new members are added each time a dog leaves the group; groups should instead shrink by attrition so the space is used in an "all in, all out" manner. For these reasons, in addition to space considerations, pair housing of dogs is often preferable to housing in small groups.

The following basic guidelines are recommended for pair or small group housing of dogs:

i) A dog's behavior should be assessed, considering any available history and observations made by staff and volunteers, to determine compatibility with other dogs generally and specifically with the proposed co-inhabitants. A thorough medical assessment is also necessary prior to housing with other dogs. Dogs who have shown or have a history of aggressive behavior toward other dogs, are fearful of other dogs, do not enjoy the company of other dogs, or are ill, injured, or in need of individual monitoring for health reasons (e.g., to measure food intake or evaluate bowel movements) are not good candidates for co-housing. As a general rule, animals with a known or suspected infectious disease concern should be housed individually, although exceptions in limited circumstances may be appropriate (e.g., co-housing two longtime companions from the same household admitted together with a mild kennel cough). Bonded housemates or compatible family groups generally benefit from being co-housed together, provided there is adequate space for them in the same enclosure. Because these dogs have come from the same environment and do not need time to get to know one another, a decision to co-house can generally be made and implemented at the time of intake even for dogs expected to have relatively short lengths of stay.

ii) Puppies under five months of age should not be co-housed with puppies from (an) other litter(s), unless there is a clear overriding benefit (e.g., placement of a young single pup with an age-matched litter). They also should not be housed with adult dogs (especially those who are recently arrived and/or have an unknown history), because apparently healthy, immunocompetent adults may be subclinical carriers of disease who are shedding pathogens that can cause active disease among more susceptible puppies.

iii) At a minimum, all puppies and dogs should receive a physical exam and be vaccinated at or prior to intake to the shelter with injectable modified-live DHPP (distemper, hepatitis, parainfluenza, and parvovirus) and intranasal *Bordetella bronchiseptica*/canine parainfluenza virus vaccines, unless they have documented proof of up-to-date vaccinations administered by a licensed veterinarian in their medical record. Dogs considered too ill for vaccination are too ill to be considered for co-housing or playgroups until they have recovered. Other non-core vaccines may be administered as determined by a veterinarian familiar with the diseases that are endemic in the area or problematic to the shelter. Puppies should be revaccinated with a DHPP vaccine every two to three weeks in a shelter environment until they reach five months of age, and dogs over five months of age at intake should receive a single repeat vaccination two to three weeks later.

iv) All dogs and puppies must be treated prophylactically with a safe dewormer effective against roundworms and hookworms to protect their health and that of the population, minimize environmental contamination, and prevent transmission to humans. They should be closely inspected for any evidence of external parasites such as fleas and ticks and be treated appropriately if any are found. Ideally, treatment with broad-spectrum antiparasiticides effective against internal and external parasites that are likely to be of concern is provided and/or a fecal examination is performed.

v) Ideally, dogs should be spayed and neutered before placement with another dog. Intact sexually mature males and females must not be co-housed with each other.

vi) Routine intake quarantines are not generally recommended, but a quarantine that encompasses the relevant incubation period(s) should be considered before co-housing dogs with known or suspected (i.e., arrival from an area with a high prevalence of infection) exposure to specific infectious diseases. In addition to allowing time to closely monitor dogs for any signs of potential infection, a quarantine period would also allow the dog to mount a full immune response to vaccinations administered at intake. However, quarantines are often impractical and counterproductive to reducing an animal's length of stay, and they may actually contribute to an increase in disease. In such instances, it may be better to house these dogs singly or with one other dog only. In the case of a disease outbreak, a veterinarian, ideally with experience in shelter medicine, should be consulted for advice about management options.

It is essential that co-housed dogs' health and behavior are closely and consistently monitored, especially during feeding and resting periods, to ensure they each have full access to food and are not being bullied. Temporary separation for feeding is recommended. Dogs should be separated if they are showing signs of infectious disease, significant injury, stress, or incompatibility. Dogs who exhibit behaviors that may annoy other members of the group or who vocalize excessively can benefit from co-housing but require close monitoring, and they may need to be removed from the pairing or

group because of the detrimental impact on other dogs (Petak 2013). In some cases, thoughtful reassignment of the dog may be possible. For example, a dog may have been a poor match to one group but thrive with another or do better paired with only one other dog. It is important to recognize that some dogs will be most comfortable when housed individually. Many shelters use playgroups in addition or as an alternative to co-housing to allow dogs an opportunity for exercise and social interaction while they remain individually housed for feeding and sleeping at night. More information on playgroups can be found in Chapter 13.

10.7 Areas for Enrichment, Exercise, and Training

Dedicated indoor and especially outdoor areas can provide substantial behavioral benefits for dogs. They can help dogs maintain or attain physical conditioning and provide psychological stimulation. They can facilitate housetraining for dogs, serve as get-acquainted areas for dogs and prospective adopters, and provide space for group dog training, agility training, and playgroups. Some shelters are also experimenting with new types of outdoor areas such as sensory gardens, which have been used in therapy for people with a variety of conditions, including dementia, autism, and special educational needs. When used in animal shelters, sensory gardens provide dogs (and other species) with access to natural environments intentionally designed to include olfactory, tactile, auditory, and visual enrichment.

Designing and building a space that is functional, safe, and limits exposure to disease and parasites is critical. Because of the difficulty in disinfecting most substrates used for outdoor areas, some degree of risk may be associated with their use, especially for young puppies and naive, newly arrived dogs at greater risk of infectious disease. It is important that the space be well maintained and attractive as well as safe and easily accessible for people and dogs. Dogs should be supervised, especially if there are multiple dogs in the area. There should be a nearby water source to provide drinking water for the dogs and to facilitate watering or cleaning of the space. When possible, locating play and training areas in public view can also showcase dogs available for adoption. Spaces should be adequately sized for the intended use(s). The number of dogs the space will accommodate, the people involved, and the specific activities that will occur all warrant consideration.

Indoor exercise and training areas should have at least one viewing window that permits someone coming to the room to look inside and determine if there are other people and dogs inside. Additional windows that allow ample natural light should be included whenever possible. The floor of the room and walls (at least 3 ft. up) should be easy to clean and disinfect. Tile, linoleum, and concrete can be slippery surfaces for dogs to run and play on. Rubber horse mats can be used over these and other surfaces to provide traction, and they can be sanitized. Depending on the location in the shelter and the intended use, sealed, textured concrete or even specialized rubber flooring may be an option. Carpet should not be used because it will absorb urine and waste and cannot be effectively disinfected. Special attention should also be paid to objects used in training or that facilitate dogs playing. Objects should either be single use or constructed of materials that can be frequently sanitized in between dogs, or protocols should be developed to limit access to dogs not likely to be particularly susceptible to or infected with a contagious disease.

Outdoor enclosures should have a secure perimeter with a fence at least 6 ft. in height with double-gated entries to prevent escape (see Figure 10.6). Overhead coverings may allow use in a range of weather conditions; the

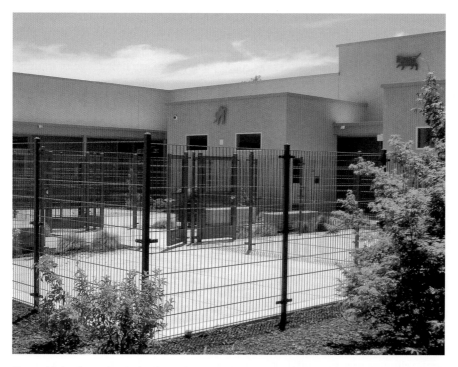

Figure 10.6 Example of a basic outdoor exercise enclosure with a concrete floor and center drain. Shade sails or similar coverings can be added to the area to provide adequate shade for dogs and people using these areas. *Source:* Reproduced with permission from S. Janeczko.

provision of shade is particularly important, especially if playgroups will be conducted. Some of the elements to be considered when designing a public dog park may also be helpful when planning outdoor areas for shelter dogs (American Kennel Club 2008). Multiple yards connected to one another or in close proximity to the dogs' housing areas are often preferable to a single, large yard, given the challenges associated with safely and securely subdividing outdoor spaces. Having multiple yards can help increase the number of dogs who are able to safely access these spaces, as dedicated spaces can be created for puppies and animals with specific infectious diseases. In addition, this can allow for a few different substrates to be used in different areas that best fit their primary use, as there are benefits and challenges with all of the available options. For example, a grassy area with wood chip/mulch walking paths may be ideal in a sensory garden, while artificial turf is likely to hold up better to heavy use by multiple dogs participating in playgroups. Materials that are specifically designed for use in dog areas, such as PetGrass® (Perfect Turf LLC, www.ptpetgrass.com) or K9 Grass® (Forever Lawn® Inc., www.k9grass.com) are increasingly available. Products that are not safe for use around dogs, such as coco mulch, must not be used. Regardless of the particular substrate chosen, the area should have adequate drainage. Feces should be removed immediately whenever possible or, at a minimum, between different dogs or groups of dogs using the area. Supplies should be readily available to keep the space clean, including waste bags, scoops, and covered garbage cans.

Basic biosecurity precautions should be developed and followed for use of these areas, including cleaning and disinfection practices, procedures to minimize environmental contamination with infectious organisms, and clear parameters outlining restrictions (if any) on which dogs may access the areas. Use of a disinfectant product that retains efficacy in the presence of organic material and has been demonstrated to reliably inactivate unenveloped viruses (i.e., canine parvovirus) is recommended. It is important to realize that natural surfaces like grass and soil cannot be disinfected, and contamination with environmentally resilient viruses or parasites may result in these areas becoming effectively "off limits" to puppies or other highly susceptible dogs. Dogs who are ill with a suspected or confirmed infectious disease or who have known exposure and are under quarantine should generally not be allowed into these areas with other dogs. Similarly, these dogs should not be allowed to use areas that cannot be adequately disinfected until they are no longer contagious or have been specifically cleared by a veterinarian for these activities and access to the specific area. Some exceptions may be possible, such as allowing a small group of dogs exhibiting mild clinical signs of infectious respiratory disease caused by *Bordetella bronchiseptica* to play together, but this should only be done on the advisement of a veterinarian familiar with shelter medicine and the animals and population in question.

The reader is directed to Chapters 12 ("Training and Behavior Modification for Shelter Dogs") and Chapter 13 ("Play and Playgroups") for information regarding compatibility, selection, and introduction of dogs to one another and about specific uses of these areas.

10.8 Initial Housing Considerations

Prompt housing decisions must be made upon admission to the shelter or shortly thereafter. Any prior history that is available, along with the physical exam findings and behavior observations gleaned from the initial interactions with the dog, should be used to guide selection of the housing unit where the dog will first be placed. This initial evaluation and pathway plan should not result in the ultimate determination of a dog's adoptability, however. As a more complete assessment of the dog's physical health and behavior is made and/or as it changes, movement to a different area of the facility or housing in an alternate style of primary enclosure may be appropriate. All dogs should also be evaluated at or prior to the time of intake and then at regular, frequent intervals thereafter (e.g., during daily rounds) to determine eligibility for and placement in a foster or adoptive home or other suitable outcome. Some key considerations for in-shelter housing selection are described in Table 10.1.

Table 10.1 Key considerations for in-shelter housing selection.

Key dog characteristic	Housing recommendation	Operational considerations
Aggressive behaviors directed to humans	• Double-sided enclosure large enough to provide enrichment and choice and to permit free movement including retreat • Secure locks to prevent escape	• Perform daily care tasks without handling or removing from the enclosure • Select enclosures in low traffic areas to reduce stimuli • Housing in proximity to exits may facilitate walks by skilled handlers, if appropriate
Exhibiting fear, anxiety, or stress	• Double-sided enclosure large enough to provide enrichment and choice and to permit free movement including retreat OR Single enriched enclosures with hiding areas • Some fearful dogs may experience less stress in smaller housing units that reduce space to evade handlers performing necessary tasks	• Perform daily care tasks without handling or removing from the enclosure • Provide hiding areas • Select enclosures in quiet, separate area to minimize stimuli • Minimize movement to new enclosures • Stick to a predictable routine • Assign consistent caregivers
Significant aggression directed to dogs	• Double-sided or single enriched enclosure • Fixed coverings on top of the enclosure and secure locks and latches to prevent escape	• Minimize visual contact with other dogs • Select enclosures near exits to reduce stimuli when entering and exiting kennel areas
Severely ill, injured, or debilitated	• House singly • Enriched cage or condo unit may facilitate temporary movement restriction	
Infectious disease	• House individually in double-compartment enclosure • House in isolation if infection is known or suspected • House in quarantine if known or likely exposure • Consider maintaining existing co-housing arrangements when animals have the same condition and adequate monitoring and treatment can be achieved without separation.	• Provide enrichment and positive human interaction while taking necessary biosecurity precautions • Use personal protective equipment appropriate to disease of concern • Limit access by public and personnel not assigned to the area
Intensive behavioral therapy	• Housing tailored to support therapeutic goal(s)	• Consider adjacency to treatment areas for dogs not able to walk on leash

10.9 Housing during Disasters

It would probably be difficult to find a shelter that has not been called upon to house animals in emergency or disaster situations that strain their capacity for care. However, attention must be paid to the individual welfare needs of these animals, who are often already distressed, diseased, or injured. They should not be placed in an environment that is detrimental to their already-fragile health and well-being. Prioritizing quality of care is especially important because despite the temporary nature of disaster situations, the need to house affected animals may persist for several weeks or months. Rescued animals who are not available for immediate adoption are usually destined for either rehousing, transportation to another location, foster care, or euthanasia.

Regardless of the challenges, every attempt must be made to house and care for rescued animals in a way that meets their needs and avoids further distress or disease transmission. Careful planning and preparation well in advance of a disaster can reduce the need to deviate from standard guidelines and best practices. The animals' needs are not suspended because of the emergency circumstances, and their needs are likely to be increased rather than decreased compared to animals in more typical shelter settings. If there is adequate capacity for care in the shelter to admit these animals, the same guidelines already outlined in this chapter should apply to their housing. Adequate personnel must be available to provide care that meets the animals' physical and behavioral needs, which will vary with the unique needs of the population. See Chapter 21, "Behavioral Care of Animals in Disasters, Cruelty Cases, and Long-Term Holds," for more information.

10.10 Conclusions

It is a significant sign of progress in the animal welfare field that animal behavior is increasingly recognized as an integral component of animal health and well-being rather than an afterthought. Application of management practices that provide opportunities for assessment, enrichment, training, and rehabilitation is now considered an essential element of a proper, humane animal shelter (Newbury et al. 2010), as is an approach to pathway planning, treatment, and outcome decision-making that balances behavioral, medical, and operational considerations. A well-designed and maintained physical facility can facilitate the development and management of an efficient and effective behavioral program in a shelter, with the quality of housing substantially impacting animal health and well-being. It is hoped that the ideas presented in this chapter, and this text in general, will benefit animal sheltering and veterinary professionals working to adapt and evolve their practices in existing facilities and inform the design and construction of new animal shelters.

References

Abrams, J., Brennen, R., and Byosiere, S.E. (2020). Trazodone as a mediator of transitional stress in a shelter: Effects on illness, length of stay, and outcome. *J. Vet. Behav.* 36: 13–18.

American Kennel Club. (2008). Establishing a Dog Park in Your Community. http://images.akc.org/pdf/canine_legislation/establishing_dog_park.pdf (accessed 30 December 2020).

Binks, J., Taylor, S., Will, A., et al. (2018). The behavioural effects of olfactory stimulation on dogs at a rescue shelter. *Appl. Anim. Behav. Sci.* https://doi.org/10.1016/j.applanim.2018.01.009.

Bowman, A., Scottish SPCA, Dowell, F.J. et al. (2017). The effect of different genres of music on the stress levels of kennelled dogs. *Physiol. Behav.* 171: 207–215.

Brayley, C. and Montrose, V.T. (2016). The effects of audiobooks on the behaviour of dogs at a rehoming kennels. *Appl. Anim. Behav. Sci.* 174: 111–115.

Cafazzo, S., Maragliano, L., Bonanni, R. et al. (2014). Behavioural and physiological indicators of shelter dogs' welfare: Reflections on the no-kill policy on free-ranging dogs in Italy revisited on the basis of 15 years of implementation. *Physiol. Behav.* 133: 223–229.

Cho, Y., Ryu, S.H., Lee, B.R. et al. (2015). Effects of artificial light at night on human health: A literature review of observational and experimental studies applied to exposure assessment. *Chronobiol. Int.* 32: 1294–1310.

Coppinger, R. and Zuccotti, J. (1999). Kennel enrichment: Exercise and socialization of dogs. *J. Appl. Anim. Welf. Sci.* 2: 281–296.

Coppola, C.L., Enns, R.M., and Grandin, T. (2006). Noise in the animal shelter environment: Building design and effects of daily noise exposure. *J. Appl. Anim. Welf. Sci.* 9: 1–7.

Garvey, M., Stella, J., and Croney, C. (2016). Auditory stress: Implications for kenneled dog welfare. Center for Animal Welfare Science, Department of Comparative Pathobiology, College of Veterinary Medicine, Purdue University. https://extension.purdue.edu/extmedia/VA/VA-18-W.pdf (accessed 28 November 2020).

Graham, L., Wells, D.L., and Hepper, P.G. (2005). The influence of olfactory stimulation on the behaviour of dogs housed in a rescue shelter. *Appl. Anim. Behav. Sci.* 91: 143–153.

Grigg, E.K., Nibblett, B.M., Robinson, J.Q. et al. (2017). Evaluating pair versus solitary housing in kennelled domestic dogs (*Canis familiaris*) using behaviour and hair cortisol: A pilot study. *Vet. Rec. Open* 4 (1): 1–14.

Hennessy, M.B., Davis, H.N., Williams, M.T. et al. (1997). Plasma cortisol levels of dogs in a county animal shelter. *Physiol. Behav.* 62: 485–490.

Hennessy, M.B., Williams, M.T., Miller, D.D. et al. (1998). Influence of male and female petters on plasma cortisol and behaviour: Can human interaction reduce the stress of dogs in a public animal shelter? *Appl. Anim. Behav. Sci.* 61: 63–77.

Hermiston, C., Montrose, V.T., and Taylor, S. (2018). The effects of dog-appeasing pheromone spray upon canine vocalizations and stress-related behaviors in a rescue shelter. *J. Vet. Behav.* 26: 11–16.

Hetts, S., Clark, J.D., Calpin, J.P. et al. (1992). Influence of housing conditions on beagle behaviour. *Appl. Anim. Behav. Sci.* 34: 137–155.

Hewison, L.F., Wright, H.F., Zulch, H.E. et al. (2014). Short term consequences of preventing visitor access to kennels on noise and the behaviour and physiology of dogs housed in a rescue shelter. *Physiol. Behav.* http://doi.org/10.1016/j.physbeh.2014.04.045.

Hiby, E.F., Rooney, N.J., and Bradshaw, J.W.S. (2006). Behavioural and physiological responses of dogs entering rehoming kennels. *Physiol. Behav.* 89: 385–391.

Houpt, K.A., Erb, H.N., and Coria-Avila, G.A. (2019). The sleep of shelter dogs was not disrupted by overnight light rather than darkness in a crossover trial. *Animals* 9: 794.

Hubrecht, R.C. (1993). A comparison of social and environmental enrichment methods for laboratory housed dogs. *Appl. Anim. Behav. Sci.* 37: 345–361.

Hubrecht, R.C. (2002). Comfortable quarters for dogs in research institutions. In: *Comfortable Quarters for Laboratory Animals* (eds. V. Reinhardt and A. Reinhardt), 56–64. Washington, DC: Animal Welfare Institute.

Hubrecht, R.C., Serpell, J.A., and Poole, T.B. (1992). Correlates of pen size and housing conditions on the behaviour of kenneled dogs. *Appl. Anim. Behav. Sci.* 34: 365–383.

Jongman, E.C., Butler, K.L., and Hemsworth, P.H. (2018). The effects of kennel size and exercise on the behaviour and stress physiology of individually-housed greyhounds. *Appl. Anim. Behav. Sci.* https://doi.org/10.1016/j.applanim.2017.11.002.

Karsten, C. (2021). Sanitation. In: *Infectious Disease Management in Animal* Shelters,

2nd ed. (eds. L. Miller, S. Janeczko, and K.F. Hurley), 166–190. Hoboken, NJ: Wiley Blackwell.

Kiddie, J. and Collins, L. (2015). Identifying environmental and management factors that may be associated with the quality of life of kennelled dogs (*Canis familiaris*). *Appl. Anim. Behav. Sci.* 167: 43–55.

Kilcullen-Steiner, C. and Mitchell, A. (2001). Platform and poster presentation AALAS national meeting Baltimore, MD abstracts. *Contemp. Top. Lab. Anim. Sci.* 40: 54–104.

Kogan, L.R., Schoenfeld-Tacher, R., and Simon, A.A. (2012). Behavioral effects of auditory stimulation on kennel dogs. *J. Vet. Behav.* 7: 268–275.

McGowan, R.T., Bolte, C., Barnett, H.R. et al. (2018). Can you spare 15 min? The measurable positive impact of a 15-min petting session on shelter dog well-being. *Appl. Anim. Behav. Sci.* 203: 42–54.

Mertens, P.A. and Unshelm, J. 1996. Effects of group and individual housing on the behavior of kennelled dogs in animal shelters. *Anthrozoös* 9: 40–51.

Myer, E.C. and Conlon, S.C. (2012). Survey of animal shelter noise levels. *Proceedings of the 41st International Congress and Exposition on Noise Control Engineering 2012, INTER-NOISE 2012,* New York, NY (19–22 August 2012). Indianapolis, IN: Institute of Noise Control Engineering.

Newbury, S., Blinn, M.K., Bushby, P.A. et al. (2010). ASV Guidelines for Standards of Care in Animal Shelters. http://www.sheltervet. org/guidelines-for-standards-of-care-in-animal-shelters (accessed 30 December 2020).

Normando, S., Contiero, B., Marchesini, G. et al. (2014). Effects of space allowance on the behaviour of long-term housed shelter dogs. *Behav. Processes.* http://doi.org/10.1016/j. beproc.2014.01.015.

Occupational Safety and Health Administration (OSHA) (2014). Occupational Noise Exposure. https://www.osha.gov/laws-regs/regulations/ standardnumber/1910/1910.95 (accessed 30 December 2020).

Patterson-Kane, E.G. and Farnworth, M.J. (2006). Noise exposure, music and animals in a laboratory: A commentary based on laboratory animal refinement and enrichment forum (LAREF) discussions. *J. Appl. Anim. Welf. Sci.* 9: 327–332.

Petak, I. (2013). Communication patterns within a group of shelter dogs and implications for their welfare. *J. Appl. Anim. Welf. Sci.* 16: 118–139.

Prescott, M., Morton, D.B., Anderson, D. et al. (2004). Refining dog husbandry and care: Eighth report of the BVAAWF/FRAME/ RSPCA/UFAW Joint Working Group on Refinement. *Lab. Anim.* 38: S1–S90.

Rooney, N., Gaines, S., and Hiby, E. (2009). A practitioner's guide to working dog welfare. *J. Vet. Behav.* 4: 127–134.

Sales, G., Hubrecht, R., Peyvandi, A. et al. (1997). Noise in dog kenneling: Is barking a welfare problem for dogs? *Appl. Anim. Behav. Sci.* 52: 321–329.

Sandri, M., Colussi, A., Giovanna Perrotta, M. et al. (2015). Salivary cortisol concentration in healthy dogs is affected by size, sex, and housing context. *J. Vet. Behav.* https:// https:// doi.org/10.1016/j.jveb.2015.03.011.

Scheifele, P., Martin, D., Clark, J.G. et al. (2012). Effect of kennel noise on hearing in dogs. *Am. J. Vet. Res.* 73: 482–489.

Schlaffer, L. and Bonacci, P. (2013). Shelter design. In *Shelter Medicine for Veterinarians and Staff,* 2nd ed. (eds. L. Miller and S. Zawistowski), 21–35. Hoboken, NJ: Wiley Blackwell.

Shiverdecker, M.D., Schiml, P.A., and Hennessy, M.B. (2013). Human interaction moderates plasma cortisol and behavioral responses of dogs to shelter housing. *Physiol. Behav.* 109: 75–79.

Siwak, C.T., Tapp, P.D., Zicker, S.C. et al. (2003). Locomotor activity rhythms in dogs vary with age and cognitive status. *Behav. Neurosci.* 117: 813–824.

Stephen, J.M. and Ledger, R.A. (2005). An audit of behavioral indicators of poor welfare in kenneled dogs in the United Kingdom. *J. Appl. Anim. Welf. Sci.* 8: 79–95.

Taylor, K.D. and Mills, D.S. (2007). The effect of the kennel environment on canine welfare: A critical review of experimental studies. *Anim. Welf.* 16: 435–447.

Taylor, S., Webb, L., Montrose, V.T. et al. (2020). The behavioral and physiological effects of dog appeasing pheromone on canine behavior during separation from the owner. *J. Vet. Behav.* 40: 36–42.

Tod, E., Brander, D., and Waran, N. (2005). Efficacy of dog appeasing pheromone in reducing stress and fear related behaviour in shelter dogs. *Appl. Anim. Behav. Sci.* 93: 295–308.

Tuber, D.S., Miller, D.D., Caris, K.A. et al. (1999). Dogs in animal shelters: Problems, suggestions and needed expertise. *Psychol. Sci.* 10: 379–386.

Wagner, D., Newbury, S., Kass, P. et al. (2014). Elimination behavior of shelter dogs housed in double compartment kennels. *PLOS ONE* 9 (5): e96254.

Walker, J.K., Waran, N.K., and Phillips, C.J. (2014). The effect of conspecific removal on the behaviour and physiology of pair-housed shelter dogs. *Appl. Anim. Behav. Sci.* 158: 46–56.

Weiss, E., Miller, K., Mohan-Gibbons, H. et al. (2012). Why did you choose this pet? Adopters and pet selection preferences in five animal shelters in the United States. *Animals* 2: 144–159.

Wells, D. and Hepper, P.G. (1992). The behaviour of dogs in a rescue shelter. *Anim. Welf.* 1: 171–186.

Wells, D.L., Graham, L., and Hepper, P.G. (2002). The influence of auditory stimulation on the behaviour of dogs housed in a rescue shelter. *Anim. Welf.* 11: 385–393.

Wells, D.L. and Hepper, P.G. (1998). A note on the influence of visual conspecific contact on the behaviour of sheltered dogs. *Appl. Anim. Behav. Sci.* 60: 83–88.

Willen, R.M., Schiml, P.A., and Hennessy, M.B. (2019). Enrichment centered on human interaction moderates fear-induced aggression and increases positive expectancy in fearful shelter dogs. *Appl. Anim. Behav. Sci.* 217: 57–62.

11

Canine Enrichment

Lisa Gunter and Erica Feuerbacher

11.1 Introduction

Despite the public's interest in companion animals, animal shelters in the United States operate under minimal federal or state regulation; consequently, dogs' experiences can vary considerably between facilities (Newbury et al. 2010). A large body of research suggests that dogs encounter a variety of potential stressors within the shelter that could negatively impact their welfare (Taylor and Mills 2007; Hennessy 2013), including but not limited to excessive noise (Sales et al. 1997; Coppola, Enns, et al. 2006; Scheifele et al. 2012; Venn 2013), spatial restriction (Hubrecht 1995; Hubrecht et al. 1995; Beerda et al. 1999), social isolation (Beerda et al. 1999), loss of owner (Hiby et al. 2006), lack of control (Hennessy et al. 1997), and absence of a daily routine (Hennessy et al. 1998).

Four to five-and-a-half million dogs enter animal shelters annually in the United States (Woodruff and Smith 2017; Rowan and Kartal 2018). In recent years considerable efforts have been made to improve outcomes for these dogs (Protopopova and Gunter 2017), resulting in substantial increases in the number of dogs adopted and returned to their owners as well as reductions in euthanasia (ASPCA 2018; Rowan and Kartal 2018). Along with

improving outcomes for animals entering shelters, organizations have increased their focus on improving the welfare of the animals in their care. One component of this approach includes the use of enrichment interventions (Taylor and Mills 2007; Hennessy 2013; Moesta et al. 2015). Yet, many procedures that are routinely used in shelters have not been experimentally tested, nor have many of the ways in which animals are cared for and housed been empirically considered.

11.2 Enrichment Interventions in the Animal Shelter

Shepherdson (1998) described enrichment as a systematic approach that attempts to understand and provide for both the "psychological and behavioral needs of captive animals." For dogs living in shelters, this could be described as their proximate or immediate welfare as they await adoption. Mellen and MacPhee (2001) further identify key additions to Shepherdson's approach that relate well to the provision of canine enrichment in animal shelters.

Enrichment programs should be proactive, taking into consideration species affinities as well as the individual's history while considering shelter resources. This chapter will

Animal Behavior for Shelter Veterinarians and Staff, Second Edition. Edited by Brian A. DiGangi, Victoria A. Cussen, Pamela J. Reid, and Kristen A. Collins.
© 2022 John Wiley & Sons, Inc. Published 2022 by John Wiley & Sons, Inc.
Companion website: www.wiley.com/go/digangi/animal

describe how these programs can be assessed and how staff and volunteer efforts can be utilized to carry out programs successfully. Like many captive environments, such as zoos or laboratories, the animal shelter is likely stressful; however, unlike these previously mentioned environments, a stay in the animal shelter is intended to be temporary. Thus, when appropriate, enrichment interventions that affect dogs' distal or ultimate welfare of leaving the shelter and living in a home, such as prolonging or reducing their length of stay, will also be discussed.

Because the focus of this chapter is on canine enrichment in the animal shelter, it does not include studies conducted on other kenneled dogs (e.g., purpose-bred dogs living in laboratories, veterinary colonies, or working dogs), rather the focus is on companion dogs that were likely once owned pets and now living under sheltering conditions. These interventions have been broadly categorized as those that provide social interaction: either with a human or canine; object enrichment; and sensory stimulation (auditory, olfactory, or visual).

11.2.1 Human Social Interaction

Our relationship with dogs is unique. Through a combination of domestication, artificial selection, and socialization, dogs have developed the ability to form bonds with us, and our social influence on them is strong (Morey 1994). When we consider this shared history with dogs, it should not be surprising that in the inherent social isolation of the animal shelter, human-animal interaction has been one of the most studied enrichment interventions (see Gunter et al. 2021 for a review).

The impact of one-time, in-shelter interactions involving 20–30 minutes of petting or play on behavioral measures and cortisol levels has been assessed in a number of studies (Hennessy et al. 1997; Hennessy et al. 1998; Menor-Campos et al. 2011; Shiverdecker et al. 2013; Dudley et al. 2015). In some of these studies, the sex of the human influenced

the impact of the petting, with women having a greater effect on cortisol reduction than men (Hennessy et al. 1997; McGowan et al. 2018). In total, these interventions report reductions in cortisol immediately following the interaction, suggesting that they decrease dogs' stress. Behaviorally, Shiverdecker and colleagues (2013) found that when dogs were left alone in a novel enclosure, they vocalized significantly more than when they were being petted, played with, or left with a passive stranger.

Willen et al. (2017) also examined the effects of 30-minute interactions across two successive days, similar to what staff or volunteers would provide in the shelter, to detect possible cumulative benefits. They found that, as demonstrated in prior studies, dogs' cortisol reduced after interacting with a person, but multiple interactions did not produce additional benefits. While cortisol decreased following 30 minutes of interaction, those reductions did not persist an hour later. Behaviorally, dogs vocalized, panted, and tried to escape the interaction room less and were seen to be wagging their tails more often in these sessions as compared to dogs that were left alone in a novel room or remained in their kennel.

More recently, McGowan et al. (2018) found that just 15 minutes with a person could decrease dogs' heart rate, increase heart rate variability (HRV), and reduce standing by the dog during the interactions. The authors found that the amount of time the dogs interacted with the volunteer was influential, such that when dogs spent less than 50% of their time in contact with the volunteer, they experienced less of a benefit from the intervention. This suggests that physical contact with the enrichment, in this case the human, is important in decreasing biological markers of stress reactivity. Willen et al. (2017) also found evidence that 15 minutes of petting reduced cortisol, but it only occurred for some dogs, notably those brought to the shelter as strays, with reductions comparable to what was found with 30-minute interactions. Dogs that were owner relinquished did not experience this effect.

It seems likely that the activity that a person engages in with the dog during these interactions affects the dogs' in-kennel behavior. Protopopova et al. (2018) examined the effects of two 15-minute-long interventions of reading and exercise that occurred daily for 2 weeks. When dogs received exercise, they moved back and forth in their kennels less often immediately preceding the intervention; but immediately after, dogs' back and forth movement increased but jumping on the kennel door lessened. For dogs that were read to by a volunteer, undesirable behaviors associated with an increased length of stay were reduced prior to the intervention. Immediately after, dogs were also moving back and forth in their kennels more often but barking and jumping on their kennel doors had decreased.

The results of Protopopova et al. (2018) are mixed in that dogs' back and forth motion in the kennel increased after both the exercise and reading interventions, a behavior previously shown to be associated with longer lengths of stay (Protopopova et al. 2014). When parsing out the interventions' positive effects, a greater reduction on door jumping was seen with exercise, but an overall larger decrease in undesired behaviors (including both door jumping and barking) was found when volunteers read to the dogs. As the authors note, more research is needed with longer observations, both before and after the interventions, to better elucidate their effects. In the meantime, shelters may consider individualizing the activity of the interaction based on the behavior of the dog, using calm interactions for dogs that need to reduce their barking, while more active dogs that are jumping on kennel doors and rubbing the walls may experience more benefit from exercise.

Interactions of 15–30 minutes occurring weekly or multiple times a week for several weeks have also been explored, such as those described by Bergamasco et al. (2010), Valsecchi et al. (2007), Normando et al. (2006), and Hennessy et al. (2002). Bergamasco et al. (2010) investigated a 25-minute intervention in

which shelter dogs played with a person and toy, were walked on leash, groomed, trained, and received food, praise, and petting three times a week for eight weeks. Although Bergamasco and colleagues found little effect of the interactions on dogs' cortisol levels or HRV, dogs' sociability over the eight-week intervention improved such that they were more likely to approach the experimenter and initiate interaction in the kennel before leaving on their leashed walk.

Valsecchi et al. (2007) tested an intervention of training, play, and petting every other day for two months and found dogs' obedience, docility, and sociability improved compared to unenriched dogs. Dogs in both the intervention and control groups showed reductions in cortisol; the authors suggested that the regular sampling and, consequently, interaction with humans may have contributed to the overall cortisol decrease. Similarly, Normando et al. (2006) reported that 15-minute, weekly interactions with a volunteer over five weeks led to changes in dogs' social behavior. Dogs receiving the intervention were out of sight less and wagged their tails more often than non-intervention dogs when the experimenter was present, and these effects persisted after the intervention ceased. Thus when considering the impacts of these interventions, it is worth noting that dogs' interest in people increases as they spend more time with us, which may aid in their likelihood of adoption and ultimate welfare of leaving the shelter and living in a home.

While interaction durations of 15 and 30 minutes have received the most attention in the literature, longer one-time interactions have also been explored. Coppola, Grandin, et al. (2006) explored the impact of a 45-minute interaction of petting, play, and grooming on dogs' cortisol levels immediately following the interaction as well as one and two days and one week later. Interestingly, Coppola and colleagues found that dogs in the contact group did not differ two hours following the interaction with the experimenter but did so when measured the following day, with no other differences observed at later time points. This study's finding of an effect on the day following human interaction remains the only evidence to date of a delayed reduction in stress for shelter dogs, suggesting the need for additional studies to determine if longer in-shelter interactions confer distinctive advantages.

Interventions in which dogs leave the shelter for few days or weeks may provide an increased benefit to dogs when compared to in-shelter interactions (Hennessy et al. 2006; Fehringer 2014; and Gunter et al. 2019). This is likely due to the prolonged nature of the interventions as well as the environment that they occur within. Hennessy et al. (2006) studied dogs fostered in a three-week prison program, during which they lived with and received obedience training and social interaction by incarcerated handlers. Post-intervention, the dogs more readily responded to cues such as sit, down, and walk. They also jumped on strangers and barked less, but yawned more, in a novel situation post-intervention than dogs that had remained at the shelter. While cortisol was relatively unaffected for both groups, the effects on behavior are cautiously optimistic evidence for the use of such programs for longer-stay dogs or those needing additional socialization.

Time in a home might confer even greater benefits to dogs awaiting adoption. Fehringer (2014) reported that placement in a foster home resulted in lower cortisol compared to in-shelter levels, and that the dogs' cortisol steadily declined over the first three days in foster care. In a recent study by Gunter et al. (2019), dogs that stayed for one or two nights in a volunteer's home were found to have lower cortisol than dogs that remained in the shelter; and while dogs' cortisol increased upon return, it was no higher than baseline levels in the shelter before fostering. Additionally, dogs' longest bouts of uninterrupted rest were highest while in the home but remained longer upon return to the shelter than before fostering. In all, these studies provide compelling evidence for the use of stays out of the shelter as an important enrichment tool with measurable benefits.

Limiting visitors in kenneling areas may also improve dogs' proximate welfare by reducing the unpredictability of human traffic, improving dogs' ability to control environmental contingencies; however, the impact on their ultimate welfare, such as reduced adoption visibility and potentially longer lengths of stay, should also be considered. Wells and Hepper (2000) found that during days with more visitors to the shelter, dogs spent more time at the front of their kennels, standing and barking. Hewison et al. (2014) prohibited potential adopter access during afternoons when the animal shelter was otherwise open for viewing dogs. They found that noise levels were over 12 dB lower during the intervention as compared to pre-intervention levels with positive changes in behavior as well. Sedentary behavior increased in both the mornings before opening and afternoons during the intervention, locomotor activity also decreased, and the frequency and duration of repetitive behaviors were reduced in the afternoon—suggesting that scheduled breaks during the day from the arousing bustle of people could afford dogs an opportunity to relax and recharge without leaving the shelter.

11.2.1.1 Human Social Interaction through Training

Thorn et al. (2006) demonstrated that dogs living in the shelter learned to sit in less than 10 minutes and performed this behavior with new people in a subsequent training session. Herron et al. (2014) provided in-kennel training for dogs twice a day and afternoon enrichment of a frozen, food-filled toy. During training, dogs were reinforced with food for making eye contact, not barking, sitting or lying down, and being at the front of the kennel. Over the course of the three-day intervention, dogs were sitting, lying down, and quiet more often and jumping less in their kennel when compared to control dogs. Additionally, control dogs showed a significant increase in barking, whining, and growling.

Training interventions in the shelter have often focused on in-kennel behavior, but changing out-of-kennel behavior can also be enriching and increase welfare, particularly if it reduces aggressive behavior. Orihel and Fraser (2008) tested a 10-day training intervention for dogs that exhibited moderate aggression toward other dogs. The intervention consisted of 30-minute sessions on leash in which a stimulus dog was presented to the dog, at decreasing distances, while the dog was cued to sit or make eye contact with the handler. Dogs were rewarded with praise and food for relaxed behavior, while behaviors such as staring or growling toward the other dog resulted in redirection of the dog's gaze by the handler. Dogs in the control group received time in an outdoor enclosure. While dogs in both groups showed similar levels of aggression pre-intervention, after 10 days of training a majority of intervention dogs showed decreases in aggressive behaviors, while dogs in the control condition showed increases in growling and muzzle licking when presented with another dog. However, when dogs in the intervention were tested one week after training had ceased, their overall aggression scores had returned to pre-intervention levels, suggesting that continued training for dogs with canine aggression is needed to make sustained behavioral change while living in the shelter.

Training in the shelter can be effective, not only with operant techniques but with simpler approaches deploying classical conditioning methods. Protopopova and Wynne (2015) demonstrated that both classical and operant conditioning can reduce undesirable in-kennel behaviors, including dogs being at the back of the kennel, facing backward, rubbing the kennel walls, and barking. The two interventions used in the study were: differential reinforcement of other behavior, whereby dogs were provided a food reward for any behavior other than the undesired ones, and non-contingent delivery of food, wherein

dogs were provided a treat regardless of their behavior. Both interventions reduced unwanted behaviors; however, the time spent training the dogs was considerably lower using classical conditioning (20 seconds per dog) than operant (2 minutes). In a follow-up study, Payne and Assemi (2017) observed that with daily pairings of a door chime with food (three to five times a week) over three weeks, kennel noise decreased by 15 dB, reducing the intensity of an established environmental stressor. In all, these studies suggest that classical conditioning is an effective, time-efficient method of training that can be more easily deployed in the shelter environment and still positively impact welfare.

11.2.1.2 Application of Evidence-Based Shelter Practices for Human Social Interaction

As evidenced by the myriad studies described here, the opportunity for shelter dogs to spend time with people consistently provides stress reduction and is the most impactful type of additive enrichment intervention. Interactions can be as short as 15 minutes, and a dog's comfort level with the person and time spent with them likely makes a difference in the beneficial effects conferred. Activities between dogs and people should be tailored to the preferences and behavior of the individual dog. For dogs to fully benefit from their time with people, it is best that interactions occur out of the kennel away from environmental stressors; and better yet, out of the shelter in foster homes as they await adoption.

Noise levels in the shelter can be extreme, sometimes exceeding 100 dB (Sales et al. 1997; Coppola, Enns, et al. 2006; Scheifele et al. 2012; Venn 2013) and surpassing the 90-dB limit set by the Occupational Safety and Health Administration for human exposure during an eight-hour period (United States Department of Labor, Occupational Health and Safety Administration 1983). This noise can be lessened by reducing in-kennel barking, and simple interventions that involve walking past the dogs' kennels and treating, regardless of behavior, can quickly accomplish this. Conversely, a scheduled break from human traffic during the day could also improve dogs' welfare, including reductions in noise and improvements in behavior, and provide a more practical option for shelters that cannot remove adopters from kenneling areas altogether. As with any unwanted behaviors, training needs to occur regularly to maintain improvement; but in general, changing behavior and learning new behaviors is possible in the shelter and is one type of human interaction that can help meet dogs' psychological and behavioral needs.

11.2.2 Canine Social Interaction

While not as well-studied as interactions with people, researchers have examined the effects of social contact with other dogs, either through housing manipulations (Mertens and Unshelm 1996; Wells and Hepper 1998; Dalla Villa et al. 2013; Walker et al. 2014) or interactions out of the kennel (Belpedio et al. 2010; Flower 2016; L. Gunter et al., work in preparation).

Mertens and Unshelm (1996) measured behavioral differences between individually and group-housed dogs and found that dogs housed together were less noisy and better behaved. In that study, dogs that were singly housed barked, whimpered, and howled more than dogs that were group-housed. The researchers observed that solo dogs were more likely to display aggressive behavior at the kennel front toward other dogs. While conflicts did arise when dogs were housed in groups (which were as large as 30 dogs), of the 211 dogs participating over the three-month study period, only five incidents occurred, resulting in what the researchers called "light wounds." Of particular interest, 10% of dogs that were singly housed during the study displayed stereotypies, while no dogs in the group-housed condition did.

Because of the need for a human presence in the group-housing condition to deescalate potential conflicts, two staff members monitored the group-housed dogs (with dogs kenneled singly at night and during feeding). Perhaps as a result of this extra human presence, dogs in this condition more often approached an unknown observer than did singly housed dogs during a behavioral test. Follow-up research is needed to address limitations of this study, including potential shelter and population differences (this study took place at two different facilities). These findings suggest that group-housing in which dogs as well as people are present could be helpful in improving sociability.

While group-housing of the size tested by Mertens and Unshelm (1996) may not be feasible for most shelters due to space, canine sociability, or staff resources, pair housing may be a viable alternative. Dalla Villa and colleagues (2013) studied the effects of group (four to five dogs in an enclosure) versus pair housing on long-stay shelter dogs and found that dogs' behavior improved under pair-housing conditions. Dogs' trotting, walking, and standing decreased in pair housing, while more lying down occurred, suggesting that dogs were spending more time resting when living together in pairs. While social behavior occurred rarely in either type of housing, agonistic behavior (i.e., defensive or threatening social behavior) was not observed between paired dogs, while such behavior made up nearly one-fifth of social interactions of group-housed dogs.

Walker et al. (2014) examined the impacts of removing one dog from a co-housed pair after the pair had been living together in the shelter for several weeks. After separation, the remaining dogs' running, changes in posture, and stretching all increased, suggestive of more activity and possible restlessness. Other behaviors that are considered stereotypic in nature and indicative of decreased welfare, such as circling and figures of eight, also increased. Many of these behaviors did begin to decline over the six-day post-separation period, although play (now without a conspecific present) remained reduced. While no changes in cortisol were found, S-IgA levels were elevated after dogs were separated from each other. Interpreting the impacts of this short-term separation on dogs' S-IgA is based on just a few studies, but the elevated levels do suggest that the acute stress of separation negatively impacted dogs' immune function. Additionally, trends for longer latencies to the middle and near negative positions in a cognitive bias test, though not significant, also support a finding that separation had a negative impact on dogs' underlying affective state. In agreement with observations by Mertens and Unshelm (1996) and Dalla Villa et al. (2013), Walker et al. (2014) found that co-housed dogs spent little time behaving agonistically (0.1%) and instead were much more affiliative (3.2%).

It is difficult to determine whether the simple presence of other dogs is, in fact, canine social interaction or merely visual stimulation, and whether such a presence is enriching to dogs or a detriment to their welfare. Wells and Hepper (1998) tested two housing conditions for dogs: one in which the dogs were able to view other dogs in directly opposing kennels versus dogs that looked out to an empty kennel row. Wells and Hepper found that dogs more often were at the front of their kennels when they were able to see other dogs and more often at the back of the kennel when they could not. No differences were observed in the dogs' behavior (i.e., standing, sitting, resting), including vocalizing.

Certainly, dogs being at the front of their kennels is helpful for adopter viewing and can lead to shorter lengths of stay (Protopopova et al. 2014). However, single housing is sometimes associated with more reactivity at the front of the kennel (Mertens and Unshelm 1996). Thus, housing dogs singly with nearby conspecific visual contact but no social interaction may have more complex effects on welfare than is currently understood, and further empirical exploration of this commonly used shelter housing arrangement is needed to inform best practices.

It is possible that social interactions outside of the kennel may be more enriching than simple visual contact. Belpedio et al. (2010) examined the effects of 30 minutes of off-leash, canine social interaction as compared to dogs remaining in their kennels. Saliva for cortisol analysis was collected each morning as a baseline as well as 30 minutes and 3 hours post-interaction, and dogs' in-kennel behavior was recorded 1 minute prior to saliva collection. The authors detected no differences in cortisol levels, but, collectively, stress-related behaviors, which included jumping, barking, and whining, occurred more frequently with dogs in the kenneled group during the study. It should be noted, though, that dogs that received social interaction did lick, pant, pace, spin and yawn more than dogs left in their kennels, suggesting a mixed effect, if any, of this particular intervention on dogs' overall welfare.

Flower (2016) investigated the impact of one-time, off-leash canine interactions on dogs' performance on a behavioral assessment with more promising results. When dogs' behavior was assessed with an unfamiliar dog on-leash, dogs that had interacted with other dogs prior to the assessment displayed more playful, submissive behavior toward the unknown dog than dogs that had not had the interaction experience. While these results are preliminary, they suggest that this type of brief social contact for dogs could be beneficial in supporting appropriate on-leash behavior when seeing other dogs in the shelter.

The benefits of canine social interaction may extend beyond positive changes in behavior. The effect of differences in housing and social contact with other dogs on cortisol and S-IgA levels has been examined (L. Gunter et al., work in preparation). Traditional kennel housing was compared to a novel housing design with smaller, glass-fronted enclosures. Two social conditions were compared within each housing type: a condition with no social contact with other dogs and a condition with three 15-minute conspecific sessions a day. Dogs experienced each of the four experimental conditions for three days. (This design provided a true control for social interaction in a given housing type.)

The authors found that dogs' S-IgA was higher when living in the novel-designed kennels (irrespective of social condition), and lower when receiving daily canine social contact regardless of housing, with no interaction effect between housing and social condition. (It is worth noting that when videos of the social contact sessions were behaviorally coded, dogs spent more time with people than the other dogs or the environment during these sessions.)

While no main effects of housing or social contact were found with dogs' cortisol values, cortisol was highest when dogs were living in novel housing and receiving no social contact and were lowest when living in traditional kennels and receiving no social contact. While these results provide evidence that dogs' contact with other dogs can influence their stress, immune function, and ultimately, welfare, more research is needed to better understand how characteristics of the social contact as well as the level of activity engaged in during these sessions can influence the intervention's impact.

11.2.2.1 Application of Evidence-Based Shelter Practices for Canine Social Interaction

While much less studied than interactions with people, dogs spending time with other dogs is likely beneficial for their welfare while living in the shelter, and efforts should be made to facilitate these interactions, particularly amongst dogs that prefer the company of other dogs. (A two-month-long survey of dogs and their conspecific skills taken at a large, open admission shelter in the Midwest found that when accounting for various medical procedures and shelter processes in which dogs would be unable to partake in off-leash interactions, less than one-third of dogs were suitable and available for interactions with other dogs on a daily basis [unpublished results].) Nevertheless, it is likely that off-leash interactions can improve dogs' behavior when seeing other dogs on-leash and can promote better welfare; however, much more research is needed to better understand how the duration of these interactions, number of dogs, methods used when managing interactions, and compatibility between the dogs contribute to these potentially positive effects.

Co-housing with another dog can likely stave off the effects of social isolation and possibly buffer the stressors of everyday life in the shelter, yet care should be taken to ensure compatibility, using paired walks and/or off-leash interactions to identify well-matched kennelmates. For dogs that are successfully co-housed with another dog, having new opportunities for social interaction identified should one of the pair be adopted would likely be helpful for the remaining dog's welfare.

11.2.3 Object Enrichment

When considering placing objects within the kennel, it is useful to revisit our definition of enrichment. Beds, chews, balls, ropes, and soft toys have varying functional value to dogs, so we must consider the species as well as the individual's history and preferences in determining how relevant an object will likely be. It is not surprising, then, that investigations into object enrichment for shelter-housed dogs have been met with mixed success (Wells and Hepper 2000; Wells 2004; Pullen et al. 2010; Kiddie et al. 2017).

Wells and Hepper (2000) explored the impacts of a bed and a suspended Nylabone® (Nylabone Products, Neptune City, NJ) chew, both placed at the front of the kennel on dogs' behavior. They found that the bed at the front of the kennel caused the dogs to spend more time there, whereas the chew did not; however, dogs' bed usage decreased when the bed was placed in the front as compared to its typical position in the back of the kennel. While dogs initially sniffed the Nylabone, fewer than 20% of the dogs were seen chewing, pawing, or tugging at it. These findings suggest that while a bed is of interest to shelter dogs, where it resides impacts use.

Subsequently, Wells (2004) provided dogs a variety of objects: squeaky and non-squeaky balls, Nylabone chews, ropes, and Boomer Balls® (Company of Animals, Broomfield, CO). In a design similar to typical shelter practices, objects were provided for longer durations, six days, with dogs' location in the kennel and behavior recorded. Overall, dogs rarely interacted with the objects (<10% of all observations) with a reduction over time, suggesting a possible habituation effect. Dogs did show a preference for the Nylabone over the other toys by spending the most time with it; and dogs moved more and stood less when provided the Nylabone, squeaky ball, and non-squeaky ball. As the author recommends, if object usage is limited and habituation likely, rotation is recommended for the highest probability of engagement.

Pullen et al. (2010) explored two categories of objects: (i) robust toys, including a Boomer Ball, rope, nylon and rubber tug, and rubber toy; and (ii) toys that are more destructible, such as a vinyl bone, soft and plush toys with squeakers, and a non-squeaky tennis ball. Robust toys were concurrently presented in combinations of hanging and on the kennel floor (trial 1), while the destructible toys were only presented alongside the robust toys, all on the floor (trial 2). Only 35% of shelter dogs interacted with the robust toys during the robust-only trial, spending on average just two minutes with them. Dogs that contacted the robust toys, spent more time interacting with them on the floor (vs. hanging) with a shorter latency to interact. When the toys were hanging, however, dogs interacted longest with the rope toy. Conversely, when shelter dogs were given the option of soft, destructible toys in trial 2, more than three-quarters of dogs spent 25% of the 15-minute session interacting with them, mainly ignoring the robust selections. They also interacted longer with the softer toys, spending

the most time with the squeaky bone, soft, and plush toys, and the least time with the tennis ball.

Kiddie et al. (2017) investigated three types of low-cost interventions to improve shelter dog behavior: partitions blocking visual contact of adjacent dogs, whole coconuts (to potentially play with, chew, or break open), or cardboard beds as possible relief from the plastic mesh bottom of a crate. Dogs were observed for two 30-minute sessions on non-consecutive days in the baseline, intervention, and post-intervention periods with each type of enrichment. While no behavioral differences were found between treatments, dogs were observed to lie down, sit, and yawn less with any enrichment (as compared to baseline and post-intervention). Of the 36 dogs in the study, all but 1 dog destroyed the cardboard bed—treating it as a chewable object rather than potential bedding. Kiddie et al. (2017) found that dogs interacted with the coconut and cardboard less over time, which could be related to their eventual deconstructed states. However, it is also probable that, as Wells (2004) found, novelty plays a role in object enrichment.

11.2.3.1 Application of Evidence-Based Shelter Practices for Object Enrichment

One of the most basic forms of enrichment shelter dogs should be provided is a bed and placing it at the back of the kennel will likely encourage its usage. When considering what toys to provide in the shelter, destructibility should be considered with unsupervised dogs, particularly those with a history of ingesting items (either in a previous home, foster care, or the shelter) and especially those that have needed medical intervention. For dogs that can be safely left alone with toys, providing objects that dogs will most likely interact with, taking into consideration species and individual preferences, is the best approach to improving welfare.

Based on the previous studies, softer objects, such as squeaky, rubber bones and plush toys, will likely be interacted with by the most dogs for longer periods of time as opposed to harder, most robust toys. Providing them on the ground will also increase the likelihood of interaction. However, individual differences exist; and simple assessments can help identify what toys dogs in your shelter prefer (which can easily be conducted during interaction sessions with volunteers or staff out of the kennel) and, along with frequent rotation, will further aid in their toy engagement.

11.2.4 Auditory Enrichment

Several studies have explored the use of auditory enrichment to change dogs' behavior and reduce noise in shelter kennels (Wells et al. 2002; Kogan et al. 2012; Bowman et al. 2015; Brayley and Montrose 2016; Bowman et al. 2017), focusing on certain genres of music or types of sound, often those that are perceived as pleasant and mood-enhancing to humans (Rickard et al. 2005).

Wells et al. (2002) investigated the impacts of classical, heavy metal, and pop music; human conversation on the radio; and a control condition of no auditory enrichment on the dogs' behavior. Each was played for four hours with dogs experiencing all music types. Dogs spent more time resting, less time standing, and more time being quiet in their kennels when classical music was played as compared to other genres of music, human conversation, or no auditory enrichment. Conversely, with heavy metal, dogs were observed barking more frequently compared to any other condition. Similarly, Kogan et al. (2012) exposed dogs to 45 minutes a day of songs from two of the same musical genres: classical and heavy metal along with a track from "Through a Dog's Ear" by Leeds and Wagner (2008), wherein classical piano music is simplified to create a more soothing rendition. Along with a control condition with no added sound, auditory stimulation was provided to the dogs three times a week for four months. As seen by Wells et al. (2002), classical music led to the most time

spent resting. Dogs vocalized more often when no music was provided and were less vocal when classical music was played, but differences were observed between classical selections. Both Wells et al. (2002) and Kogan et al. (2012) observed detrimental behavioral effects with heavy metal music, including increased body shaking, barking, and less time resting.

One consistent limitation of the aforementioned studies is the duration of the auditory intervention. Bowman et al. (2015) addressed this concern when they tested the effects of a classical music compilation compared to a no-additional-sound control. Both conditions lasted for six-and-a-half hours a day over seven days with dogs' in-kennel behavior observed twice daily for one-and-a-half hours, first in the morning and then again in the afternoon.

When classical music was played dogs spent more time sitting and laying down, with less time standing and vocalizing. While no changes in cortisol were found with the addition of music, changes in heart rate and HRV, which indicate stress reduction, were identified. Bowman et al. (2015) also investigated whether dogs habituate to auditory stimulation, another point of interest to shelters. They found that the behavioral and HRV effects of classical music began to diminish in as quickly as one day, suggesting that while classical music may be effective in improving welfare, rotating the selections that dogs are exposed to each day is important in maintaining those benefits over their stay.

In a follow-up study, Bowman et al. (2017) investigated four other genres of music in addition to classical music, using compilations of pop, soft rock, reggae, and Motown. Each of the five genres was played once for six hours with a no music (control) condition tested before and after. Regardless of genre, dogs spent more time lying down and less time standing. Barking was not impacted by any genre, but dogs were 142 times more likely to bark after the music stopped, whichever genre it was. The succession of genres in this study more closely resembles a five-day intervention of mixed genres without the inclusion of any potentially stimulating music (i.e., heavy metal)—and as such, the more meaningful comparison between music and silent control here suggests that varied, auditory enrichment is preferential to shelter noise unabated.

Brayley and Montrose (2016) tested many of the same genres in previous studies, but with the novel addition of an audiobook intervention (a more systematic version of Wells et al.'s [2002] inclusion of conversation on the radio). In two-hour presentations, dogs experienced Beethoven, 80s pop music, "Through a Dog's Ear," a reading of the *The Lion, the Witch, and the Wardrobe*, and a control condition of no additional sound. When the audiobook was played, dogs spent more time resting and less time walking, sitting, or standing compared to all other conditions. Barking and other vocalizations, such as howling, growling, and whining, also occurred least often with the audiobook, but some differences between the conditions were observed.

Considering that regular conversation tested by Wells et al. (2002) demonstrated no impact on dogs' behavior, the consistent effect of the audiobook in this study is curious. The authors suggest that the professional delivery and tempo of the book's narration may have led to greater attending by the dogs than just casual conversation.

11.2.4.1   Application of Evidence-Based Shelter Practices for Auditory Enrichment

Multiple studies support classical music as an effective intervention in the shelter, but caveats remain. Repeating the same recording across the entirety of the day, multiple days in succession (which is not uncommon in animal sheltering), has not been tested. When considering Bowman et al.'s findings, it is likely that dogs can quickly habituate to the music, reducing its calming action. At a minimum, multiple, classical music compilations should be rotated daily to potentially reduce this effect. Audiobooks are another promising form of enrichment that may increase auditory variety

while promoting behaviors associated with better welfare and could be included in the shelter's rotation of recordings.

It is unknown, however, whether dogs perceive music in a manner that is similar to us, and presumptions of a positive affect based on these recordings, such as a calming effect with classical music, may be anthropomorphic (Rickard et al. 2005). An alternate explanation for the results of these studies could be that the music is masking or changing the perception of one sound through the presence of another. In the case of the animal shelter, it's possible that classical music, more so than other types of music, may act similar to white noise, equally distributing sounds across the frequency band, masking sudden changes in sound (e.g., barking by other dogs, doors opening and closing). This may create a more consistent environment for the dogs, leading to the observed behavioral changes. Future studies exploring sound masking could help us better understand what qualities of auditory enrichment are influential in dogs' perception and their reactions in the shelter.

11.2.5   Olfactory Enrichment

Many of the reasons to explore auditory enrichment in the shelter, likely apply to olfactory interventions as well. One key feature to these interventions, however, is the species-specific relevance of olfaction in the daily lives of dogs (Nielsen et al. 2015). Over the past decade and a half, researchers have explored the impacts of odors and pheromones on the behavior and physiology of shelter dogs (Graham et al. 2005a; Tod et al. 2005; Binks et al. 2018; Hermiston et al. 2018; Uccheddu et al. 2018; Haverbeke et al. 2019).

Graham et al. (2005a) investigated lavender, chamomile, rosemary, peppermint along with a no-odor control, each diffused in front of and behind the dogs' kennels for four hours a day over five consecutive days. Exposure to both lavender and chamomile led to increases in dogs' resting and decreases in movement and vocalization. Conversely when rosemary and peppermint were diffused, resting decreased while dogs' standing, moving, and vocalizing occurred more often.

Binks et al. (2018) evaluated cloths scented with ginger, coconut, vanilla, and valerian placed in the dogs' kennels along with two control conditions: a non-scented cloth and no cloth present. For each condition, dogs' behavior was recorded for two hours a day over three successive days. With all odors, dogs vocalized and moved less and rested more compared to both controls, demonstrating a positive effect of these olfactory interventions. Moreover, dogs reclined with their eyes closed most often with coconut- and ginger-scented cloths compared to the no-cloth control. However, it is worth noting that the non-scented cloth also reduced dogs' vocalizing and movement and increased resting behavior more so than having no cloth in the kennel, suggesting more investigation may be needed to parse out the novel effect of the cloth and the odors themselves. (Use caution when implementing olfactory interventions in the shelter that involve essential oils; see resources from ASPCA's Animal Poison Control Center at www. ASPCApro.org.)

Pheromones differ from odors in that they are species-specific chemosignals that affect the behavior of conspecifics. Dog-appeasing pheromone (DAP) is a synthetic version of a pheromone produced by lactating female dogs shortly after giving birth and is processed through the canine vomeronasal organ, a specialized organ for detecting non-volatile chemosignals that is part of many species' olfactory systems. Tod et al. (2005) compared the behavioral effects of a seven-day diffuser treatment of DAP versus placebo on dogs living in separate kennel blocks at a shelter. They found that when an unknown person walked past the dogs' kennels on the final day of treatment, the average barking amplitude (loudness) of the DAP group was lower than that of the placebo; however, the peak barking amplitude did not differ, indicating that barking in both groups had similar peaks in their loudness. Likewise, when Hermiston et al. (2018) sprayed DAP directly in dogs' kennels 30 minutes prior to an unknown dog walking past the dogs' kennels, the kennel block of the DAP-treated group was more than 6 dBs lower than dogs' kennels that were untreated, a more than 30% reduction in volume. However, barking frequency and behavior did not differ between groups.

11.2.5.1 Application of Evidence-Based Shelter Practices for Olfactory Enrichment

Dog-appeasing pheromone is an impactful intervention in reducing the loudness of dog barking in the shelter. Olfactory interventions that use calming odors (i.e., lavender, chamomile, coconut, and ginger) may be a more cost-effective enrichment that affects multiple behavioral measures in addition to barking, such as increased rest and decreased movement. More stimulating odors, such as peppermint, ginger, and valerian, may be better-suited for out-of-kennel interactions where dogs can more actively engage with them. However, if costliness of intervention is not a concern, the nascent literature on DAP in the animal shelter is supportive of its effectiveness. With these types of olfactory enrichment, dispersion (and doing so in a safe manner with essential oils) is a consideration, and logistic questions, such as diffuser placement, coverage plans, and maintenance of therapeutic levels, will need to be addressed. DAP collars, while not used in these studies, have shown promise in reducing behavioral measures associated with fear and anxiety in response to a simulated thunderstorm in laboratory beagles (Landsberg et al. 2015); these may be a more appropriate mode of DAP for the shelter environment.

11.2.6 Visual Stimulation

To our knowledge, only one study has explored the effects of visual sensory stimulation, namely, television monitors, as a form of canine enrichment in the shelter. Graham et al. (2005b) investigated the impact of monitors placed at the front of dogs' kennels, with video of other dogs, unfamiliar animals, and humans as well as a blank screen, on the dogs' behavior. Each intervention type lasted four hours a day for five days. Regardless of image type, dogs' vocalizing and movement decreased with more time spent at the front of their kennel. Similar to findings on toy engagement (Wells 2004), dogs spent only 10% of their time looking at the monitors as compared to controls, and their interest waned over time, suggesting the more species-specific, interactive enrichment previously described may be preferred by dogs and provide greater welfare benefits.

11.3 Assessing Enrichment

Because enrichment can only possibly be enriching if the animal uses it, assessing enrichment interventions is essential. Not only do such practices ensure that programs are accomplishing their main goal of improving welfare, they allow shelters to make informed decisions about how they allocate their time and resources.

With this in mind, evidence-based decisions about enrichment are often made on the shelter-wide level and then on the individual dog. This helps us decide what primary enrichment programs to enact that are likely to be used by a majority of the dogs (see Section 11.2) before tailoring enrichment for smaller proportions of animals that are not engaging or benefitting from the primary enrichment the shelter provides.

Most specific decisions around efficacy will be at the individual animal level, once the primary enrichment programs have been identified, because shelters should be cognizant of the specific effects of the enrichment on the individual. At the shelter-wide level, however, a shelter could discontinue a certain type of enrichment if it is not bringing about the desired behavioral change or not used by a large proportion of dogs. They could instead opt for another enrichment type and assess it, with hopes that it will be more effective. Whether at the shelter-wide or individual level, evidence-based decisions allow the shelter to better serve all dogs, preventing shelters from spending resources on interventions that are not beneficial, and instead directing those resources to other, more effective modes of enrichment.

11.3.1 What to Measure

In terms of assessing enrichment in the shelter, there are two main classes of behavior to measure. The first is the dog's direct engagement with the enrichment. A variety of measures can be used to assess direct engagement, each answering different questions about the intervention (see Box 11.1). The other class of behavior is whether the enrichment impacts important behaviors for that individual animal, such as producing more resting behavior or a reduction in barking.

Determining if, how long, and in what way dogs engage with the enrichment is essential for determining, at a preliminary level, if that enrichment should be continued or not: is the dog engaging and in a desirable fashion? Or is the dog not engaging? If engagement is confirmed but the enrichment does not bring about the desired behavior change, one can assess if the lack of effect was due to it not impacting the behavior at all or just not to the degree desired.

Of course, one of the main goals in providing enrichment is to improve the animals' welfare and assessing the impact on dogs' behavior is critical. For example, consider a 15-minute front-of-kennel treating program, where volunteers toss hot dogs when passing by the dogs' kennels to create a positive association with visitors. To assess intervention efficacy, the shelter could measure the frequency or duration of dogs lunging or barking at the front of their kennels. A shelter that has many shy, fearful dogs might

---

Box 11.1   Key Enrichment Engagement Questions

Population Level

1) What percentage of dogs engage with a certain type of enrichment, such as a rope toy in the kennel?
   Assessment utility: Provides a shelter-wide determination of whether the item is deliverable to most dogs with a high likelihood of engagement.

Individual Level

1) Does an individual dog engage with the enrichment?
   Assessment utility: Lets a shelter tailor the individual dog's experience and ensure it includes enrichment that the dog actually uses.
2) How long did the dog engage with the enrichment?
   Assessment utility: Allows for determination of whether the intervention is sufficiently enriching or if a higher level of engagement is desired. For example, deciding to freeze a dog's stuffed KONG to increase the amount of time the dog spends interacting with it.
3) How did the dog engage with it (e.g., biting or shredding it)?
   Assessment utility: Helps determine whether enrichment is individually appropriate. For example, the dog might engage regularly with an enrichment item, but it results in bleeding gums. If that's the case, a different item may be better. This measure can also help inform decisions about objects that are often considered to be obstruction risks. If one dog is observed to shred and consume a soft toy, then the item is poorly suited for that dog; but soft toys can still be highly enriching for other dogs.

---

implement a similar program but measure behavior change differently. In this case, staff could measure dogs' frequency of approach behavior when they pass by kennels during morning rounds.

To evaluate intervention efficacy, shelters can measure behaviors before enrichment is provided and then compare those same measures afterward. This can be done on a shelter-wide level (e.g., measuring noise level in the kennels) or per individual dog (e.g., measuring the frequency or duration of barking by one dog). Tracking an individual dog's behavior daily allows us to identify changes in a dog's behavior early, which is vital in the shelter. With more knowledge sooner, more individualized interventions can be implemented sooner, such as providing an office foster for a dog that is showing initial signs of kennel reactivity. Ideally, data collection starts as soon as a dog enters the shelter. Tracking the dog's behavior can allow

detection of non-engagement with the enrichment and/or behavioral deterioration, either of which would warrant action.

Given the multifactorial nature of behavior, it is difficult to predict how quickly enrichment might affect behaviors of interest. An intervention may be effective but only after the animal has encountered the enrichment for several days or weeks. Given the time-sensitive nature of shelter work, such long observation periods are not recommended. If an intervention was implemented to counter a problematic behavior but does not produce positive behavioral change within one week at most, modifying the enrichment strategy is advised. Additionally, if no engagement is observed after even two days, changing enrichment types would be appropriate.

Ideally, shelters would assess both the engagement and the effect on behaviors of interest as they provide different information. However, engagement with some forms of enrichment can be hard to measure. For example, how would a dog's interaction with music or odors be measured? In these cases, measuring the effects of the intervention on other behavior, such as resting and activity-based behaviors, may be the only metric.

After the measurable behaviors have been selected, objective definitions are needed. Behavioral definitions should be clear and simple. They should indicate what does and does not count as a response; this is particularly important when many people are measuring. Even something as straightforward as "engaging with object" needs a definition: does chewing on it count? How about licking? Sleeping on it? An objective definition should describe what the behavior looks like and should not include subjective terms. For example, "jumping and barking with the intention of getting the person's attention" is an unsuitable definition for kennel reactivity as what the dog *meant* to do is unknown. A better definition might be: "jumping on any part of the kennel with the front two paws while simultaneously barking when a person or animal walks past." After deciding on what to measure and how to define it, the next step is deciding how to measure it.

11.3.2 How to Measure

While recording an animal and coding their behavior later is a common research practice, it is impractical for a shelter. Instead, live coding is the most feasible way to make observations. This allows staff or volunteers to integrate observations into their daily routine.

Of course, this can present challenges. It is possible that human presence alone can change the dog's behavior (known as the "observer effect"). If the behavior of interest occurs in response to a person (e.g., kennel reactivity), this might not be an issue. If the behavior is engagement with an object, though, the observer might disrupt the dog. If this is the case, clever observational skills are needed, such as observing from a greater distance or having a staff member to whom the dog is habituated (and less likely to influence the dog) record the behavior. If the shelter has the wherewithal to install cameras, remote observation reduces these observer issues significantly.

With live coding, the materials needed to record the observations can vary in their simplicity. Observations can be recorded on paper, either placed directly on the dog's kennel or in a log that the observer carries. While both are simple to implement and allow for real-time assessments of behavioral trends and enrichment decisions, observations also need to be transferred to the animal's database record, making this method more time-intensive than it may initially appear. With the ubiquity of smartphones, however, observations can be recorded directly into a shared file, eliminating the extra transfer step. Observations can be completed by staff during daily rounds or activities, or assigned to volunteers and entered in real time. Data compilation and transfer can be done on a weekly basis, if necessary, to reduce workload, as long as the data are assessed daily to allow for timely, informed decisions. For some behaviors, it is important for observations to be made when the behavior is likely to occur (e.g., measuring food guarding without food present would not be helpful).

11.3.3 Measurement Methods

There is a wide range of measurement techniques in animal behavior. The most detailed and time-intensive measurement approach is continuous measurement, in which all instances of the behavior(s) and their duration are recorded. This, however, is unreasonable for shelters. Other measurement systems that are more feasible but still provide useable data about the enrichment program should be considered. These methods include focal animal sampling, instantaneous scan sampling (ISS), interval recording (IR), momentary time sampling (MTS), and permanent products. For the purposes of our discussion, ISS, MTS, and permanent products are described in more detail in Box 11.2. For a more extensive discussion of

Box 11.2 Types of Behavioral Sampling Most Useful in the Animal Shelter

Instantaneous scan sampling. Instantaneous scan sampling (ISS) is used to quickly assess the behavior of multiple individuals, making this method very useful in sheltering. In ISS, the observer focuses on one individual and records what the dog is doing in that instant, before shifting focus to the next dog. For example, an observer might walk down a kennel aisle and mark down whether each dog is engaging with a plush toy as the observer passes the dog's kennel. Additionally, observers can record the presence or absence of a behavior. ISS can also be used to measure how frequently (percentage of observations) one dog or all dogs in a kennel row display the behavior.

Momentary time sampling. Momentary time sampling (MTS) is a blend of ISS and interval recording. In MTS, an individual animal is observed for an instant, as in ISS, but in MTS the same animal will be observed again, after a specified interval (e.g., every 20 seconds or every 10 minutes). For example, a volunteer might walk through kennels and record whether each dog was engaged with a recently delivered, peanut-butter-covered disc. Then five minutes later, the volunteer could walk through again and conduct a second observation for each dog. This observation pattern provides an estimate of behavior duration. In the example, observing the dog engaged during sample 1 and again in sample 2, with five minutes elapsing between the two, provides a six- to seven-minute estimate of engagement with the disc.

Permanent product. A permanent product is the tangible result or outcome of a behavior that can be used as a proxy for that behavior. Examples of permanent products are feces or urine in the kennel (behavior: elimination) or number of KONGs with food eaten from them (behavior: eating from stuffed KONG). We are not directly observing the behavior; we are recording the product of the behavior. Recording permanent products is often more practical because the observer does not have to be present when the behavior is occurring and can record those permanent products at the person's convenience. Instead of walking through and observing if a dog is working on a stuffed KONG, shelter staff can just note which and how many KONGs have at least some food missing when they are removed from the kennels.

Permanent products measurement for object enrichment can be easily incorporated into other daily activities. For non-consumable enrichment, being creative with what is considered a permanent product increases this technique's utility. For example, if rope toys were provided, chew marks or strings pulled from the toy could indicate interaction. For non-chewers or even rubber objects that may not show evidence of use, objects could be placed in the same location in the kennel; and if the object has moved, it is assumed the animal has touched it. This, of course, is an imperfect measure if it is accidentally moved or left in the same position after play; however, this can still provide relatively useful data with relatively low recording effort.

Permanent product measurement only works when the behavior of interest, whether interaction with an item or an undesired behavior (e.g., a furrow in the dirt from a dog that has been fence running), leaves a tangible result. Additionally, we need to be able to clearly attribute that product to an individual or group of individuals. If we are measuring whether a dog is eating its food, but the dog is co-housed and not separated when fed, we cannot necessarily attribute an empty bowl to our dog of interest.

observation and measurement techniques, see *Measuring Behavior: An Introductory Guide* (Martin and Bateson 2007) and *Applied Behavior Analysis* (Cooper et al. 2019). Appendix 11.A offers an example data sheet for monitoring engagement with enrichment.

11.4 Implementing and Maintaining an Enrichment Program

While shelters have ample enrichment options to choose from, not all programs will be appropriate, depending on the shelter's mission, population, resources, housing practices, behavioral goals, and staff and volunteer skills. As noted above, animals need to engage with the enrichment and show behavioral or psychological benefits. For this to have a chance to occur, it needs to be delivered to them, which requires consideration of human behavior and asking: (i) how are staff, volunteers, and the public engaged in preparing, delivering, and assessing enrichment? and (ii) how can enrichment be effectively and efficiently integrated into daily operations?

Obtaining the desired behavior from staff, volunteers, and the public is no different than obtaining desired behavior from our animals. There are three dimensions to pursue in this regard: (i) training, (ii) arranging the environment, and (iii) arranging consequences. When considering enrichment, shelters need to ensure that they have addressed all three of these components for their program to be successful and sustainable.

11.4.1 Training

It is essential that the personnel implementing or assessing the enrichment program have the ability to complete the tasks required of them. Just as an owner cannot expect their dog-reactive dog to be calm when another dog passes by if they have not taught an appropriate alternative response, we cannot expect our staff or volunteers to know how to implement enrichment if we have not taught them the required skills. What, then, should training entail to maximize success?

The training required will depend on the complexity of the behavior being taught. If the behavior is stuffing KONGs® (KONG Company, Golden, CO), a simple written task list, ideally with some visual aids, or a short video is likely sufficient. If the behavior is complex, such as learning to take a dog out of the kennel for a walk, then more training is required. Determining the requisite components can be determined by assessing your training: if few people are mastering the skills after training, more steps, such as modeling the behavior or breaking the behavior into smaller steps, may be needed.

Human behavioral literature indicates there are typically three components needed to produce satisfactory performances of complex behavior. First, create a task analysis of what the learner needs to do, including all necessary steps correctly ordered. A task analysis ensures that all the relevant skills are being taught and helps the mentor identify if steps are being omitted or completed incorrectly. At each step, the mentor is teaching the learner and assessing performance. By making this task analysis available to staff and volunteers (e.g., a document posted in a relevant location), it can be used for future reference. See Box 11.3.

Second, the mentor should model the behavior so that the learner can see what the full behavioral sequence looks like. Finally, the learner should perform the behavior with the mentor providing both positive feedback and negative corrective feedback. Shelters often use this type of process in new volunteer mentoring sessions or buddy dates for new dog walkers.

Howard and DiGennaro Reed (2015) examined how one shelter trained volunteers to safely take dogs from their kennels, practice polite leash skills, and work on obedience in a play yard. They found that when volunteers were trained as usual—attending a staff member's live lecture with verbal instructions and a

---

Box 11.3   Task Analysis for Harnessing a Dog

- ☐ Locate the correct kennel
- ☐ Read the information on the kennel to ensure the dog can go on a walk
- ☐ Retrieve a harness that will fit the dog, a leash, and treats
- ☐ Return to the kennel
- ☐ Throw treats to the back of the kennel to move dog away from the gate
- ☐ Open the gate the minimum amount for the dog walker to enter
- ☐ Enter the kennel
- ☐ Close the gate
- ☐ Identify the correct opening on the harness for the dog's head to go through
- ☐ Use treats to lure the dog into the harness
- ☐ Clip harness under the chest
- ☐ Assess harness and adjust so that it is not too snug or too loose
- ☐ Clip the leash to the front clip on the harness and onto the dog's collar

---

demonstration on how to do these tasks—volunteers only completed ~60% of the tasks correctly. When volunteers attended video-based training (with modules that included on-screen written instructions and images, verbal instructions corresponding to on-screen material, and a study guide), scores improved but participants failed to meet the criteria for mastery (85% of tasks completed correctly without any safety errors). Mastery was only achieved after volunteers saw the behavior modeled and received corrective feedback while they performed the tasks. Behavior modeling and feedback were also critical features of a program that trained volunteers to teach obedience behaviors to shelter dogs (Howard and DiGennaro Reed 2014).

11.4.2   Arranging the Environment

To engage staff, volunteers, and the public to successfully participate in an enrichment program, we need to arrange the environment so that it supports the desired behavior. Here is an example of insufficient environmental arrangement: a large municipal shelter had their kennel staff walk to the front office for computer data entry whenever they moved a dog to a new kennel (or keep track mentally and make notes for later). Often, this would lead to multiple staff spending at least 20 minutes each day gathered around the computer attempting to locate dogs who were not in their assigned kennels. Instead, the shelter could put a computer in the kennel area or installing install a dry erase board in the kennel area where changes could be written until they were later entered into the computer to solve this problem. Whatever the resources or desired action, it is helpful to ask: how can we arrange the workplace so that it is easy for staff and volunteers to do the right thing?

When planning an enrichment program, consider what needs to be changed in the shelter environment to facilitate correct implementation. If the program is sending dogs on field trips, have pre-packed backpacks full of treats, toys, water, and emergency numbers for the volunteer to use. If the program is using novel odors in daily olfactory enrichment, have odors pre-arranged by day in a cabinet rather than asking volunteers to search for them and figure out what was sprayed yesterday and the day before to ensure novelty.

How enrichment is scheduled during the day will also impact whether delivery actually occurs. While enrichment programs were historically viewed as optional activities when time allowed, they are now understood to be essential components of providing appropriate care to and maintaining the welfare of the animals in our custody. Though personnel time needs to be considered, many enrichment programs can add very little work and, in some cases, even reduce labor. If the enrichment program makes care easier and improves animals' lives through reducing behavioral issues, it can be sustained with little external input (i.e., providing praise, gift cards, or other additional reinforcers).

Mapping out the typical day of personnel involved in implementing enrichment programs can identify potential opportunities and challenges. For example, sending dogs on sleepovers when staff are cleaning kennels might be difficult if those staff are also responsible for bringing dogs out for these getaways. A better option may be sending dogs beforehand, so that the dogs are out of their kennels when cleaning occurs. Similarly, putting dogs' rations in buckets on their kennels for the public and volunteers to dispense throughout the day can provide many occasions for enrichment while not adding to staff duties as it actually eliminates the need to distribute and retrieve bowls from inside kennels.

Along with making implementation easy to do correctly, indicating that the enrichment has been delivered needs to be straightforward. Checking a box on a small dry erase board on the kennel could indicate the dog received a chewable item or recently spent time with a person. Additionally, tracking enrichment usage should be quick and simple; this is why using permanent products works well (see Box 11.2). Solutions will vary by shelter; however, talking to impacted staff and volunteers about what would make delivering and tracking the enrichment easiest will likely yield some creative solutions from the people who have probably been thinking about these issues. Finally, the enrichment and behavioral records need to be evaluated by a team member who is tasked with making data-based enrichment decisions, and the records should be entered into the dog's record, so that its preferences for enrichment and its behavior changes can be used by all personnel.

11.4.3 Arranging Consequences

The final piece of successfully managing human behavior is arranging reinforcement contingencies that support the desirable behavior. As much as it would be wonderful if everyone just "did the right thing," that is, unfortunately, not how behavior works,

especially if we are asking staff or volunteers to do extra work or change their procedures to implement an enrichment program. A brief overview of tactics that can be employed to help maintain enrichment delivery and assessment is presented below. For more in-depth discussions on behavior-based ways to bring about top performances from people, we refer readers to *Performance Management* (Daniels and Bailey 2014) and *Human Competence*: *Engineering Worthy Performance* (Gilbert 2007).

This first tactic requires a quick definition: a reinforcer is *by definition* a stimulus, which, when delivered following a behavior, increases the future likelihood of that behavior (see Chapter 3 for more information on learning theory). Positive reinforcers, such as money or praise, may be effective. While money is a powerful reinforcer, its accessibility in the limited-resource environment of most animal shelters makes it an unlikely option. However, shelters do have other valuable reinforcers at their disposal such as praise, which is free to give and is one of the most underused positive reinforcers (Flora 2000). Simply recognizing when someone has done well (even if it is their job to do that task) can be highly effective. Praise should be made publicly and should explicitly indicate the behavior for which it is being given. With the advent of social media, praising staff, volunteers, and members of the public is even easier, although delivering the praise in person is still important.

The social stimulation that staff and volunteers receive from interacting with each other can also be reinforcing. Volunteer satisfaction can be significantly enhanced by connectedness to other volunteers, especially to more experienced volunteers or volunteers from whom they can learn new skills (Zappa and Zavarrone 2010). In the authors' experience, very active volunteers often create their own social networks in the shelter, both with staff and other volunteers. Rather than waiting for this to occur organically, shelters can foster these types of interactions by having new volunteers shadow kennel staff and work collaboratively with them to reduce their workload. Enrichment programs can be designed with a team component where volunteers or a staff member and a volunteer work together to deliver and assess the enrichment.

Another category of potential reinforcers is professional development, which can advance staff and volunteer skills, knowledge, and responsibility. These opportunities can be contingent on completing certain desirable activities, such as delivering enrichment for a certain number of days. In fact, providing staff with increased responsibility within their organization can reduce absenteeism (Fried et al. 1972; Hammer et al. 1981). Setting up these opportunities not only provides the occasion to reinforce desirable performances, it allows shelters to develop the skilled staff and volunteers they need.

Reinforcement contingencies can be set in place to maintain all parts of an enrichment program. For example, volunteers could earn a $2 voucher to the shelter store after preparing 50 toilet rolls filled with kibble. Staff could earn extra time on the following day's lunch break after all dogs receive three types of enrichment the day before. Members of the public could earn shelter t-shirts after taking 10 dogs on field trips or 5 dogs on sleepovers. Staff could receive raffle tickets for a weekly drawing, if they record the enrichment usage of all the dogs in the shelter one day during their workweek.

11.4.4   Using Staff for Effective Enrichment Programs

While enrichment programs should be developed by staff that are skilled in behavioral principles, the management and delivery of the program does not need to be restricted. Even for shelters that have behavior teams, these teams likely do not have the human resources to carry out daily interventions. Instead, having animal care staff (or as we prefer it more holistically described: animal experience staff) manage these programs, with

enrichment delivery by staff and volunteers, can be particularly impactful as these staff usually spend the most time with the dogs.

Animal care staff can use their many observations throughout the day to identify dogs that are showing concerning behaviors (e.g., kennel reactivity or catatonia) and need additional support, and provide enrichment if they have responsibility for delivery decisions, or relay the information to the person(s) in the shelter that does. This allows dogs to benefit from interventions sooner and empowers all staff to make decisions about how they can improve dogs' lives. The opportunity for animal care staff to engage with the animals beyond daily maintenance (i.e., cleaning and feeding) can be used as a reinforcer for their more mundane tasks. Furthermore, being part of the enrichment program's design, such as when dogs are enrolled or objects are delivered, can improve the success of organizational programs (Lawler and Hackman 1969), such as increasing the likelihood that the enrichment will be carried out correctly and regularly.

For administrative staff without regular interaction with dogs, participating in interventions that directly affect the dogs can be reinforcing. One particular program that can be a great collaboration is an office foster program. The behavior team can work together with medical and operational staff to curate the list of dogs, and animal care staff or morning volunteers can deliver the dogs to the offices. Administrative staff can provide their availability via shared calendar or respond to a daily sign-up email. Many shelters have informal office fostering, but formalizing the program allows dogs to reap the benefits of consistent human interaction, and staff with less daily dog contact can participate in their care.

11.4.5   Engaging the Public for Effective Enrichment Programs

The public can be employed in various capacities depending on the enrichment program. Visiting groups (4-H, Girl Scouts, or corporate teams) can participate in one-time volunteering opportunities preparing object enrichment, such as stuffed KONGs or toys (e.g., braided ropes). Placing an enrichment preparation station in the shelter lobby captures an audience that may not have considered volunteering when they walked through your doors. To do this successfully, have the necessary materials ready for assembly and make a photo guidebook (task analysis) about the enrichment's preparation, such as how to braid a rope toy or create a snuffle mat.

Delivery of enrichment can also be accomplished through public engagement. Visitors can easily deliver food or toy enrichment as long as the instructions are simple and explicit. For example, dogs' daily rations of food can be placed in a bucket on the dog's kennel. Kibble can then be dropped into a delivery tube or directly into the kennel throughout the day, allowing potential adopters to interact in desirable ways with the dogs. This can create positive associations with new people and reduce barking in the kennels (Protopopova and Wynne 2015; Payne and Assemi 2017).

Typically, shelters implement walking programs, shelter dog training classes, and in-kennel reading programs to provide human interaction to the dogs. More recently, shelters have created field trip (Gunter et al. 2021) and sleepover programs (Gunter et al. 2019) with public options for community participation. Shelters can tailor dogs' eligibility based on behavior, allowing both the dog and person to enjoy the interaction while reducing risk and increasing the likelihood of continued participation in the program. Finding ways to reduce barriers for the public to interact with the shelter and improve the welfare of the dogs can be an excellent tool in recruiting new volunteers and increasing the overall reach of the organization in the community.

11.5 Conclusions

While the provision of enrichment is necessary for dogs living in animal shelters, so is the assessment of engagement and determination of benefits, namely, creating the desired change we want to see in the dogs' behavior. There are a wide range of sampling and measurement techniques for monitoring enrichment usage and its behavioral effects. Choosing the right one for your shelter will rely on which behaviors are being measured and the resources available to record those measures. Both enrichment delivery and enrichment tracking must be easy and straightforward to do for those who are doing it, but such efforts are only worthwhile if the data being collected are used. Once enrichment programs are in place, data-informed decisions about which enrichment types are provided, on both the shelter-wide and individual dog levels, must be consistently re-evaluated based on the current population of dogs. In total, this will allow shelters to most usefully employ their resources and best serve the dogs in their care.

Please visit the companion website for video clips and downloadable resources associated with this chapter.

References

American Society for the Prevention of Cruelty to Animals (ASPCA). (2018). Pet Statistics. https://www.aspca.org/animal-homelessness/shelter-intake-and-surrender/pet-statistics (accessed 1 December 2019).

Beerda, B., Schilder, M.B., Bernadina, W. et al. (1999). Chronic stress in dogs subjected to social and spatial restriction. II. Hormonal and immunological responses. *Physiol. Behav.* 66 (2): 243–254.

Belpedio, C., Buffington, L., Clusman, C. et al. (2010). Effect of multidog play groups on cortisol levels and behavior of dogs (*Canis lupus familiaris*) housed in a humane society. *J. Appl. Comp. Anim. Behav.* 4 (1): 15–27.

Bergamasco, L., Osella, M.C., Savarino, P. et al. (2010). Heart rate variability and saliva cortisol assessment in shelter dog: Human–animal interaction effects. *Appl. Anim. Behav. Sci.* 125 (1): 56–68.

Binks, J., Taylor, S., Wills, A. et al. (2018). The behavioural effects of olfactory stimulation on dogs at a rescue shelter. *Appl. Anim. Behav. Sci.* 202: 69–76.

Bowman, A., Dowell, F.J., Evans, N.P. et al. (2017). The effect of different genres of music on the stress levels of kennelled dogs. *Physiol. Behav.* 171: 207–215.

Bowman, A., Scottish SPCA, Dowell, F.J. et al. (2015). "Four Seasons" in an animal rescue centre; Classical music reduces environmental stress in kennelled dogs. *Physiol. Behav.* 143: 70–82.

Brayley, C. and Montrose, V.T. (2016). The effects of audiobooks on the behaviour of dogs at a rehoming kennels. *Appl. Anim. Behav. Sci.* 174: 111–115.

Cooper, J.O., Heron, T.E., and Heward, W.L. (2019). *Applied Behavior Analysis*. London, UK: Pearson.

Coppola, C.L., Enns, R.M., and Grandin, T. (2006). Noise in the animal shelter environment: Building design and the effects of daily noise exposure. *J. Appl. Anim. Welf. Sci.* 9 (1): 1–7.

Coppola, C.L., Grandin, T., and Enns, R.M. (2006). Human interaction and cortisol: Can human contact reduce stress for shelter dogs? *Physiol. Behav.* 87 (3): 537–541.

Dalla Villa, P., Barnard, S., Di Fede, E. et al. (2013). Behavioural and physiological responses of shelter dogs to long-term confinement. *Vet Ital.* 49 (2): 231–241.

Daniels, A. and Bailey, J.S. (2014). *Performance Management*. Atlanta, GA: Performance Management Publications.

Dudley, E.S., Schiml, P.A., and Hennessy, M.B. (2015). Effects of repeated petting sessions on leukocyte counts, intestinal parasite prevalence, and plasma cortisol concentration of dogs housed in a county animal shelter. *J. Am. Vet. Med. Assoc.* 247 (11): 1289–1298.

Fehringer, A.A. (2014). Stress in shelter dogs and the use of foster care to improve animal welfare. Baccalaureate dissertation. Pennsylvania State University.

Flora, S.R. (2000). Praise's magic reinforcement ratio: Five to one gets the job done. *Behav. Anal. Today* 1 (4): 64.

Flower, S. (2016). The effect of play group on the behavior of shelter dogs. Master's thesis. City University of New York.

Fried, J., Weitman, M., and Davis, M.K. (1972). Man-machine interaction and absenteeism. *J. Appl. Psychol.* 56: 428.

Gilbert, T.F. (2007). *Human Competence: Engineering Worthy Performance*. Hoboken, NJ: Pfeiffer Publishing.

Graham, L., Wells, D.L., and Hepper, P.G. (2005a). The influence of olfactory stimulation on the behaviour of dogs housed in a rescue shelter. *Appl. Anim. Behav. Sci.* 91 (1): 143–153.

Graham, L., Wells, D.L., and Hepper, P. G. (2005b). The influence of visual stimulation on the behaviour of dogs housed in a rescue shelter. *Anim Welf.* 14 (2): 143–148.

Gunter, L.M., Feuerbacher, E.N., Gilchrist, R. et al. (2019). Evaluating the effects of a temporary fostering program on shelter dog welfare. *Peer J.* 7: e6620.

Gunter, L.M., Gilchrist, R.J., Blade, E.M. et al. (2021). Investigating the impact of brief outings on the welfare of dogs living in US shelters. *Animals* 11 (2): 548.

Hammer, T.H., Landau, J.C., and Stern, R.N. (1981). Absenteeism when workers have a voice: The case of employee ownership. *J. Appl. Psychol.* 66 (5): 561.

Haverbeke, A., Uccheddu, S., Arnouts, H. et al. (2019). A pilot study on behavioural responses of shelter dogs to olfactory enrichment. *Vet. Sci. Res. J.* 1 (1): 29–34.

Hennessy, M.B. (2013). Using hypothalamic–pituitary–adrenal measures for assessing and reducing the stress of dogs in shelters: A review. *Appl. Anim. Behav. Sci.* 149 (1): 1–12.

Hennessy, M.B., Davis, H.N., Williams, M.T. et al. (1997). Plasma cortisol levels of dogs at a county animal shelter. *Physiol. Behav.* 62 (3): 485–490.

Hennessy, M.B., Morris, A., and Linden, F. (2006). Evaluation of the effects of a socialization program in a prison on behavior and pituitary–adrenal hormone levels of shelter dogs. *Appl. Anim. Behav. Sci.* 99 (1): 157–171.

Hennessy, M.B., Voith, V.L., Young, T.L. et al. (2002). Exploring human interaction and diet effects on the behavior of dogs in a public animal shelter. *J. Appl. Anim. Welf. Sci.* 5 (4): 253–273.

Hennessy, M.B., Williams, M.T., Miller, D.D. et al. (1998). Influence of male and female petters on plasma cortisol and behaviour: Can human interaction reduce the stress of dogs in a public animal shelter? *Appl. Anim. Behav. Sci.* 61 (1): 63–77.

Hermiston, C., Montrose, V.T., and Taylor, S. (2018). The effects of dog-appeasing pheromone spray upon canine vocalizations and stress-related behaviors in a rescue shelter. *J. Vet. Behav.* 26: 11–16.

Herron, M.E., Kirby-Madden, T.M., and Lord, L.K. (2014). Effects of environmental enrichment on the behavior of shelter dogs. *J. Am. Vet. Med. Assoc.* 244 (6): 687–692.

Hewison, L.F., Wright, H.F., Zulch, H.E. et al. (2014). Short term consequences of preventing visitor access to kennels on noise and the behaviour and physiology of dogs housed in a rescue shelter. *Physiol. Behav.* 133: 1–7.

Hiby, E.F., Rooney, N.J., and Bradshaw, J.W. (2006). Behavioural and physiological responses of dogs entering re-homing kennels. *Physiol. Behav.* 89 (3): 385–391.

Howard, V.J. and DiGennaro Reed, F.D. (2014). Training shelter volunteers to teach dog compliance. *J. Appl. Behav. Anal.* 47: 344–359.

Howard, V.J. and DiGennaro Reed, F.D. (2015). An evaluation of training procedures for animal shelter volunteers. *J. Organ. Behav.* 35: 296–320.

Hubrecht, R.C. (1995). Enrichment in puppyhood and its effects on later behavior of dogs. *Lab. Anim. Sci.* 45 (1): 70–75.

Hubrecht, R., Wickens, S., and Kirkwood, J. (1995). The welfare of dogs in human care. In: *The Domestic Dog* (ed. J. Serpell), 180–198. Cambridge, UK: Cambridge University Press.

Kiddie, J., Bodymore, A., and Dittrich, A. (2017). Environmental enrichment in kennelled pit bull terriers (*Canis lupus familiaris*). *Animals* 7 (4): 27.

Kogan, L.R., Schoenfeld-Tacher, R., and Simon, A.A. (2012). Behavioral effects of auditory stimulation on kenneled dogs. *J. Vet. Behav.* 7 (5): 268–275.

Landsberg, G.M., Beck, A., Lopez, A. et al. (2015). Dog-appeasing pheromone collars reduce sound-induced fear and anxiety in beagle dogs: A placebo-controlled study. *Vet. Rec.* 177 (10): 260.

Lawler, E.E. and Hackman, J.R. (1969). Impact of employee participation in the development of pay incentive plans: A field experiment. *J. Appl. Psychol.* 53: 467.

Leeds, J. and Wagner, S. (2008). *Through a Dog's Ear: Using Sound to Improve the Health and Behavior of Your Canine Companion*. Boulder, CO: Sounds True.

Martin, B. and Bateson, P. (2007). *Measuring Behavior: An Introductory Guide*. Cambridge, UK: Cambridge University Press.

McGowan, R.T., Bolte, C., Barnett, H.R. et al. (2018). Can you spare 15 min? The measurable positive impact of a 15-min petting session on shelter dog well-being. *Appl. Anim. Behav. Sci.* 203: 42–54.

Mellen, J. and MacPhee, M.S. (2001). Philosophy of environmental enrichment: Past, present, and future. *Zoo Biol.* 20 (3): 211–226.

Menor-Campos, D.J., Molleda-Carbonell, J.M., and López-Rodríguez, R. (2011). Effects of exercise and human contact on animal welfare in a dog shelter. *Vet Rec.* 169 (15): 388.

Mertens, P.A. and Unshelm, J. (1996). Effects of group and individual housing on the behavior of kennelled dogs in animal shelters. *Anthrozoös* 9 (1): 40–51.

Moesta, A., McCune, S., Deacon, L., and Kruger, K.A. (2015) Canine enrichment. In: *Animal Behavior for Shelter Veterinarians and Staff* (eds. E. Weiss, H. Mohan-Gibbons, and S. Zawistowski), 160–171. Oxford, UK: Wiley Blackwell.

Morey, D.F. (1994). The early evolution of the domestic dog. *Am. Sci.* 82 (4): 336–347.

Nielsen, B.L., Jezierski, T., Bolhuis, J.E. et al. (2015). Olfaction: An overlooked sensory modality in applied ethology and animal welfare. *Front. Vet. Sci.* 2: 69.

Newbury, S., Blinn, M.K., Bushby, P.A. et al. (2010). *Guidelines for Standards of Care in Animal Shelters*. Apex, NC: Association of Shelter Veterinarians.

Normando, S., Stefanini, C., Meers, L. et al. (2006). Some factors influencing adoption of sheltered dogs. *Anthrozoös* 19 (3): 211–224.

Orihel, J. S. and Fraser, D. (2008). A note on the effectiveness of behavioural rehabilitation for reducing inter-dog aggression in shelter dogs. *Appl. Anim. Behav. Sci.* 112 (3–4): 400–405.

Payne, S.W. and Assemi, K.S. (2017). An evaluation of respondent conditioning procedures to decrease barking in an animal shelter. *Pet Behav. Sci.* (3): 19–24.

Protopopova, A. and Gunter, L.M. (2017). Adoption and relinquishment interventions at the animal shelter: A review. *Anim Welf.* 26 (1): 35–48.

Protopopova, A., Hauser, H., Goldman, K.J. et al. (2018). The effects of exercise and calm interactions on in-kennel behavior of shelter dogs. *Behav. Process.* 146: 54–60.

Protopopova, A., Mehrkam, L.R., Boggess, M.M. et al. (2014). In-kennel behavior predicts length of stay in shelter dogs. *PLOS ONE* 9 (12): e114319.

Protopopova, A. and Wynne, C.D. (2015). Improving in-kennel presentation of shelter dogs through response-dependent and response-independent treat delivery. *J. Appl. Behav. Anal.* 48 (3): 590–601.

Pullen, A.J., Merrill, R.J.N., and Bradshaw, J.W.S. (2010). Preferences for toy types and presentations in kennel housed dogs. *Appl. Anim. Behav. Sci.* 125: 151–156.

Rickard, N.S., Toukhsati, S.R., and Field, S.E. (2005). The effect of music on cognitive performance: Insight from neurobiological and animal studies. *Behav. Cogn. Neurosci. Rev.* 4 (4): 235–261.

Rowan, A. and Kartal, T. (2018). Dog population & dog sheltering trends in the United States of America. *Animals* 8 (5): 68.

Sales, G., Hubrecht, R., Peyvandi, A. et al. (1997). Noise in dog kennelling: Is barking a welfare problem for dogs? *Appl. Anim. Behav. Sci.* 52 (3–4): 321–329.

Scheifele, P., Martin, D., Clark, J.G. et al. (2012). Effect of kennel noise on hearing in dogs. *Am. J. Vet Res.* 73 (4): 482–489.

Shepherdson, D.J. (1998). Tracing the path of environmental enrichment in zoos. In: *Second Nature: Environmental Enrichment for Captive Animals* (eds. D.J. Shepherdson, J.D. Mellen, M. Hutchins), 1–12. Washington, DC: Smithsonian Institution Press.

Shiverdecker, M.D., Schiml, P.A., and Hennessy, M.B. (2013). Human interaction moderates plasma cortisol and behavioral responses of dogs to shelter housing. *Physiol. Behav.* 109: 75–79.

Taylor, K.D. and Mills, D.S. (2007). The effect of the kennel environment on canine welfare: A critical review of experimental studies. *Anim. Welf.* 16 (4): 435.

Thorn, J.M., Templeton, J.J., Van Winkle, K.M. et al. (2006). Conditioning shelter dogs to sit. *J. Appl. Anim. Welf. Sci.* 9 (1): 25–39.

Tod, E., Brander, D., and Waran, N. (2005). Efficacy of dog appeasing pheromone in reducing stress and fear related behaviour in shelter dogs. *Appl. Anim. Behav. Sci.* 93 (3): 295–308.

Uccheddu, S., Mariti, C., Sannen, A. et al. (2018). Behavioural and cortisol responses of shelter dogs to a cognitive bias test after olfactory enrichment with essential oils. *Dog Behav.* 2: 1–14.

United States Department of Labor, Occupational Health and Safety Administration. (1983). Occupational noise exposure: Hearing Conservation Amendment, final rule. *Federal Register*, 48: 9738–9785.

Valsecchi, P., Pattacini, O., Beretta, V. et al. (2007). Effects of a human social enrichment program on behavior and welfare of sheltered dogs. *J. Vet Behav.* 2 (3): 88–89.

Venn, R.E. (2013). Effects of acute and chronic noise exposure on cochlear function and hearing in dogs. PhD dissertation. University of Glasgow.

Walker, J.K., Waran, N.K., and Phillips, C.J. (2014). The effect of conspecific removal on the behaviour and physiology of pair-housed shelter dogs. *Appl. Anim. Behav. Sci.* 158: 46–56.

Wells, D.L. (2004). The influence of toys on the behaviour and welfare of kennelled dogs. *Anim. Welf.* 13 (3): 367–373.

Wells, D.L., Graham, L., and Hepper, P.G. (2002). The influence of auditory stimulation on the behaviour of dogs housed in a rescue shelter. *Anim. Welf.* 11 (4): 385–393.

Wells, D.L. and Hepper, P.G. (1998). A note on the influence of visual conspecific contact on the behaviour of sheltered dogs. *Appl. Anim. Behav. Sci.* 60 (1): 83–88.

Wells, D.L. and Hepper, P.G. (2000). The influence of environmental change on the behaviour of sheltered dogs. *Appl. Anim. Behav. Sci.* 68 (2): 151–162.

Willen, R.M., Mutwill, A., MacDonald, L.J. et al. (2017). Factors determining the effects of human interaction on the cortisol levels of shelter dogs. *Appl. Anim. Behav. Sci.* 186: 41–48.

Woodruff, K.A. and Smith, D.R. (2017). An estimate of the number of dogs in US shelters. *Proceedings of the NAVC Conference Small Animals Edition*, Orlando, Florida (4–8 February 2017). Gainesville, FL: North American Veterinary Community.

Zappa, P. and Zavarrone, E. (2010). Social interaction and volunteer satisfaction: An exploratory study in primary healthcare. *Int. Rev. Econ.* 57: 215–231.

Appendix 11.A Data Sheet

Time Sampling

Put an "x" in the box if the dog was engaging with the enrichment item as you passed the kennel. Alternatively, put an S for sniffing, C for chewing, E for eating, L for licking, or N for not engaging with the enrichment item

KENNEL	MON Item:	TUES Item:	WED Item:	THURS Item:	FRI Item:	SAT Item:	SUN Item:
1							
2							
3							
4							
5							
6							
7							
8							
9							
10							
11							
12							
13							
14							
15							

12

Training and Behavior Modification for Shelter Dogs
Pamela J. Reid and Tristan Rehner-Fleurant

12.1 Introduction

The number of dogs entering shelters is declining across the United States (Hawes et al. 2019; Rowan and Kartal 2018). In the first edition of this text, Reid and Collins (2015) noted that shelter professionals were expressing concern that, with the continued success of spay-neuter and other safety net programs, shelter populations would soon consist primarily of animals presenting with medical and behavior problems that jeopardize their adoption. While the reasons animals end up in shelters are varied and complex, problematic behavior continues to figure as a top cause of relinquishment (see Chapter 6) and, anecdotally, shelter professionals across the United States describe dealing with an increasing percentage of incoming animals with behavior problems, as well as more extreme and varied behavior problems.

Furthermore, as Reid and Collins pointed out in 2015, a strengthening of state and federal laws and the resulting heightened attention on animal cruelty crimes by law enforcement agencies have led to an increase in the confiscation of animals from abusive and neglectful situations, poorly run commercial breeding facilities, hoarders, overpopulated sanctuaries, and dogfighters. As an example, since the ASPCA first partnered with the New York City Police Department in 2014, animal cruelty investigations have increased 200% over pre-partnership years, when only a small number of animal control officers were responsible for the five boroughs. The victims of animal cruelty tend to be poorly socialized to humans, fearful, and in the case of fighting dogs, aggressive to other animals. Thus, agencies sheltering confiscated animals are experiencing an increased need for behavioral intervention in these populations—to ward off decline during long-term legal holds, to improve quality of life, and to help the animals become appropriate candidates for adoption (see Chapter 21).

The growing demand for specialized behavioral interventions has figured prominently in the animal sheltering field's push toward a more holistic approach to care. A holistic approach elevates the importance of psychological well-being and emphasizes the parity of medical and behavioral health care (Washington Post n.d.). Dr. Jacklyn Ellis and Melissa Shupak of Toronto Humane Society concur, stating that "it is possible that as a greater spotlight is being shone on behaviour problems and psychological well-being more generally in animal sheltering, behaviour problems are simply being identified and taken more seriously" (personal communication).

Animal Behavior for Shelter Veterinarians and Staff, Second Edition. Edited by Brian A. DiGangi, Victoria A. Cussen, Pamela J. Reid, and Kristen A. Collins.
© 2022 John Wiley & Sons, Inc. Published 2022 by John Wiley & Sons, Inc.
Companion website: www.wiley.com/go/digangi/animal

Thus, more and more shelters are establishing programs dedicated to providing specialized training and behavior modification to their animals. In this chapter, the authors describe a variety of interventions and protocols shared by a sampling of North American organizations with well-developed behavior programs.

12.2 Structured Training Programs

Many shelters offer obedience training classes to the public. Fees generated from these classes contribute to the shelter coffers, but the primary aim is to keep owned dogs out of shelters and to prevent the return of adopted dogs by improving behavior in the home (Patronek et al. 1996; see Chapter 6). Shelters, particularly those with an average length of stay beyond 7–10 days, often extend basic obedience training to include shelter dogs prior to adoption. The goals of in-shelter training programs are to improve dogs' adoptability and psychological quality of life and to prevent behavioral decline while dogs are in the shelter.

Shelter training programs for dogs up for adoption emphasize basic manners, such as "sit," "down," "wait," "four on the floor," loose-leash walking, interacting with people without jumping on them, and sitting at the front of the kennel to greet people. An example protocol for teaching "four on the floor" appears in Box 12.1. Some shelters teach additional behaviors intended to facilitate positive

---

Box 12.1   Four on the Floor

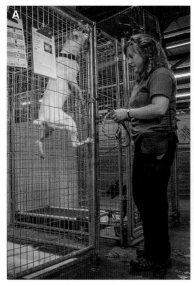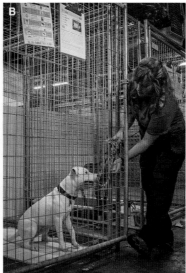

Time commitment: 10 minutes

Purpose: Teach dogs to sit or stand for leashing

Pointers:

- Reward for four on the floor intermittently throughout the day.
- For some dogs, this may have to be broken into even smaller steps. The general idea is to stop the process of removing the dog from the kennel any time the dog's feet come off the ground. When all four feet are on the ground, the process can resume.

Steps:

1) Approach the kennel door, open the latch, set up proper control of the kennel door, and ready your leashing equipment.
2) Begin shaping the behavior you would like by opening the kennel door slightly.
3) If the dog jumps up, close the door immediately and look away from the dog. Wait until she resumes four on the floor.
4) When all four feet are on the floor again, look at the dog and begin to open the kennel door again.
5) Repeat steps 2–4 until you can open the door enough to leash the dog without the dog jumping.
   - Once the door is open reasonably wide with the dog maintaining four feet on the floor, give a treat at nose level to encourage the dog to keep all four feet on the floor while you slip the leash on.
6) Once leashed, some dogs may be able to exit the kennel without jumping. If this is the case, allow the dog to exit the kennel.
7) If the dog jumps once leashed, close the door immediately and look away from the dog. Wait until she resumes four on the floor.
8) Repeat this until you can open the door wide enough for the dog (already on leash) to walk through while maintaining four on the floor.
   - It may be more effective for some dogs only to expect four on the floor for the leashing and then immediately open the door for them to exit so the contingency is very clear (rather than shutting the door on them if they jump again once the leash is applied).
   - To prevent frustration in select dogs, it may also be beneficial (initially) to maintain a high rate of reinforcement with treats at nose level, starting with leash application and continuing until the dog has exited the kennel.
9) Once the dog readily offers four on the floor in this context, begin working backward, requiring four on the floor for touching the kennel latch (after the latch has been opened), then four on the floor for kennel latch opening, then for carabiner removal on the latch, then for the handler's approach to kennel.
10) You can also build in rewards for sitting or backing up behavior if the dog readily offers one of these as opposed to four feet on the floor at the kennel door.

Source: Based on ASPCA Anti-Cruelty Behavior Team's Four on the Floor Protocol developed for cruelty case dogs held in a temporary shelter.

interactions with potential adopters, such as name recognition, eye contact, hand targeting, and trick training (e.g., "shake"). Some shelters that house dogs for longer periods also include more complex behaviors like "stay," walking past other dogs without reacting, waiting to eat food or pass through doorways until released with a cue, settling into a crate or onto a bed or mat, "drop it," "leave it," and sitting automatically in front of doors/gates or when people approach. Ideally, training occurs while dogs remain available for adoption so that they don't miss out on opportunities to be seen by potential adopters. However, shelters such as Kanawha-Charleston Humane Association, have found it beneficial to send their more rambunctious dogs to a 10-week prison program for intensive one-on-one training. The return rate for adopted dogs who completed the prison program is only 4%, compared to 16% for the rest of their dog population (J. Hypes, personal communication).

Increasingly, shelters employ dedicated behavior staff who focus exclusively on training, behavior modification, and coaching sheltering staff and volunteers to promote good psychological quality of life for dogs. However, many shelters, particularly municipal agencies, lack the budget to hire specialized behavior staff and rely instead on volunteers to conduct training, often within the context of walking and socialization sessions. A popular model is to offer a tiered volunteer program (Bright and Hadden 2017). Lower-level volunteers focus on socialization and teaching simple tasks, such as sitting and lying down on cue. In contrast, higher-level volunteers employ their advanced skills to take on sophisticated training projects, including agility, nosework and cooperative care training for low-stress handling and husbandry, or to work with more behaviorally challenged dogs (see Box 12.2 for an example of teaching body targeting). Shelters can also establish mutually

---

Box 12.2   Body Targeting for Low-Stress Handling

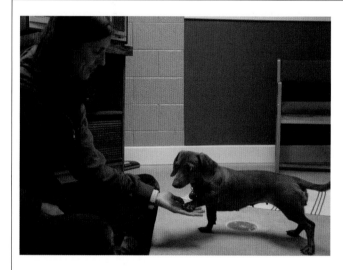

Time commitment: 15 minutes

Purpose: Teach basic body targeting for low-stress handling

Pointers:

- Teaching body targeting facilitates low-stress handling because little to no restraint is needed and the dog can withdraw and take a break at any time. It is important to pay attention when the dog withdraws and not try to grab the dog or hold her there.
- If the dog appears stressed but is not taking a break on her own, incorporate breaks into your session.
- It can be helpful to practice this with a second person present, who can slowly begin to touch the dog as if completing an exam or applying medication. Break this down into similar criteria as listed in the protocol below. This helps generalize to a vet or vet tech being the one to do most of the handling, while you maintain the target/stationing, deliver the reinforcement, and insert breaks as needed.
- Don't forget to teach the targeting from both sides of the dog (right and left).

Paw target:

1) Begin by cueing the dog to sit. Mark and reward.
2) Place a treat in your hand and close your hand into a fist.
3) Show the dog your fist—let her smell it.
4) Once she smells the food, hold your fist a few inches in front of the sitting dog.
5) Wait until the dog paws at your hand. Mark and reward by opening your hand and let the dog have the treat.
6) If the dog does not paw at your hand after a few tries, you may have to break it down into smaller steps and shape lifting the paw and, ultimately, the pawing at your hand.
7) Repeat steps 2–6 until the dog is consistently and purposefully pawing at your hand when you present it. Occasionally reward with a treat from your other hand instead of giving the dog the treat hidden in your fist.
8) Discontinue putting a treat in your fist. When the dog paws your hand, mark and consistently reward with a treat delivered from your free hand.
9) Next try presenting an open hand, marking and rewarding each time the dog touches your palm with her paw.
10) Repeat until the dog is consistently and purposefully performing the behavior.
11) Add duration starting with 1 second, then mark and reward. Then 2 seconds, mark and reward. Increase duration up to 10 seconds.
12) Gradually introduce paw handling once the dog has learned to hold her paw on your hand:
    a) Touch the dog's paw with your thumb (incorporate adding duration after each new criterion).
    b) Close your hand around the dog's paw lightly.
    c) Touch the paw with your other hand.
    d) Lightly feel between the dog's toes.
    e) Manipulate the paw as if washing or applying a skin medication.
13) Add in the cue *"paw"* just before you present your hand, so the dog learns to give you his paw when you ask.

Source: Based on ASPCA Behavioral Sciences Team's Body Targeting Protocol developed for cruelty case dogs held in a temporary shelter.

beneficial relationships with local dog trainers, who donate their time to help shelter dogs and, at the same time, acquire experience training a variety of dogs. Shelters can maximize the benefits to dogs by having behavior specialists and trainers provide direct coaching to their volunteers, as Howard and DiGennaro Reed (2014) showed that in-person coaching by a trainer is superior to written or video instructions for effectively teaching volunteers how to train basic manners.

Since the first edition of this textbook, the trend toward using reward-based techniques for training new skills and discouraging unwanted behaviors has continued. The popularity of such methods is in line with repeated findings that dogs are less stressed by, and, in some cases, more responsive to training procedures that use appetitive over aversive incentives. (For a review of studies comparing training methods, see Guilherme Fernandes et al. 2017; Ziv 2017.) Reward-based training is also thought to foster more positive relationships between dogs and people (Deldalle and Gaunet 2014; Rooney and Cowan 2011), although Vieira de Castro et al. (2019) found no significant difference in dogs' attachment to their owners as a function of training method in the Ainsworth Strange Situation Test. While an in-depth discussion of the appropriateness of exclusive reliance on reward-based methods is beyond the scope of this chapter, the authors feel strongly that shelter dogs deserve access to effective and efficient interventions that are intended to improve overall quality of life. Adhering to this philosophy may sometimes mean the judicious, careful use of aversives.

Food is the most common form of reward used in shelters—with good reason, as Feuerbacher and Wynne (2012) demonstrated that social interaction (praise and petting) was an ineffective reinforcer for shelter dogs. Conditioned rewards (a "marker," such as a clicker or a specific word paired with food) are used by some. Thorn et al. (2006) observed quicker responsiveness and better retention with the use of a verbal marker over the clicker when teaching shelter dogs to sit. However, Dorey et al. (2020) found that preceding rewards with either a clicker or praise did not enhance learning of a simple behavior (wave) in shelter puppies and may, in fact, have impaired subsequent acquisition of the "stay" behavior.

Whether shelter dog training programs have the desired effect of staving off behavioral deterioration is still an open question. Numerous studies have confirmed that, at least in the short term, shelters are stressful environments for dogs (Coppola et al. 2006; Hennessy et al. 2001; Hiby et al. 2006; Passantino et al. 2014). However, some dogs do seem to adapt to the shelter within a few days to weeks, thus evidence of decline while in the shelter for lengthy periods of time is mixed. (For reviews, see Protopopova 2016 and Chapter 21.) Nevertheless, regular human contact in the form of socialization, play, and obedience training is clearly beneficial for many shelter dogs (Conley et al. 2014; Coppola et al. 2006; Hennessy et al. 2002; Menor-Campos et al. 2011; Tuber et al. 1996). To improve quality of life in the shelter and facilitate adjustment to a new home, Tuber et al. (1999) recommend daily human contact in a "real-life room," combined with teaching dogs to relax quietly in crates and to sit when people approach their kennels (Figure 12.1).

Studies focused on how the behavior of shelter dogs influences adopters continue to produce conflicting findings. Some have found that, for shelter dog adopters, physical appearance trumps behavior (Luescher and Medlock 2009; Protopopova et al. 2012;

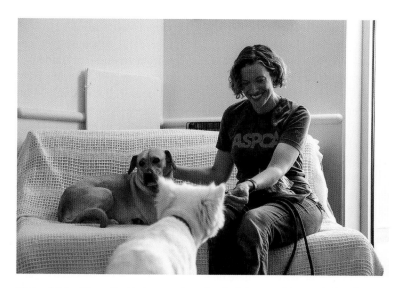

Figure 12.1 These timid dogs are learning to interact with people in a home-like real-life room.

Protopopova and Wynne 2016; Protopopova and Gunter 2017). However, Wells and Hepper (1992) report that when choosing a dog to adopt, people say they would place more emphasis on the dog's behavior than on its appearance. The respondents said they would prefer dogs that come to the front of the kennel, sit, interact, and refrain from barking (Wells and Hepper 1992). In a study with just three shelter dogs, undergraduate students viewed video footage and rated the dogs as more adoptable after the dogs completed a training program in which unruly behavior in the kennel and pulling on-leash were replaced with a sit response (Winslow et al. 2018). Weiss et al. (2012) discovered that some adopters were even attracted to dogs that jumped up on them. Although it seems logical to assume that teaching basic manners to shelter dogs will make them more appealing to adopters, some "impolite" behaviors that can be interpreted as affectionate gestures may actually be desirable in a shelter dog. It might be advantageous for staff to avoid discouraging any inherently social behavior.

Some studies, however, have demonstrated that training programs, in conjunction with other interventions, improve dogs' chances of adoption. Braun (2011) reported that the number of dogs remaining long-term in one Viennese shelter was reduced by half after the shelter instituted a dog-walking program. The volunteers who walked the dogs were coached by a professional trainer, which suggests that the dogs probably received training during their walks. Certainly, the rise in adoptions could also have been due to increased exposure to potential adopters or changes in behavior resulting from the social interactions, sensory enrichment, and physical exercise experienced by the dogs during walks. Similarly, in Italy, implementing a program that included training and socialization, a public campaign to promote shelter dogs, and pre- and post-adoption counseling resulted in 27.5% more adopted dogs than a comparable shelter that did not implement the program (Menchetti et al. 2015).

After determining that the behaviors of lying next to potential adopters and playing with them during out-of-kennel interactions were more likely to lead to decisions to adopt (Protopopova and Wynne 2014), Protopopova et al. (2016) employed a structured meet-and-greet process. First, potential adopters were taken to a small outdoor area and encouraged to invite the dog to play using the dog's favorite toy. Then, the experimenter rewarded the dog for lying near or at least staying in proximity to the adopter. Control dogs met potential adopters in a large outdoor enclosure containing various toys while the experimenter stood passively by the gate. Dogs in the structured meet-and-greet group were 2.5 times more likely to be adopted than control dogs. Unfortunately, after training staff in nine US shelters on the structured meet-and-greet program, Protopopova et al. (2020) discovered significant deviations in protocol implementation several months post-training, and there was no demonstrable increase in adoptions compared to the period before protocol introduction.

Other studies have also failed to find higher adoption rates or shorter lengths of stay as a result of training shelter dogs. Reasoning that social, friendly dogs would appeal to adopters, researchers at a Florida shelter looked at the effect of teaching dogs to make eye contact with people (Protopopova et al. 2012). Dogs received 15-minute daily sessions over the course of six days from 10 different trainers to encourage generalization. Although researchers confirmed that dogs in the training group learned the eye contact response, they were no more likely to be adopted than control dogs. There was also no effect on their length of stay in the shelter.

Dogs at an Ohio shelter were taught a set of desirable behaviors, such as sitting, making eye contact, and coming to the front of the kennel, while undesirable behaviors, such as jumping up and barking, were discouraged. Confirming that the training was successful, these dogs were more likely to sit and lie down and less likely to jump up or bark than control dogs. However, like the previous study, this study failed to demonstrate any impact of training on adoption rates (Herron et al. 2014).

Perry et al. (2020) compared adoption rates between dogs that received walks plus 15–20 minutes/day of manners training (sit, down, loose-leash walking) and dogs that received one of three types of daily enrichment (walks, walks plus a food-filled KONG® [KONG Company, Golden, CO] toy or walks plus a petting and massage session). They found no difference in the percent of dogs adopted or the length of stay across the groups. However, this result is likely due to the fact that almost all (98%) of the dogs participating in the study were adopted, 80% within the first day they were available.

Many shelters provide basic training to all of their dogs but target specific subgroups for more intensive training. Dogs with minor or moderate behavior concerns, such as those prone to jumping up, becoming highly aroused, or mouthing people, are the ones most likely to be assigned to training programs. Some shelters choose instead to focus on dogs that are challenging to place for reasons unrelated to behavior, such as pit bull type dogs (Cain et al. 2020). Patronek and Glickman (1994) proposed that increasing public demand for dogs more than one year of age would have the most significant impact on adoption rates. A public relations example is the Animal Protective Association of Missouri's Grown-Ass Adult campaign to showcase adult and senior pets (Animal Rescue Site by Greater Good n.d.). If Patronek and Glickman (1994) are correct, shelters with training programs might be wise to focus on older adolescents and adults.

Studies that examine the impact of training programs on adoption rates for specific subgroups may yield more compelling results to support the role of training to enhance adoptability. Conversely, rather than look at adoption rate or length of stay, it might be most informative to evaluate the effect of training programs on return rates. Few of the shelters we surveyed explicitly compare return rates for dogs that received intensive training before adoption with those that did not (P. Reid, ASPCA, New York, unpublished data). Dogs that are more challenging to place may also be at greater risk of re-relinquishment after adoption, but few researchers have looked at the relationship between basic manners training and the likelihood of returns (Wells and Hepper 2000).

12.3 Behavior Modification Programs within the General Shelter Environment

Shelter dog populations can present with the full gamut of behavior problems. Information about a dog's behavioral tendencies should be obtained from the owner at intake, if available, and by everyone interacting with the dog during the dog's stay in the shelter (Chapter 9). Shelter professionals report aggression to people as the most serious behavior problem when it comes to limitations for adoption (D'Arpino et al. 2012). In an informal email survey of shelters with behavior programs, few shelters reported working with dogs that are offensively aggressive to people (P. Reid, ASPCA, New York, unpublished data). One notable exception is mild to moderate food guarding, which, while often highly responsive to treatment, seems to not be a significant concern for adopters (Marder et al. 2013; Mohan-Gibbons et al. 2012). In addition, food guarding in the shelter does not appear to be predictive of food and/or chew bone guarding in the adoptive home (Marder et al. 2013; McGuire et al. 2020). Finally, choosing not to assess for food guarding in the shelter does not pose an increased safety risk to staff or volunteers (Mohan-Gibbons et al. 2018). For these reasons, few shelters bother to modify food guarding but instead make food-guarders available with full disclosure to potential adopters.

David and Woytalewicz (2017) described a rehabilitation program for shelter dogs with a bite history to either humans or dogs. The program's treatment plans were intensive and lengthy. The behavior modification protocols, which had to be executed by highly experienced behavior staff, involved desensitization and counter-conditioning (DSCC) to triggering stimuli, teaching safety and warning cues, and training alternative behaviors and bite inhibition. Of the three case studies they presented (from nearly 300 dogs that went through the program), the shortest length of stay was one year and the longest was three years. Overall, they claimed an 87% success rate, as defined by adoption with no subsequent report of biting. For the three case studies, the shortest follow-up was six months and the longest was two years (David and Woytalewicz 2017). In addition to the potential ethical and liability concerns with treating and placing dogs like these, most organizations simply can't devote their limited resources to treating serious human-directed aggression, which might take years to resolve.

In terms of safety risk, resource requirements, and prognosis for improvement, it is the authors' opinion that problems such as intraspecific aggression, excessive arousal, and fear are more feasible to treat in the shelter environment.

12.3.1 Intraspecific Aggression

Dogs that show aggression toward other dogs pose a significant challenge. They can be difficult to manage in the shelter environment and they require special placement considerations to ensure that adopters are willing and able to accept the responsibility of owning a dog-aggressive dog. According to a survey conducted by the Center for Shelter Dogs, aggression toward other dogs ranks in the top three reasons why private shelters refuse admittance to dogs (D'Arpino et al. 2012). Respondents to a survey of 43 Canadian animal shelters indicated that 20–49% of dogs entering their shelters exhibited intraspecific aggression (Orihel et al. 2015).

Many shelters do not attempt to modify aggression toward other dogs, but those that do often rely on obedience training techniques that will allow adopters to manage the behavior. Dogs are taught to walk calmly on-leash and/or to maintain eye contact with a handler while in the presence of other dogs. Some shelters go one step further by using DSCC to condition dogs to relax and anticipate good things when other dogs are near. Variants on this approach, such as Behavior Adjustment Treatment (Stewart 2016) and Play Way (Cook 2017), merge gradual exposure to stimulus dogs with some combination of extinction and reinforcement contingencies. In addition to rewards, such as the opportunity to explore the environment or to engage in play with people, the aggressive dog may also receive negative reinforcement in the form of moving away from the (presumably aversive) stimulus dog for brief periods when they perform the desired, non-reactive response.

Orihel and Fraser (2008) remain the only researchers to have published empirical data on the effectiveness of a DSCC program for intraspecific aggression in shelter dogs. They identified 16 dogs who exhibited aggression to other dogs in a standardized behavior evaluation. Nine treatment dogs received daily 30-minute sessions in an outdoor area. During each session, the dogs were repeatedly approached by stimulus dogs and rewarded for sitting or making eye contact with their handler. Aggressive behaviors were interrupted using a leash and a head halter (Halti Headcollar, Company of Animals, Broomfield, CO) to direct the dog's head and body away from the stimulus dog. Seven control dogs spent 30 minutes each day in the same outdoor area; they were simply released into the area with toys and a person present but received little or no interaction from the person. After 10 days, all dogs were reassessed by an observer who was not blind to whether the dog had been in the treatment or control condition. However, a naïve observer also rated a random selection of video footage from both before and after treatment as a means of detecting potential bias, and none was reported. Seven of the nine treatment dogs were rated as less aggressive on retest, whereas five of the seven control dogs were significantly more aggressive. Twelve dogs that were still in the shelter 1 week later were retested again and, unfortunately, there was no sustained reduction in aggression once treatment was ceased. While this report suggests that the severity of dog-directed aggression can be reduced or at least not worsened with behavior modification, continued treatment is necessary to maintain any improvement in behavior. Regrettably, 30-minute daily sessions that require two handlers are infeasible for many shelters, and there is no guarantee that adopters will continue the treatment.

Some shelters address dog-directed aggression problems by implementing a playgroup program, such as Dogs Playing for Life™. Providing shelter dogs with repeated socialization opportunities is thought to teach them to relax, interact, and sometimes even play with other dogs, while also reducing the incidence of stress-related behaviors while they are in their kennels (Belpedio et al. 2010). Dogs that are potentially aggressive to other dogs often need a gradual introduction to playgroups. They are first exposed to carefully selected dogs that are especially tolerant and resilient. They may require correction for inappropriately pushy or threatening behaviors, and they may need to be muzzled, at least initially, to ensure safety. The goal is for socializing with dogs to become so reinforcing that the dog is no longer motivated to behave aggressively (Dogs Playing for Life n.d.). To date, there is no systematic analysis of the efficacy of the playgroup experience for resolving intraspecific aggression. See Chapter 13 for a detailed discussion of playgroups for shelter dogs.

12.3.2 Excessive Arousal

Increasingly, shelter behavior professionals report that excessive or high arousal is a significant behavior concern leading to increased length of stay and reduced likelihood of adoption. The term "excessive arousal" is often used interchangeably with "impulsivity," "hyperactivity," "hyperarousal," or "reactivity" and is generally characterized by a dog's increased responsiveness to stimuli in the environment, exaggerated emotionality and reduced behavioral inhibition (Sforzini et al. 2009; Wright et al. 2011). Behaviorally, these terms are applied to a suite of potentially problematic behavior, including repetitive behavior in the kennel (pacing, circling, spinning, bouncing, barking) and unruly, rambunctious behavior when exiting or outside of the kennel (jumping up on people; mouthing or play-biting people; grabbing and/or tugging on the leash, people's clothes or objects; pulling on the leash; crashing into or leaping onto things; snatching treats and toys). Certain dogs are also inclined to redirect aggression toward nearby people or animals when in a high state of arousal. In addition to these behaviors being undesirable to potential adopters and potentially unsafe for shelter staff, they can have a deleterious effect on other animals' shelter experience. Barking, in particular, is highly "contagious" and, therefore, disruptive to the entire shelter population (Coppola et al. 2006). Behaviors consistent with excessive arousal are believed to be indicative of poor well-being (Coppola et al. 2006; Cussen and Reid 2020).

Over their first five days in Australian shelters, a sample of 38 owner-surrendered dogs were observed to engage in high arousal behaviors, encompassing 15% of the total time the dogs were monitored (Clay et al. 2019). However, it is unclear the extent to which excessive arousal in shelter dogs is an artifact of the environment. Admittedly, shelters are considered inherently stimulating. However, some dogs more than others seem to become physiologically and behaviorally aroused by the shelter environment, and we don't know if these same dogs exhibit problematic behavior outside of the shelter. Engaging in highly active, repetitive behavior in their kennels may simply be a tactic that some dogs adopt for coping with confinement and stimulation (Denham et al. 2014).

We do know that high arousal behaviors are not observed solely in shelters. Hyperactivity and arousal are reported reasons for owners surrendering dogs (Clay et al. 2019). Some dogs are described as highly impulsive by their owners—for instance, they are reported to "act without thinking," are prone to overreacting, and persist with a behavior even in the face of punishment (Shabelansky and Dowling-Guyer 2016; Wright et al. 2011). Small dogs, such as terriers, and young dogs tended to be described as impulsive more often than toy breeds and mature dogs. In another study of owned dogs, adolescents, especially, were found to be more active, intolerant of frustration, and prone to impulsive behavior (McPeake et al. 2019). Even though age appears to be a risk factor (Brady et al. 2018), Riemer et al. (2014) reported evidence to suggest that impulsivity may be a stable trait in dogs, persisting over the six years their dogs were studied.

The good news is that shelter dogs were no more likely to be rated as impulsive by their owners than dogs acquired from breeders (Wright et al. 2011). However, this study did not control for the possibility that dogs exhibiting high arousal in the shelter were never adopted. And, given the reported increase in problematic behavior in shelter dog populations, this finding may not be representative of current shelter dog populations.

Few published studies have focused exclusively on preventing or reducing high arousal behavior in the shelter. Amaya and her colleagues (Amaya et al. 2020a, 2020b) compared the effect of three types of enrichment (lavender, dog-appeasing pheromone, and music) on arousal behaviors in kenneled shelter dogs and found that slow tempo piano or violin music resulted in less barking, more resting, and increased heart rate variability, implying reduced arousal and stress.

The two types of enrichment activities often recommended for reducing high arousal behavior in kennels can seem paradoxical because on the one hand, dogs are encouraged to engage in energetic behaviors and, on the other, they are encouraged to behave calmly. One line of reasoning is that if exercise provides a physical outlet for energy, daily exercise outings should result in dogs that are calmer in their kennels afterward because they are fatigued. Alternatively, providing calm, quiet interaction with people is also thought to encourage relaxed behavior in kenneled dogs. Protopopova et al. (2018) compared the impact of these two activities on in-kennel behavior before and after daily enrichment sessions. Some dogs were exercised by playing retrieve games or running on leash for 15 minutes each day. (Bear in mind that 15 minutes of exercise is unlikely to fatigue most dogs.) Other dogs were taken to a quiet room to spend 15 mins with a person who did not engage with the dog but simply read aloud from a book. Regardless of the type of intervention, dogs engaged in what adopters report as desirable behavior (less moving back and forth and more facing forward; Wells and Hepper 1992) when the experimenter stood in front of their kennels prior to the sessions. After the sessions, however, behaviors in the kennels that Protopopova et al. (2014) found to be correlated with longer lengths of stay and lower adoption rates increased. Dogs that had been exercised were more active, spending more time moving back and forth, in the presence of the experimenter in front of their kennel. Dogs that had been read to exhibited a mix of desirable and undesirable behaviors that suggested they found the experimenter less interesting. They were less likely to face the experimenter or spend time at the front of the kennel, and they were less likely to jump on the front of the kennel and bark at the experimenter. The researchers propose that these enrichment interventions might be most beneficial at the end of the day so potential adopters see the more social pre-session behavior rather than the more active or asocial post-session behavior.

Luescher and Medlock (2009) did not target high arousal behavior per se but instead taught randomly selected shelter dogs to approach the front of their kennel and sit when people approached. These dogs were 1.4 times more likely to be adopted than untrained dogs, although there was no effect on length of stay. Protopopova and Wynne (2015) compared the effectiveness of two different procedures intended to reduce undesirable in-kennel behavior. One, a response-independent procedure commonly known as "drive-by treats," paired the presence of a person in front of the dog's kennel with food. The other was a response-dependent procedure in which the person waited for the dog to refrain from exhibiting undesirable behavior (leaning against or jumping up on the walls, facing backward or staying in the back of the kennel, barking, etc.) before giving a treat. They found that both procedures were equally effective at reducing undesirable kennel behavior (Protopopova and Wynne 2015). In a subsequent study, though, they discovered that adopters were just as likely to choose control dogs that had not been exposed to the response-independent drive-by treats

procedure (Protopopova and Wynne 2016). In an effort to encourage calm, quiet behavior in their dogs, some shelters have incorporated an automated treat delivery device, called Pet Tutor™ (Smart Animal Training Systems, Indianapolis, IN), but as yet no efficacy data have been published (Figure 12.2).

Treatment interventions for out-of-kennel arousal behavior typically include a combination of enhanced environmental enrichment, including physical activity, such as shelter dog running programs (Lausch 2014) and treadmill running, along with impulse control/frustration tolerance exercises, such as tug-and-release, delayed-reward training, and reinforcement for calm behavior (i.e., Click to Calm, Parsons 2012). Applied research on effective treatment and management interventions for excessive arousal in the shelter is a ripe area for future work.

12.3.3 Fearfulness

It is the authors' experience that the most insidious behavior concern among shelter dogs is fear because, even though fear can result in severe suffering, it may be overlooked by shelter staff. Fearful dogs are often behaviorally inhibited or

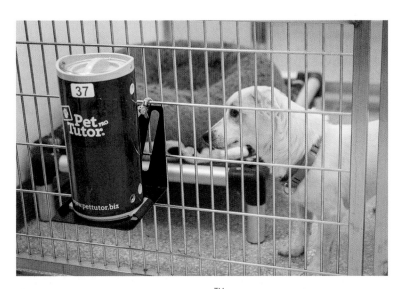

Figure 12.2 A dog waits for the Pet Tutor™ to deliver food. *Source:* Reproduced with permission of San Diego Humane Society.

even completely shut down in the shelter, which means that they can be relatively easy to care for and may not garner as much attention. The term "fear" encompasses many manifestations of social and non-social fear and anxiety, including fear of being handled or restrained, fear of people, fear of other dogs, fear of being alone (isolation distress or separation anxiety), fear of certain environments, activities, or objects, fear of loud noises, and fear of anything unfamiliar (neophobia). Fearful responses include trembling, panting, freezing, withdrawing, hiding, attempting to escape, and defensive aggression (Gähwiler et al. 2020; Voith and Borchelt 1996b). Chronic fearfulness can have devastating effects on a dog's quality of life, health, and even lifespan (Cussen and Reid 2020; Dreschel 2010; McMillan 2013).

Shelter interventions for fearfulness consist of various behavior modification procedures, including DSCC, operant conditioning, and occasionally flooding. DSCC works to change a dog's response to a frightening stimulus by repeatedly presenting the stimulus at such a low level that fear is kept to a minimum, thereby setting the dog up to tolerate the exposure, and by pairing the stimulus with something the dog likes, such as food, play, or enjoyable touch. The fearful responses that were originally elicited are "countered" as the dog comes to anticipate the new, pleasurable outcome. The goal of operant conditioning is to train the dog to perform specific behaviors when in the presence of a feared stimulus or while enduring a feared experience. Flooding involves prolonged exposure to a feared stimulus or experience until the dog eventually habituates to it (in learning theory lingo, until the dog's fear extinguishes). Concrete examples of interventions for specific fears are provided in various applied animal behavior texts (Landsberg et al. 2012; Lindsay 2005; Voith and Borchelt 1996a).

Simple forms of behavior modification that may benefit fearful dogs can be administered across the board to all dogs in a shelter. Conley et al. (2014) introduced an additional two minutes of human socialization to the daily husbandry routine of cleaning and feeding for a group of small breed shelter dogs. The person engaged in quiet interaction with the dog in their kennel; some dogs were also encouraged to play with a toy. These dogs were subsequently more likely to approach familiar and unfamiliar people standing outside of their kennel than control dogs who didn't receive the socialization sessions.

Most of the shelters informally surveyed by the authors treat dogs with fearfulness, and those with more robust behavior programs even dedicate a quieter section of their housing— usually five to seven runs—for these dogs (P. Reid, ASPCA, New York, unpublished data). A group of researchers in Turkey (Demirbas et al. 2017) moved eight adult dogs, formerly free ranging in an urban environment before being captured and placed in the shelter, into a separate area for focused behavioral treatment. Four of the dogs exhibited fearful or defensively aggressive behaviors toward people at the beginning of treatment, while the other four were either friendly or neutral. The standardized treatment plan consisted of one week to habituate and then six weeks of daily social interactions, basic obedience training and acclimatization to a home-like environment. One extremely fearful dog required additional DSCC to people before the standardized protocols. At the end of the program, one of the defensively aggressive dogs still reacted aggressively toward unfamiliar people. The extremely fearful dog was still unwilling to approach familiar or unfamiliar people. None of the four fearful dogs was comfortable in the home-like environment, which is not surprising given that these were urban street dogs. However, all the dogs were judged to have improved behavior and welfare in the shelter over the course of treatment.

The ASPCA Cruelty Recovery Center devotes a separate area to dogs on legal hold that need treatment for moderate to extreme fearfulness (Zverina and Cussen 2020). Despite it being a makeshift emergency shelter (see Chapter 21), this area has specially designed kennels, treatment spaces, and play yards that minimize the need for leashing and handling. Human activity in the area is limited, and handling of the dogs is restricted to designated handlers who specialize in low-stress interactions. Social and environmental enrichment is provided daily. Behavior modification sessions involving standardized treatment protocols developed at the ASPCA Behavioral Rehabilitation Center (BRC) are conducted by skilled behavior staff. Under the guidance of a veterinary behaviorist and staff veterinarians, the dogs are also on a consistent regimen of fluoxetine and gabapentin. During the period 2017–2019, 66 fearful dogs were enrolled in the program; no more than 10–12 dogs at a time. The dogs were seized as evidence in animal cruelty cases, including institutional hoarding (sanctuary) (n = 19), backyard breeder (n = 15), dogfighting (n = 13), individual hoarding (n = 11), and puppy mills (n = 8). Twenty-four dogs (36%) improved to the extent that they met adoptability guidelines and, once their legal hold was up, were adopted into homes. Another 29 dogs (44%) showed improvement but still needed intensive treatment at the BRC before being successfully adopted. Dogs that were likely to benefit the most from treatment at the emergency shelter were classified as moderately fearful; the extremely fearful dogs needed transfer to the BRC for intensive treatment at a facility dedicated to the rehabilitation of fearful dogs.

Increasing numbers of shelters are using psychotropic medications to treat dogs suffering from moderate to extreme fear. Indeed, all the shelters the authors interviewed incorporate psychopharmaceuticals into their behavior treatment plans in anywhere from 10–90% of their cases (P. Reid, ASPCA, New York, unpublished data). However, the value of this type of intervention remains unclear. Monitoring the effectiveness of drug therapy can be more challenging in the shelter environment than in a home because subtle changes in behavior are harder to detect and undesirable side effects may go unnoticed (Marder 2013). Drug therapy should always be used in conjunction with other strategies, such as behavior modification and environmental modifications (e.g., the use of visual barriers, the provision of a hiding spot or relocation to a quieter kennel area). But that means that with these other variables in play and a reliance on non-blinded reports from staff, assessing the efficacy of a specific medication can prove impossible. Furthermore, depending on the choice of drug, dogs may not be held in the shelter long enough to experience the full benefits (Marder 2013). Finally, some shelters will not put dogs up for adoption until they have undergone a proper weaning procedure—a policy that increases length of stay for medicated dogs but, in many cases, may be warranted in order to predict quality of life post-adoption. For an in-depth discussion of the use of behavioral pharmacology in shelter animals, see Chapter 22.

12.4 Success of Behavior Modification in Shelters

Little research exists on the effectiveness of behavior modification for shelter animals. Few shelters have the staff resources to collect and publish objective data on behavior change. Likewise, following up with adopters to determine if behavioral improvements stick is not a simple task. Follow-up calls or home visits are time intensive. If adopters are reached, owner reports are not considered highly reliable because the layperson's interpretation of a question about behavior often does not match the interviewer's intent. However, the use of a validated questionnaire, such as the Canine Behavioral Assessment and Research Questionnaire (C-BARQ), should alleviate this worry (Hsu and Serpell 2003).

Fortunately, shelters with longstanding rehabilitation programs suggest that the majority of owners don't ask for support and report being satisfied with their adopted pets (Center for Shelter Dogs 2021). Some owners relate never experiencing the original problem behavior at all post-adoption, while others report dealing with the concern during the first weeks after adoption but rarely after the 3-month mark (A. Marder, personal communication). Follow-up conducted by the ASPCA also confirms that few owners regret the decision to adopt behaviorally rehabilitated dogs (P. Reid, ASPCA, New York, unpublished data). This dedication may reflect shelter staff's early identification of potential adopters truly committed to taking on a pet with problems. We know that many owners do not consider behavior problems, even serious concerns such as aggression, justification for relinquishing or returning a pet (Marder et al. 2013; Zawistowski and Reid 2017). The concern still exists, however, that some adopters, even though they are committed to keeping these dogs, continue to experience the behavior problem to such a degree that their lives are negatively impacted.

Most shelters do not separate out return rates for dogs who had received behavior modification from the regular adoption population. The few that do, however, report mixed results. Some acknowledge that their return rate is higher, while others report fewer returns of their treated animals. Dr. Alicia Buttner, Director of Animal Behavior for the Nebraska Humane Society, says, "One might expect that dogs needing behavior modification would be more likely to be returned, but we don't see that in our shelter. In fact, we see the same or slightly lower return rates compared to dogs in our general adoption program, depending on the time frame. We screen adopters to ensure the dog is a good fit for their home, then provide specialized behavior counseling at the time of adoption and provide post-adoption support. We are transparent with the dog's behavioral issues and needs, and we do whatever we can to support them once the dog is in their home" (personal communication). Rhea Moriarity, Training and Behavior Department Manager for Longmont Humane Society, reports that for 2019, 1% of dogs that had received behavior modification were returned, as compared with a general return rate of 16% (personal communication). Could it be that adopters of rehabilitated dogs are more tolerant of problems? Or perhaps the additional screening and extra attention paid to special adoptions result in a reluctance for owners to report to the original shelter when they have given up on an animal? It is possible that behaviorally challenged dogs are relinquished to a different shelter, rehomed, or euthanized at a rate comparable with general shelter dogs. Of course, the hope is that behavior modification of behaviorally challenged dogs is successful in significantly reducing or eliminating behavior that, before treatment, prevented adoption. At this point in time, we simply do not know.

12.5 Dedicated Behavior Rehabilitation Facilities

While still rare, a handful of shelter and rescue organizations in the United States have dedicated behavior staff and special facilities for housing and rehabilitating dogs with severe behavior problems. After a successful pilot study, the ASPCA's BRC in Weaverville, North Carolina, opened its doors in 2018. The authors believe this to be the first shelter facility specifically designed and dedicated solely to the treatment of undersocialized, fearful dogs. The dogs originate primarily from cruelty and neglect cases nationwide. Criteria for acceptance into the program are as follows: the dogs' fearful behavior is severe enough to restrict placement options and/or to impair their ability to function as a companion animal; they are physically healthy; they do not have additional behavior problems such as resource guarding, separation-related anxiety or offensive aggression toward people or dogs. Manifestations of fear that dogs display on intake range from moderate responses such as avoidance, immobility, and mild defensive aggression to extreme responses such as anal gland expression, escape behavior, and catatonia.

Specially trained staff conduct targeted behavior modification sessions. Each dog receives one 15-minute treatment session per day, five days a week starting two weeks after their arrival. Interestingly, the project's pilot study revealed that delaying treatment by two weeks resulted in dogs needing fewer treatment sessions to complete the program than dogs who started treatment immediately (although incorporating the delay resulted in the same length of stay for these dogs) (K. Collins, ASPCA, New York, unpublished data). Treatment protocols focus on four categories: fear of people, fear of handling, fear of leashing and leash walking, and fear of novelty. Sessions take place in the dogs' kennels, in rooms designed to resemble normal household environments ("real-life rooms"), in outdoor and indoor play yards, on walking paths, and

in other outdoor areas. As dogs progress, they are taken offsite to experience typical suburban surroundings and interactions.

Dogs learn to make positive associations with people through a variety of procedures performed in multiple contexts. Initially, behavior modification sessions are conducted by a limited number of behavior specialists who become familiar to the dogs. Access to motivators such as food and interactions with other dogs is restricted to behavior treatments so those things can be paired predictably with people. Confident, social "helper" dogs are involved in behavior modification sessions, especially early in the program, to provide social support to the dog in treatment and facilitate affiliative behavior toward people. Box 12.3 contains a protocol on implementing a helper dog playgroup. For an in-depth

---

Box 12.3   Helper-Dog Playgroups

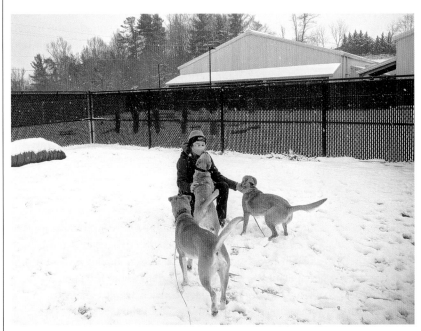

Source: Courtesy of Tim Molina.

Time commitment: 15–30 minutes

Purpose: To help dog-friendly fearful dogs feel more comfortable around people

Steps:

1) If needed, clean and disinfect the playpen floor. Place supplies in the pen for spot cleaning. Break some treats into bite-sized pieces and put them in your pocket. Grab a few toys and scatter them around the pen. Finally, ask another handler to assist you with the session.
2) Choose a confident, friendly dog (your "helper dog") and a fearful dog. With the other handler, take the pair to the pen.
3) If the dogs have not met before, do a quick on-leash introduction.
   - Keep leashes loose during the greeting.
   - If the dogs do not get along, choose a different helper dog or switch to a different exercise instead.
   - If the dogs do seem to like each other, let the play begin! Both handlers should stay in the playpen to supervise the session. If the dogs are small enough to physically manage alone, one handler can supervise.
4) Stay seated on the floor in the middle of the pen for the duration of the session.
   - Interact freely with the helper dog. Play with toys, pet her, and feed her small treats.
   - Every once in a while, toss a treat to the fearful dog. Otherwise, ignore her completely. Playing "hard to get" is the most effective strategy when working with scared animals. If the dog approaches, you can let her sniff you and feed her some treats, but do not look at her or try to touch her.
5) End the session after 10–25 minutes. Try your best to make collecting the fearful dog as stress-free as possible.
6) Over several sessions, you can start interacting with the fearful dog when she approaches you—but wait until you feel that she is really "asking" for your attention. (Watch for things like pawing; solicitous barking; repeated play bowing; relaxed body language; and initiating physical contact by rubbing against you, playfully mouthing, or climbing into your lap.) Go slow and back off immediately if she seems fearful. NEVER force contact. Try engaging the dog in play with a toy. If the dog looks tempted but too afraid to approach, toss it away from you at first. Eventually, you can work up to gently stroking her, as long as the touch does not make her retreat. If you are unsure about how she feels, stop touching her and see what she does. If she moves toward you or stays close, touch her again. If she moves away, offer treats or a toy instead.

Source: Based on ASPCA Behavioral Rehabilitation Center's Helper-Dog Playgroups Protocol developed for undersocialized, fearful dogs.

discussion of social learning, see Whiten and Ham (1992).

Operant conditioning of behaviors such as targeting hands with various body parts, using both positive and negative reinforcement contingencies (including increasing distance and decreasing social pressure), is incorporated to encourage interaction during the early stages of treatment and is expanded upon as dogs develop a positive response to familiar people. As dogs' fear of people diminishes and they choose to remain in proximity to people, handling protocols are introduced using counterconditioning, DSCC, and body target training.

Many of the dogs at the BRC react with fear when people reach toward them to attach a leash and/or when they feel the pressure of a leash. Leash treatments begin with teaching dogs to tolerate the application of both a slip lead (the most common leash-walking tool used in shelters) and a clip lead. (See Box 12.4 for a slip lead DSCC protocol.) Dogs are first

---

Box 12.4   Slip Lead Desensitization and Counter-Conditioning

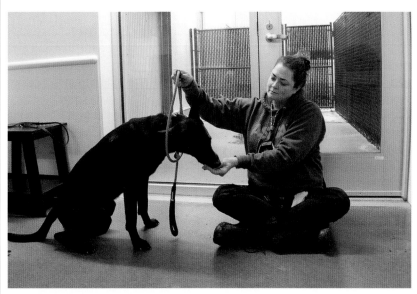

Source: Courtesy of Christine Young.

Time commitment: 10 minutes

Purpose: Reduce fear of people putting a slip lead over the dog's head

Pointers:

- DSCC reminder: Stimulus first, treat second. Don't present your stimulus and food at the same time. There should be a distinct order. The stimulus should predict the delivery of the treat.
- Do a warm-up. At the beginning of each session, do a couple of easy reps at a previous level/step.
- Throw in some easy reps. As you progress, throw in a rep or two that the dog will find really easy to tolerate.
- Make sure the dog is moving toward you for the treats. Sit still and remain quiet. Do not attempt to move the leash toward the dog until she is ready.

Steps:

1) Sit on the floor with the side of your body facing the dog in a non-threatening manner.
2) Begin by making a loop with the slip lead and place it on the floor with a pile of treats in the middle. Note that the dog doesn't have to do anything but learn to expect something good right when the slip lead is revealed. This exercise focuses on the use of classical conditioning alone. If the dog moves away from you, make a note to adjust your behavior during the next rep, but still deliver the treat. Your goal is not to reward desired behavior; your goal is to build a new association and a new conditioned response.
3) Once the dog is readily eating the treats, you can now move to operant conditioning. Gradually raise the loop of the slip lead off the floor inches at a time until the dog will put her head through the loop to eat treats that are on the floor (or in your hand) on the other side of the loop. Do not move onto the next step until the dog is eating treats from your hand.

- If the dog becomes nervous or stops eating, make the exercise easier by raising the portion of the slip lead closest to your hand while leaving the rest of the loop flat on the ground.
4) Continue to lift the slip lead gradually further off the ground. Once the dog is reliably moving her head through the loop to eat treats from your hand, start to fade the lure and give the treat after the dog has offered the behavior.
  - If the dog does not offer the behavior as you start to fade the lure, hide a treat in a closed fist and deliver it after the dog puts her head through. Slowly fade out all lures (i.e., visible food, closed fist, etc.). The dog should see the slip lead and put her head through in hopes of getting a reward (i.e., food treat or exit from the kennel).
5) Once you can put the slip lead on, don't forget to incorporate counter-conditioning to your body movement. Slight position change = tossed treat. Remember to keep the dog's fear level under threshold.

Source: Based on ASPCA Behavioral Rehabilitation Center's Helper-Dog Playgroups Protocol developed for undersocialized, fearful dogs.

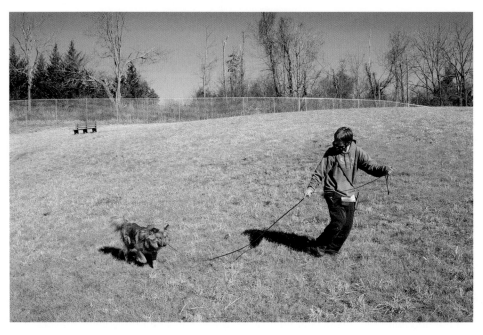

Figure 12.3 An ASPCA Behavioral Rehabilitation Center staff member walks a fearful dog on a long line. *Source:* Courtesy of Christine Young.

walked in a restricted space on a long line, so that they can distance themselves from the handler without experiencing leash pressure, and then the line is gradually shortened to 6 ft. (see Figure 12.3). Box 12.5 provides an example protocol for teaching "Follow Me," which is an initial step in the leash-walking process. Once they are comfortable walking close to people (or, if a dog seems particularly sensitive to leash pressure, outside the context of performing the "Follow Me" behavior first), dogs are acclimated to increasing gentle leash

Box 12.5 Follow Me

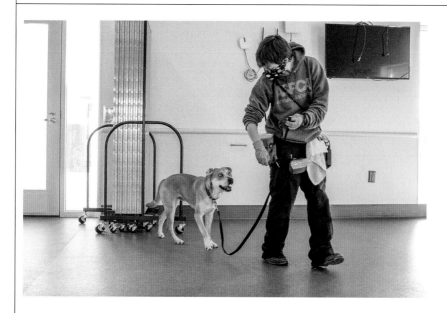

Time commitment: 10 minutes

Purpose: Help fearful dogs enjoy going on walks and coming when called

Pointers:

- This protocol can be started in the dog's kennel if the dog can walk on leash. If the dog is transported via crate, then you can start this protocol in an area where the dog is comfortable.
- If the fearful dog likes other dogs, first do this protocol in the presence of a people-friendly "helper dog." Begin to walk away from the treatment dog, holding onto the helper dog's leash so she will follow you. Give your helper dog a few treats once in a while so that she enjoys the experience and follows you readily. The fearful dog will typically follow along. Once the fearful dog has done a few sessions with the helper dog, try a session without a helper dog present.
- Remember to keep your body language non-threatening. Keep your body turned away from the dog at all times. If you speak to the dog, keep your voice soft and soothing. Stop talking altogether if it appears that verbal encouragement doesn't help—or makes the dog even more nervous.
- This protocol uses a combination of negative and positive reinforcement methods. When the dog moves forward, you move forward to increase the distance between you and her (R-), and she gets to eat a treat (R+).

Steps:

1) Bring the dog into a large enclosed indoor area or outdoor pen. Clip a drag line on the dog's collar (if you're able to safely do so) and let it drag so that you can collect her more easily when the session is over.
   - Implementing this protocol in a large area doesn't work for all dogs—sometimes a smaller area works better. Shrink the space if you think this will set the dog up for better success— use portable exercise pens as needed.

2) Turn your body away from the dog and squat down. Extend a hand low, close to the ground and behind you toward the dog, showing her that you're holding a couple of treats.
3) Wait five seconds. If the dog doesn't move toward you, drop the treats, slowly stand, and walk about 5–10 ft. away. Keep your body turned away and wait for the dog to approach and eat the treats on the ground.
4) Repeat step 3 until successful. Eventually, the dog should start to move toward you when you squat and extend your treat hand. The instant she stops, drop the treats and walk away.
5) When the dog approaches within 6 ft. of you a few times, try feeding her the treats from your hand. If she doesn't take them within 5 seconds, drop them and move away.
6) Once the dog is consistently approaching to take treats from you while you're squatting, try standing and offer her a treat.
   - If standing is too scary for the dog, consider the intermediate step of kneeling.
7) If you use a helper dog at first, repeat steps 1–6 without the helper dog.

Follow Me—Picking Up the Leash—Let's Go
Start this portion of the protocol when the dog is successful with the steps above.

Steps:

1) With a lightweight long line attached to the dog's collar, slowly take the end of the long line, being careful not to create any tension in it. Practice several reps, tossing or handing the dog treats when she follows you.
   - If you or the dog accidentally create tension, immediately drop the line and give the dog a break. If the dog has trouble recovering, toss treats. If the dog is still having a difficult time recovering, stop and work on hand feeding until she recovers.
2) Once the dog is 80% consistent with following you when you begin to walk, add the cue "*Let's go*" just before you take your first step forward. The moment the dog steps forward, say, "*Yes!*" and reward her with a treat. While keeping the leash loose, encourage the dog to move along beside or behind you. You can use treats to lure the dog or toss treats onto the ground in front of the dog. Keep your body language as unthreatening as possible and use a quiet tone when you speak to the dog. Reward any movement in the right direction.
   - If the dog is having a difficult time when tension is put on the lead, stop walking and work on counter-conditioning to leash tension. Change your body position from sitting or squatting to standing. Once the dog remains under threshold with leash tension with you standing, begin your walk again.
3) When the dog remains under threshold and can easily take one step, gradually increase the number of steps the dog must take before earning her reward.
4) Once she is reliably moving forward with the verbal cue, move to intermittent reinforcement, keeping in mind that the walk itself might be the best reward.
5) As the dog becomes more relaxed with this exercise with you holding the long line, start counter-conditioning to very light leash pressure while walking. Apply brief, mild leash pressure, then toss treats. Keep her fear level under threshold. Take breaks as needed—intersperse your reps if that sets her up for better success.
6) Once the dog seems to be relaxed with leash pressure, begin to gradually shorten the line. Take breaks as needed.
   - If the dog's fear increases, take a step backward, or take a break. However, on occasion, and depending on the dog's learning history and level of resilience, it might be appropriate to see if the dog is able to cope through the stressful situation and recover. This must be decided on a case-by-case basis.

7) When the dog has reached 80% consistency and reliability on a shortened long line, try the exercise on a 6-ft. leash. Once she can walk on a regular-length leash, start to walk her in other familiar environments with a helper dog.

8) Once the dog is able to walk in familiar environments while remaining under threshold, incorporate counter-conditioning to your body movement and positions. Slight position change = tossed treat. Remember to keep the dog's fear level under threshold. When the dog is walking nicely, work on positional changes such as standing still, sitting on a bench, on the ground, or squatting down.

Source: Based on ASPCA Behavioral Rehabilitation Center's Follow Me Protocol developed for undersocialized, fearful dogs.

pressure. They are then introduced to short walks in quiet, familiar areas before progressing to longer walks in unfamiliar places and more heavily trafficked environments. The final step is ensuring that dogs can walk by themselves, without the support of a helper dog.

As dogs become less fearful in general, DSCC is used during exposure to regular household objects, such as furniture and televisions in real-life rooms, to household sounds, and to everyday experiences. They learn to navigate stairs, walk calmly through doorways and gates, enter and relax in crates, and load into vehicles (see Figure 12.4). They learn to engage in interactive play with familiar people and to tolerate the presence of unfamiliar people, eventually approaching and interacting with them. As they progress, they learn to allow a variety of people, including strangers, to leash and walk them, initially in familiar areas but ultimately in novel environments as well, including a typical suburban neighborhood and a park. As soon as dogs behave as though they enjoy being touched by familiar people, unfamiliar people are incorporated into social play and handling sessions, including vehicle loading. During the final stages of the program, sessions are conducted without helper dogs.

In consultation with a veterinary behaviorist and a staff veterinarian, dogs in the BRC program are put on a daily regimen of fluoxetine and gabapentin. As they near graduation, all

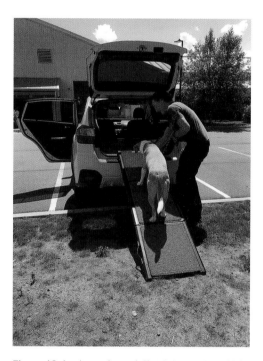

Figure 12.4 An undersocialized dog at the ASPCA Behavioral Rehabilitation Center learning to load into a vehicle. *Source:* Reproduced with permission of ASPCA. *Source:* Courtesy of Deidre Franklin.

dogs are fully weaned to ensure that medication is not required to maintain fear reduction and to ensure a good quality of life.

The BRC team carefully documents all procedures and collects performance data during treatment sessions and regularly scheduled behavior assessments. At the most recent data analysis, 441 dogs were enrolled into the program during a pilot phase conducted from

2013–2017 at St. Hubert's Animal Welfare Center in Madison, New Jersey, and, more recently at the permanent BRC facility in Weaverville, North Carolina (from 2018 on). Three hundred and eighty dogs have graduated, requiring a mean of 78 treatment sessions (SD = 46.7) spanning an average of 96 days in treatment (SD = 54.7). This constitutes a success rate of 86.2% (380 of 441 dogs). Graduating dogs are primarily transferred to partner shelters for placement. Outcomes were confirmed for 301 dogs, of which 297 dogs were successfully adopted into homes (K. Collins, unpublished data).

Aside from the severity of fear at intake, data analyses to date have not yet identified additional factors predictive of successful rehabilitation (K. Collins, unpublished data). Ultimately, additional scientific findings and BRC treatment protocols will be shared with the animal welfare and scientific communities so that more animals can be rehabilitated and placed in adoptive homes.

In 2017, the Canine Center Florida (CCF), operated by Aimee Sadler of Dogs Playing for Life, opened its doors to homeless dogs with severe behavior problems. The board-and-train center sits on 13 fenced acres and houses 36 dogs in indoor/outdoor kennels. There are numerous fenced play yards, a covered event pavilion for outdoor training, a large open space for off-leash exercise, and a set of dormitories for staff and students. At the time of this writing, 201 dogs from 33 North American animal welfare organizations have been enrolled in the program. These dogs were determined to have such serious behavior concerns that their chances for successful adoption were slim to none. Their presenting behavior problems consisted primarily of various forms of aggression: intraspecific aggression, aggression toward people, handling aggression, resource guarding, territorial aggression, redirected aggression, and predatory behavior. Other problems included fearfulness, excessive arousal, and separation anxiety. Only dogs with extensive and severe bite histories are excluded from the program (A. Sadler, personal communication).

Each dog experiences daily in-kennel enrichment, playgroups (for eligible participants), at least twice daily out-of-kennel activities, one-on-one and group training sessions and a customized treatment program to address their specific behavior problem(s) (see Figure 12.5). The specially trained CCF staff employ a wide range of tools and techniques to achieve the desired behavior change. Mentees and shadow students are incorporated into generalization training when the dogs are ready. As dogs progress through the program, they are exposed to more normal pet dog experiences, including offsite field trips, sleepovers in the dormitories, and foster "test drives."

Thus far, 179 of 201 enrolled dogs completed the CCF program, requiring on average 140 days of treatment. Four were successfully placed in working roles: one service dog, two narcotics detection dogs, and one arson detection dog (see Figure 12.6). The rest were either returned to their original shelter or transferred to placement partners for adoption; on average, the dogs were adopted within 19 days. The CCF staff track outcomes for all dogs in the program and provide extensive post-adoption follow-up support. Three adopted dogs were subsequently euthanized (two for aggression to people, one for unknown reasons). Twenty-five dogs were humanely euthanized while still in the program: six for medical reasons and the remainder for unresolvable aggression to people or dogs. Overall, the program boasts a success rate of 87.6% (A. Sadler, personal communication).

In addition to the need for highly trained, knowledgeable staff to minimize the risk of injury from aggressive dogs and to provide post-adoption support, a significant limitation of CCF is its sustainability. As one example, they charge hefty fees for dogs coming into the program, which means their services are out of reach for most shelters. Indeed, when a sample of sheltering organizations was surveyed, 83% reported that they would like to use CCF's

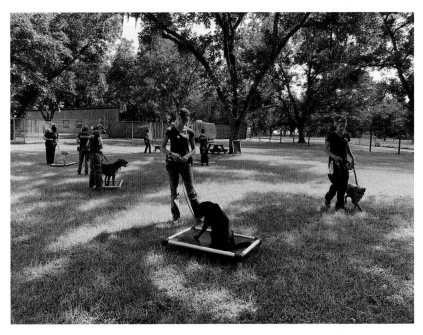

Figure 12.5 A group training session at the Canine Center Florida in which dogs are learning to stay in place while other dogs move around the area. *Source:* Reproduced with permission of Canine Center Florida.

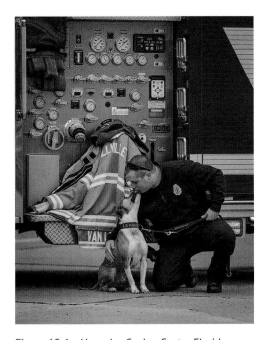

Figure 12.6 Hansel, a Canine Center Florida graduate, working as an arson detection dog. *Source:* Reproduced with permission of Throw Away Dogs Project.

services but only 27% could afford it. A specialized behavior program like CCF can best serve the animal welfare community when sponsors step up to subsidize the cost of treatment and by focusing the program on treating dogs with a reasonable prognosis for improvement.

12.6 Conclusions

An increasing number of shelters and rescue groups recognize the importance of caring holistically for their animals, emphasizing both behavioral AND physical health in maintaining animals' overall well-being in the shelter. Of course, some organizations have more resources to devote to the development and implementation of training and behavior modification programs than others. The authors' communications with sheltering organizations reveal wide variation in different organizations' priorities. Several choose to work with more complex cases involving anxiety, fear, and aggression, while others focus their efforts on basic training designed to make their shelter dogs more attractive to potential adopters. Most use reward-based methods. All share the goals of improving quality of life, increasing adoptability, and preventing behavioral deterioration in long-stay animals. Scientific evidence to support the efficacy of specific strategies to achieve these goals is still sparse, and the authors encourage shelters and rescue groups to devote time to collecting treatment data and tracking post-placement outcomes. Recognizing which behavior problems need treatment and identifying the most efficient, effective ways to provide that treatment in a shelter setting will not only save more lives in a direct sense—it also has the potential to reduce length of stay, allowing organizations to get the most out of available resources and ultimately help a greater number of animals. Gaining and sharing this kind of knowledge through research and collaboration will continue to play a significant role in the coming years, as the animal welfare community strives to resolve treatable behavior problems, ultimately improving shelter dogs' quality of life and making their successful adoption possible.

Please visit the companion website for video clips and downloadable resources associated with this chapter.

References

Amaya, V., Paterson, M.B.A., Descovich, K. et al. (2020a). Effects of olfactory and auditory enrichment on the heart rate variability in shelter dogs. *Animals*. http://doi:10.3390/ani10081385.

Amaya, V., Paterson, M.B.A., and Phillips, C.J.C. (2020b). Effects of olfactory and auditory enrichment on the behaviour of shelter dogs. *Animals*. http://doi:10.3390/ani10040581.

Animal Rescue Site by Greater Good. (n.d.). https://blog.theanimalrescuesite.greatergood.com/apa-adoption-center-posters/ (accessed 20 February 2021).

Belpedio, C., Buffington, L., Clusman, S. et al. (2010). Effect of multidog play groups on cortisol levels and behavior of dogs (*Canis lupus familiaris*) housed in a humane society. *J. Appl. Comp. Anim. Behav.* 4: 15–27.

Brady, K., Cracknell, N., Zulch, H. et al. (2018). A systematic review of the reliability and validity of behavioral tests used to assess behavioral characteristics important in working dogs. *Front. Vet. Sci.* http://doi:10.3389/fvets.2018.00103.

Braun, G. (2011) Taking a shelter dog for walks as an important step in the resocialization process. *J. Vet. Behav.* 6: 100.

Bright, T.M. and Hadden, L. (2017). Safewalk: Improving enrichment and adoption rates for shelter dogs by changing human behavior. *J. Appl. Anim. Welf. Sci.* 20: 95–105.

Cain, C.J., Woodruff, K.A., and Smith, D.R. (2020). Phenotypic characteristics associated with shelter dog adoption in the United States. *Animals*. http://doi:10.3390/ani10111959.

Center for Shelter Dogs at Cummings School of Veterinary Medicine at Tufts University (2021). Special Adoptions. https://centerforshelterdogs.tufts.edu/dog-behavior/special-adoptions/ (accessed 29 June 2021).

Clay, L., Paterson, M., Bennett, P. et al. (2019). Early recognition of behavior problems in shelter dogs by monitoring them in their kennels after admission to a shelter. *Animals*. http://doi:10.3390/ani9110875.

Conley, M.J., Fisher, A.D., and Hemsworth, P.H. (2014). Effects of human contact and toys on the fear responses to humans of shelter-housed dogs. *Appl. Anim. Behav. Sci.* 156: 62–69.

Cook, A. (2017). What Is the Play Way? http://playwaydogs.com/about-the-play-way/ (accessed 15 February 2021).

Coppola, C.L., Grandin, T., and Enns, M. (2006). Human interaction and cortisol: Can human contact reduce stress for shelter dogs? *Physiol. Behav.* 87: 537–541.

Cussen, V. and Reid, P.J. (2020). Mental health issues in shelter animals. In: *Mental Health and Well-Being in Animals*, 2nd ed. (ed. F. McMillan). Oxfordshire, UK: CAB International.

D'Arpino, S., Dowling-Guyer, S., Shabelansky, A. et al. (2012). The use and perception of canine behavioral assessments in sheltering organizations. *Proceedings of the American College of Veterinary Behaviorists/American Veterinary Society of Animal Behavior Veterinary Behavior Symposium*, San Diego, CA (3 August 2012). American Veterinary Society of Animal Behavior.

David, S. and Woytalewicz, K. (2017). Case study of methods for the rehabilitation of dogs that have bitten: Shelter dogs. In: *Dog Bites: A Multidisciplinary Perspective* (eds. D.S. Mills and C. Westgarth), 368–378. Sheffield, UK: 5M Publishing.

Deldalle, S. and Gaunet, F. (2014). Effects of 2 training methods on stress-related behaviors of the dog (*Canis familiaris*) and on the dog-owner relationship. *J. Vet. Behav.* 9: 58–65.

Demirbas, Y.S., Safak, E., Emre, B. et al. (2017). Rehabilitation program for urban free-ranging dogs in a shelter environment can improve behavior and welfare. *J. Vet. Behav.* 18: 1–6.

Denham, H.D.C., Bradshaw, J.W.S., and Rooney, N.J. (2014). Repetitive behaviour in kenneled domestic dog: Stereotypical or not? *Physiol. Behav.* 128: 288–294.

Dogs Playing for Life. (n.d.). https://dogsplayingforlife.com/dpfl-manual/ (accessed 30 April 2021).

Dorey, N.R., Blandina, A., and Udell, M.A.R. (2020). Clicker training does not enhance learning in mixed-breed shelter puppies (*Canis familiaris*). *J. Vet. Behav.* 39: 57–63.

Dreschel, N.A. (2010). The effects of fear and anxiety on health and lifespan in pet dogs. *Appl. Anim. Behav. Sci.* 125: 157–162.

Feuerbacher, E.N. and Wynne, C.D.L. (2012). Relative efficacy of human social interaction and food as reinforcers for domestic dogs and hand-reared wolves. *J. Exp. Anal. Behav.* 98: 105–129.

Gähwiler, S., Bremhorst, A., Tóth, K. et al. (2020). Fear expressions of dogs during New Year fireworks: A video analysis. *Sci. Rep.* http://doi.org/10.1038/s41598-020-72841-7.

Guilherme Fernandes, J., Olsson, I.A.S., and Vieira de Castro, A.C. (2017). Do aversive-based training methods actually compromise dog welfare? A literature review. *Appl. Anim. Behav. Sci.* 196: 1–12.

Hawes, S.M., Camacho, B.A., Tedeschi, P. et al. (2019). Temporal trends in intake and outcome data for animal shelter and rescue facilities in Colorado from 2000 through 2015. *J. Am. Vet. Med. Assoc.* 254: 363–372.

Hennessy, M.B., Voith, V.L., Hawke, J.L. et al. (2002). Effects of a program of human interaction and alternations in diet composition on activity of the hypothalamic-pituitary-adrenal axis in dogs housed in a public animal shelter. *J. Am. Vet. Med. Assoc.* 22: 65–71.

Hennessy, M.B., Voith, V.L., Mazzei, S.J. et al. (2001). Behavior and cortisol levels in dogs in a public animal shelter, and an exploration of the ability of these measures to predict problem behavior after adoption. *Appl. Anim. Behav. Sci.* 73: 217–233.

Herron, M.E., Kirby-Madden, T.M., and Lord, L.K. (2014). Effects of environmental enrichment on the behavior of shelter dogs. *J. Am. Vet. Med. Assoc.* 244: 687–692.

Hiby, E.F., Rooney, N.J., and Bradshaw, J.W.S. (2006). Behavioural and physiological responses of dogs entering re-homing kennels. *Physiol. Behav.* 89: 385–391.

Howard, V.J. and DiGennaro Reed, F.D. (2014). Training shelter volunteers to teach dog compliance. *J. Appl. Behav. Anal.* 47: 344–359.

Hsu, Y. and Serpell, J.A. (2003). Development and validation of a questionnaire for measuring behavior and temperament traits in pet dogs. *J. Am. Vet. Med. Assoc.* 223: 1293–1300.

Landsberg, G., Hunthausen, W., and Ackerman, L. (2012). *Behavior Problems of the Dog and Cat*, 3rd ed. London, UK: Elsevier.

Lausch, B. (2014). Find Your New Running Partner at a Dog Shelter. https://www.runnersworld.com/runners-stories/a20839910/find-your-new-running-partner-at-a-dog-shelter/ (accessed 2 April 2021).

Lindsay, S.R. (2005). *Handbook of Applied Dog Behavior and Training*, vol. 3. Ames, IA: Blackwell.

Luescher, U.A. and Medlock, R.T. (2009). The effects of training and environmental alterations on adoption success of shelter dogs. *Appl. Anim. Behav. Sci.* 117: 63–68.

Marder, A. (2013). Behavioral pharmacotherapy in the animal shelter. In: *Shelter Medicine for Veterinarians and Staff*, 2nd ed. (eds. L. Miller and S. Zawistowski), 569–576. Hoboken, NJ: Wiley Blackwell.

Marder, A.R., Shabelansky, A., Patronek, G.J. et al. (2013). Food-related aggression in shelter dogs: A comparison of behavior identified by a behavior evaluation in the shelter and owner reports after adoption. *Appl. Anim. Behav. Sci.* 148: 150–156.

McGuire, B., Orantes, D., Xue, S., et al. (2020). Abilities of canine shelter behavioral evaluations and owner surrender profiles to predict resource guarding in adoptive homes. *Animals.* https://doi.org/10.3390/ani10091702.

McMillan, F.D. (2013). Quality of life, stress, and emotional pain in shelter animals. In: *Shelter Medicine for Veterinarians and Staff*, 2nd ed. (eds. L. Miller and S. Zawistowski), 83–92. Hoboken, NJ: Wiley Blackwell.

McPeake, K.J., Collins, L.M., Zulch, H. et al. (2019). The Canine Frustration Questionnaire—Development of a new psychometric tool for measuring frustration in domestic dogs (*Canis familiaris*). *Front. Vet. Sci.* 6: 152. http://doi:10.3389/fvets.2019.00152.

Menchetti, L., Mancini, S., Catalani, M.C. et al. (2015). RandAgiamo™, a pilot project increasing adoptability of shelter dogs in the Umbria Region (Italy). *Animals.* http://doi:10.3390/ani5030383.

Menor-Campos, D.J., Molleda-Carbonell, J.M., and López-Rodriguez, R. (2011). Effects of exercise and human contact on animal welfare in a dog shelter. *Vet. Rec.* 169: 388–391.

Mohan-Gibbons, H., Dolan, E.D., Reid, P. et al. (2018). The impact of excluding food guarding from a standardized behavioral canine assessment in animal shelters. *Animals.* http://doi:10.3390/ani8020027.

Mohan-Gibbons, H., Weiss, E., and Slater, M. (2012). Preliminary investigation of food guarding behavior in shelter dogs in the United States. *Animals* 2: 331–346.

Orihel, J.S. and Fraser, D. (2008). A note on the effectiveness of behavioural rehabilitation for reducing inter-dog aggression in shelter dogs. *Appl. Anim. Behav. Sci.* 112: 400–405.

Orihel, J.S., Ledger, R.A., and Fraser, D. (2015). A survey of the management of inter-dog aggression by animal shelters in Canada. *Anthrozoös* 18: 273–287.

Parsons, E. (2012). *Click to Calm: Healing the Aggressive Dog*. Waltham, MA: KCPT/Sunshine Books, Inc.

Passantino, A., Quartarone, V., Pediliggeri, M.C. et al. (2014). Possible application of oxidative stress parameters for the evaluation of animal welfare in sheltered dogs subjected to different environmental and health conditions. *J. Vet. Behav.* 9: 290–294.

Patronek, G.J. and Glickman, L.T. (1994). Development of a model for estimating the size and dynamics of the pet dog population. *Anthrozoös* 7: 25–41.

Patronek, G.J., Glickman, L.T., Beck, A.M. et al. (1996). Risk factors for relinquishment of dogs to an animal shelter. *J. Am. Vet. Med. Assoc.* 209: 572–581.

Perry, P.J., Scarlett, J.M., Houpt, K.A. et al. (2020). A comparison of four environmental enrichments on adoptability of shelter dogs. *J. Vet. Behav.* 35: 1–7.

Protopopova, A. (2016). Effects of sheltering on physiology, immune function, behavior, and the welfare of dogs. *Physiol. Behav.* 159: 95–103.

Protopopova, A., Brandifino, M., and Wynne, C.D.L. (2016). Preference assessments and structured potential adopter-dog interactions increase adoptions. *Appl. Anim. Behav. Sci.* 176: 87–95.

Protopopova, A., Brown, K.M., and Hall, N.J. (2020). A multi-site feasibility assessment of implementing a best-practices meet-and-greet intervention in animal shelters in the United States. *Animals.* http://doi:10.3390/ani10010104.

Protopopova, A., Gilmour, A.J., Weiss, R.H. et al. (2012). The effects of social training and other factors on adoption success of shelter dogs. *Appl. Anim. Behav. Sci.* 142: 61–68.

Protopopova, A. and Gunter, L.M. (2017). Adoption and relinquishment interventions at the animal shelter: A review. *Anim. Welf.* 26: 35–48.

Protopopova, A., Hauser, H., Goldman, K.J. et al. (2018). The effects of exercise and calm interactions on in-kennel behavior of shelter dogs. *Behav. Process.* 146: 54–60.

Protopopova, A., Mehrkam, L.R., Boggess, M.M. et al. (2014). In-kennel behavior predicts length of stay in shelter dogs. *PLOS ONE*: e114310. http://doi:10.1371/journal.pone.0114319.

Protopopova, A. and Wynne, C.D.L. (2014). Adopter-dog interactions at the shelter: Behavioral and contextual predictors of adoption. *Appl. Anim. Behav. Sci.* 157: 109–116.

Protopopova, A. and Wynne, C.D.L. (2015). Improving in-kennel presentation of shelter dogs through response-dependent and response-independent treat delivery. *J. Appl. Behav. Anal.* 48: 590–601.

Protopopova, A. and Wynne, C.D.L. (2016). Judging a dog by its cover: Morphology but not training influences visitor behavior toward kenneled dogs at animal shelters. *Anthrozoös* 29: 469–487.

Reid, P.J. and Collins, K. (2015). Training and behavior modification in the shelter. In: *Animal Behavior for Shelter Veterinarians and Staff*, 2nd ed. (eds. E. Weiss, H. Mohan-Gibbons, and S. Zawistowski), 172–190. Hoboken, NJ: Wiley Blackwell.

Riemer, S., Mills, D., and Wright, H. (2014). Impulsive for life? The nature of long-term impulsivity in domestic dogs. *Anim. Cogn.* 17: 815–819.

Rooney, N.J. and Cowan, S. (2011). Training methods and owner-dog interactions: Links with dog behaviour and learning ability. *Appl. Anim. Behav. Sci.* 132: 169–177.

Rowan, A. and Kartal, T. (2018). Dog population and dog sheltering trends in the United States of America. *Animals.* https://doi.org/10.3390/ani8050068.

Sforzini, E., Michelazzi, M., Spada, E. et al. (2009). Evaluation of young and adult dogs' reactivity. *J. Vet. Behav.* 4: 3–10.

Shabelansky, A. and Dowling-Guyer, S. (2016). Characteristics of excitable dog behavior based on owners' report from a self-selected study. *Animals.* https://doi.org/10.3390/ani6030022

Stewart, G. (2016) *Behavior Adjustment Training 2.0*. Wanatchee, WA: Dogwise Publishing.

Thorn, J.M., Templeton, J.J., Van Winkle, K.M.M. et al. (2006). Conditioning shelter dogs to sit. *J. Appl. Anim. Welf. Sci.* 9: 25–39.

Tuber, D.S., Miller, D.D., Caris, K.A. et al. (1999). Dogs in animal shelters: Problems, suggestions and needed expertise. *Psychol. Sci.* 10: 379–386.

Tuber, D.S., Sanders, S., Hennessy, M.B. et al. (1996). Behavioral and glucocorticoid responses of adult domestic dogs (*Canis familiaris*) to companionship and social separation. *J. Comp. Psychol.* 110: 103–108.

Vieira de Castro, A.C., Barrett, J., de Sousa, L. et al. (2019). Carrots versus sticks: The relationship between training methods and dog-owner attachment. *Appl. Anim. Behav. Sci.* http://doi.org/10.1016/j.applanim.2019.104831.

Voith, V.L. and Borchelt, P.L. (1996a). *Readings in Companion Animal Behavior*. Trenton, NJ: Veterinary Learning Systems.

Voith, V.L. and Borchelt, P.L. (1996b). Fears and phobias in companion animals. In: *Readings in Companion Animal Behavior* (eds. V.L. Voith and P.L. Borchelt), 140–152. Trenton, NJ: Veterinary Learning Systems.

Washington Post (n.d.). Rethinking the Role of the Animal Shelter. https://www.washingtonpost.com/brandstudio/purina/rethinking-the-role-of-the-animal-shelter/ (accessed 19 January 2021).

Weiss, E., Miller, K., Mohan-Gibbons, H. et al. (2012). Why did you choose this pet? Adopters and pet selection preferences in five animal shelters in the United States. *Animals*. https://doi.org/10.3390/ani2020144.

Wells, D.L. and Hepper, P.G. (1992). The behaviour of dogs in a rescue shelter. *Anim. Welf.* 1: 171–186.

Wells, D.L. and Hepper, P.G. (2000). Prevalence of behaviour problems reported by owners of dogs purchased from an animal rescue shelter. *Appl. Anim. Behav. Sci.* 69: 55–65.

Whiten, A. and Ham, R. (1992). On the nature and evolution of imitation in the animal kingdom: Reappraisal of a century of research. *Adv. Stud. Behav.* 21: 239–283.

Winslow, T., Payne, S.W., and Massoudi, K.A. (2018). Functional analysis and treatment of problem behavior in 3 animal shelter dogs. *J. Vet. Behav.* 26: 27–37.

Wright, H.F., Mills, D.S., and Pollix, P.M.J. (2011). Development and validation of a psychometric tool for assessing impulsivity in the domestic dog (*Canis familiaris*). *Int. J. Comp. Psychol.* 24: 210–225.

Zawistowski, S. and Reid, P. (2017). Dogs in today's society: The role of applied animal behavior. In: *The Domestic Dog: Its Evolution, Behaviour and Interactions with People*, 2nd ed. (ed. J. Serpell), 227–244. Cambridge, UK: Cambridge University Press.

Ziv, G. (2017). The effects of using aversive training methods in dogs—A review. *J. Vet. Behav.* 19: 50–60.

Zverina, L. and Cussen, V. (2020). Report on a program to improve outcomes for fearful dogs: The ASPCA in-shelter mini-rehabilitation center. Poster presented at the Animal Behavior Society Conference, Virtual (28–31 July 2020).

13

Play and Playgroups
Lindsay R. Mehrkam

13.1 Introduction

There is perhaps no other animal species so characteristically associated with play than the domestic dog. This is true not only of dogs who live in our homes as pets; it is also true when it comes to choosing a companion from the shelter. In our society, play is often synonymous with our view of dogs. For example, when dogs reject play initiation from a potential adopter in an out-of-kennel setting, they are less likely to be adopted (Protopopova and Wynne 2014). Shelters routinely share photos and videos of dogs engaging in fun, playful behaviors to promote interest in adoption. Parks are constructed specifically to promote off-leash play between dogs and their owners, as well as with other dogs. As many owners and professionals know, there is no question that dogs engaging in healthy play with one another is one of the most engaging sights to observe. Not surprisingly, as shelter management practices continue to evolve, playgroups have become a widely popular and useful practice in many shelters. In a 2018 nationwide survey, approximately 83% of responding shelters in the United States reported using playgroups in some way (Shabelansky and Segurson 2018).

Playgroups may be defined as organized opportunities for multiple dogs to interact off leash in an area outside of their kennels, usually in a designated fenced yard or indoor space. Beyond this definition, however, playgroups vary widely in both their form and function.

It may come as somewhat of a surprise to many, however, that the concept of allowing dogs to engage in off-leash play with one another in both public outdoor settings (e.g., dog parks) and shelter settings is somewhat controversial. Some argue that dogs do not need to play to have a good quality of life. Even more contentious topics include how to best manage play in dogs, how much and how often play should be a part of a shelter dog's life, how play contributes to a dog's quality of life in the shelter, and whether play impacts adoptability. As animal care professionals, we are guided by evidence-based management techniques, tools, and practices, and playgroups should be no exception.

This chapter will first examine the scientific literature on the benefits of play for dogs' well-being and provide evidence to inform professionals on both the rationale for incorporating playgroups and how to best do so. Throughout this chapter, a number of operational concepts essential to successful playgroups will be discussed. Terms defined include "consent," "aversives," "flooding," "punishment," "healthy play," and "reinforcing." These are all terms rooted in behavioral science, with specific definitions, and they have important applied value in playgroup contexts.

Animal Behavior for Shelter Veterinarians and Staff, Second Edition. Edited by Brian A. DiGangi, Victoria A. Cussen, Pamela J. Reid, and Kristen A. Collins.
© 2022 John Wiley & Sons, Inc. Published 2022 by John Wiley & Sons, Inc.
Companion website: www.wiley.com/go/digangi/animal

13.2 The Science of Play

Ask anyone what the function of predatory behavior is, and they will probably respond "to eat," or what the function of copulation is, and we will hear "to produce offspring." The answers about the function of play tend to produce a bit more diversity, such as "for fun," "to expel excess energy," "to practice," or "to strengthen social bonds." However, the purpose of play remains a bit of a mystery to scientists. In addition, because the structure of play appears frivolous and incomplete relative to other more "necessary" behaviors (e.g., aggression, mating, foraging), play hasn't been the subject of much serious study for scientists in animal behavior and was once considered to be a sort of "behavioral fat" (Muller-Schwarze et al. 1982), which animals only engage in to expend surplus energy. However, given that play occurs in so many individuals and species, we know it must have a biologically relevant function. For this reason, play has received renewed interest from scientists. It can incur immediate costs to the participants, including an increased risk of injury and predation (Fagen 1981; Harcourt 1991; Burghardt 2005) and loss of energy (Palagi 2007). Thus, it follows that because play has costs, it must also afford benefits (Hinde 1974; Bekoff and Byers 1981; Fagen 1981; Smith 1982). But what are they?

Play is difficult to define, consists of a relatively small portion of an individual's full behavioral repertoire, and does not appear to have a readily observable behavioral function. The apparent absence of proximate causes of play have led scientists to suggest that the primary benefits gained from play are delayed (over the span of a lifetime, developmental stages, or across generations of a species), rather than immediate (accessible in the direct environment and within a developmental stage).

Several theories propose explanations for the evolutionary functions behind social play. One of the earliest is surplus resource theory (SRT), which states that animals use the excess resources and energy afforded to them during juvenile periods to explore their environment (Burghardt 2005; Pellegrini et al. 2007). SRT also attempts to specify the conditions necessary for play to develop in different species. Such conditions may include sufficient parental care, long periods of immaturity, and the ability to thermoregulate and engage in and recover from vigorous activity. From this view, play can be observed in animal species with surplus resources or at times of the year when resources are abundant.

There is relatively little known about the immediate benefits of play to an animal (Bekoff and Byers 1998; Hall 1998), but continued research provides new clues and theories. Play can afford opportunities for behavioral and cognitive innovation and subsequent practice of newly developed behaviors and strategies (Bateson 2005; Bjorklund and Rosenberg 2005; Bruner 1972; Stamps 1995). It has also been proposed that "play is for practice" (Burghardt 2005); that is, social play affords opportunities for social learning and allows organisms to develop the physical and psychological skills needed to cope with stressful or unexpected situations (Spinka et al. 2001; Dugatkin 2014).

Play has now become a behavior of great interest and value to many scientists and practitioners, although there is still not a clear scientific consensus about its benefits. In actuality, play may have multiple functions, depending on the species and the individual.

13.2.1 Social Play in Canids

Although play can take different forms, social play has been of particular interest to scientists. It is usually the focus of research on playful species because not only is it often considered an easily recognizable form of play, but it is also generally performed more frequently and for longer periods of time than object play (Burghardt 2005). Social play may be defined as play behaviors directed at conspecifics (Burghardt 2005), although social play between members of different species has also been documented (e.g., humans and dogs; Rooney et al. 2001). It may lead to the forging of long-lasting social bonds among animals (Carpenter 1934), including primates (Mendoza-Granados and Sommer 1995), and may serve to provide young males with coalition partners who may be important in their adult life (de Waal 1992). Social play may also promote opportunities to fine-tune behaviors integral to successful competition, foraging, and mating, all of which have clear survival value for all species. Some have suggested that the function of rough-and-tumble play is to assert "dominance" due to "a variety of social and social/physical challenges [that] arise in the course of these activities" (McCune 1998). It has also been suggested that social play may aid in the development of cognitive skills (Bekoff 2000, 2004) by providing opportunities for the "self-assessment" of developmental progress as compared to conspecifics (Thompson 1996). For example, play fighting in male rats may be beneficial to individuals by testing the propensity of potential competitors to fight (Smith et al. 1999), and courtship play in primates may help overcome female reluctance to mate with males (Pellis and Iwaniuk 1999). Immediate adaptive motor benefits, such as increasing the versatility of motor responses, have also been suggested in primates (Palagi 2007). It is well known that play is most common in larger-brained vertebrates (Pellis and Iwaniuk 2004; Burghardt 2005). Various forms of play— including social, solitary, and object play— have been documented most widely in chimpanzees (Matsusaka 2004; Palagi et al. 2006), gorillas (Palagi et al. 2007), bonobos (*Pan paniscus*) (Palagi et al. 2006; Palagi 2008; Palagi and Paoli 2007), rats (Panksepp et al. 1985), domestic dogs (Bekoff 1974; Bauer and Smuts 2007; Ward et al. 2008), and wolves (Cordoni 2009).

Many canid species are social, and spending time among conspecifics provides more opportunities for social play (Bekoff 1972; Fagen 1981;

Burghardt 2005; Horowitz 2009). Occurrences of social play have been reported frequently in captive wolves (Fox 1970; Cordoni 2009), and it has been reported that captive animals play more than wild animals, presumably because they have the surplus energy required to engage in play behavior. The characteristic playfulness of domestic dogs may support this presumption; dogs afford rich opportunities for researchers to study a variety of species-typical play behaviors and how the physical and social environment affect play.

Dogs are in many ways an ideal model for understanding play both structurally (how it looks) and functionally (why it occurs, why it has evolved, and what it achieves for the individual animal and/or species). Relative to most other species, dogs have been identified as a species with characteristically high levels of interspecific and intraspecific play (Bauer and Smuts 2007; Ward et al. 2008; Cordoni 2009) and furthermore engage in high levels of play not only as juveniles but also long into adulthood. Generally, dogs have been selectively bred to be playful with humans as well as other dogs, as these are often considered desirable traits. In addition, home environments, rich with toys and ample space, often permit and promote play.

Both exogenous and endogenous factors can influence play in dogs. The motivation to engage in play, for example, may reflect a breed's propensity for exhibiting predatory motor patterns/sequences (Coppinger and Coppinger 2001). For example, Mehrkam et al. (2017) found that livestock guarding dogs (LGDs) were less motivated to play with a toy compared to herders and retrievers. Solitary play with a toy involves looking at and following the toy's movement (e.g., orient, eye, stalk, chase) and possibly picking up the toy (grab-bite). Herders and retrievers both exhibit intact but truncated predatory sequences, which have been selected for in these breed types so they can successfully perform their respective working roles (Coppinger and Coppinger 2001; Udell et al. 2014). By contrast, breeders select for the inhibition of motor patterns later in the sequence to enable LGDs to successfully perform their working roles. These findings suggest that there may be motivators of both social and solitary play that correspond with breed types and that correspond with breed-typical motor patterns, as proposed by Coppinger and Coppinger (2001). Additional biological factors may influence dogs' motivation to engage in play—as well as what motivates them to play with conspecifics. Mehrkam et al. (2017) found that neuter status predicted the occurrence and duration of social play: dyads containing dogs of mixed neuter-status type (e.g., neutered and intact individuals) engaged in social play at higher levels than did dyads containing dogs of the same neuter status (e.g., two intact males or two intact females).

Of the three breed types tested by Mehrkam et al. (2017) (LGDs, herders, and retrievers), no breed was significantly more likely to engage in play overall; environmental factors (i.e., which stimuli were presented prior to play) were a significantly better predictor of play levels than breed. Though this is somewhat contrary to Coppinger's hypothesis, it is important to acknowledge that play, like many behaviors, is influenced by a combination of breed type, neuter status, and environmental factors. Across breeds, social play was no more likely to be facilitated by nonsocial stimuli (e.g., toys or release from brief confinement/separation) than by social stimuli (e.g., direct human attention); by contrast, solitary play was more likely to be facilitated by nonsocial stimuli than by social stimuli. Social play may thus reflect a motivation or function to "test" or reinforce social bonds between conspecifics when a valued resource (e.g., toy, human attention) is present. Strong motivators of human-dog play may include toy-related stimuli regardless of breed type (Mehrkam et al. 2017).

Given the presence of human handlers in playgroups, an understanding of human-dog play is also important to their successful management. The presence of an attentive familiar human caregiver has been repeatedly shown to facilitate social play between familiar dogs (Mehrkam et al. 2017; Mehrkam and Wynne 2021). Passive handlers can still influence social play levels as well, but not nearly as much. There can be different approaches and styles of handlers during playgroups, and this can likewise have differential effects on playgroup success. Following from both anecdotal observations as well as the literature, well-timed and moderate vocal praise from handlers during appropriate dog-dog play can further promote play without leading to conflict or aggression.

13.2.2 Psychological Benefits of Play

Aside from its theoretical importance in the field of animal behavior, play has practical importance as well. It is well established that play can be an indicator of good welfare in animals (Held and Spinka 2011). For example, play has been associated with reduced cortisol in a variety of species and occurs in the absence of fitness threats (Spinka et al. 2001). Engaging in play may be self-rewarding to the organism and produce pleasurable emotional experiences or afford other private (i.e., unobservable) benefits (i.e., animals play "for fun," Held and Spinka 2011; Pellegrini and Smith 2008). It is also associated with positive emotions in animals and in humans as well as increased endogenous opioids in the brain (i.e., increased mental stimulation and reward activation) in animal models (Vanderschuren et al. 1997). Social play is associated with increased oxytocin in owned dogs (Romero et al. 2015), and opportunities to engage in toy play after a training session have also been associated with improved training outcomes (Affenzeller et al. 2017). Although much research is continuing in this area, there is ample evidence to support the notion that various play types may be reliable indicators of good welfare in a range of animal species, including dogs.

Given these findings, dogs who have an opportunity to participate in well-run play-groups may experience much-needed psychological benefits that may help them to cope with stressful shelter environments. Although animals may reduce play during times of potential conflict or stress among the group (e.g., wolves in Cordoni 2009) or when there are limited resources, it has been reported that play may also occur during these times as a way to regulate stress. For example, Palagi (2007) found that play in primates seems to occur in anticipation of forthcoming stress associated with feeding. In addition, play has been suggested as a potential way to regulate stress associated with competition for owner attention in domestic dogs (Mehrkam et al. 2017; Mehrkam and Wynne 2021). Collectively, these findings offer an important reminder that just because dogs may engage in play doesn't necessarily mean that they are free from stressful contexts; in contrast, it may be that play opportunities with other dogs are even necessary to regulate or respond to the stress of being in the shelter and that the occurrence of play may indicate successful coping or resiliency. This only further underscores the importance of having playgroups in shelter operations and behavior programs, as well as the resources to support them.

The incorporation of well-integrated play-groups into shelter enrichment programs may improve quality of life for dogs during their stay in the shelter—and also get them into homes more quickly, which is also expected to benefit their psychological well-being. Adopters often report that play is a desirable behavior (Dogs Playing for Life n.d.; Protopopova and Wynne 2014). In addition, access to a play session with preferred toys before training sessions improved performance in training in pet dogs (Affenzeller et al. 2017). Whether social play with other dogs—rather than toys—also promotes improvement in performance in training is an interesting but currently unexplored question. The benefits of

social play in dogs have only recently been examined in the context of environmental enrichment.

13.2.3 Playgroups as Enrichment

One way quality of life for shelter dogs may be improved is through enrichment or, more specifically, *environmental enrichment.* Environmental enrichment may be formally defined as an animal husbandry strategy that seeks to enhance physical and psychological well-being by providing stimuli that promote species-typical behaviors, novel sensory stimulation, and behavioral choice (Shepherdson 1998). Today, playgroups are becoming more widely accepted as a social enrichment strategy for shelter dogs, but do all playgroups always meet these goals? To assess scientifically whether any enrichment strategy is effective, it must produce the intended behavioral effects on the animal being exposed to the intervention.

While environmental enrichment strategies may have a common definition, they can come in many different forms. Different types of enrichment may include feeding, object-based or tactile, visual, olfactory, structural, and social components. When implemented, playgroups are typically intended as a social enrichment strategy. By definition, social enrichment involves opportunities to solicit and access interactions with conspecifics, as well as with staff and volunteers. In addition, playgroups can provide increased exploratory opportunities and increased sensory stimulation (e.g., structural, olfactory, or visual enrichment). Remember that access to dogs, for many—but not all—is a primary reinforcer. However, sometimes, food—another primary reinforcer—will compete with a dog's motivation to engage with conspecifics, thereby disrupting play. Enrichment should also promote behavioral choices and control without overwhelming the animals, which is especially relevant when it comes to playgroups. To ensure playgroups are enriching, the S.P.I.D.E.R. framework for enrichment programs can be applied (Mellen and MacPhee 2001). Originally developed by behavioral scientists at Disney's Animal Kingdom zoological institutions, which implement robust enrichment programs, the components of this framework apply to shelter playgroups as well and include: Setting Goals, Planning, Implementation, Documentation, Evaluation, and Readjustment (see animalenrichment.org for more information).

Social enrichment may be defined as strategies that promote the provision of conspecific interactions (Hoy et al. 2010), although interactions with other species (e.g., humans) have been recently suggested to meet these criteria as well. Increased opportunities for play, species-typical social interactions, companionship, physical exercise, and socialization with both other dogs and people may occur through successful, well-run dog-dog playgroups. In addition, depending on how the playgroup handlers coordinate and manage inter-dog interactions, playgroups can also afford increased opportunities for training and bonding to handlers and potential adopters. For example, Shabelansky and Segurson (2018) reported that most respondents from US shelters believed playgroups improve knowledge of a dog's behavior (97%), improve quality of life/welfare (96%), and reduce stress (96%). Other perceived benefits included improvement of staff morale (87%) and reduction in length of shelter stay (70%).

Species-typical behaviors are those we would expect to see all individuals within a species perform in their natural habitat. Certainly, it can be somewhat tricky to define what a species-typical behavior is for a domestic animal, as their "natural habitat" can be hard to define. Despite this challenge, the scientific literature suggests that inter-dog play is indeed a species-typical behavior for domestic dogs. In the absence of highly pressured artificial selection, free-roaming village dogs engage in play behavior, as do New Guinea singing dogs (Dwyer and Minnegal 2021). Although certainly age, general health, and experiential factors (such as inadequate socialization) can impact an individual dog's development of play, as a species, dogs do play. Therefore, playgroups as an environmental enrichment strategy do provide opportunities for species-typical, natural behaviors.

Mehrkam et al. (2014) explored whether human interaction from familiar caregivers could be a form of social enrichment for pair-housed wolves and wolf-dog crosses in a private sanctuary. The researchers measured levels of conspecific affiliation, including social play, and human-directed affiliation, as well as general activity levels and stereotypic behavior. The results indicated that human interaction was enriching, evidenced by significant increases in conspecific affiliation (including social play) and human-directed affiliation, increases in activity levels, and reductions in stereotypic pacing as compared to baseline sessions in which human interaction was not provided. Later, Mehrkam and Wynne (2021) replicated this procedure with pet dogs who lived in the same home and observed similar increases in social play during conditions in which owner attention was available compared to conditions in which the owner was absent or was present but ignoring their dogs. Thus, attention from caregivers, which often includes social and verbal praise and tactile stimulation, may facilitate positive emotional responses in captive canines (Mehrkam et al. 2014; Mehrkam et al. 2017; Mehrkam and Wynne 2021). In addition, play did not escalate to aggression in any of the dyads studied during experimental sessions, despite high-intensity social play being regularly observed. Therefore, when conducting playgroups, handlers should be encouraged to deliver verbal praise and, when appropriate, petting to facilitate healthy play, especially among dogs who are familiar with one another. It is reasonable to assume that similar effects might be observed with dogs in playgroups who may be relatively unfamiliar with one another and their handlers; however, future research is needed to confirm this assumption.

As with any enrichment or behavior modification strategy, there may be medical reasons why playgroups may not be approved or may be limited for an entire shelter's population, a subset of the population, or an individual animal. Any candidates for playgroups should be selected only following the clearance of veterinary staff. In addition, although inter-dog play is certainly a species-typical behavior, one should not assume that all dogs are suited for dog-dog playgroups or find play with other dogs positively reinforcing. It is important to remember that while some dogs may be reactive to other dogs across time and situations, other dogs in the population may exhibit discomfort or conflict toward other dogs due to behavioral deterioration experienced as a result of being in the shelter environment. Dogs may exhibit increased stereotypic behaviors and increased withdrawal or loss of interest in social contact with people and/or other dogs, as well as increased aggression and reactivity toward other dogs (Protopopova 2016). In some situations, dogs housed in a shelter may appear to be reactive toward other dogs due to the presence of a barrier but may not exhibit reactivity in a playgroup context. Thus, while it is necessary to select dogs carefully, shelters must also be careful not to exclude dogs who may benefit from playgroup based on easily modifiable problems or for reasons that may be simply artifacts of the shelter environment.

Research on enrichment preferences in a variety of species demonstrates that although a strategy may indeed be species-appropriate, individual learning history and experience must also be considered; not all individuals of a species may find the same enrichment strategy highly reinforcing/enriching or highly preferred, if preferred at all (Mehrkam and Dorey 2014; Mehrkam and Dorey 2015). This lesson also applies to playgroups, as a variety of lifetime experiences (e.g., lack of socialization with other dogs, stress, injury or trauma, or other aversive interactions with dogs and/ or people) may lead individual dogs to find

play with other dogs unenjoyable. It is worth noting that, over time, this could change with proper positive experiences/conditioning, but whether a shelter wants to pursue this will depend on resources and length of stay. Identifying appropriate candidates for playgroups is of great importance to success and will be discussed in more detail later in this chapter.

13.3 Tools and Terminology

The science of learning and behavior analysis is clear: tools are *stimuli*. Stimuli can be defined as any environmental change or event that can be perceived by an individual. To be conceptually systematic, it is best to think of these tools in this way, rather than as rewards, reinforcers (positive or negative), punishers (positive or negative), corrections, or interrupters. Scientifically, for stimuli to be *reinforcers*, they must cause an observed increase in the future likelihood of a behavior. Likewise, for stimuli to be *punishers*, they must cause an observed decrease in the future likelihood of a behavior. Furthermore, reinforcers and punishers are categorized by whether they were added (i.e., positive) or removed (i.e., negative) to the environment to have their effect on the organism. Therefore, whether we call the tools we use *aversives, rewards, reinforcers* or *punishers, interrupters, or corrections* depends on how they affect the future probability of that behavior, no matter how tempting it may be for us to use those labels beforehand or to make the error of assuming that just because we intend to use a tool for a certain reason, the intended effect will follow.

Tools that are used often in playgroups include vocal praise, vocal corrections, treats, toys, break and/or pig boards, leashes, collars, harnesses, muzzles, carabiners (to lock or secure gates), water spray bottles, shake cans, compressed air, and air horns. Certainly, other dogs are used in practice as live "tools" to help facilitate play and other social interactions between other dogs. In a nationwide survey of playgroup practices, vocal corrections were the most common (86%), followed by verbal praise (82%), "leash-on" (leaving the leash attached to the dog) (77%), and "body/social pressure" (71%). Use of control poles, prong or pinch collars, and electronic collars were least reported (Shabelansky and Segurson 2018). These tools can be used as interventions and combined with other techniques, including recall and obedience training, differential reinforcement, and timeouts or planned ignoring by handlers (see Figure 13.1).

When determining which tools to use in playgroups, shelter professionals should keep in mind that reliance on aversives can lead to the association of both people and other dogs with unpleasant occurrences in off-leash contexts, particularly if playgroups are the only contexts in which dogs would interact freely with people or dogs in the shelter environment. In addition, overinvolvement of handler interventions intended to interrupt undesired behaviors can be disruptive to healthy play interactions. This can also be further negatively reinforcing to the handler because intervening can remove the possibility of a potential conflict. Handlers should be cautious when correcting or interrupting dogs during play and ensure that they are only doing so for behaviors that are indicative of negative outcomes. Although preventing conflicts or fights is important for dog welfare, it should not come at the expense of sufficient opportunities for healthy social play.

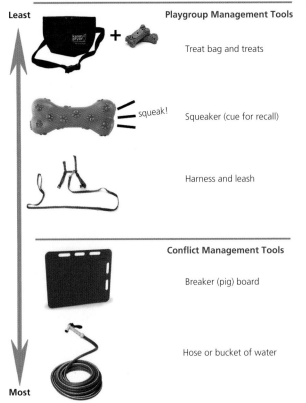

Shelter Playgroup Alliance Playgroup Tools: Least to Most Intrusive

Least

Playgroup Management Tools

Treat bag and treats

squeak! Squeaker (cue for recall)

Harness and leash

Conflict Management Tools

Breaker (pig) board

Hose or bucket of water

Most

Figure 13.1 Recommendations for least intrusive to most intrusive stimuli used to manage shelter dog playgroups. *Source:* Courtesy of Mara Velez.

13.4   Shelter Playgroup Models

Currently, there are two formal models with a specific structure for conducting playgroups, including written protocols and guidelines, published manuals, and associated training opportunities for shelter professionals. The first one established was the Dogs Playing for Life (DPFL) model, which incorporates a wide variety of tools and techniques to efficiently conduct playgroups. The second is the model advocated by the Shelter Playgroup Alliance (SPA) that emphasizes a LIMA-based approach to playgroups (least intrusive, minimally aversive). Both models emphasize the role of playgroups as enrichment strategies aimed at promoting shelter dog quality of life and offer in-person workshops in which representatives come to a shelter and help shelter staff and volunteers develop and implement playgroups or refine/consult on existing playgroup programs. Both DPFL and SPA emphasize treating each dog as an individual. Both emphasize a holistic approach to maintaining a good quality of life for shelter dogs, including meeting dogs' physical, behavioral, and emotional needs. The two models differ substantially on the goals of the playgroup, what constitutes healthy play, the range of tools used to manage dog-dog play, and the type of intervention methods used.

Rather than adopting and strictly following the guidelines of one of these models, the vast majority of shelters run a modified version of one or a combination of the two. In a nationwide US shelter survey study by Shabelansky and Segurson (2018), the majority (83%) of responding organizations use playgroups and with some frequency (71% had more than three per week). However, the average number of dogs in each playgroup was small, indicating that most organizations do not provide the majority of their dog population with the opportunity to play with other dogs on a regular basis. Participating shelters indicated that their playgroups use both large and small groups of dogs and aversives/interrupters as

well as treats, toys, and vocal praise. In practice, shelters should adapt their playgroups based on their resources (including staff and volunteers), population of dogs (and needs of individual dogs), and shelter environment. A playgroup may not follow either model with perfect integrity. In addition, a successful and enriching playgroup program is one that will continuously ensure a balance of both the physical and behavioral needs of the dogs.

13.4.1   Dogs Playing for Life

Dogs Playing for Life (DPFL) is a nonprofit organization developed by Aimee Sadler in 1998 at the Southampton Animal Shelter in Southampton, New York. It is the longest-running and most widely used organized playgroup model in the United States. DPFL describes their program as a "training and behavior modification program for shelter dogs featuring play groups" (DPFL n.d.). DPFL emphasizes maximizing the efficiency of playgroups, using them with the goal of not only providing physical and mental enrichment but with the added goal and function of using playgroups as an operational and behavioral assessment tool to assist with both daily shelter operations and behavioral evaluations of dogs. Typically, relatively large playgroups (six or more dogs at any one time) are recommended (though this somewhat depends on the shelter) and widely used to maximize efficiency and allow for a range of conspecific interactions.

In addition, handlers monitor inter-dog interactions but generally intervene only when a fight is occurring. When intervening, handlers use a wide range of tools to deliver warnings and corrections to dogs and typically do not use toys, treats, or verbal praise often if at all. The DPFL model advocates an "every dog, every day" approach to playgroups and aims to use playgroups as a way to maximize operational efficiency, socialize the dogs, and expend excess energy in a healthy and interactive way." The DPFL website states that playgroups are the foundation for teaching dogs to "behave in an appealing and attractive way for volunteers and adopters" (DPFL n.d.).

One of DPFL's main goals is to promote and increase the number of play and other species-typical opportunities for as many dogs in a shelter as possible. Often, playgroups following a DPFL model will be larger (containing more dogs) than what appears to be the typical group size used by shelters (DPFL, personal communication). For example, the DPFL manual (n.d.) states that one of their longest-running and most successful collaborating shelters averages approximately 60 dogs overall in playgroups within the 2.5 hours playgroups are run every morning. They note that "a handler can attend to many more dogs through offering playgroups, rather than attempting to leash walk each individual dog for a short period of time." DPFL's manual is available on their website (www.dogsplayingforlife.com).

One main advantage of the DPFL model may be maximizing the efficiency of shelter resources. The DPFL playgroup model also allows for a potentially wider range of species-typical behaviors, including agnostic and exploratory behaviors. DPFL encourages handlers to allow dogs to "have altercations or interactions that they can work out on their own" and "to learn from each other what is and isn't appropriate" (DPFL n.d.). The emphasis is placed on monitoring the dogs' behavior holistically in the context of the entire social interaction, rather than on discouraging specific problematic behaviors or precursors to aggression.

The DPFL model has been widely successful in terms of implementation at a wide number of shelters. However, it is important to note that the methods used in the DPFL model may have a greater potential for flooding if dogs in the playgroup find other dogs aversive. One dog could find the presence of other dogs aversive for any number of reasons—fear, territoriality, pain, or guarding of an area of the yard/another play partner/a

handler. In addition, since DPFL encourages a relatively more hands-off approach to managing playgroups, inter-dog conflict may be more likely to occur, even if that conflict does not often lead to serious fights. For example, it is not encouraged that DPFL handlers intervene in response to behaviors in isolation, even if they are indicative of higher arousal or potential conflict. Such behaviors might include pinning the ears back, holding the tail erect, raising hackles, mounting, growling, or showing teeth, even though many of these behaviors do occur during conflict. An additional disadvantage may be the level of experience/training/skill needed by handlers to safely manage a large group, recognize when it is appropriate to intervene, and know how to do so effectively and humanely. Together, these challenges could result in relatively limited generalizability of this approach across shelters or even across personnel within the same shelter. The use of aversives (e.g., verbal reprimands, spraying) are considered to be easier to immediately implement than delivering treats or praise for acceptable behavior; given the well-documented power of aversives to suppress behavior, this may lead to a higher likelihood of staff relying on these tools, despite potentially harmful side effects on a dog's learning history. The DPFL manual provides a summary of potential disadvantages of each training tool used in the DPFL program.

There is some preliminary research to support the efficacy of the DPFL model. For example, stress-related in-kennel behaviors were observed to decrease in shelter dogs randomly assigned to a DPFL-model playgroup compared to dogs in the same shelter randomly assigned to an on-leash walk for the same duration of time per day across four days (Belpedio et al. 2010). This may be somewhat supported by Mehrkam and colleague's most recent study, as they did not find significant differences in physiological stress measures between DPFL and control dogs overall (Mehrkam et al., unpublished results).

13.4.2   Shelter Playgroup Alliance

The Shelter Playgroup Alliance (SPA) is a nonprofit organization founded by Mara Valez and includes shelter staff and behavior experts who developed a framework that emphasizes "a least intrusive, minimally aversive (LIMA)-based approach." The mission of SPA is to provide animal welfare organizations with education and tailorable guidelines and support materials that facilitate healthy inter-dog interactions. The SPA describes itself as a model that promotes "safe and healthy play, limits the use of aversives, and minimizes the risk of injury and behavioral fallout." In addition, an important feature of SPA is that it also emphasizes the use of strategies outside of playgroups in their enrichment programs for shelter dogs. In this way, playgroups are viewed as only one part of a shelter enrichment program. SPA's shelter playgroup guidelines aim to promote choice and control for shelter dogs, as well as adherence to the ethical guidelines adopted by certifying bodies such as the International Association of Animal Behavior Consultants (IAABC 2018) and Certification Council for Professional Dog Trainers.

The SPA Inter-Dog Playgroup Guidelines (2019) recommend much smaller playgroups (two to six dogs per playgroup). The SPA guidelines also state that "LIMA-based playgroups are devoted to providing dogs with opportunities to consent, physical and mental safety, and avoid the use of aversives." The LIMA ethical standard was conceptualized to provide competency-based criteria for animal behavior professionals. Trainers and consultants who follow the LIMA ethical standard often refer to the Humane Hierarchy created by Dr. Susan Friedman. In particular, this involves maintaining low levels of arousal, limiting the number of dogs in playgroup, maximizing handler-to-dog ratios, and prescribing alternate enrichment strategies for dogs in addition to or instead of playgroups. The SPA guidelines further state that "LIMA-based playgroups control the environment in a way that sets the stage for dogs to be successful, while utilizing tools that increase desired behaviors, rather than those that temporarily suppress unwanted behaviors." The SPA guidelines also emphasize that handlers consider the body language of the dogs throughout the entire interaction to ensure that all dog participants are enjoying inter-dog play.

Specifically, the SPA guidelines recommend groups of two to three dogs and a 2:1 dog-to-handler ratio for "low-risk tolerance" organizations. For "higher-risk tolerance" organizations, the guidelines recommend four to six dogs per playgroup with a 3:1 (or greater) dog-to-handler ratio. SPA does recommend that a 3:1 ratio can be a low-risk option if the group consists of a stable population whose dog skills are well established. In addition, introducing dogs through protected contact and with leashes on is recommended. The use of food and toys during playgroup is also permitted, so long as the delivery of both food and toys are kept under good handler control during the playgroup and appropriate for the individual dogs in the group (e.g., no guarding history) as well as the density of dogs in the play area. The SPA guidelines acknowledge that "while tools that discourage behaviors may be necessary in some situations, LIMA-based playgroups aim to minimize their use rather than rely on them." LIMA-based playgroups include dogs that find spending time with other dogs positively reinforcing and removes dogs that do not for reasons that might include becoming fearful, overaroused, or stressed or showing behavior indicative of a desire to leave. Like DPFL, SPA also offers workshops and mentorships for shelter professionals wanting to learn more about how to successfully implement their playgroup model at their organization.

An advantage of the SPA playgroup model includes aiming to limit stimuli that may be potentially aversive or punishing to an animal. Although it can be argued that experiencing unpleasant consequences is a natural part of any organism's learning history (Vollmer 2002), there is also ample evidence to show the negative effects such stimuli can have on both dogs and their trainers, especially when applied repeatedly (Casey et al. accepted for publication; Cooper et al. 2014). In addition, the SPA model maximizes stimuli that are intended to be rewarding or reinforcing; importantly, such reward-based training practices have been shown to be beneficial for dogs, ranging from pet dogs to shelter and working dogs (Blackwell et al. 2008; Cooper et al. 2014; Protopopova and Wynne 2015; Ziv 2017), among other species (Ferguson and Rosales-Ruiz 2001).

The disadvantages of the SPA playgroup model may include reduced efficiency due to fewer dogs per playgroup and greater need for resources (e.g., proper harnesses, treats, treat pouches), increased staff and/or volunteer demand, and reduced opportunities for both off-leash exercise and a wide range of species-typical social behaviors, including play. Thus, high-intake shelters may have a difficult time implementing this model; however, SPA states that their 66-page guidelines (available at www.shelterdogplay.org) were developed based on behavioral science with input from well-educated animal behavior and training professionals with experience in open- and limited-admission shelters and that "the guidelines are intended to be flexible to meet the needs of each shelter."

Most recently, a multi-site study by Mehrkam et al. (unpublished results) found that shelter dog playgroups that utilized treats and vocal praise from handlers and used a LIMA-based approach resulted in improved in-kennel behavioral welfare, improved indicators of adoptability, and significantly lower cortisol levels than either a control shelter not using playgroups and two shelter playgroups that used aversives regularly. Furthermore, the researchers found that post-playgroup salivary cortisol levels were higher only in dogs that participated in a small (two-to three-dog) playgroup that used aversives; interestingly, dogs in the control group, large playgroup with aversives, and small playgroup with treats and vocal praise all exhibited decreased salivary cortisol levels after playgroup. This suggests that the increased rate of aversives used per dog in the small playgroup using aversives may have contributed to increased physiological stress in these dogs. With respect to behavioral outcomes, only the small playgroup using rewards significantly improved indicators of behavioral welfare and adoptability in the kennel. In contrast, the control (no playgroup) dogs exhibited significantly decreased behavioral welfare and adoptability. It is important to note that there was substantial within-shelter variation in cortisol and behavior across individual dogs, suggesting that shelter dogs may indeed respond to playgroups differently based on individual experiences. The results of this study suggest that playgroups—especially reward-based playgroups such as those recommended by the SPA model—may include reduced inter-dog conflict, improved behavioral outcomes, and lower stress levels for dogs.

13.5 Canine Playgroups in Shelter Settings

Although social play is a natural, species-typical behavior for most dogs, playgroups in the shelter are surprisingly controversial—both in terms of whether playgroups are effective in promoting shelter dog welfare and also what is the best way to run them. There is also concern about the relative risks of increased inter-dog aggression and disease transmission. Part of this debate is due to the fact that every shelter is unique, and what may work well in one shelter may be extremely challenging in another. A shelter that has limited volunteers, high turnover, or frequent disease outbreaks, for example, may not feel confident in its ability to effectively and safely run playgroups seven days per week. The results of an online nationwide survey by

Maddie's Fund suggest that playgroups in US shelters are generally safe for dogs and people (Shabelansky and Segurson 2018) and fights, bites, and injuries are not as prevalent as some critics of shelter playgroups might argue. This is also consistent with research in dog parks, although fights in dog parks seem to occur more frequently, likely due to less oversight or intervention observed in dog parks. For example, one study found that less than 5% of all dog-dog play interactions in two dog parks were intervened in by owners, including interactions that led to serious altercations (Mehrkam et al., unpublished results). Playgroups can provide needed enrichment, social interaction, and exercise for a large number of dogs efficiently, and thus are a particularly attractive tool for high-dog-intake shelters.

Interaction among dogs brings unavoidable risk, and, accordingly, one should not assume that play comes without potential harm. Inter-dog play has the propensity to escalate into minor altercations fairly often, although the evidence suggests that severe fights resulting in injury or even death are relatively rare. Shabalensky and Segurson (2018) appear to report that 12% of shelters, however, do report two to five bites to people during the course of a year. It is important to note that such severe outcomes tend to be relatively rare; nonetheless, they should be accepted as a potential outcome and risk of a play-group—or, truly, any time multiple dogs occupy the same space. Despite the risks, the potential benefits of playgroups are many, and, as described by the Association of Shelter Veterinarians (ASV), they should be considered "when the benefits can be maximized and the risks adequately addressed" (ASV 2019).

13.5.1 Setting Goals for a Successful Playgroup Program

As is best practice for enrichment programs, "successful" must be operationally defined by identifying behavioral goals. Playgroups generally should not be implemented at a shelter unless the behavioral goals are agreed upon by all team members and include input from key behavior, medical, and operations staff. Some goals might include the following:

- To assess behavior
- To provide social enrichment and promote species-typical behaviors (conspecific social behavior, interspecific social behavior, or both)
- To bring shy or fearful dogs "out of their shell" (i.e., reduce fearful or shy behaviors)
- To acquire and/or practice appropriate communication skills between dogs
- To maximize the use of resources (e.g., as a strategy to exercise dogs and get them out of kennels during cleaning)

Certainly, more than one goal may be selected for any one playgroup, and, moreover, the same shelter may aim for a different goal per group of dogs—or even for individual dogs within a group.

Once goals are agreed upon, it is time to plan the playgroup program. First, acknowledge that whenever multiple dogs interact in a confined space there are potential risks. A plan for conflict or fights should be planned, prepared for, and articulated among the shelter staff *before* play-group begins. Should a fight or incident occur, such events should be clearly communicated verbally within the relevant teams of the shelter and documented in writing, ideally along with a contingency plan. Everyone involved in playgroups, whether staff or volunteer and regardless of role, should be on the same page to ensure consistency. This can be accomplished by ensuring that personnel (i) have reviewed the playgroup protocols and incident reports, (ii) had an opportunity to contribute to the writing and/or to comment on the plan when it was being created, (iii) are held accountable for following the plan, and (iv) have the ability to give feedback on the plan and recommend adjustments after implementation. Active planning includes antecedent arrangements for both the physical and social environment.

13.5.2 Arranging the Physical Environment

First and foremost, play areas should be safe, secure (e.g., with high fences), and large enough to promote play among multiple dogs. Equally important is that play areas have places for dogs to avoid interaction, rest, or engage in other species-typical behaviors (e.g., sniffing, digging) if they choose. Shelters may consider elevated platforms or other structures with ramps and/or stairs, which afford the opportunity for dogs to both climb to an elevated position out of reach of other dogs and hide underneath. Benches, picnic tables, and kiddie pools are also useful options regularly used in these ways by dogs in playgroup. Ideally, play areas should be multiple connected areas rather than a single area so they can be closed off if needed, and they should have separate entrance and exit pens to reduce conflict and promote safe interactions between dogs during greetings, as well as clear pathways for dogs and handlers to avoid unnecessary altercations or confusion among handlers. It is also recommended that play yards contain gates that swing both ways, containers to place toys in that are out of reach to dogs (to reduce resource guarding), carabiners to secure dogs to fences in emergency situations, and interruption tools (air horns, break sticks, spray bottles) in weather-resistant containers. Play areas should be regularly inspected and well maintained to prevent injuries and escapes and to promote sanitation.

There is some debate about whether toys or treats should be in the play area. For example, DPFL recommends against toys or treats "or any other valued resource since they can become a potential distraction or issue." However, it is possible that treats and other appetitive stimuli can be used safely if kept securely contained in a treat pouch attached to the handler and delivered intentionally and directly to specific dogs at appropriate times. Handlers should not, for example, give treats to dogs when they are mobbing or jumping on them, but can provide treats as a reinforcer for

successful recalls to the handler or taking breaks during play. In fact, shelter dogs who participated in playgroups that primarily utilized rewards such as food and vocal praise had significantly lower cortisol levels, lower behavioral indicators of stress, and higher behavioral indicators of adoptability (Mehrkam et al., unpublished results). Resource guarding can also be maintained by a variety of consequences, depending on the individual dog's history (Mehrkam et al. 2020). For example, dogs may exhibit resource guarding not only to retain access to the guarded item (positive reinforcement), but also to remove the perceived threat via negative reinforcement. (This is, in part, why animals sometimes guard items or areas that no longer contain food, water, or toys.)

It is recommended that flat, washable collars without buckles and quick-release snaps are used during playgroup to prevent entanglement between dogs. Staff should ensure that collars are fitted properly on each dog prior to playgroup. Muzzles (basket and nylon are most recommended) should also be used regularly as a precaution for any dogs who may have exhibited reactivity toward other dogs or handlers but may still be considered potential candidates for playgroup. Six-foot rope, nylon, or leather leashes, as well as BioThane® (BioThane Coated Webbing Corp., North Ridgeville, OH) longlines (to prevent tangling), are also all recommended. Gentle Leader® headcollars (PetSafe®, Knoxville, TN) are not recommended during playgroups as they can create quick and intense pressure on the dog's head and neck and present an immediate danger to the dog if the leash gets caught or stuck on an object in the play yard.

Other tools include two-way radios (e.g., for handlers to communicate across a large play yard over the sound of many dogs, to communicate with other staff inside the shelter, or to move dogs in and out of playgroup), an airhorn, compressed air, citronella deterrent spray, shake cans, spray water bottles, stainless steel water bowls used to make a loud, clanging sound, and squeaky toys. Shock or electronic collars should never be used in playgroups; a growing body of research has indicated they are no more effective than reward-based training and also lead to welfare concerns (e.g., Cooper et al. 2014).

13.5.3   Arranging the Social Environment

In a playgroup, the social environment consists of the handlers and other dogs, and, sometimes, adopters or other community members or dogs walking outside of the play area. Given the various aspects of the playgroup environment, attributing roles is key before entering the play yard, with one group leader per play area.

One of the most common recommendations made for best practices in managing dog-dog play interactions is with respect to size. Size considerations are relevant in two ways: the first consideration is the quantitative size of the playgroup (i.e., number of dogs present), and the second consideration is whether to allow dogs to be in playgroups together based on their physical size.

There is no optimal or universally agreed upon number of dogs to include in any one playgroup at a single time. It is estimated that the average playgroup size for most shelters is eight dogs (Shabelansky and Segurson 2018). Johnson et al. (2013) reported that dogs that participated in three-dog playgroups (n = 24) and dogs that participated in five-dog playgroups (n = 12) both showed improvements across behavioral measures of in-kennel arousal and excitability between pre- and post-playgroup observations at the shelter. More specifically, the researchers reported that dogs in the three-dog playgroup showed improvements across all measures except for position in kennel, where no change was observed. While it should be noted that the authors conducted very brief (approximately 10s) behavioral observations, they also acknowledged that future research on playgroups should be conducted to more comprehensively assess if playgroups do improve

in-kennel behavioral arousal levels resulting in improved adoptability and overall dog well-being.

Inter-dog play most often occurs between two dogs (Käufer 2014). DPFL does not generally recommend restrictions on size limits of playgroups or handler-to-dog ratios. SPA recommends a maximum of four to six dogs per playgroup, with a 2:1 ratio of dogs to handlers, and also recommends ensuring that a minimum of two handlers be present at all times. There is an increased risk of aggression in dog parks when more than two dogs are involved in a play interaction (Mehrkam et al., unpublished results). Interestingly, however, there appears to be no correlation between average size of the typical playgroup and an increased risk of fights or injuries (Shabelansky and Segurson 2018). Mehrkam et al. (unpublished results) found there was no significant overall effect of size of playgroup alone on behavioral welfare indicators.

It may actually be the case that playgroups larger than two or three dogs offer more choice and control to individual dogs because they have more potential play partners to choose from (including if one dog doesn't reciprocate play solicitation or engagement from another dog), so long as space is sufficient for dogs to avoid an interaction or to engage in other exploratory behaviors if they prefer. Overall, the ideal-sized playgroup is one that matches the space and number of handlers available while considering the composition of dogs present in the playgroup as well as the shelter's population. In other species, including humans, crowding may increase the likelihood of aggressive interactions and should be avoided. It is recommended that the number of dogs per playgroup should be determined based on (i) the number of experienced, trained handlers available to manage the playgroup, (ii) the physical size of the play space to prevent crowding effects and mobbing, and (iii) the tools and methods used to manage the dogs. According to the ASV, handlers should optimize human and animal safety by limiting the number of dogs in playgroups based on staff/volunteer training, skillset, and shelter resources. In addition, the nature of the dogs themselves (e.g., age, disposition, temperament, physical ability) is essential to consider. A playgroup consisting of older calm dogs or a group of juvenile small, playful dogs may be able to be substantially larger than a group of rowdy medium or large juvenile dogs.

Playgroups can be beneficial for dogs of all physical sizes. There is some debate, however, as to whether dogs of different relative sizes should be part of the same playgroup. Healthy dog-dog play is possible between dogs of different relative sizes and has been observed in both playgroup, dog park, and in-home settings (Mehrkam et al., unpublished results); however, it is estimated that fewer than half of shelters utilizing playgroups allow dogs of various weights and sizes in one playgroup (Shabelansky and Segurson 2018). One reason for this is that incidents between small and large dogs do occur. When they do, such incidents can pose a high risk of serious injury, especially to the smaller dog. Predatory aggression is a possibility when there is a substantial size difference, and the risk of injury can increase in off-leash settings. Given that this behavior can result in serious injury or death to smaller dogs, pairing up unfamiliar large and small dogs may not be worth the risk. In addition, dog owners who experienced conflicts in dog parks reported that large dogs sustained physical bites more often than small dogs (J. Berg, personal communication). Clearly, this suggests that large dogs can also be at risk of physical injury in off-leash settings. These risks should be kept in mind by handlers if they plan to combine dogs of different relative sizes together in playgroups. The SPA and the ASV both recommend matching or pairing dogs based on their size or considering relative size when selecting playgroup participants.

Nonetheless, it could be harmful to withhold a potentially enriching interaction between two potentially successful play partners based on size alone. In addition, it has been observed that dog owners do discourage play between dogs of different relative sizes more frequently than play between dogs of the same relative size, even when the probability of play-induced aggression is not significantly different (Mehrkam and Wynne, unpublished data). Therefore, if handlers do combine small and large dogs together, handlers should be aware that they are not discouraging or interrupting healthy play or other social interactions solely because of this potential size bias.

While only 48% of shelters allowed dogs of various weights/sizes in one playgroup, dog size was one of the least commonly reported reasons for exclusion from shelter playgroups, so this may not present a major barrier to their implementation (Shabelansky and Segurson 2018). Nonetheless, it may be a precautionary strategy to hold separate large and small dog playgroups, even if there is truly no empirical difference in risk factor, especially if it makes handlers more confident in their ability to adequately manage playgroups (see Figure 13.2). In addition, by controlling/eliminating the variable of size from perceptions of whether social play is healthy or leading into dangerous territory, handlers may have one fewer aspect to consider in a constantly dynamic scenario. Systematic study of this issue is certainly warranted.

13.5.4 Selecting Playgroup Candidates

Playgroups can be beneficial for dogs of all ages, sizes, breeds, and temperaments. However, it is important for handlers and other shelter staff to evaluate whether each individual dog is willing to participate in playgroup and finds the experience enriching or reinforcing; such evaluations are sometimes referred to loosely as "consent tests," or, more scientifically, "choice tests" or "preference assessments" (see Box 13.1). Inclusion in playgroups will depend on the individual dog. Dogs should not be excluded due to blanket restrictions, such as breed. Dogs that display on-leash reactivity or barrier

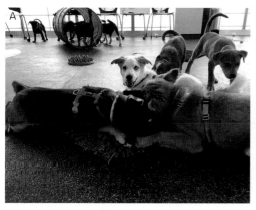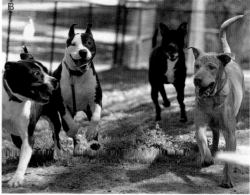

Figure 13.2 Small (A) and large (B) dog playgroups. Shelter playgroups can vary widely in their form and function. *Source:* Courtesy of Rachel Cohen-Maso (A) and Dogs Playing for Life™ (B).

reactivity can still be candidates for playgroups. Those behaviors are not considered accurate predictors of aggression or sociability in an off-leash scenario such as playgroups (DPFL n.d.), although this is largely based on anecdotal observations. This would be a worthwhile and important claim to verify in future research on playgroups, especially given the increasing attention on the validity of shelter behavior assessments.

Shabelensky and Segurson (2018) gathered useful data on playgroup population metrics. For example, they found that, on average, 50%

of a shelter's dog population participated in playgroups. The percentage of dogs taken out to participate in playgroups was significantly higher in low-intake shelters versus high-intake shelters. The most common reasons why dogs were not allowed in playgroup activity were aggression to other dogs (78%) and being post-surgical (73%), followed by being "in quarantine" (58%), "lack of dogs with matching play styles" (56%), and illness (54%). Hyperactivity, dog size, and breed restriction were least commonly reported as reasons for exclusion. In addition, if a dog has shown

---

Box 13.1   A Word About "Consent"

It is excellent practice for handlers to assess each dog's willingness to participate in an inter-dog interaction in protected or limited contact prior to introducing them into a playgroup. Often, these assessments may be described as "consent tests" or brief, momentary observations to determine if a dog "consents" to being in a playgroup setting or interacting with another dog. Although the use of this term is motivated by good intentions, it is not scientifically accurate to use "consent" in this context. When this term is used in a psychological, research-based, or legal sense, the participant who "consents" fully understands

the risks and benefits of the activity (American Psychological Association 2020). In addition, inferring that an animal "consents" may run the risk of not attending to subtle cues indicating that the interaction should be intervened in or terminated (e.g., averting gaze, stiffening body, change in tail position). This is not to say that animals do not have the capacity to consent but that in most playgroup settings, it is more accurate, parsimonious, and practically helpful to state that animals are given a *choice* to be in playgroup and a *choice* to leave. It is possible to assess whether all individuals want to continue to participate without ascribing "consent."

offensive aggression to dogs in the past (e.g., ignoring cues of other dogs, pursuing a dog that is actively retreating and/or hiding, seeking out opportunities to aggress when not provoked), they should be eliminated as a playgroup candidate (DPFL n.d.). Dogs who are extremely fearful, do not show signs of progressing socially with repeated playgroup experiences, and/or are deteriorating as a result of the playgroup experience should also be excluded from playgroups. In these cases, such dogs may show clear behavioral indicators of not enjoying the playgroup experience (e.g., hiding throughout the duration of playgroup, cowering, staying in corners, showing reluctance to enter the play yard after repeated exposures, increasing defensive behaviors in response to play). Finally, it is possible that human and personnel factors (e.g., availability of sufficiently trained staff, access to training resources) may also play a role in why the majority of dogs in most shelter populations are not included in playgroup.

'Helper dogs' may be described as social, behaviorally tolerant dogs who also are reliably motivated to engage in play or are tolerant with a wide range of dogs and play styles, including mildly inappropriate behavior from other dogs (DPFL n.d.). As a result, helper dogs may be used in playgroups often or for multiple playgroups. Often, handlers rely on these dogs to "warn or correct obnoxious or aggressive behavior proportionally" (DPFL n.d.). Helper dogs can be overused and may display higher than usual stress levels relative to the average for their playgroup; instead, a playgroup team should make a special effort to identify multiple tolerant dogs to rotate through this role if possible. Overusing helper dogs may also put them at increased risk of injury or physical or behavioral fatigue. In addition, overreliance on helper dogs can sometimes (i) condition handlers to not respond or intervene when needed because of the expectation that the helper dog will deliver the warnings or corrections or (ii) create a reluctancy in handlers to create playgroups made up of new individuals. This

is another reason why carefully rotating the individuals in the group is encouraged.

13.5.4.1 Physical Health Considerations

Playgroups can provide opportunities for physical exercise, which may dramatically reduce stress and disease susceptibility and also improve body condition and other physical health outcomes. When considering *any* enrichment program—not just playgroups—a veterinarian or member of the shelter's medical team should perform a complete physical examination and evaluate the candidate against preestablished selection criteria. Medical staff may need to impose temporary limitations on playgroups when risk of infectious disease is high (e.g., during a disease outbreak, especially in young puppies or other vulnerable populations). Dog-dog playgroups pose a potential risk to the entire shelter population if medical or biological issues are not assessed. Some considerations include the following:

- Dogs who develop or exhibit signs of contagious illness, particularly respiratory disease, should not be considered for playgroup.
- Dogs who have any injuries or painful conditions should not be considered for playgroup. Not only does this pose the risk of worsening a present or potential injury, but it can also reduce a dog's emotional threshold and increase the probability of negatively reinforced aggression toward other dogs.
- Any medications that a dog is on that could have behavioral effects (e.g., psychopharmaceuticals, corticosteroids, pain medications) should be considered and may need to inform how the playgroup should run and the participants included, if the dog is to be included.
- Neuter status, age, weight, size, and sex should be considered when putting dogs into groups, but none of these factors alone should automatically disqualify a dog from being a playgroup candidate.
- If medically cleared, puppies should be included in playgroups, including those with adult dogs who are socially appropriate

(playful, tolerant). This can be critical for teaching puppies bite inhibition and play behavior; puppy-only playgroups or pairings should be supervised to prevent the rehearsal of undesirable behaviors.

In a nationwide survey of US shelters, very few respondents reported that they suspected playgroups contributed to the spread of parvovirus (<1%), distemper (0%), or canine influenza (1%), however, playgroups were occasionally suspected of spreading kennel cough (19%) (Shabelansky and Segurson 2018). To maximize benefits and mitigate risks, the ASV recommends that shelter staff and volunteers follow standard operating procedures and protocols designed with input from the shelter veterinarian to minimize disease transmission. Such protocols should include screening for infectious diseases, medical conditions impacting participation, and other risk factors (e.g., age, vaccination status), as well as implementation of biosecurity practices for dogs, play yards, toys, and equipment. Reporting and tracking of negative outcomes (e.g., bites, injuries, undesirable or detrimental behaviors, and disease transmission) should occur in a formal and transparent manner (ASV 2019).

Physical injuries are an obvious medical concern as well. Fortunately, the incidence of dog-dog aggression—including serious fights—within playgroups appears to be lower than what many might fear. It is possible that control over behavioral and environmental conditions minimizes the risk of inter-dog injury. For example, shelter playgroup rules may include limiting the number of dogs in a play area and carefully selecting dogs who participate in playgroups.

13.5.4.2 Behavioral Health Considerations

When run successfully, playgroups can provide not only physical health benefits, but also behavioral health benefits. These include opportunities for enrichment, behavioral assessment, olfactory stimulation, training, and behavior modification. Quality of playgroups should be emphasized over quantity. It is important to ensure that playgroups do not exceed a higher handler-to-dog ratio than the facility can support or the carrying capacity of the play area. In general, handlers should be able to see the entirety of each dog's body at all times to accurately observe interactions and body language. There should be enough room and space for a dog to not only engage in vigorous, healthy play, but also to escape or avoid an interaction if possible, as well as to use the play yard to perform other enriching behaviors that they may have limited opportunities to do easily in a kennel (smelling, exploring, scent marking, urinating, defecating, etc.). Not only can playgroups lead to calmer behavior and potentially increased motivation and/or attentiveness for training due to expelling extra energy, but also playgroup coordinators who use toys, treats, and praise can capture opportunities for successful recalls and check-ins with the handler, as well as pauses in dog-dog play to reinforce self-regulation of play (e.g., promoting opportunities for the dogs to learn to pause and take breaks during play without handler intervention). Finally, by being among conspecifics, there is also more opportunity for social learning across dogs that can promote positive social interactions.

As with medical history, an individual dog's behavioral history and background must also be considered when determining suitable shelter playgroup candidates. A history of previous serious inter-dog offensive aggression should warrant exclusion. Caution is also warranted when assessing playgroup candidates from dogfighting backgrounds given the prevalence of conspecific aggression in this population. Cautious assessment through protected contact and/or the use of muzzles for a probationary period may be necessary.

One important reminder is that there is such a thing as behavioral flexibility. Through learning and experience, behaviors can come into contact with other sources of reinforcement in the environment and acquire other functions beyond their species-specific purposes. Mounting is an excellent example; it can manifest as a displacement behavior (induced by frustration or a high motivation to engage in a different behavior that is not currently possible). However, it can also be reinforced by conspecific attention, as well as interspecific attention, and may culminate in play. For this reason, for the majority of dogs, no one behavior or historical report should determine their behavioral eligibility to participate in playgroups.

13.5.5 Implementation of Playgroups

The implementation of a successful playgroup can take a wide range of forms. A successful playgroup can be large, small, use toys, use treats, or none of the above. Importantly, individual dogs may respond differently to the same type of playgroup intervention. Playgroups are a dynamic and fluid conversation between dogs and handlers. One should not assume that just because one method of playgroup was successful for a group of dogs one day that it will always be successful, because the players and the context are rarely constant.

For example, the use of any tool that immediately inflicts (or has the potential to inflict) physical pain or discomfort is not consistent with the LIMA principle that anything other than mild aversives should not be used as a first-line or routine intervention, except in cases of imminent safety concerns. If punishment is warranted (e.g., to stop one dog from lunging at, attacking, or injuring another), it will better set the dog up for success if a replacement behavior can also be trained using a reinforcement-based method (e.g., to recall the dog back to the handler after the event). Doing so will not only allow the dog to still obtain reinforcement in the playgroup context, but also help establish and maintain more adaptive behavior rather than simply suppressing the punished behavior (which may also establish handlers as conditioned aversive stimuli). All behaviors—no matter how annoying, aversive, or potentially harmful to humans or other dogs—have a function if they are increasing the future frequency or likelihood of a behavior (reinforcement theory). In addition,

although the term "interrupter" is used often in practice to refer to a stimulus that temporarily prevents or stops a behavior from continuing, it should be noted that this is not necessarily a scientific term in behavioral psychology.

The specific strategies used within the LIMA hierarchy may be different across individual dogs and highly context-specific. For example, water spray bottles may not be effective punishers or disruptors for all dogs. In these cases, stronger aversives may need to be used more quickly. Antecedent interventions (i.e., arranging the animal's environment beforehand) can be accomplished in the form of appropriately matching dogs based on their preferred play styles prior to introducing the dogs to the playgroup setting or walking a dog prior to entering the playgroup. In addition, motivating operations to engage in play should be considered. For example, whether a dog has had an opportunity to appropriately eliminate prior to entering the play yard may affect the dog's motivation to initiate or reciprocate play with conspecifics. Similarly, helper dogs who may participate in several playgroups per day (sometimes back-to-back) may eventually experience a decreased motivation to play or interact with other dogs in successive playgroups. In many cases, dogs who are perfectly tolerant but do not at first appear interested in playing upon arrival to the playgroup often do initiate play following elimination. This is an example of appropriately arranging antecedent interventions and motivating operations to promote and maximize play interactions. In addition, providing opportunities in the environment for dogs to self-regulate their play interaction can be highly enriching as well.

It is worth noting that the application of LIMA in shelter playgroup contexts is debated amongst some shelter professionals. Because LIMA is typically applied to behavior interventions intended to modify behavior over time, it is reasonable to ask whether the use of LIMA is appropriate in shorter-term situations where staff may need to manage behavior without long-term access to the animal. Whether LIMA can be applied successfully in one's facility is an important discussion that shelter professionals should have among behavior teams. These discussions should include a careful consideration of the advantages and disadvantages of each type of playgroup model or when it is appropriate to use a combination of tools. This may include considerations of each individual dog's length of stay in the shelter, the relative likelihood of the dog having access to play and other enriching interactions in the play yard if corrections cannot be used, the number of dogs in the shelter relative to the available staff time, and operations restrictions (e.g., limited time to clean kennels). While humane and ethical management choices must be made, shelter professionals should also be honest with themselves about whether their organization's physical and social environment can support the philosophical preferences or ideals. Well-intended aims must not come at the expense of the functionality of the organization or of providing physical exercise and enrichment opportunities to dogs. Shelters should make the decision that has the greatest overall benefit to the dog's well-being and adoptability, both during their stay in the shelter as well as post-adoption.

Although following a framework and standard protocols is considered best practice for promoting consistency among staff and volunteers, just because staff may be using one model does not mean the playgroup will always be equally enriching or equally restrictive for all dogs participating. Models are arbitrary to the dogs, after all; what they respond to are specific antecedents, behaviors, and consequences (whether internal/physiological or external/environmental), how their environment is arranged, and, of course, individual biological variables. These are the factors relevant in determining what behavioral, physical, and emotional responses the dogs experience during playgroup and will inform shelter professionals whether each individual dog perceives their playgroup experience as an enriching event.

13.5.5.1 Defining and Visualizing "Healthy Play"

As previously mentioned, playgroups are often intended to be a social enrichment strategy for dogs in shelters. Therefore, handlers typically want to observe and promote opportunities for healthy dog-dog play during playgroups. In addition, facilitating appropriate interactions between dogs—if play doesn't occur—would still meet the goals of effective social enrichment. In other words, the opportunity to interact with other dogs in various ways outside of play (e.g., greeting interactions, mutual exploration, mutual resting, and even successfully resolved agonistic interactions) could still be enriching for dogs in playgroups.

Healthy social play in dogs may be defined as simultaneous, reciprocal affiliation between conspecifics that includes at least one of the following components: self-handicapping, inhibited biting, rough-and-tumble play (e.g., wrestling), chasing, and exaggerated predatory behaviors. Self-handicapping occurs when one individual voluntarily uses less advantageous strategies (e.g., inhibition of behaviors) that result in the maintenance or continuation of the interaction (Bekoff and Allen 1998; Burghardt 2005). Examples of these strategies may include a dog choosing to be the target of another dog's chase or positioning their body underneath another dog during wrestling. In addition, agonistic interactions should occur at a very low rate, if at all, during healthy play. Inhibited biting may be defined as oral contact on a conspecific's body without causing injury or distress vocalizations (e.g., whining, yelping). Play wrestling can defined as continuous bodily contact between conspecifics that may include inhibited biting and shaking, growling, and forceful movement that does not result in injury or obvious distress. Notably, this type of activity is often reciprocated by the play partner. Play chasing is defined as running alongside or directly behind a conspecific with a concurrent absence of observable signs of aggression (e.g., snarling, teeth baring with lip curled, raised hackles) or fear or distress (e.g., tail tucking, yelping, whining) from the individual being chased. Finally, low-intensity predatory behavior may include low-intensity and/or incomplete predatory motor patterns (e.g., stalk, chase, bite) that may occur out of sequence, in the absence of observable non-predatory aggressive behaviors, and do not result in intentional injury.

The research on dog-dog play has long fascinated animal behaviorists, evidenced by decades of research on the topic. It is well established that play signals exist in conspecific (dog-dog) social play. Social play can be distinguished by its self-restraint, use of play signals, self-handicapping, and role reversals. There is an inaccurate assumption that play needs to be entirely reciprocal or even appropriate at all times to be true, healthy play. However, in play between adult dogs, older/larger and more dominant dogs rarely self-handicapped and typically adopted "winning" roles more than 50% of the time (Smuts 2014). Most dog play seems to occur in pairs, but in both puppies and adults, third parties sometimes intervene in dyadic play for various reasons (e.g., to gain attention from conspecifics, to prevent an altercation). Smuts (2014) also reported that previous observations at a dog daycare showed that the majority of dog dyads may not always exhibit formal dominance signals in off-leash interactions; however, groups of dogs have been observed to use the same formal dominance signals as those seen in wolves (e.g., high posture by dominant individuals and muzzle licking by subordinate individuals). Smuts (2014) also accurately summarizes that multiple studies of dogs interacting in dog-park-like settings reported the absence of biting, perhaps in part because dogs reconcile to prevent escalation to more severe conflicts. Another reason may be because owners whose dogs engage in such severe aggression may proactively self-select their dogs out of opportunities to engage in off-leash interactions. Although biting may certainly occur without offensive aggression, owners and handlers may nonetheless be

overly cautious about it occurring during play because it is a behavior that can cause physical injury to another dog if applied with sufficient force.

When looking structurally at dog play (i.e., the form of the play), there are some behaviors that have been observed as reliable play signals, including play bows. Play bows are visual signals in dogs originally hypothesized to signal playful intent to another dog, or that whatever behavior was to follow was play (Bekoff 1995). Indeed, in an eight-month study involving two public dog parks, approximately 98% of the play bow occurrences were during play bouts that ended without conflict (Mehrkam et al., unpublished data). More recently, Byosiere et al. (2016) gathered data on 414 play sessions that included play bows between dyads of 16 dogs and found that play bows can function to keep play going but also to allow dogs to pause in a way or posture that affords flexible outcomes. Thus, after a play bow occurs and has been preceded by a pause, more active behavior is likely to follow (Horowitz 2009). It is also possible, as Bekoff (1995) observed, to see increased offensive behavior following a play bow. Byosiere et al. (2016) furthermore suggested that the play bow gives the dog exhibiting the bow a physical advantage to better perform offensive or escape behavior (e.g., by exhibiting a posture that allows the dog to easily change direction).

13.5.5.2 Recognizing Dog-Dog Conflict

Recognizing dog-dog conflict and its precursors is perhaps the most important role of the handler to ensure healthy, "welfare-positive" playgroups. These are playgroups that are enriching to the dogs participating in them by reducing abnormal behaviors or those indicative of stress and promoting opportunities for psychological stimulation and physiological health. Differentiating agonistic or aggressive behaviors from social play requires knowledge of canine ethology and experience managing inter-dog interactions in person, as well as knowledge of context-specific factors that contribute to high-arousal situations. Because play involves patterns that may include agonistic, predatory, sexual, and/ or predator-avoidance behavior (Fagen 1981; Bekoff 2001), recognizing accurate precursors immediately is a challenge and an acquired skill. In fact, Tami and Gallagher (2009) found that owners, trainers, and other experienced animal professionals were unable to accurately distinguish between play and aggression in videos of dog-dog interactions, and, furthermore, were not significantly more accurate than non-owners. Specifically, piloerection, biting, herding, standing over, and showing teeth in the play video were mainly interpreted incorrectly as aggressive cues; in contrast, barking, bouncing, ears held erect and forward, and tail-wagging were often incorrectly interpreted as playful cues. Therefore, improving the ability of people—including those who have professional experience with dog behavior—to accurately recognize behavioral precursors and know the likelihood that a particular behavior will lead to play or aggression is important to maintaining dog welfare.

Though certainly a distinct setting, behavioral research in dog parks can offer information on how play-induced conflict and aggression can be observed when no management or intervention occurs. Of all play types, observational studies show that play wrestling has the highest probability of play-induced aggression, followed by social locomotor play and social object play; nonetheless, all play types pose some level of risk. There are countless resources available on behavioral "red flag" precursors to aggression and/or conflict available. It should be noted, however, that many such resources available may not necessarily be science-based or statistically supported (see Box 13.2 for evidence-based precursors to conflict and/or aggression).

In addition, it is important to acknowledge that dogs may not display overt aggression or fighting but may still display signs of conflict, stress, or discomfort. In these cases, it would also be appropriate to intervene by redirecting

---

> **Box 13.2   Evidence-Based Precursors to Dog-Dog Conflict and/or Aggression During Play**
>
> - Tucked or raised, elevated tail (above body level)
> - Full-body hackles (raised from base of neck to base of tail) combined with a visibly stiff body
> - Fixed stare, accompanied by low growls, lunging, and bite attempts

---

the dog still soliciting play or social interaction (so as to positively reinforce them for social interaction). If possible, both dogs can be redirected simultaneously. This will also help to reinforce the dog that is uncomfortable to check in with a handler or seek a safe space away from the dog. One dog should not be playing at the expense of another. Handlers should pay particular attention to tail position (particularly a tail hanging down or a tucked tail), cowering or hiding under a structure or near a handler/owner, trembling, and one dog repeatedly physically displacing others. It should also be remembered that although play and conflict signals are species-typical, individual dogs will likely have different propensities for showing them depending on their own reinforcement histories.

It is important to keep in mind that no one behavior will be a predictor of a fight 100% of the time, nor will any one behavior always be a predictor of non-aggression. The probability of any one behavior to be an indicator of a fight varies based on the individual dogs involved in a playgroup, the knowledge and skill of the handlers, and each dog's reinforcement history for each behavior. Behavior is highly fluid and dynamic, and while it is helpful to know relative probabilities, behaviors should be thought of as *indicators* of an outcome in a playgroup environment rather than an automatic prescription for how to intervene. Precursors should not necessarily be evaluated in isolation, and the playgroup environment must be evaluated holistically. Nonetheless, consistency is important—in the way dogs are introduced, when tools are employed and how they are used, and the mission and goals within a single playgroup event or dynamic.

As a final note, while even the most successful and enriching playgroups in shelter settings do not come without potential risks, observational and experimental data both in dog parks and in comparing playgroups confirm similar estimates of serious inter-dog fights. Shabelansky and Segurson (2018) found that serious fights that were difficult to break up or resulted in wounds requiring medical attention occurred as follows: 21% reported one serious fight, 33% reported two to five, and 7% reported more than five during the one-year study period. Bites to people also occurred, with 10% of responding shelters reporting one bite and 12% reporting two to five bites during the study period. Despite these findings, the benefits of well-run playgroups overall do appear to outweigh the risks in most shelters.

See Chapter 8 for information on how to safely manage dog-dog and dog-human conflict.

13.5.5.3 Handler Roles and Interventions

It is worth noting the effect that handler roles and interventions can have on the outcome of dog play interactions and the ability to run successful playgroups. Handlers should be astute observers of behavior, be able to implement the playgroup protocol with consistency, and have proficient handling skills. Scientific studies on human-dog play are well established and ever-growing, with evidence of well-recognized play signals between people and dogs as well as between dogs. Understanding human-dog play is still highly relevant to shelter professionals who manage playgroups.

First, the mere presence of a handler attending to the dogs is likely to have an effect on dog-dog social dynamics. Mehrkam et al. (2014) demonstrated that human interaction significantly increased positive social interactions, including social play, between pair-housed wolves and wolf-dog crosses in a sanctuary compared to baseline conditions in which human interaction was not available. In addition, attention from both owners and a less familiar person successfully facilitated social play in working breeds of dogs (Mehrkam et al. 2017).

Handlers should be aware that *specific* behaviors they exhibit during playgroup could potentially be perceived as play invitations by dogs to engage in human-dog play. Although there are clearly obvious play signals that humans can engage in to purposively evoke play in dogs that we may not consider appropriate for playgroup (e.g., bowing or lunging toward the dog), it is important to be aware of more subtle handler behaviors that could evoke play, such as as patting a floor/surface, whispered vocalization, clapping, and chasing/running away, which are all play signals commonly used by dog owners (Rooney et al. 2001). According to Rooney and colleagues, thigh slaps, clicking fingers, pointing, laughing, quickly moving hands ("shoo hands"), stamping feet, shuffling feet, and vertical bows (bending forward and downward until torso is horizontal with waist) were all behaviors exhibited by human handlers that also might occur during human-dog play, albeit these were observed less frequently and were relatively ineffective at evoking play in dogs; nonetheless, these behaviors may be commonly observed by handlers during playgroups. Horowitz and Hecht (2016) analyzed videos of dogs and their owners playing; out of 187 play bouts, they found a diverse range (more than 30 identifiable types) of human-dog play and found that "tease" (defined as a set of actions involving both parties acting in response to each other in a playful manner), "feigning toss" (pretending to toss a ball or a toy), lightly pushing or tapping the dog, "ruffle" (vigorous petting), and vocalizations ("get/got," "play," "yes") all promoted positive affect in pet dogs.

Regardless of whether these function as play signals, it should be acknowledged that these behaviors (among others) could get the dogs' attention and potentially evoke human-dog play and reduce dog-dog play. This in itself is not inherently a problem, especially as human-dog play can increase the enriching value of the playgroup; however, it could compete with a dog's motivation to engage in dog-dog play opportunities during playgroups. This is important to consider if promoting conspecific play opportunities is a major goal of an organization's playgroup program. One could make the argument that the probability of a handler evoking these signals in a playgroup setting is relatively low compared to owners in their homes with their pet dogs. Although dogs who were strays may be suspected to not find humans as relevant or reinforcing, human-dog play is observed in free-roaming village dogs in Mexico (Ruiz-Izaguirre et al. 2014), with 85% of male dogs engaging in play with humans compared to 55% of female dogs. Therefore, dogs with limited training and experience with in-home owners can still be influenced and responsive to human play signals even if the person identified themselves as just a caretaker rather than an owner. We must also be aware that dogs—whether owner surrenders or strays—likely have prior reinforcement histories resulting from playing with humans.

When implementing playgroups, handlers must be careful not to miss red flags or indicators of conflict and intervene appropriately. However, handlers can easily *overmanage* social interactions between dogs during playgroup in ways that may prevent or disrupt healthy play. Incorrect perceptions of dog body language can lead to "false positives" and inappropriate redirection; in this way, being too risk-averse can prevent normal social interactions. For example, Tami and Gallagher (2009) found that play and aggression were the two behaviors that people most often incorrectly reported when viewing videotaped dog-dog interactions. Furthermore, the experience level of the participant (e.g., whether they were dog owners, dog show judges, trainers, veterinarians, or behaviorists) did not significantly affect their accuracy in categorizing inter-dog interactions.

Human handlers must resist the urge to impart their own anthropomorphic perceptions of dog behavior at the expense of enriching play opportunities. Preventing the occurrence of non-harmful species-typical and communicative behavior can lead to frustration, redirected aggression onto another dog or a handler, or simply the loss of a valuable opportunity for exercise and enrichment. Trainers should be aware of these possible intervention effects.

13.5.5.4 Documentation and Evaluation

When monitoring interactions, shelters should consider having their teams document the playgroup dynamics. Documenting and evaluating can be a daunting task, especially when managing multi-dog groups. It is therefore often overlooked or ignored due to time and sometimes the anxiety of not knowing how to best do so or what to look for. Evaluation of any enrichment program, including playgroups, is key to demonstrating its safety and efficacy. Evaluation can come in many different forms, and one does not need to be a PhD-level scientist to do meaningful data collection, documentation, and evaluation of playgroups! At the same time, monitoring the dynamics of the dogs' behavior in the moment is obviously the first priority, so data collection should only be done simultaneously during playgroups when there is a low dog-to-handler ratio. The use of technological tools, such as surveillance cameras or voice-to-text apps on a portable device (phone, tablet, palm pilot, etc.), may also facilitate real-time documentation.

This is where the identification of playgroup goals plays such a helpful and important role. Most playgroup programs aim to provide safe off-leash social interactions for dogs in the population. Assess how many dogs or what percent of the population is included, as well as any incidents of serious conflict or injuries as a start. One might also begin to assess the instances of play that occur. The SPA Inter-Dog Playgroup Guidelines has example summary logs available at www.shelterdogplay.org along with other helpful resources.

When running smaller playgroups and/or when additional staff or volunteers are available for observation, focal samples can also be considered. Focal samples involve observing one or more than one individual continuously and recording everything they do. There can also be value in taking more momentary data. This is a more common approach in field settings where there are lots of individuals and behaviors to observe (as would be the case in a large playgroup). To do this, one could scan the playgroup every minute (or every couple of minutes) and record the number of dogs playing as well as the number of dogs engaging in other behaviors. At first, the dynamics of dog-dog playgroups can make it seem impossible to collect data or document interactions; however, with a bit of practice and patience (and a willingness to readjust as needed) any shelter professional can master this skill. In addition, behavioral scales can be developed to record different dimensions or aspects of inter-dog play (intensity/arousal, duration, quality of play, type of play, etc.).

It is important to realize that some of the greatest benefits of playgroups may not come as snapshots, but in terms of behavior change or progress over time. Therefore, it is good practice to monitor individual dogs' behaviors multiple times and each time they are in playgroups in order to get a continuous understanding of how they are responding and to ensure playgroups remain enriching for each individual dog.

Realistically, shelters are most likely not going to be able to videotape all sessions and meticulously code behaviors as is done in a laboratory setting. However, if possible, shelters might consider mounting surveillance cameras and reviewing them only in cases when a fight or serious injury occurs to dogs or humans. In those cases, replay the video and try to identify antecedents and consequences in order to minimize their likelihood of recurrence.

As with all enrichment, it is essential that shelters are using their evaluations to readjust their playgroup programs as needed. As dynamic as playgroups are (considering the constant influx of dogs in and out of the shelter, as well as temporal changes in behavior and physical needs of individual dogs as they stay in the shelter), no two playgroups may ever be alike. Even if the same dogs are playing, both internal and external factors may be at play that affect the nature and picture of the social relationship for both dogs. In addition, staff and volunteer changes may require adjustments to handler-dog ratios or tools used to ensure all handlers involved are comfortable and well trained in correctly managing playgroups. Operational changes, as well as any changes to the physical environment, may also be needed to adjust the time of day, duration, and location in which playgroups are run so that they are most efficient and most likely to be successful for the organization and specific facility. Psychological flaws in thinking (e.g., belief perseverance, confirmation bias, negativity bias, hindsight bias, and our own reinforcement histories) can all lead us to the temptation to adopt a one-size-fits-all approach, to think one method is inherently better than another, or to resist the need to constantly readjust. It is critical, but challenging, for effective enrichment programs to be flexible and adapt to changes in industry and ethical standards to best meet the needs of the animals they are intended to serve.

13.6 Evaluating Quality of Life and Adoptability

Behaviors indicative of a dog's quality of life in the shelter, while there is some overlap, are not necessarily the same behaviors that correlate or predict length of stay in the shelter (or adoptability). Lying with head down, stretching, and yawning in the kennel have been positively associated with low cortisol levels (Hekman et al. 2021; Gunter et al. 2021), whereas being in the front of the kennel and attending to a person (both of which are associated with shorter length of stay) had no relation to salivary cortisol (Mehrkam et al, unpublished results). In contrast, barking, lip licking, licking self, and standing were all positively correlated with higher salivary cortisol concentrations (Mehrkam et al., unpublished results). One exception to this is play initiation; ignoring play initiation from a potential adopter has been found to be correlated with increased length of stay (Protopopova and Wynne 2014) and may also be a negative indicator of a dog's quality of life.

Anecdotally, it is often claimed that playgroups promote adoptability. For example, DPFL states on their website that two open admission shelters that have successfully implemented DPFL have a live release rate in excess of 95% (DPFL n.d.). Indeed, this effect is easy to imagine, though it is important to remember that correlation does not mean causation. As previously discussed, higher live release rates and shorter lengths of stay do not necessarily mean that dogs possess a higher quality of life during their time in the shelter. Mehrkam et al. (unpublished results) tested whether a pit bull-type dog viewed in playgroup via video was perceived as being more adoptable and having higher welfare compared to the same dog viewed alone in its kennel and in the play yard but interacting with a person with other dogs present. Respondents indicated that they all had an affinity for dogs and more than half indicated they were considering adopting a dog in the near future. Surprisingly, the results showed that the same dog had lower adoptability ratings when viewed in a playgroup than when the dog was viewed in the play yard but interacting with a staff member or when the dog was viewed displaying sociable behaviors in

the kennel (e.g., gazing, tail wagging, rubbing against kennel door, and soliciting interaction). However, participants gave the highest welfare ratings in the playgroup condition, suggesting that playgroups may help potential adopters view a dog as healthier and happier within their shelter environment. Importantly, this may increase positive perceptions of the shelter, but it may also unintentionally decrease a person's inclination to adopt that dog if they perceive them as content in the shelter environment. Collectively, these results suggest that perceptions of adoptability and welfare are distinct measures in their own right. Although programs that improve both adoption and quality of life outcomes for an individual dog are always desired and indeed possible, shelter professionals must keep in mind that the two may not always automatically be improved together. We should be aware that a strategy that improves a potential adopters' perception of the dog's welfare state may not necessarily increase the adopter's likelihood to adopt the dog.

As the industry emphasizes high welfare states and socially conscious sheltering over live release and euthanasia rates, shelters should ensure they are meeting both goals and industry standards for adoptability and welfare. Successful playgroups can be a useful way to address both measures.

13.7 Conclusions

While some of the recommendations in this chapter are evidence-based, there is still so much that remains unknown about the science of playgroups. One interesting aspect that has not yet been fully investigated is how playgroups may affect the wellness of shelter staff and volunteers. Exploring whether or not shelters that run playgroups differ in their levels of employee and volunteer satisfaction, retention, compassion fatigue, burnout, and knowledge and skills related to canine behavior would be an area worthy of future study.

The best playgroup style is the one that matches a shelter's resources, staff knowledge, consistency, and dog population dynamics. Furthermore, assessing staff and/or volunteer availability, skills, and other resources should take place across medical, behavior, and operations teams. It is important to accept and recognize that there is no such thing as a zero-risk playgroup. All playgroups come with some level of risk, but much of that can be prevented by skilled handlers who are knowledgeable about the ethology and structure of behaviors in dogs, as well as how dogs learn about the consequences of their behaviors in individual, dynamic playgroups. Rather than identifying a specific model, it may be more practical for shelter professionals to identify specific goals for a playgroup targeted to the individual dog,

dyad, or group. There is truly a science, but also an art, to running playgroups. It is important for shelters to have easy, manageable ways to evaluate their programs that do not compromise staff time. Playgroups are dynamic, and the method that works for one dog may not work for all. Each dog will respond individually to the set of circumstances and opportunities in the playgroup environment. The right combination of learning principles, experience, knowledge of dog body language, and an awareness of all potential triggers/antecedents and outcomes will help foster the best way to run playgroups.

Please visit the companion website for video clips and downloadable resources associated with this chapter.

References

Affenzeller, N., Palme, R., and Zulch, H. (2017). Playful activity post-learning improves training performance in Labrador retriever dogs (*Canis lupus familiaris*). *Phys. Behav.* 168: 62–73.

American Psychological Association. (2020). APA Dictionary of Psychology: Consent. https://dictionary.apa.org/consent (accessed 26 September 2021).

Association of Shelter Veterinarians. (2019). Playgroups for Shelter Dogs. https://www.sheltervet.org/assets/PDFs/ASV%20Play%20Group%20Position%20Statement%202019.pdf (accessed 26 September 2021).

Bateson, P. (2005). The role of play in the evolution of great apes and humans. In: *The Nature of Play: Great Apes and Humans*. New York: Guilford Press.

Bauer, E.B. and Smuts, B.B. (2007). Cooperation and competition during dyadic play in domestic dogs, *Canis familiaris*. *Anim Behav* 73 (3): 489–499.

Belpedio, C., Buffington, L., Clusman, C. et al. (2010). Effect of multidog play groups on cortisol levels and behavior of dogs (*Canis lupus familiaris*) housed in a humane society. *J. Appl. Comp. Anim. Behav.* 4 (1): 15–27.

Bekoff, M. (1972). The development of social interaction, play, and metacommunication in mammals: An ethological perspective. *Q. Rev. Biol.* 47 (4): 412–434.

Bekoff, M. (1974). Social play and play-soliciting by infant canids. *Amer. Zool.* 14 (1): 323–340.

Bekoff, M. (1995). Play signals as punctuation: The structure of social play in canids. *Behav.* 132 (5–6): 419–429.

Bekoff, M. (2000). Animal emotions: Exploring passionate natures: Current interdisciplinary research provides compelling evidence that many animals experience such emotions as joy, fear, love, despair, and grief—we are not alone. *Bioscience* 50 (10): 861–870.

Bekoff, M. (2001). Social play behaviour. Cooperation, fairness, trust, and the evolution of morality. *J. Conscious. Stud.* 8 (2): 81–90.

Bekoff, M. (2004). Wild justice and fair play: Cooperation, forgiveness, and morality in animals. *Biol. Phil.* 19 (4): 489–520.

Bekoff, M. and Allen, C. (1998). Intentional communication and social play: How and why animals negotiate and agree to play. In: *Animal Play: Evolutionary, Comparative, and*

Ecological Perspectives (eds. M. Bekoff and J.A. Byers), 97–114. Cambridge, UK: Cambridge University Press.

Bekoff, M. and Byers, J.A. (1981). A critical reanalysis of the ontogeny and phylogeny of mammalian social and locomotor play: An ethological hornet's nest. In: *Behavioral Development: The Bielefeld Interdisciplinary Project* (eds. K. Immelmann, G.W. Barlow, L. Petrinovich et al.), 296–337. Cambridge, UK: Cambridge University Press.

Bekoff, M. and Byers, J. (1998). *Animal Play: Evolutionary, Comparative, and Ecological Perspectives*. Cambridge, UK: Cambridge University Press.

Bjorklund, D.F. and Rosenberg, J.S. (2005). The role of developmental plasticity in the evolution of human cognition: Evidence from enculturated, juvenile great apes. In: *Origins of the Social Mind: Evolutionary Psychology and Child Development* (eds. B.J. Ellis and D.F. Bjorklund), 45–75. New York: Guilford Press.

Blackwell, E.J., Twells, C., Seawright, A. et al. (2008). The relationship between training methods and the occurrence of behavior problems, as reported by owners, in a population of domestic dogs. *J. Vet. Behav.* 3 (5): 207–217.

Bruner, J.S. (1972). Nature and uses of immaturity. *Am. Psychol.* 27 (8): 687.

Burghardt, G. (2005). *The Genesis of Animal Play*. Cambridge, MA: MIT Press.

Byosiere, S.E., Espinosa, J., and Smuts, B. (2016). Investigating the function of play bows in adult pet dogs (*Canis lupus familiaris*). *Behav. Proc.* 125: 106–113.

Carpenter, C.R. (1934). A field study of the behavior and social relations of howling monkeys. In: Comparative Psychology Monographs, 1905–1975. Baltimore, MD: Johns Hopkins Press.

Casey, R.A., Mendl, M.T., and Blackwell, E.J. (accepted for publication). Dogs are more "pessimistic" if their owners use two or more aversive training methods. *Sci. Rep.*

Cooper, J.J., Cracknell, N., Hardiman, J. et al. (2014). The welfare consequences and efficacy of training pet dogs with remote electronic training collars in comparison to reward based training. *PLOS ONE* 9 (9): p.e102722.

Coppinger, L. and Coppinger, R. (2001). *Dogs: A New Understanding of Canine Origin, Behaviour and Evolution*. Chicago, IL: University of Chicago Press.

Cordoni, G. (2009). Social play in captive wolves (*Canis lupus*): Not only an immature affair. *Behav.* 146: 1363–1385.

de Waal, F.B.M. (1992). Appeasement, celebration, and food sharing in the two *Pan* species. In: *Topics in Primatology*, vol. 1, *Human Origins* (eds. T. Nishida, W.C. McGrew, P. Marler et al.), 37–50. Tokyo, Japan: University of Tokyo Press.

Dogs Playing for Life. (n.d.). Dogs Playing for Life Manual. https://dogsplayingforlife.com/dpfl-manual/ (accessed 26 September 2021).

Dugatkin, L.A. (2014). *Principles of Animal Behavior*, 3rd ed. New York: W.W. Norton.

Dwyer, P.D. and Minnegal, M. (2021). Relationship between wild-living and village-living dogs in New Guinea. *Proc. Natl. Acad. Sci.* https://doi.org/10.1073/pnas.2020432118.

Fagen, R. (1981). *Animal Play Behavior*. New York: Oxford University Press.

Ferguson, D.L. and Rosales-Ruiz, J. (2001). Loading the problem loader: The effects of target training and shaping on trailer-loading behavior of horses. *J. Appl. Behav. Anal.* 34 (4): 409–423.

Fox, M.W. (1970). A comparative study of the development of facial expressions in canids: Wolf, coyote and foxes. *Behav.* 36: 49–73.

Gunter, L.M., Gilchrist, R.J., Blade, E.M. et al. (2021). Investigating the impact of brief outings on the welfare of dogs living in US shelters. *Animals* 11 (2): 548.

Hall, S. (1998). Object play by adult animals. In: *Animal Play: Evolutionary, Comparative, and Ecological Perspectives* (eds. M. Bekoff and J. Byers), 45–60. Cambridge, UK: Cambridge University Press.

Harcourt, R. (1991). Survivorship costs of play in the South American fur seal. *Anim. Behav.* 42: 509–511.

Hekman, J.P., Karas, A.Z., and Dreschel, N.A. (2012). Salivary cortisol concentrations and behavior in a population of healthy dogs hospitalized for elective procedures. *Appl. Anim. Behav. Sci.* 141 (3–4): 149–157.

Held, S.D.E. and Spinka, M. (2011). Animal play and animal welfare. *Anim. Behav.* 81: 891–899.

Hinde, R.A. (1974). *Biological Basis of Human Social Behaviour*. New York: McGraw-Hill.

Horowitz, A. (2009). Attention to attention in domestic dog (*Canis familiaris*) dyadic play. *Anim. Cogn.* 12 (1): 107–118.

Horowitz, A. and Hecht, J. (2016). Examining dog–human play: The characteristics, affect, and vocalizations of a unique interspecific interaction. *Anim. Cogn.* 19 (4): 779–788.

Hoy, J.M., Murray, P.J., and Tribe, A. (2010). Thirty years later: Enrichment practices for captive mammals. *Zoo Biol.* 29 (3): 303–316.

International Association of Animal Behavior Consultants. (2018). IAABC Statement on LIMA. https://m.iaabc.org/about/position-statements/lima/ (accessed 26 September 2021).

Johnson, A.K., Dougherty, H.C., Sunday, P. et al. (2013). Independent study 490A: Do play groups for shelter dogs reduce in-kennel arousal and excitability levels? *Iowa State University Animal Industry Report* 10 (1).

Käufer, M. (2014). *Canine Play Behavior: The Science of Dogs at Play*. Wenatchee, WA: Dogwise Publishing.

Matsusaka, T. (2004). When does play panting occur during social play in wild chimpanzees? *Primates* 45 (4): 221–229.

McCune, L. (1998). Immediate and ultimate functions of physical activity play. *Child Dev.* 69 (3): 601–603.

Mehrkam, L.R. and Dorey, N.R. (2014). Is preference a predictor of enrichment efficacy in Galapagos tortoises (*Chelonoidis nigra*)? *Zoo Biol.* 33 (4): 275–284.

Mehrkam, L.R. and Dorey, N.R. (2015). Preference assessments in the zoo: Keeper and staff predictions of enrichment preferences across species. *Zoo Biol.* 34 (5): 418–430.

Mehrkam, L.R., Hall, N.J., Haitz, C. et al. (2017). The influence of breed and environmental factors on social and solitary play in dogs (*Canis lupus familiaris*). *Learn. Behav.* 45 (4): 367–377.

Mehrkam, L.R., Perez, B.C., Self, V.N. et al. (2020). Functional analysis and operant treatment of food guarding in a pet dog. *J. Appl. Behav. Anal.* 53 (4): 2139–2150.

Mehrkam, L.R., Verdi, N.T., and Wynne, C.D. (2014). Human interaction as environmental enrichment for pair-housed wolves and wolf–dog crosses. *J. Appl. Anim. Welf. Sci.* 17 (1): 43–58.

Mehrkam, L.R. and Wynne, C.D. (2021). Owner attention facilitates social play in dog–dog dyads (*Canis lupus familiaris*): Evidence for an interspecific audience effect. *Anim. Cogn.* 24 (2): 341–352.

Mellen, J. and MacPhee, M.S. (2001). Philosophy of environmental enrichment: Past, present, and future. *Zoo Biol.* 20 (3): 211–226.

Mendoza-Granados, D. and Sommer, V. (1995). Play in chimpanzees of the Arnhem zoo: Self-serving compromises. *Primates* 36 (1): 57–68.

Muller-Schwarze, D., Stagge, B., and Muller-Schwarze, C. (1982). Play behavior: Persistence, decrease, and energetic compensation during food shortage in deer fawns. *Science* 215 (4528): 85–87.

Palagi, E. (2007). Play at work: Revisiting data focusing on chimpanzees (*Pan troglodytes*). *J. Anthropol. Sci.* 85: 63–81.

Palagi, E. (2008). Sharing the motivation to play: The use of signals in adult bonobos. *Anim. Behav.* 75 (3): 887–896.

Palagi, E., Antonacci, D., and Cordoni, G. (2007). Fine-tuning of social play in juvenile lowland gorillas (*Gorilla gorilla gorilla*). *Dev. Psychobiol.* 49 (4): 433–445.

Palagi, E., Tommaso Paoli, T., and Borgognini Tarli, S. (2006). Short-term benefits of play behavior and conflict prevention in *Pan paniscus*. *Int. J. Primatol.* 27 (5): 1257–1270.

Panksepp, J., Siviy, S., and Normansell, L. (1985). The psychobiology of play: Theoretical and methodological perspectives. *Neurosci. Biobehav. Rev.* 8 (4): 465–492.

Pellegrini, A.D., Dupuis, D., and Smith, P.K. (2007). Play in evolution and development. *Develop Rev.* 27 (2): 261–276.

Pellis, S.M. and Iwaniuk, A.N. (1999). The problem of adult play-fighting: A comparative analysis of play and courtship in primates. *Ethology* 105: 783–806.

Pellis, S.M. and Iwaniuk, A.N. (2004). Evolving a playful brain: A levels of control approach. *Int. J. Comp. Psychol.* 17: 92–118.

Protopopova, A. (2016). Effects of sheltering on physiology, immune function, behavior, and the welfare of dogs. *Physiol. Behav.* 159: 95–103.

Protopopova, A. and Wynne, C.D.L. (2014). Adopter-dog interactions at the shelter: Behavioral and contextual predictors of adoption. *Appl. Anim. Behav. Sci.* 157:109–116.

Protopopova, A. and Wynne, C.D. (2015). Improving in-kennel presentation of shelter dogs through response-dependent and response-independent treat delivery. *J. Appl. Behav. Anal.* 48 (3): 590–601.

Romero, T., Nagasawa, M., Mogi, K. et al. (2015). Intranasal administration of oxytocin promotes social play in domestic dogs. *Commun. Integr.* 8 (3): p.e1017157.

Rooney, N.J., Bradshaw, J.W.S., and Robinson, I. H. (2001). Do dogs respond to play signals given by humans? *Anim. Behav.* 61 (4): 715–722.

Ruiz-Izaguirre, E., Bokkers, E.A., Ortolani, A. et al. (2014). Human–dog interactions and behavioural responses of village dogs in coastal villages in Michoacán, Mexico. *Appl. Anim. Behav. Sci.* 154: 57–65.

Shabelansky, A. and Segurson, S. (2018). The Use, Safety and Perception of Dog Playgroups in Animal Shelters. https://www.maddiesfund.org/dog-playgroups-in-animal-shelters.htm (accessed 26 September 2021).

Shelter Playgroup Alliance. (2019). Inter-Dog Playgroup Guidelines. https://www.shelterdogplay.org/shelter-playgroup-alliance-guidelin (accessed 26 September 2021).

Shepherdson, D.J. (1998). Tracing the path of environmental enrichment in zoos. In: *Second Nature: Environmental Enrichment for Captive Animals.* (eds. D.J. Shepherdson, J.D. Mellen, and M. Hutchins), 1–12. Washington, DC: Smithsonian Institution Press.

Smith, L.K., Fantella, S.-L.N., and Pellis, S.M. (1999). Playful defensive responses in adult male rats depend on the status of the unfamiliar opponent. *Aggress. Behav.* 25 (2): 141–152.

Smith, P.K. (1982). Does play matter? Functional and evolutionary aspects of animal and human play. *Behav. Brain Sci.* 5: 139–184.

Smuts, B. (2014). Social behaviour among companion dogs with an emphasis on play. In: *The Social Dog: Behavior and Cognition* (eds. J. Kaminski and S. Marshall-Pescini), 105–130. Cambridge, UK: Academic Press.

Spinka, M., Newberry, R.C., and Bekoff, M. (2001). Mammalian play: Training for the unexpected. *Q. Rev. Biol.* 76 (2): 141–168.

Stamps, J. (1995). Motor learning and the adaptive value of familiar space. *Am. Nat.* 146: 41–58.

Tami, G. and Gallagher, A. (2009). Description of the behaviour of domestic dog (*Canis familiaris*) by experienced and inexperienced people. *Appl. Anim. Behav. Sci.* 120 (3–4): 159–169.

Thompson, K.V. (1996). Play-partner preferences and the function of social play in infant sable antelope, *Hippotragus niger. Anim. Behav.* 52: 1143–1152.

Udell, M.A.R., Ewald, M., Dorey, N.R. et al. (2014). Exploring breed differences in dogs (*Canis familiaris*): Does exaggeration or inhibition of predatory response predict performance on human-guided tasks? *Anim. Behav.* 89: 99–105.

Vanderschuren, L.J., Niesink, R.J., and Van Pee, J.M. (1997). The neurobiology of social play behavior in rats. *Neurosci. Biobehav. Rev.* 21 (3): 309–326.

Vollmer, T.R. (2002). Punishment happens: Some comments on Lerman and Vorndran's review. *J. Appl. Behav. Anal.* 35 (4): 469–473.

Ward, C., Bauer, E.B., and Smuts, B.B. (2008). Partner preferences and asymmetries in social play among domestic dog, *Canis lupus familiaris*, littermates. *Anim. Behav.* 76 (4): 1187–1199.

Part IV

Cats in the Shelter

14

Handling Shelter Cats

Brenda Griffin

14.1 Introduction to Safe and Humane Handling

When it comes to handling cats in the shelter, handler safety must always be a high priority. Many shelters receive large numbers of cats with unknown health histories, including individuals that display aggressive behaviors. These animals can be challenging to handle and pose substantial safety risks to untrained and unskilled staff who attempt to do so. Not only are bites and scratches painful, a variety of serious zoonotic diseases are associated with cat-related injuries. Transmission of diseases such as rabies and cat scratch fever may occur, and cat bite wounds frequently result in serious bacterial infections, all of which may be life-threatening. For these reasons, the use of handling techniques that protect the handler by minimizing the risk of scratches and bites is essential.

Historically, a variety of techniques have been used to handle cats in shelters, ranging from gentle handling of tractable cats to the routine use of cat tongs and rabies poles for moving or restraining cats. The "pole and boot" technique was a particularly aggressive method used by some shelters to restrain cats at the time of euthanasia. It involves placing and tightening the loop of a rabies pole around a cat's neck or thorax, using the pole to pull them from their enclosure to the floor, and finally stepping on their hindquarters to restrain them while injecting euthanasia solution into the cat's chest. Methods such as this might be safe for the handler if executed without error, but certainly are neither safe nor humane for the cat and should never be used today. In particular, forceful handling must always be avoided, and rabies poles should never be used for capture or handling because they can cause serious, even fatal, injuries as well as emotional distress to cats. "Scruffing" cats is a more widely used restraint technique. With this method, the handler grasps the cat by the scruff of the neck with one hand while holding their hind feet in the opposite hand. The cat is then stretched out longways on their side across a table or other surface (see Figure 14.1). Though less extreme than the "pole and boot" technique, many cats experience unnecessary fear and stress when restrained in this manner, increasing the odds of defensive aggression and handler injury. Techniques such as this are still taught and used today, yet they are rarely necessary or appropriate, and their use should be avoided.

Over the past three decades, science has greatly expanded our understanding of cat behavior, which has led to the development

Animal Behavior for Shelter Veterinarians and Staff, Second Edition. Edited by Brian A. DiGangi, Victoria A. Cussen, Pamela J. Reid, and Kristen A. Collins.
© 2022 John Wiley & Sons, Inc. Published 2022 by John Wiley & Sons, Inc.
Companion website: www.wiley.com/go/digangi/animal

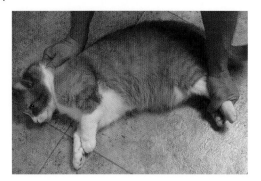

Figure 14.1 A handler restrains a cat on his side by holding the scruff of his neck and hind feet while leaning over him. With no control in his current situation, this cat is experiencing stress and fear as reflected by his facial tension, large round pupils, and twitching tail. In this state, he is more likely to struggle and fight to attempt to escape—posing a safety risk to the handler and himself. Restraint such as this should not be used.

Box 14.1   Benefits of "Low-Stress" or "Fear-Free" Handling

- Enhances animal care by reducing animal stress and fear
- Improves handler safety
- Reduces handler stress
- Improves animal safety and welfare
- Improves tractability with repeated handling of animals
- Facilitates adoption
- Enhances community reputation and relations

and use of improved handling techniques. We now understand that cats commonly experience fear, anxiety, stress, and frustration in animal shelters. These negative emotional states are the reasons that they struggle and resist restraint or behave aggressively when they are handled. In contrast, cats that are not highly stressed or afraid remain relatively calm during handling and are less likely to struggle, scratch, and bite. For this reason, handling techniques that minimize fear, anxiety, stress, and frustration (often referred to as "low-stress" or "fear-free" methods) improve handler safety. Of note, when handling is minimally stressful for animals, they are more likely to accept and respond positively to repeated handling over time. This is a crucial consideration in shelters, where animals may require frequent handling, and further enhances staff safety as well as animal welfare and adoptability. Box 14.1 contains a list of benefits of these techniques.

The term "low-stress handling" was originally coined by the late Dr. Sophia Yin, a veterinarian and animal behaviorist who was an expert and pioneer in developing and disseminating information on these techniques. The term "Fear Free" was coined by Dr. Marty Becker, a veterinarian and founder of an educational company by the same name, which provides online training courses related to decreasing fear, anxiety, and stress in pets in numerous contexts where animals are handled. Of particular note, the Fear Free Shelter Program (https://fearfreeshelters.com) provides online training and resources at no cost to shelter staff and volunteers. Some education companies and several professional organizations also provide online educational resources aimed at reducing cat stress associated with care and handling, including the American Association of Feline Practitioners (AAFP), the American Society for the Prevention of Cruelty to Animals, the International Society of Feline Medicine, and the CATalyst Council (see Box 14.2). Finally, some professional organizations as well as a number of authors have published guidelines, journal articles, and book chapters describing techniques and methods to reduce feline stress and fear during handling and care (Carney et al. 2012; Ellis et al. 2013; Ellis and Sparkes 2016; Griffin 2020; Griffin 2011; Griffin and Hume 2006; Hammerle et al. 2015; Herron and Shreyer 2014; Lloyd 2017; Overall et al. 2004; Rodan 2010; Rodan et al. 2011; Yin 2009).

Box 14.2   Online Educational Resources and Videos

American Association of Feline Practitioners (https://catvets.com)
  Feline Friendly Practice Program educational resources and videos https://catvets.com/education/online/videos

American Society for the Prevention of Cruelty to Animals (http://aspcapro.org)
  Humane handling videos and webinars available by searching this site

International Society of Feline Medicine (https://icatcare.org)
  Cat Friendly Clinic Program educational resources and videos
  https://catfriendlyclinic.org/vets-nurses/handling-of-cats/

CATalyst Council (http://www.catalystcouncil.org)
  Cat Friendly Practice educational resources and videos
  http://www.catalystcouncil.org/resources/health_welfare/cat_friendly_practices/

Fear Free Shelter Program (https://fearfreeshelters.com)
  Complimentary comprehensive online courses and resources for shelter staff and volunteers including recommendations for Fear Free handling, housing, behavioral care, monitoring, and more

Low Stress Handling University (www.lowstresshandling.com)
  Fee-based certification in low-stress handling, developed by Sophia Yin, DVM

Minimizing fear, anxiety, stress, and frustration in animals should always be a high priority for shelters. Indeed, safe and humane handling is a key requirement for animal health and well-being. Although it is not possible to completely eliminate animals' negative emotional reactions, a great deal can be done to promote a "low-stress" or "fear-free" environment. It may be tempting to think that creating such an environment would be too time-consuming, difficult, or expensive in the context of a busy shelter. To the contrary; there are many simple, practical, and inexpensive approaches that can make a huge difference in terms of reducing animal stress and fear, enhancing comfort, and making cats easier to handle, work with, and care for in the shelter.

For these reasons, shelters should have protocols in place to minimize feline stress beginning prior to their arrival at the shelter and continuing throughout their stay. Staff should be trained to be proactive and encouraged to always think ahead to minimize stress and fear. Even small changes in a shelter's practices and its environment have the potential to dramatically impact the well-being and behavior of cats. Shelters should have policies and protocols in place for environmental management of animal stress and fear, including safe and humane handling of cats. Of course, there will always be some individuals for which reducing stress and fear is more difficult. Therefore, in addition to general protocols, special protocols should also be established for those animals displaying signs of severe stress and fear, including feral-behaving animals. Protocols should be flexible enough to allow staff to meet the needs of individual cats whenever possible. Staff training should include working with animal models to practice using handling techniques and tools before attempting to use them on cats.

This chapter briefly reviews common triggers for fear, anxiety, stress, and frustration in shelter cats and the impact on their health and behavior. In particular, it describes how cats perceive the environment and how they communicate their emotional feelings. With regard to handling cats in the shelter, concepts, guidelines, techniques, and tools for reducing these negative emotional states are presented and discussed, including environmental management and handling cats of varying levels of tractability and socialization during routine movement, intake procedures, daily care, and euthanasia. The time invested in learning these concepts and techniques will ultimately lead to safer, more humane, and more efficient animal care. The best possible results will be achieved when the entire shelter team embraces and implements stress reduction protocols and humane handling techniques.

14.2 Triggers for Stress, Fear, and Other Negative Emotional States in the Shelter

Admission to any shelter is a stressful event because of the sudden and dramatic change in environment. The strange sights, smells, and sounds combined with the presence of unfamiliar people and animals trigger stress, which is often accompanied by feelings of fear, anxiety, and even frustration. Virtually all cats experience at least some degree of stress when they enter a shelter. Triggers for stress, fear, and other negative emotional states in the shelter include transport; confinement in a new environment; social isolation; strange smells; noises; other animals; diet changes; handling; restraint; irregular caregiving schedules; unpredictable events; crowding; changes in temperature, light pattern, and/or ventilation; illness; the absence of familiar human contact; and the presence of unfamiliar human contact. In fact, anything unfamiliar to a cat can trigger the stress response. In addition, when cats are housed in shelters, stress and frustration frequently arise from the lack of opportunities they

possess for engaging in activities that would help them to feel better or cope. For example, a cat may be motivated to retreat to a quiet spot for a nap but have no option to do so. She may be unable to move to a comfortable location where she could feel safe and escape the sounds of barking dogs.

14.2.1 Impact on Health and Behavior

Stress and related negative emotional states can have a profound influence on both health and behavior. Acutely, these negative emotional states are accompanied by catecholamine (also known as adrenalin) release, which prepares the body for "fight" or "flight." Catecholamine release increases heart and respiratory rate, as well as blood pressure, while influencing behavioral responses. When acutely stressed, cats may hide, refuse to eat, attempt to escape, or behave aggressively. On occasion, they may temporarily freeze, and some may remain frozen, immobile, and "shut down" in a catatonic-like state of helplessness—in this state, they may be unable to move or respond as a result of overwhelming stress and fear. For some, a single traumatic event such as forceful handling results in a learned negative association, which could make handling and care much more difficult in the future. In contrast, if stress and fear are minimized, animals are calmer and more tractable, facilitating the delivery of efficient quality care. If chronically stressed, cats may develop serious, ongoing behavior problems and remain difficult to handle throughout their shelter stay.

In addition to affecting the emotional health and well-being of cats, stress and related negative emotional states can have a significant impact on physical health (Sparkes et al. 2016; Horwitz and Rodan 2018). Acute stress is known to reduce appetite, induce gastrointestinal upset, and exacerbate existing medical conditions including heart disease, hormone imbalances, urinary tract disease, and allergies. Stress is intimately related to immunity, and when stress persists, it compromises the immune system, lowering resistance to infection. The link between stress and feline respiratory disease (especially infection with feline herpesvirus-1) is well known. Simply stated, stressed shelter cats are more likely to develop upper respiratory disease—and take longer to recover—compared to those who experience less stress. Indeed, reducing stress not only improves the behavior of shelter cats, it also reduces the incidence and severity of respiratory disease, further facilitating handling, care, and adoption.

14.2.2 Understanding Cat Communication Signals and Emotions

Communication is the transfer of information from one individual to another when an individual sends or emits a signal that may modify another individual's behavior. Signals carry information that the individual wants to convey as well as information about the internal state of the signaler (Landsberg et al. 2013). Cats use auditory, visual, olfactory, and tactile signals to communicate. Carefully observing what cats are and are not doing is key to understanding their communication signals. Caregivers must strive to understand feline communication so that they can respond properly to the different signals emitted by cats (Landsberg et al. 2013).

Individual cats display a wide variety of emotional reactions in the shelter environment depending on their genetic makeup, personality, level of socialization, and past experiences. In other words, what one cat finds distressful, versus positively stimulating or even relaxing, will be different from one individual to the next. With training and experience, staff can ascertain a great deal about a cat's emotional state by observing their behavior: behavior is a reflection of emotional state. Cats actively communicate how they are feeling through a constant stream of signals, the most obvious of which involve changes in their body postures and vocalizations. When they experience stress

and fear, they generally become tense—their bodies stiffen, and tension can also be seen in their faces. As stress/fear increase, their pupils become increasingly large and round, their eyes widen more and more, and their ears tend to flatten and shift sideways or rotate back. Some individuals remain silent, while others may growl, hiss, or even scream.

In addition to active communication, cats also communicate passively. Passive communication includes behavioral inhibition or "lack of behavior" such as freezing in place, avoiding contact, or failing to perform routine maintenance behaviors such as eating and grooming, and physiologic changes that one might discover through careful observation or physical examination. For example, one might notice rapid breathing and dilated pupils in a fearful cat. Excessive shedding is also common when cats are nervous or otherwise stressed. A careful observer can deduce what an individual animal is experiencing emotionally by accurately interpreting body language and vocalizations, as well as by understanding these more passive forms of communication.

It is important to recognize that there are many ways that cats communicate stress and related emotional states—behavioral responses will vary among individuals. The "four Fs" are used to describe common types of behaviors associated with stress and fear: fight, flight, fret/fidget, and freeze behaviors. Some cats display "fight" behaviors including struggling, growling, hissing, scratching, or biting. Such aggressive behavior is their attempt to drive away a perceived threat. Others display "flight behaviors." In this case, they may cower, look away, and move away as they attempt to escape or hide, or otherwise try to avoid or evade contact. Still others display "fret or fidget" behaviors— they might move restlessly, pacing or shifting about. A careful observer might notice their eyes scanning the environment or that they nervously lick their lips. Finally, some display "freeze" behaviors. These cats should not be mistaken as relaxed, instead they are tense and frozen. Many stressed and fearful cats display a mixture of fight, flight, fret/fidget, and freeze behaviors. The presence of these behaviors tells us that the cat is stressed and fearful, and not that they are "mean," "nasty," or unsocialized. When one sees these behaviors, they should respond with compassion, adjusting their interactions with the animal to reduce their perception of a threat, for example by moving away from them and giving them more space. In addition, an attempt should be made to ascertain additional triggers in the environment that may be contributing to the cat's stress and fear so that steps can be taken to reduce or eliminate them as soon as possible.

14.2.3 Environmental Management

The goal of environmental management is to minimize environmental triggers for stress and fear in order to help cats stay calmer and more relaxed. The calmer the cat, the easier they will be to handle. By reducing cat fear and stress, the handler optimizes safety and increases the odds of safe and humane ("low-stress") interactions with the cat. Safe and humane handling begins with understanding the potential impact of the shelter environment on cat behavior. Staff can learn to prevent and minimize negative emotional responses by carefully considering how cats are likely to perceive the environment and making adjustments to avoid or mitigate potential stressors and fear inducing stimuli. When staff are observant and in tune with how the environment, as well as their own actions, impact cat stress, they can take simple, practical steps to mitigate it.

Not only does a cat's response to environmental stimuli depend on their unique self, it also depends on the severity and number of given environmental stressors, as well as their duration of exposure to them. Obviously, the more severe the stress and the longer it lasts, the more difficult it is for cats to cope and the

more likely they will be to suffer harmful effects from it. When stress is perceived as inescapable, uncontrollable, or unpredictable, it is especially severe. That said, cats can cope with new and novel stimuli provided that fear responses are not overwhelming or sensitizing. It is especially helpful for staff to critically consider the environment from the cats' perspective. Thinking in terms of what they are experiencing—what they are hearing, smelling, seeing, and feeling—is a key to environmental management for stress reduction and successful handling.

14.2.3.1 Cats' Senses and Perceptions
The ways in which cats hear, smell, taste, and see, as well as their sense of touch, influence their perception of the world around them and greatly influence how they feel emotionally and how they behave. Understanding how cats' senses contribute to their perceptions goes a long way toward helping staff manage the environment so that it is less intimidating and more relaxing for them. Chapter 2 provides a detailed review of the uniquely specialized senses of cats. Box 14.3 contains a brief summary of cats' senses and perceptions and highlights simple means of management.

14.3 Keys to Successful Handling

Safe and humane handling and restraint of cats of varying ages, personality types, social experiences and stress/fear levels requires skill, knowledge of normal feline behavior and communication, and flexibility. Knowing when to ask for help and when and how to properly use tools or equipment for handling is also essential. Staff members should be well trained to recognize signs of stress and fear in cats and to mitigate them through environmental management, positive, calming interactions, and the use of appropriate distractions and rewards. Cat savvy caregivers who are

---

Box 14.3   Understanding Cats' Senses and Managing Their Perceptions

Hearing

- Highly sensitive to sounds: loud and novel noises including the sounds of other animals, such as barking, increase stress and fear.
- Keen sense of hearing—they may hear things we do not.
- Management: minimize loud and sudden noises; use white noise to blunt loud sounds.

Smell

- Highly sensitive to odors: strong and noxious odors increase stress and fear. Odors and pheromones from other animals may also increase stress and fear.
- Keen sense of smell—they may smell things we do not.
- The smell of tasty treats can help them feel better.
- Management: avoid strong and noxious odors. Provide pleasant odors. Spot clean to preserve familiar scent.

Taste

- Especially attracted to meats including fish and liver: both taste and smell make these pleasant and rewarding.
- Management: offer delicious foods to entice, distract, and reward cats.

Vision

- Highly sensitive to motion: rapid movements increase stress and fear.
- Greater peripheral vision: they may see things around them that we do not.
- Management: move slowly, calmly, and deliberately; avoid threatening postures; block stressful visual stimuli (e.g., close doors to block outside activity or gently place a towel over a cat to provide a visual shield)

Touch

- Highly sensitive to approach and touch. They may feel threatened if we lean over them, approach head on, or get too close too fast.
- Certain areas of the body tend to be especially sensitive including the feet, mouth, genitals, and belly.
- Management: use slow, steady contact while avoiding rapid stroking, sudden manipulations, or overly restrictive restraint; avoid contact with areas of the body that tend to be most sensitive.

---

comfortable around cats and who are patient and creative may find that they are particularly adept at working with cats in a safe and humane manner.

In all cases, success begins with developing a clear, scientifically valid understanding of why and how cats behave and respond as they do in the context of being handled in a shelter. Once this is well understood, one can then understand and apply key concepts of safe and humane handling. These key concepts involve reducing feline stress and fear by:

- Going slow when working with cats
- Ensuring that cats maintain a sense of control and perceive that escape or hiding is possible
- Minimizing physical restraint
- Continually observing body language, apprising behavior, and adjusting handling accordingly.

By applying the following knowledge and concepts, shelters can successfully reduce cat stress and fear, while optimizing handling safety.

14.3.1 Understanding Feline Stress and Fear Responses

Imagine what it would be like if your body automatically released adrenaline into your blood stream anytime you experienced something the least bit new or unusual. Suddenly, when you least expected it, you might find your heart pounding in your chest, your cheeks flushing, your respiratory rate increasing, and your palms sweating. With all of that adrenaline coursing through your system, you might be jumpy, defensive, or otherwise reactive. And, if your adrenaline continued to flow while you were uneasy, you just might begin to panic. This is what it feels like to be a cat in the unfamiliar, unpredictable environment of a shelter. Compared to many other domestic species, cats have heightened fight or flight responses. They are biologically programmed to release epinephrine (adrenaline) into their bloodstream when they feel even the least bit apprehensive, fueling their bodies for fight or flight on a moment's notice. When stress or fear is triggered, cats are literally hardwired for escape or defense. If they feel threatened and perceive that they cannot escape the threat, their response is heightened even more, and they are much more likely to behave aggressively.

When working with cats, it is crucial to keep in mind that aggressive responses do not occur simply because a particular cat is "mean," "nasty," poorly socialized, or feral. They occur because cats are sensitive and responsive to perceived danger regardless of their level of socialization. Indeed, experiencing apprehension, stress, or fear is not a willful act. These involuntary emotional reactions result in epinephrine (adrenaline) release, and the behavior that follows is the result of biochemical activation of the stress response. As such, it is crucial not to take the behavior of cats personally. Instead, we must remember that behaviors associated with stress and fear are involuntary expressions. It is our job to help cats feel safe and comfortable in the shelter because when they do, they are much easier to handle.

14.3.2 Handling Concepts

Working with cats requires patience. The expression "you can't rush a cat" is true: rushing increases stress and resistance. Safe and humane handling must aim to keep cats as comfortable and relaxed as possible during handling. Going slow is an important means of doing this. Ultimately it is not only safer, it is more efficient because the cat will be much more likely to accept handling when the handler proceeds in a slow, calm, and deliberate manner.

In some instances, appraisal of a cat's behavior may indicate that selection of a more private and quiet environment will be the key to providing a safe and humane handling experience. For cats that appear stressed or fearful from the time of initial contact, providing even a short period of time for them to acclimate to new surroundings and calm down prior to handling is often rewarding. This is especially important for cats because once highly stressed or provoked, they often remain reactive for a prolonged time and may become more reactive if they are stimulated again before they have been allowed a period of time to calm down.

As previously stated, when stress is perceived as inescapable, uncontrollable or unpredictable, it is especially severe. When cats are faced with situations in which they perceive that they have no control and no ability to escape, their stress responses will be heightened, and defensive behaviors will be more likely. This is because a sense of control is very important to cats: it helps them cope and "keep it together" in stressful situations. In and of itself, handling can be stressful and fear invoking for cats. Many cats will be teetering on the edge of defensive aggression during handling.

By avoiding force and using the minimal amount of restraint necessary to manipulate them, cats are less likely to struggle, resist or to behave aggressively. Although it is not possible to know precisely what an individual cat is experiencing during handling, we can critically presume that cats will feel less threatened and maintain more of a sense of control when we handle them in non-forceful ways and restrict them as little as possible. By simply allowing cats to assume preferred postures when we work with them, and to remain in comfortable positions and in locations where they feel safe, we can provide them with the control they need to stay adequately calm and to accept (or at least tolerate) handling. For example, a cat might choose to sit up rather than lie down during microchip scanning. Or, a cat might prefer to remain in the bottom of the carrier while being examined and vaccinated. These are two simple, yet powerful examples of how small accommodations can help cats cope and accept handling rather than displaying fight or flight behaviors.

For cats, the ability to escape, hide, or otherwise shield themselves from a stressful situation is a powerful means of coping because it gives them some sense of control over unpleasant stimuli. When cats perceive that they can escape if need be, or that they are somehow shielded or hidden, they can cope much more effectively with stressful or fear inducing experiences. Remember that they are hardwired for escape or defense: when they view a stressor as inescapable, they are much more likely to struggle and resist. The ways in which we approach and handle them can alter their perception of and response to the situation. It is fair to presume that if they perceive that escape is somehow possible, they will feel more of a sense of control and will therefore remain calmer and be more likely to tolerate or accept our presence and handling. For example, if we scan them for a microchip by standing behind them, this will be much less threatening than if we face them directly and move the scanner over their head. Alternately, some cats will

remain more relaxed if you cover them with a towel or let them nestle under your arm while working with them, presumably because they feel safer if they perceive they are hiding.

In contrast, the traditional restraint technique of scruffing cats and stretching them out on their sides (see Figure 14.1) increases cats' stress and fear response because it completely takes away their freedom of movement and sense of control. This type of restraint is seldom necessary and frequently serves to increase reactivity and defensive behavior. It certainly does not help cats to relax and accept handling more readily in the future. Alternatively, using light restraint while allowing a cat to remain in a more comfortable position and distracting and comforting them with gentle massaging or scratching of their head or neck can help cats to relax and accept handling and is much less likely to trigger an aggressive reaction.

Finally, carefully observing cats' body language during interaction and handling is crucial. Their behavior can change very rapidly. In particular, watch for increasing tension in their body and keep a close eye on their face. A sudden increase in the size of the pupils, flattening or rotation of the ears, and/or twitching of the tail are all signs of increasing stress/fear. It may be tempting to increase restraint when such signs are noted, however this will only serve to increase fear and resistance, making it more likely that the cat will panic and respond defensively in an attempt to escape. Instead, easing restraint and making adjustments such that the cat is allowed some sense of control, freedom of movement, or security will decrease stress/fear and resistance. When cats can be made to feel more comfortable, they will continue to tolerate handling rather than fighting it. Handlers that attempt to prove they can manhandle a fractious cat are handlers that are frequently scratched and bitten.

Indeed, minimal, gentle restraint should always be the goal. This is supported by scientific evidence that indicates gentle human contact can lessen adverse effects of unpleasant stimuli, eliminate fear responses, and even relieve signs of pain in animals (McMillan 2002). Most cats respond best to gentle restraint and react negatively when "over-restrained." In many instances, creative management and patient, skillful handling will avoid the need for additional physical restraint, improving animal and staff safety while reducing stress. When physical restraint is necessary to avoid human injury or injury to an animal, it should be of the least intensity and duration necessary (Newbury et al. 2010). Proper equipment in good working order and adequate staff should be readily available in the event they are needed to ensure safe and humane handling.

14.4 General Guidelines for Safe and Humane Handling

The following guidelines for safe and humane handling provide general directions and recommendations for staff designed to keep cats gently under control while minimizing cat stress and fear and ensuring the safety of both the cat and the handler(s). These guidelines emphasize minimizing stress and fear because the more successful handlers are at keeping cats calm, the more they will succeed in safely and humanely handling them in the short term and positively impacting their behavior in the future.

14.4.1 Before Initiating Contact: Observe, Assess, and Plan

Before attempting to handle any cat, take a few moments to assess the situation. Observe the cat. Ask yourself: Where is the cat? In a cage or carrier, in the front or back? What is the cat doing? What is the cat communicating through her body language and behavior? Are signs of stress and fear present? If so, what is likely triggering them? Is it safe to proceed at this time?

Also consider the environment. Are you in a safe location? If the cat were to get away from you, could the cat escape from the immediate area or retreat somewhere that would make it difficult to safely and humanely retrieve them? Capturing an escaped cat can be very stressful for both the cat and the handler and increases the risk of injury for both. Are there doors or windows that could be closed prior to opening the cat's enclosure? Doing so is an imperative part of safe and humane handling. Are there potentially stressful stimuli in the environment? What can you do to mitigate them? Are there noises or activities that can be curtailed or otherwise blocked before proceeding? If you are going to be transporting the cat, do you have the proper equipment (such as a top loading carrier) available and ready? If you are going to be doing something else (such as an intake exam and vaccinations), do you have everything you need to proceed?

Finally, take a moment to pay attention to yourself. Do you feel comfortable handling this cat in this situation? What do you need to feel comfortable? Do you need to ask for help? By assessing the cat, the environment, and your own comfort and ability with handling the cat in the given situation, you will be able to address concerns proactively and optimize the odds of successfully handling the cat. Always develop a well thought out plan based on these assessments before initiating contact with an animal. A little thoughtful planning goes a long way toward a successful outcome. Planning and preparation take time, but it is time well spent because handling is much more efficient when everything goes smoothly.

14.4.2 Start Off on the Right Foot: Initiating Contact

Whether working with people or animals, first impressions are powerful. To start off on the right foot with someone, we must be polite and considerate by taking into account their point of view and choosing our actions carefully and deliberately in the hopes of receiving a positive response from them. With cats, this means carefully considering how they are likely to perceive us, including both our actions and emotions, as well as how they are likely to perceive the environment, given their point of view.

In terms of emotions, it is important to recognize that how we feel influences the way others feel. Our behavior and body language affect those around us—including animals (Spinka 2012). For example, if we are nervous and jumpy, those around us may begin to feel this way too. Conversely, if we are calm and relaxed, this can help those around us to feel the same way as well. Therefore, in order to optimize the odds of "a good first impression" and successful handling of a cat, we must strive to stay as calm and relaxed as possible when interacting with them because this can help them to feel calm and relaxed too.

Handlers and caregivers must be aware of their body postures when preparing to approach a cat. Instead of approaching head on, approach from one side or the other because this will be less threatening. Similarly, instead of staring directly at them, gazing off to one side is likely to be better received. And, rather than approaching quickly, aim to give them time to adjust to your presence. Movements should always be slow and smooth; avoid reaching over or leaning over them.

Handlers must also make the environment feel as calm and safe as possible. This includes minimizing noise and strong odors. The number of people present, especially strangers, should be limited to only those necessary for the tasks at hand. Likewise, traffic in and out of the work area should be eliminated if possible, or at least limited to the extent possible, and doors should be closed to block visual stimuli outside of the area. Finally, a variety of highly palatable treats should be on hand to create a pleasant aroma and to entice, distract, and/or reward the cat as much as possible.

Another important aspect of initiating contact with a cat is to consider how and where to first touch them. It is especially important to proceed very slowly with touching cats that are displaying signs of fear and discomfort: these cats often require extra time to accept

the presence of handlers and may be especially slow to warm up to being touched. To understand a cat's point of view, consider what your own reactions would be to a stranger who immediately reached out and abruptly touched you.

When initiating contact with a cat, begin with an appropriate greeting. Calmly offering a cat tasty treats by gently placing them within easy reach can serve as a good icebreaker for some cats. Talking to them in a calm and friendly tone may also be perceived as inviting by some cats. For others however, remaining silent may be more calming (Liu et al. 2020). Provided the cat does not appear highly stressed/fearful or defensive, the next step is to offer a hand to them and allow them a moment or two to sniff and respond. It's best if the cat chooses to initiate appropriate social contact with the handler. Forced interactions should always be avoided and whenever possible, the handler should wait for the cat to come to them. In many cases, the cat will accept an offered hand and the handler can then begin gently touching them by rubbing and scratching the sides of their face and neck—areas where most cats enjoy being petted (see Figure 14.2). The handler should always aim to start out by touching the cat in such areas where the cat is unlikely to be sensitive. As the handler makes contact, they should take care to slowly move their hand and apply steady pressure as they touch the cat. The handler should aim to maintain continuous contact, rather than lifting their hand on and off the cat over and over again. This will help the cat to relax and, for some individuals, to enjoy being touched, rather than increasing their discomfort.

For example, if one were to initiate contact with a cat in a cage, they would calmly approach the cage front, standing sideways (not leaning or staring). After pausing for a moment, they might greet the cat in a calm, friendly voice before opening the cage door. They might pause briefly again to see if the cat takes a step forward toward them. Next, they

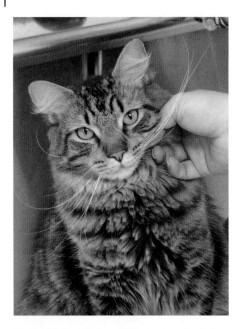

Figure 14.2 Most socialized cats enjoy being rubbed and scratched around their face and neck—these areas are generally not sensitive and are good areas to start out touching when initiating contact with a cat. This cat accepts the handler's hand: his relaxed face and small oblong pupils relate that he is comfortable with this contact.

might offer a hand to the cat while maintaining a sideways stance. If the cat chose to readily accept the hand, they might then begin scratching and rubbing the side of the cat's face and neck. Similarly, a useful method of offering a hand to a cat is to use a "finger-nose technique" to engage them. In this case, the handler simply slowly advances their outstretched index finger toward the cat and then holds it in front of their face. Many cats will initiate contact by rubbing the offered index finger, after which the handler can then proceed by rubbing the sides of the cat's face and/or scratching the chin and neck while using calm, steady pressure. As the cat continues to relax, she will likely be ready to accept additional handling.

If a cat is contained in a carrier, the handler could try to initiate contact by opening the carrier door and allowing the cat a few moments to become oriented to the situation. Many cats will watch and sniff as they consider whether to come out or not. The handler might offer their hand or perhaps wave their fingers near the carrier door to encourage the cat to come forward and exit the carrier. As always, the handler should refrain from looming over the cat in the carrier. Instead, greeting the cat by offering treats and verbal encouragement may help her feel calm and comfortable enough to come out. If a cat is not comfortable enough to leave the carrier, the handler should never pull or dump the cat out. Instead, the handler should be respectful of the cat's need to remain there and remove the top half of the carrier in order to initiate contact. The handler should be prepared to calmly place a towel over the cat as soon as the top is removed so that the cat continues to feel comfortable and safe. This can also help to protect the handler should the cat become defensive. To keep the cat comfortable in her chosen place, the handler can allow the cat to remain in the bottom half of the carrier while performing the care needed. If the cat prefers, the handler should allow her to hide under the towel while care is provided. If the handler needs to lift the cat, the towel could be used to cover the cat while the handler slowly and deliberately lifts her, providing gentle but firm support. Wrapping a cat in a towel to lift them out of a carrier or cage can be a useful technique to enhance calm behavior and safety. As always, the least amount of restraint necessary should be used. Once swaddled in the towel, the cat should be held gently, but snugly, against the handler's body. One hand can be placed loosely around the neck, which is gently scratched to comfort and distract the cat, while maintaining safe control of the cat. Alternatively, the towel can be gently but snugly held in place around the cat's neck for safe control (see Figure 14.3A). This technique is useful for lifting a cat out of their enclosure and moving them within a room, however cats should never be carried through the shelter in this manner because the risk of escape is too great.

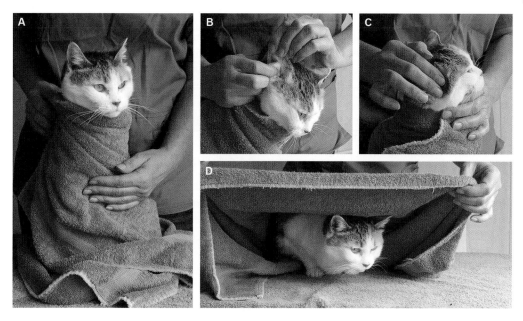

Figure 14.3 This series of photos illustrates the use of a towel wrap to facilitate cleaning a cat's ears. The towel wrap is used as an aid in gentle restraint and also provides the cat with privacy when she is periodically afforded a brief break during the process. A. A towel has been wrapped around the cat's neck like a cape in order to gently restrain her and to prevent her from scratching at her ears with her hind feet while the handler cleans them. Note that the handler is behind the cat in a non-threatening position. B. While holding the cape in place, the handler gently holds the earflap in an upright position as she applies ear cleaner using a soaked cotton ball. C. After applying the ear cleaner, the handler gently massages the ear before releasing the cape to free the cat. D. The handler holds the towel over the cat's head as she provides her with a break to give her control for a few moments to shake her head and cope with the procedure. After a brief break, the cape is reapplied, and the process is repeated until both ears have been cleaned.

If the cat needs to be transferred to a cage, the handler should proceed by replacing the top of the carrier and then placing the carrier in the cage so that the cat can choose to come out in her own time. Remember: a cat should never be dumped or dragged out of a carrier. Doing so would completely remove any sense of control the cat might have and would increase stress/fear, making escape or defensive behaviors much more likely. Space-permitting, the carrier can remain available in the cat's enclosure for the cat to retreat and hide if they choose. If the carrier will be left in the cage with the cat for any length of time, the door should either be secured in an open position or removed to prevent it from accidentally closing and preventing the cat from being able to change locations in the cage. Draping a towel over the cage front will provide additional privacy and reduce visual stimuli for the cat as she adapts to her new situation.

14.4.3 During Contact: Observe, Assess, and Adjust

Handlers should always take a few moments to observe a cat before approaching or handling them. In addition, they should continue to carefully observe them during their approach and throughout the time they are working with them. By recognizing how the cat is feeling, the handler can adjust their actions and techniques, taking into account the cat's current level of stress and discomfort in the given situation. Keep in mind that some cats will be teetering on the edge of defensive aggression.

If they are pushed beyond their ability to cope, they will respond with fight or flight behaviors. If instead the handler helps them to maintain some sense of control and safety, this will increase the odds that the cat will continue to tolerate handling. The cat may not be able to fully relax, but at the same time the cat will remain steady enough for the handler to complete necessary examination or care. If at any time the handler recognizes that stress and fear are increasing based on the cat's body language, they should take a break by lightening restraint in order to provide the cat with time and space to relax. If the cat begins to relax, the handler can adjust their approach and try again. With this in mind, a useful rule of thumb when working with cats is the "two second rule." If a cat begins to resist handling, the handler must never allow them to struggle for more than a couple of seconds before stopping to take a break. This rule is important because stress and fear in cats can escalate to aggression very rapidly. Once a cat becomes highly defensive, they often remain in a state of agitation for quite some time from which it will take them much longer to calm down. In addition, they may be even less likely to accept handling in the future. For cats that continue to resist and struggle for more than two seconds, the handler should stop and take a brief break to further observe, assess, and adjust. In some instances, giving a cat a break and adjusting positions will be all that is needed to successfully continue. In other instances, it may be necessary to completely reevaluate the handling plan, delay the procedure, or ask others for help. In cases where cats are increasingly stressed/fearful, delaying the procedure to another time may be best. Alternatively, behavior medications or sedation may be necessary to calm the cat.

As always, constantly observe and assess the cat's body language and vocal signals during handling. If the cat's tension eases up, it is reasonable to elect to continue handling them carefully and ever watchfully. However, if the cat's fear/stress escalates a second time, it is time to stop. Repeatedly continuing in the face of increasing stress/fear will certainly result in the cat having a bad experience, and it is unsafe for the handler(s). In addition, the cat may become sensitized to handling, which will make it even more difficult to work with them in the future.

14.4.4 Don't Use Punishment

In the past, it was sometimes taught that an animal should not be allowed "to get away with" aggressive behavior and that they should be punished for it instead. This is erroneous. The truth is that you can't punish fear: attempting to punish a fearful, defensive cat will only serve to reinforce their fear/stress, resistance to handling, and aggression. It will also substantially increase the odds of handler injury. When a cat lashes out defensively, handlers sometimes become angry—but they should remember that such behavior is the result of the animal's stress and fear; it is not malicious. A handler should never respond in anger nor should they use force or punishment to handle a cat (Newbury et al. 2010). Physically restraining a struggling animal is neither humane nor safe.

14.4.5 Try Tasty Treats

It is not possible to punish fear, but it can be counter conditioned. In other words, the way a cat feels in a given situation can be changed. Changing the way a cat feels will also change the way the cat behaves. Food can sometimes be a powerful means of overcoming negative emotions. For example, if a cat is uneasy, they may become much more comfortable if offered a very tasty treat. For example, offering a fearful, resistant kitten some delicious food may result in them quickly warming up to their handler's presence.

Tasty treats often put animals at ease in new situations. They can also be used to distract or redirect nervous or fidgety animals during handling, including both cats and dogs. Dogs are often more likely to partake of treats—as opposed to many cats—but treats should still be tried because for some cats, they can make a big difference by diffusing stress, decreasing the amount of physical restraint necessary, and increasing the cat's tolerance of handling. Little bits of canned cat food, tuna fish, soft cheese spread, or freeze-dried liver are favorites for many cats. Finding the right treat can make a big difference in how well a cat tolerates handling. It is best to have a variety of treats available to maximize the odds of finding one that a given cat will respond well to. For example, a cat may refuse dry kibble, but be very eager to eat bits of tuna!

Examples of using food to distract cats and promote positive associations with handlers include feeding tasty treats during routine examination and procedures such as microchip scanning, administration of vaccines or other injections, or the application of a topical parasite control product. Food can also be used to facilitate administration of oral medications should they be prescribed during a cat's shelter stay. Canned foods, soft cheese spreads, and commercially available treats designed to cover oral tablets or capsules as well as flavored liquids can all simplify administration of medication. Treats work best when they are used before a cat becomes highly stressed. As stress increases, cats are less likely to accept treats. Upon returning a cat to their enclosure, always place a treat inside for them as a reward. This may serve to distract the cat as the handler exits and closes the door—and if they do not eat it right away, they may eat it after the handler leaves. It's always a good idea to reward tolerance/acceptance of handling!

14.4.6 Handling for Examination and Procedures

When examining cats and performing necessary animal care procedures, handling and restraint should always be gentle and supporting. Using positive, consistent, and predictable

human-cat interactions helps cats cope with necessary care. Assessment and planning should take location and timing of examinations and procedures into consideration. Procedures should be prioritized from the most important and necessary items down to those items that can wait if the cat is highly stressed and resistant to handling. Techniques will obviously differ depending on the individual cat's behavior and tolerance of handling. Cats that are highly fearful and reactive, including those that are poorly socialized, will require additional consideration to ensure safe and humane handling.

For cats that are tractable, procedures should be performed in a place and position in which the cat is likely to be comfortable. This might be on a soft towel on an exam table, in their bed in their housing enclosure, or even on a towel in your lap. Every effort should be made to help the cat stay as calm and comfortable as possible. By preventing heightening of stress and fear, safe and humane handling can be accomplished.

During examination and procedures, always allow the cat to face away from you. This is far less threatening and is safer for the handler because the cat's claws and teeth will be facing away as well; it also allows the cat to look around the environment, which may provide a sense of control. Within the overall prioritization of importance, always perform the least stressful parts of examination or procedures first. In instances where you must position the cat to allow access to a particular area of their body, consider how they will feel most comfortable. For example, if you need to examine the cat's abdomen, rather than flipping the cat onto her back, try lifting up her front end so that she is standing on her hind legs. If you need to look under the tail, rather than cranking up on the tail, try gently scratching and rubbing the top of the cat's rump—most cats will stand and lift their tails when this is done, allowing easy visual inspection of this area. If access to a leg is needed for drawing blood, instead of forcing the cat to lie on her side, allow the cat some control to sit up while you gently and slowly extend the leg as necessary to gain access.

Here is an example of providing thoughtful, flexible care for a cat showing marked signs of stress and fear at the time of intake. Principles of infectious disease control and shelter medicine indicate that vaccinating cats as close to the time of intake as possible is crucial to providing the best possible protection against disease. However, if a cat is markedly fearful and reactive at the time of intake, it may be best to allow a brief period of time for them to calm down before proceeding with intake vaccination. Instead of risking staff safety and compromising cat welfare by vaccinating them when they are highly fearful and reactive, cover the carrier containing the cat and place it in an enclosure in a quiet, dimly lit room for 30–60 minutes. After that period of time, many cats will be calmer, and at this point, staff may be able to remove the top of the carrier, cover the cat with a towel, and proceed with vaccination. If the cat's stress/fear begin to increase with handling, the remainder of the intake procedures could be delayed until the following day to allow the cat additional time to adjust to their new environment. A flexible protocol such as this will successfully facilitate safety, timely vaccination, and humane care.

14.4.7 Using Handling Tools and Equipment

Numerous tools and types of equipment are available to facilitate handling cats. The goals of using any such tools or equipment should always be to reduce the amount of physical restraint necessary to control the cat and to limit the cat's exposure to fear-inducing stimuli. Ultimately, they should be used to help reduce cat stress and fear while enhancing handler and cat safety. The *ways* in which tools or equipment are used is crucial to ensure that they mitigate and limit stress versus increase the risk of physical or emotional harm. Improper or forceful use of any tool or technique can escalate a high stress situation rather than diffuse it, compromising animal welfare and creating an unsafe situation for both animals and people.

Techniques or equipment suitable for one animal or situation may be inappropriate for another, thus a "one size fits all" approach must be avoided. Instead, several different tools and types of equipment should be available and selected based on the appraisal of the individual and the situation. For example, towel wraps are useful aids for handling many cats because they can reduce stress and enhance handler safety. A towel placed correctly around an animal's neck can increase control of the head while avoiding the use of more intense physical restraint. With cats that like to hide, towel wrap techniques may provide for a more pleasant handling experience. They can also be used as both an aid in gentle restraint during procedures as well as a respite for the cat during breaks in handling (see Figure 14.3). In other instances, Elizabethan collars can be useful and humane tools for protecting the handler from cat bites while reducing the cat's visual field to help mitigate stress. In some situations, it may be necessary to administer "chemical restraint" using a hands-off approach with humane restraint equipment such as cage nets or squeeze devices. In contrast, tools such as control poles should never be used to restrain cats because they can easily cause substantial, even life-threatening physical injury, as well as profound emotional trauma. Likewise, the routine use of slip leads, cat tongs, or any restraint device that can cause significant compression of the neck or thorax must be avoided (see Figure 14.4). Tools that completely thwart a cat's sense of control (such as a cat bag) should likewise be avoided. In all cases, regardless of the tools or type of equipment used, deliberate, calm handling is essential.

Figure 14.4 Commercially available cat tongs. Tools such as cat tongs, control poles, slip leads, or any restraint device that can cause significant compression of the neck or thorax should never be used to restrain cats because they can easily cause substantial, even life-threatening physical injury as well as profound emotional trauma. Likewise, use of any tool that completely thwarts a cat's sense of control must be avoided.

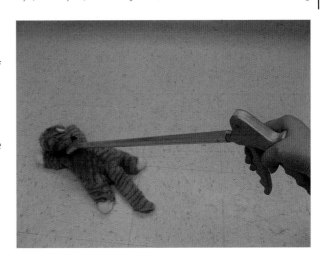

14.5 Tips, Techniques, and Tools for Stress Reduction and Humane Handling

Keeping cats calm is crucial for safe and humane handling, therefore a comprehensive approach to preventing, reducing, and managing feline stress in the shelter is essential. First and foremost, handling techniques must always take stress reduction into account, therefore recommendations for humane handling must include broad based approaches for stress reduction. The following tips, techniques, and tools for stress reduction and humane handling are meant to serve as starting points for working with cats. Cats are individuals and will respond as such—handlers must therefore be flexible and observant so that they are prepared to adjust their methods and plans according to the needs of individuals. This will ensure the safest and most humane outcomes.

14.5.1 Provide Information to the Public Prior to Shelter Admission

For cats that will be relinquished to the shelter, planning their admission to the extent possible, including providing key information to their caregivers in advance, can significantly reduce their stress during the process. Instruct relinquishers to always use carriers for transporting

cats to the shelter. Advise them to secure the carrier in the car to prevent it from turning over during transport. Placing the carrier on the floorboard in front of the passenger seat is often the safest and most secure location for transport. Suggest that they place bedding inside the carrier to improve the cat's comfort and security as well as to reduce slipping. Wire carriers should be covered loosely with a towel to visually shield the cat from scary sights and noise should be minimized.

Whenever possible, staff should find out in advance if a cat tends to be highly nervous or has a history of behaving aggressively in new situations. If this is the case, then an effort should be made to have the cat brought in at a quiet time of day when staff will have more time to admit them. Alternatively, staff might ask them to keep the cat contained outside until ready to receive them. Cats and their caregivers will also benefit from knowing what to expect when they arrive at the shelter. In many instances, information can be made readily available through the shelter's website or via volunteers.

14.5.2 Maintain Calm Admission Areas

Admission areas can be busy, crowded, and stressful for animals, shelter staff, and the public. Whenever possible, scheduling and planning for most admissions will result in much calmer admissions areas, which then allows the process to go more smoothly. Scheduling should strive to alleviate bottlenecks and minimize wait times. Ideally, cats and dogs should be received in separate admissions areas—or admitted at different times of day whenever possible. Staff should always take care to maintain a calm demeanor during the admission process by working in a quiet, steady manner and talking in calm and soothing tones. Simply taking care to minimize noise and rapid movements will go a long way to making everyone feel more comfortable. Weather permitting, leaving animals in cars until such time that someone is available to perform intake care right away and transport them directly to housing areas will minimize congestion and stress. Providing elevated surfaces, such as counter tops or shelving, on which to rest carriers containing cats is a simple but powerful means of reducing stress because cats instinctively feel more secure when they can perch at a high vantage point, "out of a predator's reach." Avoid placing carriers at floor level and keep them away from dogs and other cats to the greatest extent possible. For example, towels or sheets can be provided in the waiting room for covering carriers containing cats immediately upon entry, shielding them visually from dogs and other stress-invoking stimuli.

14.5.3 Use Carriers to Move Cats

Moving cats while they are contained in transport carriers offers many advantages. Carriers can be covered to reduce exposure to environmental stimuli that may trigger fear as they are moved through the shelter. This is especially important for cats because their behavior can change rapidly when fear is triggered. They can go from a state of relaxation to a state of panic in only a few seconds. If a handler is carrying a cat in their arms and fear is triggered, a risk of escape and injury is suddenly created for both the cat and handler. Transporting them instead in a covered carrier will keep them calmer and is safer for

everyone. Whenever possible, use carriers designed to open from the top or from which the top half is easily removed: this makes it easier to move the cat in and out of the carrier in a non-stressful manner.

The way in which the carrier is held and carried also impacts the experience of the cat inside. Holding it by the handle and carrying it beside your leg like a briefcase places the cat at eye level of any dogs that you must pass (see Figure 14.5). In addition, the carrier will likely be in motion because it will probably swing to and fro as you walk, and this motion can create additional stress for the cat inside. Instead, it is best to hold a carrier containing a cat in front of your body (see Figure 14.6). Holding it close to your chest with both hands will ensure that it is away from any potential on-looking dogs, as well as reducing motion as the cat is transported. In the case of feral-behaving cats in traps, holding a wire trap against your body is not recommended as a matter of safety. Traps should always be covered, and they should be held as level and as stable as possible to minimize motion from swinging when carried.

Before moving a cat, remember to consider the environment. What sights, sounds, and scents will you be passing? Take action to minimize the cats' exposure to potential triggers for stress and fear. Be aware of other people and animals. When needed, ask for assistance to open doors or to look ahead to ensure that the path ahead is clear and calm.

14.5.4 Separate Cats from Other Species

The presence and sounds of unfamiliar dogs is extremely distressing and fear invoking for cats. As such, from the time they arrive at the shelter and continuing throughout their stay, care should be taken not to place cats within spatial, visual, or auditory range of dogs whenever possible. In fact, different species should routinely be separated from one another to the extent possible. Dog wards should be separate from cat wards; and for shelters that house other species, they should be separated, too. For

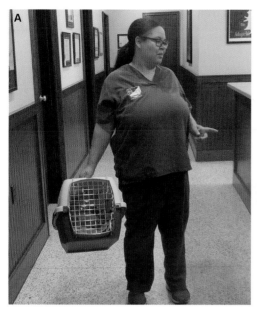
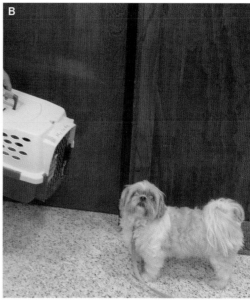

Figure 14.5 The way in which a cat carrier is held and carried impacts the experience of the cat inside. A. The handler is holding the carrier like a briefcase. B. This places the cat at eye level of dogs along her path and creates a "to and fro" motion while she walks, adding additional stress for the cat inside.

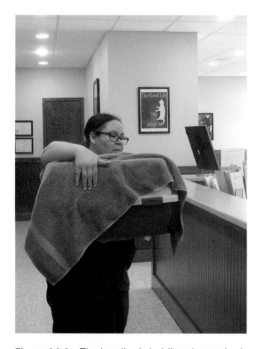

Figure 14.6 The handler is holding the carrier in front of her body close to her chest with both hands. This ensures that the cat does not encounter any on-looking dogs and reduces motion as it's carried. Note that the carrier is also covered to visually shield the cat during transport.

example, birds should be housed separately from dogs and cats; rabbits and other small mammals should be housed in areas away from birds, dogs, and cats, and so forth.

14.5.5 Control Noise

As previously stated, minimizing loud and sudden noises, including barking, is a crucial component of environmental management to reduce cat stress and promote calm behavior. Soundproofing systems can help. Noise can be also be blunted by using background sounds such as soothing music, water fountains, or white noise machines. A radio playing soft music at a low volume may provide a welcome distraction and prevent cats from being startled by loud noises. Importantly, most caregivers enjoy listening to the radio, and happy caregivers positively contribute to a relaxed environment. Staff and volunteers should refrain from loud talking and always take care to minimize noise during the course of their duties. For example, staff should avoid clanging metal gates, cage doors, and food bowls.

Many shelters use inexpensive paper trays for feeding, which can aid in noise reduction as well as saving time.

14.5.6 Control Odors and Consider Using Pheromones

Good air ventilation and routine sanitation protocols are important means of reducing stress-triggering odors in the environment. Using enzymatic cleaners and other products designed to eliminate odors as part of a shelter's routine sanitation protocols will help ensure a more pleasant environment for animals and people alike. Cleaning well between animals will decrease potential stressful odors from others. Noxious odors, such as the smell of isopropyl alcohol or strong fumes from cleaning and disinfectant products, should be avoided. In addition, staff and volunteers should refrain from wearing strong smelling perfumes or lotions during work hours.

Cats may respond positively to the potentially calming effects of commercially available diffusers containing synthetic analogues of naturally occurring feline facial pheromones (Pereira et al. 2016). These products can be sprayed onto towels and bedding—but this should be done at least 30 minutes prior to exposing the cat. The recommended 30-minute wait time after spraying allows the alcohol, which is the typical carrier for the pheromone in the spray, to diffuse or evaporate. Where resources are limited, the best use of pheromones might be in wards designated for housing cats displaying marked signs of stress and fear (see Chapter 17).

14.5.7 Reduce Visual Stimuli

As previously described, blocking visual stimuli in the environment can be a very effective means of reducing patient stress and fear. Avoiding bright lights, closing doors to block outside activities, covering carriers containing cats, and draping a towel over a cat to block their vision during a procedure are all examples.

14.5.8 Ensure Secure Footing

Many cats may be uncomfortable standing or moving on slippery surfaces such as stainless-steel cages or tables. Ensuring secure footing can ease stress and fear, promote comfort, and facilitate handling and examination. Examples include using bedding in enclosures, placing a non-slip mat on a scale, or a towel or a few sheets of soft newspaper on a slick exam surface.

14.5.9 Provide Consistent Housing Designed for Stress Reduction

Housing design and operation should enhance the comfort and safety of cats while minimizing stress and fear. Cats should be housed consistently in the same enclosures, which must provide adequate space for them to move about and change positions and locations as well as space for feeding and resting areas that are well separated from litter areas (see Chapter 16). Soft bedding should be available not only for comfort but so that animals may establish a familiar scent that aids in acclimation to a new environment. In order to preserve the familiar scent, bedding should not be changed unless it becomes soiled. Cats will also benefit from being cared for by consistent, familiar people whenever possible. Every cat needs a comfortable area to rest, hide, and perch. To provide a refuge, a secure hiding place must be available for all cats so that they can remove themselves from things they perceive as stressful. In fact, the ability to "escape" from stressful stimuli by hiding dramatically decreases stress in cats (Carlstead et al. 1993). A sturdy cardboard box can be placed in the cage to provide a hiding place as well as a perch. There are also a variety of purpose made hiding boxes for cats (such as cat dens) that are commercially available. For those cats who are severely stressed or reactive, covering the cage front, in addition to providing a hiding box, and posting signage to allow the cat time to calm down or "chill out" for several hours or even a few days can facilitate adaptation to their new environment.

14.5.10 Use Cat Dens

Cat dens are designed as secure boxes and are equipped with a guillotine-style door on one end and a portal–style door on one side (see Figure 14.7A). They make excellent hiding boxes for cats, and their design facilitates safe and humane handling. The guillotine door is usually secured in the closed position when the den is used as a hiding box within a cage, while the portal door is left open (see Figure 14.7B). Conveniently, dens take up less floor space in a cat's enclosure than most cat carriers and can also be used to transport cats. For example, if a cat is moved from a holding ward to an adoption ward, the cat den can be used as a transport carrier. Placing the den with its familiar scent in the new enclosure with the cat will hasten adjustment to the new ward. Cat dens are also very useful for decreasing stress and fear during daily cleaning procedures. Rather than moving the cat to a different cage, which is inherently stressful, the cat is allowed to simply stay in their den. The portal door is closed to contain the cat while their cage is quietly tidied and replenished around them as needed.

14.5.11 Use Behavior Medications: Gabapentin and Trazodone

Administration of the oral behavior medications gabapentin and trazodone can be very helpful for calming cats (Stevens et al. 2016; Pankratz et al. 2017; van Haaften et al. 2017). These drugs should not be reserved only for cats with severe stress/fear—cats with mild to moderate stress/fear will also benefit greatly from their use. When stress is mitigated by such drug therapy, cats are more likely to respond to good environmental management and behavioral care. Both of these medications are widely available, highly cost-effective, and have a wide margin of safety. Of note, their use does not preclude the use of additional (injectable) sedative medications if needed. See Chapter 22 on Behavioral Pharmacology.

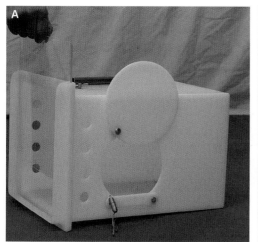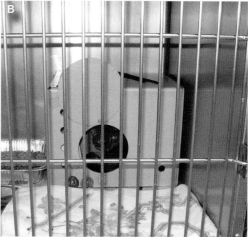

Figure 14.7 A. A commercially available cat den (Tomahawk Live Trap, Hazelhurst, WI). Note the guillotine-style door on the front of the den and a portal-style door on one side. B. A commercially available cat den (Animal Care and Equipment Services [ACES], Boulder, CO) serves as a secure hiding place for a cat. The den's circular portal door can be closed from a safe and non-threatening distance while the cage is spot cleaned as needed. The cat can also be securely transported in the den.

14.5.12 Develop Protocols for Cats with High Levels of Stress and Fear

Protocols for cats with high levels of stress and fear must be flexible and should afford a variety of options. Protocols should begin with recognition of cats exhibiting marked stress and fear at the time of entry. Such cats should be housed in specially designated quiet areas away from other animals and foot traffic. As previously explained, delaying a procedure to allow a cat time to relax in a quiet environment before handling is often the best option when urgent intervention is not necessary. The precise means by which any particular cat is handled will depend on the individual: handling methods must be approached and tailored according to the individual's needs and responses. Forceful handling and restraint must be avoided. Administration of oral doses of trazodone or gabapentin is ideal whenever possible. For cats that require contact but remain unsafe to humanely handle, "chemical restraint" should be used under the order of a veterinarian to limit stress and ensure the safety of everyone involved. Stress and pain during injections of sedatives and anesthetic agents should be mitigated by using humane handling techniques, small gauge needles, and changing needles prior to injection to ensure they are as sharp and smooth as possible.

14.5.12.1 Tools for a Hands-Off Approach

For cats that cannot be safely touched, a hands-off approach should be used. A variety of tools can be used for hands-off handling including cat dens, squeeze cages, nets, and trap dividers. Keep in mind that how humane various tools are will depend on how they're used and the skill of the user. Handlers must be calm, gentle, deliberate, and efficient in their application to provide the least stressful experience possible for both the cat and themselves. Developing this ability takes practice, skill, and finesse.

In addition to their use as hiding boxes and transport carriers, cat dens can be used to facilitate the safe transfer of cats to or from other enclosures with guillotine-style doors.

For example, if a cat arrives at the shelter in a box trap, she can be safely transferred to a cat den in a considerate, hands-off way. To accomplish this, the two containers are aligned, and the guillotine doors are both raised (see Figure 14.8). If the goal is to administer an injection, the cat can be transferred to a commercially available squeeze cage via the guillotine door of the cat den. By gently sliding the squeeze cage apparatus toward the cat until it is in light contact with their body, the handler can inject through the bars of the cage without unnecessarily physically compressing the cat (see Figure 14.9). Alternatively, a commercially available "hand shield" can be used to facilitate injection of a cat in a den (see Figure 14.10). Transferring a cat from a carrier or other container with a swinging door rather than a guillotine-style door is not recommended because of the risk of escape.

A net is another potentially useful tool for handling highly stressed cats. Several commercially available cat nets are available. In some cases, the design allows the user to close the opening of the net using a special sliding mechanism on the handle (see Figure 14.11). This type of net (often called a cage net) is designed for use when a cat is enclosed in a cage or other confined space. Once a cat is securely netted, "chemical restraint" may be administered through the netting. Covering the cat with a thick towel or blanket will aid in safe and humane restraint while an injectable anesthetic is administered. As soon as the cat is relaxed and immobilized, she should be removed from the net. When used properly, nets minimize stress, prevent injury of the animal, and ensure staff safety. In contrast, commercially available cat tongs should never be used for routine movement or restraint of cats because of the risk of injury to the cat.

14.5.12.2 Special Considerations for Community Cats

When community cats enter the shelter, they should be placed in the quietest ward available away from other animals and foot traffic. They

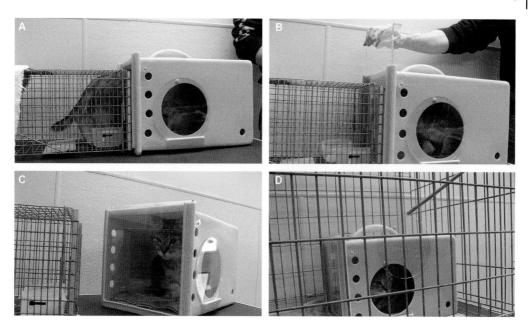

Figure 14.8   A cat is safely and humanely transferred from a box trap to a cat den. A. The two containers are aligned and the guillotine doors are raised. The towel, which was initially covering the trap to visually shield the cat, has been pulled back to expose the cat, and the handler has stepped out of the cat's sight—the cat is responding to being exposed by moving into the den. B. Next, the handler calmly replaces the guillotine door of the den by carefully and quietly sliding it into place. Note that the handler is considerably out of the cat's view while accomplishing this. C. Once the cat is safely secured in the den, it can then be covered with a towel to visually shield the cat and gently carried to an appropriate ward, where it can be placed inside an enclosure. D. Once inside the enclosure, the den's portal door can be easily opened from a safe distance such that the cat can use the den as a hiding place.

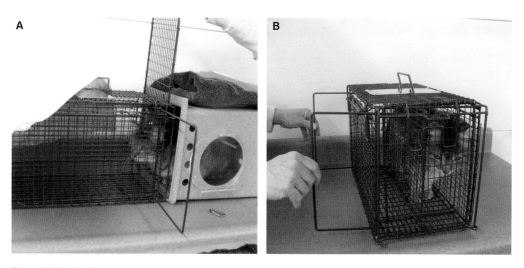

Figure 14.9   A. By raising and lowering the guillotine doors, a cat is safely and humanely transferred from a cat den to a squeeze cage for restraint. Note the use of a cloth to cover the cage. B. The design of the squeeze cage allows the cat to be gently pushed over to one side to facilitate injection through the bars of the cage. Following injection, the cage can be covered with the cloth to reduce stress by visually shielding the cat.

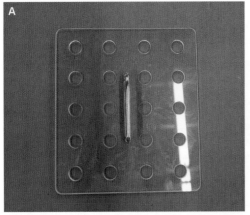
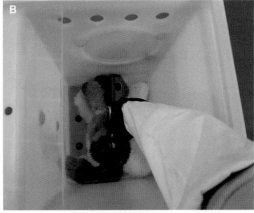

Figure 14.10 A. Commercially available "hand shield" for use with a cat den (Tomahawk Live Trap, Hazelhurst, WI). B. An injection can be administered through one of the circular holes in the durable transparent plastic shield while the handler uses it to gently confine the cat in the back of the den. Note that the cat den is positioned on its end and that the handler is wearing protective gloves for added safety.

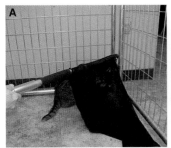
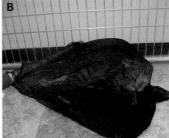
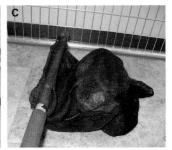

Figure 14.11 A Freeman cage net (Animal Care and Equipment Services [ACES], Boulder, CO) is used to humanely handle a cat in an enclosure. The design of the net allows the user to close the opening to the net using a special sliding mechanism on the handle of the pole. A. The net is placed over the cat. B. As the handler moves closer, the cat moves farther into the net and the net is closed. C. The handler calmly and gently rolls the net onto the pole to confine the cat securely, preventing thrashing. A towel can then be used to cover the cat while an anesthetic injection is administered.

should be housed for the briefest amount of time for assessment and trap-neuter-return. Cats that are truly feral should never be confined long term in a shelter. Because of their lack of socialization, capture and handling is extremely stressful for them. Although it is impossible to eliminate fear responses in feral cats, caregivers can help these cats to cope during the time they must be confined to undergo spay-neuter procedures by actively working to create the least stressful environment possible and by limiting their exposure to people and other stimuli as much as possible. Environmental management

should include previously described practices to minimize and mitigate cat stress and fear. A calm and quiet environment is essential, and cats should be left undisturbed to the extent possible. Only when necessary for proper care and monitoring, should caregivers disturb cats in any way. In addition to environmental management, proper education of caregivers and veterinary staff on the use of equipment to facilitate a "hands-off" approach is key to minimizing feline stress and fear, while keeping caregivers and cats safe. In most instances, cats should be humanely trapped using commercially available live traps

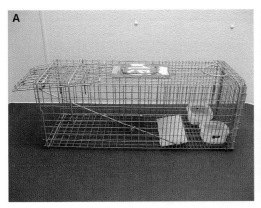 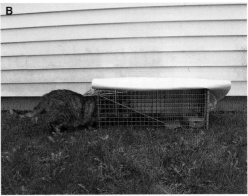

Figure 14.12 A. A commercially available box trap (Tomahawk Live Trap, Tomahawk, WI). When a cat steps on the spring-loaded foot plate to reach the food bait, the trap door will close and lock. B. A cat enters a commercially available humane box trap (Tomahawk Live Trap, Hazelhurst, WI). Covering the trap serves to make it more inviting. In addition, it will help to reduce stress and fear by providing cover and security, helping to calm the cat once captured.

(see Figure 14.12). For those cats that are elusive, a drop trap is a humane alternative but generally requires substantial time and patience (see Figure 14.13). Once captured, cats may be securely held short term in their covered traps while awaiting surgery (one to two days maximum). Transferring them to larger enclosures increases the risk of human injury as well as cat escape, and most cats will successfully escape if afforded any opportunity to do so. Recapturing escaped cats can be extremely difficult and poses substantial safety risks to personnel. In addition, escaped cats can be destructive as they attempt to hide and resist recapture. Keeping cats confined in traps not only reduces stress and the risk of escapes, it facilitates administration of anesthetics. With the cat confined in a trap, this can be done without extensive handling, minimizing

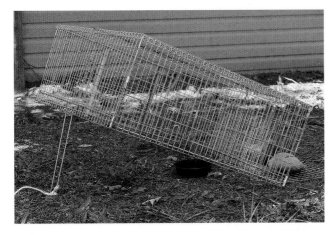

Figure 14.13 Commercially available drop trap, which is fully collapsible for ease of transport (Tomahawk Live Trap, Hazelhurst, WI). A drop trap can be used to humanely capture cats that will not enter a box trap. Strong-smelling food is placed on the ground beneath the trap, and the caregiver waits covertly nearby until the cat takes the bait. From the remote location, the caregiver pulls a string to remove the prop stick, causing the trap to drop, capturing the cat. A guillotine-style transfer door is used to safely transfer the cat from the drop trap into a regular box trap or transfer cage for transport.

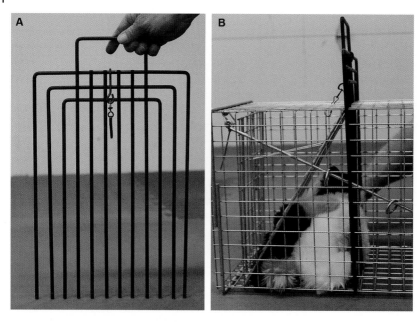

Figure 14.14 A. Commercially available trap divider (Tomahawk Live Trap, Hazelhurst, WI). B. The trap divider is used to humanely restrict a cat in a box trap in a safe, hands-off manner to facilitate intramuscular injection of an anesthetic agent.

stress, and enhancing safety for both cats and personnel. This is accomplished by using a commercially available "trap divider" to more tightly confine the cat. This allows an injection of anesthesia to be administered to the cat between the trap's wire bars (see Figure 14.14). In this way, cats are kept in their traps and only removed once they have been heavily sedated or anesthetized. Then, at the completion of surgery and before awakening, they can be returned to their traps for recovery. With this system, cats are never handled while conscious, and there are no opportunities for escape or injury. And, importantly, they do not sustain any additional stress from unnecessary handling (Griffin 2011).

14.5.12.2.1 *Gabapentin for Community Cats*

In addition to environmental management and hands-off handling techniques, administration of oral gabapentin may further attenuate cat fear responses during the process of trap-neuter-return. A recent study demonstrated that it can be safely and humanely administered to confined cats using a tomcat catheter and that dosages of 50–100 mg per cat

were safe and not associated with increased sedation (Pankratz et al. 2017). To administer an oral suspension to a cat in a trap, a trap divider should be used to temporarily restrict the cat to one end of the trap. Immediately following restriction of the cat, the end of an open tomcat catheter, which is attached to a dosing syringe, is slowly and deliberately inserted into the corner of the cat's mouth to deliver the suspension (see Figure 14.15). Alternatively, capsule contents can be mixed directly into highly palatable food at the time of trapping and with subsequent feedings.

14.6 Recommendations for Handling Cats during the Process of Euthanasia

When the decision has been made to euthanize a cat (or any animal), the process must be conducted with the highest degree of respect and with the goal of providing the most humane death possible (Leary et al. 2020;

Figure 14.15 An oral suspension of gabapentin is administered to a community cat in a trap using an open tomcat catheter attached to a dosing syringe. Note the use of a trap divider to confine the cat to one end of the trap, facilitating administration. *Source:* Courtesy of College of Veterinary Medicine, North Carolina State University.

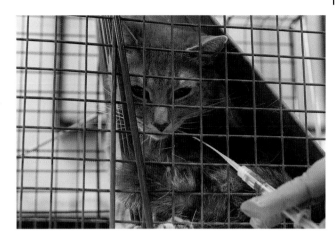

Newbury et al. 2010). This means minimizing pain, distress, and all other negative effects to that animal during the process. Any technique used should result in rapid loss of consciousness followed by cardiac or respiratory arrest and, ultimately, a loss of brain function. At the same time, animal handling should minimize fear and distress experienced by the animal prior to loss of consciousness. Even though it may not always be possible to completely eliminate all anxiety and pain, the process of euthanasia should always be carried out in such a way to minimize these as much as possible. Furthermore, as a general rule, a gentle death that takes longer to accomplish is preferable to a rapid, but more distressing death (Rhoades 2002; Leary et al. 2020). Because emotional and behavioral responses vary considerably among cats, the selection of euthanasia techniques must be tailored to the needs of individual cats. They must also take into account the technical skills and proficiency of the personnel carrying out the procedures. Personnel must be technically proficient with both euthanasia techniques as well as methods for safe and humane handling. This requires organizational commitment to providing ongoing professional training and support for staff performing these procedures (Leary et al. 2020; Newbury et al. 2010). Emphasis on the application of the following concepts is required in order to make the

process of euthanasia as humane as possible (e.g., free of pain and distress).

1) Always strive to euthanize animals within their physical and behavioral comfort zones and provide the calmest environment possible. For virtually all animals (including cats), being placed in a novel environment is stressful; therefore, a euthanasia approach that can be applied in familiar surroundings reduces stress (Leary et al. 2020).

2) Personnel involved should be prepared to adjust handling and euthanasia methods and techniques based on the behavior of individual cats. Oral administration of behavior medications may be helpful for calming cats to mitigate stress during the euthanasia process. Sedation and/or anesthesia may assist in achieving the best conditions for euthanasia of some animals and may be necessary when struggling during capture or restraint may cause pain, injury, or anxiety to the animal or danger to personnel (Leary et al. 2020). In some instances, it may be possible to reduce handling stress by administering sedatives and anesthetic agents orally.

3) For cats accustomed to human contact, gentle handling using minimal restraint in a familiar and safe environment is often the best approach (Leary et al. 2020) (provided

of course that they are comfortable being handled in the shelter).

4) Cats that are highly stressed/fearful, including those that are feral, injured, or otherwise distressed require special consideration regarding handling and restraint and the euthanasia technique selected must allow for this. A hands-off approach to handling (see previous section) combined with a method of administration that will result in the least distress possible is the best general approach.

5) Keeping highly stressed/fearful individuals in familiar environments for the process and minimizing visual, auditory, and tactile stimulation are important means of mitigating stress and distress.

14.6.1 Environment

Euthanasia is often performed in a dedicated, single purpose room. A euthanasia room should be quiet, clean, orderly, well-lit, stocked with proper equipment, and have sufficient space (Rhoades 2002). Animals should not be permitted to observe or hear the euthanasia of other animals or permitted to view the bodies of dead animals whenever possible, with few exceptions. To assure a smooth, dignified and safe operation, only the people directly involved in the process should be present during procedures. The room should be a sacred and peaceful place to provide a calm, respectful death. Interruptions must be avoided, and signage should be used to direct other staff members not to enter when procedures are in process. That said, it is crucial to recognize that all animals tend to be stressed by novel environments. The simple act of taking a cat from a familiar environment into a novel room can induce considerable stress. Although maintaining a single purpose euthanasia room is important, when cats have already been housed in the shelter and are acclimated to their housing area, it can be very stressful to transport them from where they are residing to a novel room. For

this reason, electing to perform euthanasia in the ward where that animal resides is a decision that should be made on a case-by-case basis because a familiar environment may reduce stress. The physical layout of the shelter is a practical consideration. For instance, cats should never be transported through a kennel of barking dogs to the euthanasia room. All of the recommendations in this chapter that pertain to environmental management for stress reduction are profoundly important at the time of euthanasia.

14.6.2 Microchip Scanning Prior to Euthanasia

It is important to keep in mind that all cats should be systematically scanned for a microchip prior to euthanasia. The ability to carry this out in a thorough and low-stress manner must be considered when determining the best handling and euthanasia techniques to use for an individual cat. In order to achieve proper scanning, cats must be removed from carriers to prevent interference during the scanning process that would prevent chip detection. When scanning on a stainless-steel table, a towel (or paper) should be placed under the cat not only for the cat's comfort but also to prevent interference that could reduce the likelihood of chip detection (Lord et al. 2008). Cats that will not accept handling must be heavily sedated prior to euthanasia so that proper scanning can be performed.

14.6.3 Euthanasia Techniques and Handling Methods

Humane euthanasia should be achieved through the administration of a sodium pentobarbital solution (often called "euthanasia solution"). For cats, acceptable routes of administration for injection of euthanasia solution include intravenous (IV) and intraperitoneal (IP). For cats that are unconscious or anesthetized prior to injection, intracardiac (IC) or intrarenal (IR) routes are also acceptable (Newbury et al. 2010;

AAFP 2021). Each of these routes of administration has advantages and disadvantages. In all instances, using a new needle of the smallest gauge possible will serve to reduce pain and discomfort during administration. Diluting euthanasia solution with saline or sterile water makes it easier to inject through a small needle (i.e., 25 gauge in very small kittens and 23 gauge in average-size cats).

Intravenous injection is theoretically very desirable because it results in rapid loss of consciousness and death (generally only seconds for each). However, reliably administering an IV injection in a low-stress manner is often difficult in cats that have not been sedated unless they are profoundly lethargic as a result of physical illness. Intravenous injections are also technically difficult to perform especially in very small cats and kittens, as well as those with poor venous access due to dehydration or other causes of poor peripheral perfusion. Pre-euthanasia sedation can be used to facilitate IV administration of sodium pentobarbital solution. However, such sedation may also make it more difficult to access peripheral veins. When pre-euthanasia drugs are used, subcutaneous injection (rather than intramuscular injection) is recommended because it is less painful for the animal. It is also easier to accomplish with less restraint compared to intramuscular injection and is equally effective within virtually the same amount of time. If pre-euthanasia drugs result in loss of consciousness, then an IC injection can be performed. Like IV administration, IC administration results in rapid death. An additional advantage of IC administration is that it can be used to verify death if the needle and syringe are left in place following injection. Cessation of visual motion of the syringe verifies cardiac standstill. Intracardiac (or IR) injections are unacceptable unless it has been reliably verified that the animal is unconscious, comatose, or anesthetized (i.e., lack of deep pain/toe withdrawal reflex) (Newbury et al. 2010).

For tractable cats, it is often much easier to administer an IP injection with minimal handling and restraint. Of note, with IP injection

the time to loss of consciousness is delayed compared to IV or IC injection. It typically takes at least a couple of minutes for a cat to lose consciousness following injection, and respiratory and cardiac arrest typically do not occur until 10–15 minutes post-injection.

There are a number of crucial keys to optimize the process of euthanasia using IP administration of sodium pentobarbital. Firstly, the dosage of euthanasia solution required is much higher than with IV, IC, or IR administration—at minimum, the dosage should be three times the recommended dosage of these routes. Using an even higher dose (such as five times the IV dose) will result in more rapid loss of consciousness, which is desirable. IP injection can be used in cats and kittens up to 15 lbs of body weight. The one exception is cats in an advanced state of pregnancy because it is difficult to avoid inadvertent injection into the uterus instead of the peritoneal cavity. In this case, IV or IC injection should be performed. IP injection is not recommended for very large cats (15 or more pounds) because of the high likelihood of excitement prior to the loss of consciousness.

When performed well, IP euthanasia results in cats passing peacefully into unconsciousness and death with few exceptions. In contrast, when the process of IP injection is performed poorly many cats will experience delayed loss of consciousness and heightened excitement during this time. With IP injection, care should be taken to avoid inadvertently injecting into the spleen or other organs, which could induce additional pain and excitement (Grier and Schaffer 1990). For this reason, injections may be best administered in the right lower quadrant of the abdomen or on the ventral midline. In addition, aspiration should be used to confirm negative pressure (as would be expected if the needle is in the peritoneal cavity) prior to injection. Using at least three times the IV dose (or more) will hasten loss of consciousness. Warming the solution prior to injection may also improve comfort. In terms of easily recognizable landmarks for IP injection, aim for the

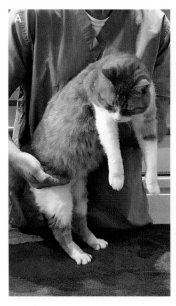
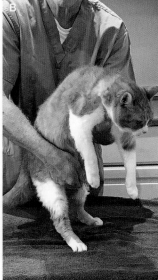
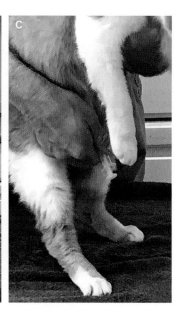

Figure 14.16   A. This cat is standing on his hind legs as the handler uses his left hand under the cat's chest to gently lift his front end off the table. The handler's right hand indicates the landmark for IP injection "just in front of the cat's leg." Note that the handler approaches the cat from behind to avoid leaning over him or facing him head on, which could be perceived by the cat as threatening. B. The handler demonstrates the technique for IP injection. C. Note the placement of the syringe on the midline with the hand holding the syringe just in front of the cat's leg.

midline (or to the right of the midline) just in front of the cat's hind leg (see Figure 14.16A). Following aspiration to verify negative pressure, the solution is injected without delay and the needle is then withdrawn from the abdomen.

To ensure that cats pass peacefully, humane handling is crucial: cats must be kept calm before, during, and after IP injection. In addition, a quiet, dimly lit environment is highly recommended. Tractable cats need only very light restraint and should be allowed to remain in a natural position rather than being flipped onto their side or back for injection. Personnel should allow the cat to stand while facing away from the handler, who then can gently lift them off of their front legs by placing a hand under their chest in order to perform the injection (see Figure 14.16B). All handling recommendations included in this chapter, including those for initiating contact should be used and the cat should be petted and soothed afterwards. Rather than injecting directly from the syringe itself, another option

is to use extension tubing to facilitate injection. For cats that are more active, one handler can pet and distract the cat while the needle is placed in the abdomen attached to a short piece of extension tubing with the syringe at the opposite end to inject the solution. Flushing the line with saline is necessary to ensure delivery of the entire volume of euthanasia solution. A new needle should be used for each animal, but tubing can be reused between cats.

Following IP injection, tractable cats may be swaddled securely in a towel with only their head and neck exposed. The handler can then rub their face and neck, soothing them until they lose consciousness. Another humane option is to immediately return the cat to their familiar enclosure with their hiding box, and to cover their box as well as the front of their cage with a towel to keep the environment as quiet, calm and peaceful as possible. If not in their housing ward, then the cat should be returned to their transport carrier, which is then covered and kept in a quiet area. Following IP injection, cats should never be placed on the floor or left unattended on a table and noise and light must be minimized. Cats should remain confined in a quiet, calm, dimly lit environment and must be monitored, which is best accomplished by listening as opposed to handling or otherwise disturbing the cat as they begin to lose consciousness. Cats should remain quiet without vocalization or struggling or other signs of excitement as they gradually lose consciousness. The goal is always to avoid excitement and to promote a smooth loss of consciousness during which the cat experiences minimal distress. Once unconscious, cats must continue to be monitored until they have progressed to respiratory and cardiac arrest.

In some cases, IP injection can be performed with the cat in a wire transport carrier. For cats that resist handling, this can be a good method to accomplish the injection with little stress. To perform IP injection, place the carrier on an exam table in a quiet room and keep the top and sides loosely covered with a towel. The cat will usually crouch quietly in the bottom. Gently slide the carrier off one side of the table, taking care to keep it level and steady. Slide it far enough off the table so that the wire floor supporting the cat's ventral abdomen is no longer on the table. A long needle (usually 1.5 inch) can then be gently introduced to accomplish the IP injection through the wire bars without otherwise touching the cat. When performed slowly and deliberately, most cats will remain calm and steady during this procedure. Highly reactive and feral cats generally must be sedated prior to euthanasia for microchip scanning. This should be done using a hands-off approach to make it as low stress as possible (see previous section). With regards to assessing chosen euthanasia techniques and handling methods, if cats are passing peacefully into unconsciousness, then the techniques and methods are likely to be good. If not, the selected techniques and methods should be reconsidered and adjusted to ensure the gentlest death possible. For more information on euthanasia techniques, refer to the chapter on euthanasia in *Shelter Medicine for Veterinarians and Staff*, 2nd ed. (Miller and Zawistowski 2013).

14.7 Conclusions

Techniques for safe and humane handling aim to keep cats gently under control while minimizing their stress and fear and ensuring the safety of both the cat and their handler(s). To accomplish this, actively reducing cat stress and fear through environmental management is essential. With training, experience, and a willingness to work together, shelter staff can create a calm environment for cats, which will result in smoother and safer handling and care. Successful safe and humane handling also requires patience, practice, good timing, finesse, and the ability to continuously apprise and assess the animals' signals and situation and adjust accordingly. Importantly, how cats are handled in the shelter not only impacts how they respond and behave, it also impacts the shelter's professional image. Ultimately, the way in which cats are handled affects the welfare of the cats themselves as well as that of those who handle them. By using a holistic approach to reducing cat stress and fear during care and handling, staff can create a safer and more pleasant work environment for everyone—animals and humans alike.

Please visit the companion website for video clips and downloadable resources associated with this chapter.

References

American Association of Feline Practitioners (AAFP). (2021). Euthanasia Process. https://catvets.com/end-of-life-toolkit/euthanasia-process (accessed 14 December 2021).

Carlstead, K., Brown, J.L., and Strawn, W. (1993). Behavioral and physiological correlates of stress in laboratory cats. *Appl. Anim. Behav. Sci.* 38: 143.

Carney, H., Little, S., Brownlee-Tomasso, D. et al. (2012). AAFP and ISFM feline-friendly nursing care guidelines. *J. Fel. Med. Surg.* 14 (5): 337–349.

Ellis, L.H., Rodan, I., Carney, H.C. et al. (2013). AAFP and ISFM feline environmental needs guidelines. *J. Fel. Med. Surg.* 15: 219–230.

Ellis, S. and Sparkes, A. (2016). International Society of Feline Medicine Guide to Feline Stress and Health. https://icatcare.org/shop/publications/isfm-guide-feline-stress-and-health (accessed 21 September 2020).

Grier, R.L. and Schaffer, C.B. (1990). Evaluation of intraperitoneal and intrahepatic administration of a euthanasia agent in animal shelter cats. *J. Am. Vet. Med. Assoc.* 197 (12): 1611–1615.

Griffin, B. (2011). Care and control of community cats. In: *The Cat: Clinical Medicine and Management* (ed. S. Little), 1290–1309. St. Louis, MO: Elsevier.

Griffin, B. (2020). Strategies to reduce stress and enhance patient comfort during the spay-neuter process. In: *High-Quality, High-Volume Spay and Neuter and Other Shelter Surgeries* (ed. S. White), 103–124. Hoboken, NJ: Wiley Blackwell.

Griffin, B. and Hume, K.R. (2006). Recognition and management of stress in housed cats. In: *Consultations in Feline Internal Medicine V* (ed. J.R. August), 717–734. St. Louis, MO: Elsevier.

Hammerle, M., Horst, C., Levine, E. et al. (2015). 2015 AAHA canine and feline behavior management guidelines. *J. Am. Anim. Hosp. Assoc.* 51 (4): 205–221.

Herron, M. and Shreyer, T. (2014). The pet-friendly veterinary practice: A guide for practitioners. *Vet. Clin. North Am. Small Anim. Pract.* 44 (3): 451–481.

Horwitz D.F. and Rodan I. (2018). Behavioral awareness in the feline consultation: Understanding physical and emotional health. *J. Fel. Med. Surg.* 20, 423–436.

Landsberg, G., Hunthausen, W., Ackerman, L. (2013). Developmental, social, and communicative behavior. In: *Behavior Problems of the Dog and Cat*, 3rd ed. (eds. G. Landsberg, W. Hunthausen, and L. Ackerman), 13–28. St. Louis, MO: Saunders Elsevier.

Leary, S., Underwood, W., Anthony, R. et al. (2020). AVMA Guidelines for the Euthanasia of Animals: 2020 Edition. https://www.avma.org/sites/default/files/2020-01/2020-Euthanasia-Final-1-17-20.pdf (accessed 15 August 2020).

Liu, S., Paterson, M., Camarri, S. et al. (2020). The effects of the frequency and method of gentling on the behavior of cats in shelters. *J. Vet. Behav.* 39: 47–56.

Lloyd, J. (2017). Minimising stress for patients in the veterinary hospital: Why it is important and what can be done about it. *Vet. Sci.* 4 (22): 1–19.

Lord, L.L., Pennell, M.L., Ingwersen, W. et al. (2008). Sensitivity of commercial scanners to microchips of various frequencies implanted in dogs and cats. *J. Am. Vet. Med. Assoc.* 233 (11): 1729–1735.

McMillan, F.D. (2002). Development of a mental wellness program for animals. *J. Am. Vet. Med. Assoc.* 220: 965.

Miller, L. and Zawistowski, S. (2013). *Shelter Medicine for Veterinarians and Staff*, 2nd ed. Hoboken, NJ: Wiley-Blackwell.

Newbury, S., Blinn, M.K., Bushby, P.A. et al. (2010). *Guidelines for Standards of Care in Animal Shelters*. Apex, NC: Association of Shelter Veterinarians.

Overall, K.L., Rodan, I., Beaver, B.V. et al. (2004) Feline Behavior Guidelines from the American Association of Feline Practitioners. https://catvets.com/guidelines/practice-guidelines/behavior-guidelines (accessed 20 July 2020).

Pankratz, K.E., Ferris, K.K., Griffith, E.H. et al. (2017). Use of single-dose oral gabapentin to attenuate fear responses in cage-trap confined community cats: A double-blind, placebo-controlled field trial. *J. Fel. Med. Surg.* 20 (6): 1–9.

Pereira, J.S., Fragoso, S., Beck, A. et al. (2016). Improving the feline veterinary consultation:

The usefulness of Feliway spray in reducing cats' stress. *J. Fel. Med. Surg.* 18 (12): 959–964.

Rhoades, R.H. (2002). The euthanasia area. In: *The Humane Society of the United States Euthanasia Training Manual*, 21–30. Washington, DC: Humane Society of the United States.

Rodan, I. (2010). Understanding feline behavior and application for appropriate handling and management. *Top. Companion Anim. M.* 25 (4): 178–188.

Rodan, I., Sundahl, E., Carney, H. et al. (2011). AAFP and ISFM feline-friendly handling guidelines. *J. Fel. Med. Surg.* 13 (5): 364–375.

Sparkes, A., Bond, R., Buffington, T. et al. (2016). Impact of stress and distress on physiology and clinical disease in cats. In: *International Society of Feline Medicine Guide to Feline Stress and Health* (eds. S. Ellis and A. Sparkes), 39–52. Wiltshire, UK: International Society of Feline Medicine.

Spinka, M. (2012). Social dimension of emotions and its implication for animal welfare. *Appl. Anim. Behav. Sci.* 138: 170–181.

Stevens, B.J., Frantz, E.M., Orlando J.M. et al. (2016). Efficacy of a single dose of trazodone hydrochloride given to cats prior to veterinary visits to reduce signs of transport- and examination-related anxiety. *J. Am. Vet. Med. Assoc.* 249 (2): 202–207.

van Haaften, K.A., Eichstadt, L.R., Stelow, E.A. et al. (2017). Effects of a single pre-appointment dose of gabapentin on signs of stress in cats during transportation and veterinary examination. *J. Am. Vet. Med. Assoc.* 251 (10): 1175–1181.

Yin, S. (2009). *Low Stress Handling, Restraint and Behavior Modification of Dogs and Cats.* Davis, CA: Cattle Dog Publishing.

15

Feline Behavioral Assessment
Jacklyn J. Ellis

15.1 Introduction

The life history, quality of previous experiences, and temperament of individual cats will greatly influence their behavior and how they should be managed while in the shelter system. Identifying individual differences and tailoring pathways and management plans is a crucial component of providing appropriate care to meet their behavioral needs. The Association of Shelter Veterinarians recommends regular behavior assessment of animals starting at intake through the duration of their stay as a critical part of maintaining behavioral health and mental well-being (Newbury et al. 2010). Behavior assessments can help to determine the propensity for undesirable behavior, to match cats with appropriate adopters, and to monitor their well-being while in the shelter (Siegford et al. 2003; Weiss et al. 2015; McCobb et al. 2005). It is commonly recommended that these assessments should be conducted as soon as possible after the animal arrives at the shelter in order to avoid prolonging length of stay (Scarlett et al. 2017). Results of behavior assessments are often used to make decisions about which animals are considered "adoptable," which require behavior modification, and which require interventions for stress alleviation. However, the process of conducting these behavior assessments

can be unclear. There are several frameworks that can be used by shelters to assess behavior. Their suitability may vary based on the goal of the assessment and the resources of the shelter. As trap-neuter-return efforts have increasing success, shelter intake rates are dropping (Levy et al. 2014), and staff is now able to work with cats with behaviors that would not have been considered for placement in the past. As shelter populations change, behavioral interventions and management may play a larger role in shelter programs, and understanding how behavior assessments can be used by shelters is crucial in this transition.

This chapter aims to (i) outline frameworks for assessing behavior, (ii) define the purposes for conducting behavior assessments in shelters, and (iii) guide shelters in how to use behavior assessments most effectively.

15.2 Frameworks for Assessing Behavior

Cats exhibit a range of discernible behaviors (e.g., grooming, hissing, sitting). Patterns of these behaviors are interpreted as traits (e.g., "fearful," "affectionate," "aggressive"). The goal of a behavior assessment is to infer which traits are being expressed through

Animal Behavior for Shelter Veterinarians and Staff, Second Edition. Edited by Brian A. DiGangi, Victoria A. Cussen, Pamela J. Reid, and Kristen A. Collins.
Companion website: www.wiley.com/go/digangi/animal

Table 15.1 Advantages and disadvantages of frameworks for assessing behavior.

Potential advantages of frameworks of assessing behavior	Structured behavioral test	Scan samples	Ad libitum behavior observation	Trait rating	Qualitative behavior history
Provides quantitative data set	✓	✓	✗	✓	✗
Conducted under controlled conditions	✓	✓	✗	✗	✗
Not impacted by shelter-induced stress	✗	✗	✗	✗	✓
Does not cause added stress	✗	✓	✓	✓	✓
Not subject to bias	✓	✓	✗	✗	✗
Assessment can be completed quickly after intake	✓	✗	✗	✗	✓
Assessment does not require additional space	✗	✓	✓	✓	✓
Assessment does not require significant training	✗	✓/✗	✓	✓	✓
Can be used for cats of all intake types	✓	✓	✓	✓	✓/✗
Assesses constructs directly	✗	✓/✗	✗	✓	✓

observation of these behaviors. There are several methodological frameworks in which this assessment can take place. Each presents advantages and disadvantages for use in shelter environments (see Table 15.1).

15.2.1 Structured Behavioral Test

Under this framework, an animal is exposed to one or more stimuli under controlled conditions during a predetermined timeframe and their behavioral response is measured. Conventionally, these tests are administered only once, but repeat testing can be conducted as well. The stimuli presented are usually selected to reflect stimuli that may be encountered in a traditional home environment. For example, a hypothetical test to assess if a cat is prone to inter-cat aggression could involve holding a second cat 1 ft. from the focal cat's cage for one minute and measuring the behaviors associated with aggression or affiliation exhibited by the focal cat. The method of

measuring these behaviors varies, but could include the presence or absence of a behavior (e.g., hissing), an ordinal rating of the severity of the behavior (e.g., 1 = pupils not dilated to 5 = pupils fully dilated), and the frequency, duration/proportion, or latency of a behavior (e.g., meowed four times, was in hiding box for 60% of test period, approached after 37 seconds). The conditions controlled within the testing environment usually include the characteristics of the room, the behavior of the tester, and the order in which the stimuli are presented, but controlling additional conditions may be requested as well. For example, a test may require a quiet room with no windows, the tester refrain from acknowledging the animal, and that animal be presented first with a novel object, then being pet with a stick, and finally introduced to an unfamiliar animal.

This framework has the advantage of producing a quantitative data set. If shelters set clear criteria for what results classify an "adoptable' animal, this framework facilitates easy decision-making, thereby reducing the time required to debate each case and reducing the burden of guilt often associated with rejecting an animal (UC Davis Koret Shelter Medicine Program 2019). These quantitative results can also be compared across individuals to understand how performance in these tests differs between variables such as intake type, sex, and reason for surrender. Findings could be used to generate a greater understanding of the different needs of these demographic categories, or within individuals to compare response to different stimuli (e.g., male or female handlers) to contribute to ideal placement recommendations.

Unfortunately, this framework has several disadvantages. Standardized behavior tests can use a lot of shelter resources (e.g., staff time, space for testing). It is also difficult (if not impossible) to present stimuli and conditions that adequately recreate real world situations, thus bringing into question the validity of results. Take for example, the hypothetical test to assess if a cat is prone to inter-cat aggression given above. Introducing a new cat to a resident cat in a home setting is often stressful for one or both cats. However, a responsible owner will ensure this introduction is gradual and paired with positive stimuli. In the hypothetical test situation this introduction is instantaneous, and the shelter setting presents additional stressors (e.g., barking dogs, confinement) likely not present in a home. It is not difficult to imagine that this trigger-stacking may result in a reaction that is not representative of how this cat would react to meeting a new cat in a home environment. Furthermore, while the controlled conditions limit the variability expected in the results (by reducing confounding factors), this may limit the ability to generalize the results outside of the confines of the test. For example, a test may be designed to assess tolerance of petting by measuring the presence/absence of swatting in response to touch, and the control conditions might stipulate that it is always conducted by the same handler to reduce

variability in approach style. However, results of that test may not be generalizable to other handlers with different approach styles. Finally, the stimuli presented in these tests are often purposefully provoking, resulting in a high degree of false positives (Patronek and Bradley 2016). Patronek and Bradley (2016) demonstrate mathematically that behavioral tests designed to identify aggressive behaviors in dogs provide results that are "no better than flipping a coin."

15.2.2 Scan Samples of Behaviors

This framework involves an observer approaching an animal's enclosure and recording the presence or absence of specific behaviors or behavioral indicators. To be most impactful, this would be conducted at multiple time-points, ideally on a regular schedule. Within a shelter this could be scheduled in association with other regular tasks, such as before cleaning/feeding. The regular schedule could therefore help in standardizing the conditions (e.g., before shelter is open to the public, before feeding/cleaning). Specified behaviors could include indicators of both positive (e.g., approach cage front, playing) and negative (e.g., hiding, hissing) emotions. Other indicators linked to stress could also be recorded, for example food intake (Ellis et al. 2014; Tanaka et al. 2012) or sickness behaviors (Stella et al. 2013; Tanaka et al. 2012). Certain behaviors could also be assessed on a continuum, such as pain (Epstein et al. 2015) or stress (e.g., the Cat-Stress-Score; Kessler and Turner 1997). These assessments require behavioral definitions and training of observers, but do not require previous experience with the individual animal.

This framework produces an ordinal data set and thus scores could be associated with specific criteria that can be used for decision-making or to monitor progress in behavior modification. The system also produces information about the cat's behavior daily, so information can be gathered quickly, problems can be identified early, and progress can be monitored easily. Unlike standardized behavioral tests, it does not use many resources (since assessments are conducted in the cat's home environment and can be done alongside regular shelter activities), is collected at multiple time points by design (eliminating the risk of making interpretations based on a single data point that could be anomalous), and is not in response to purposefully provoking stimuli.

Unfortunately, behaviors observed under this framework would also be influenced by the inherently stressful conditions of the shelter. This means that behaviors observed may not reflect how the cat would behave in a home environment. Additionally, these scans are best suited to monitor chronic problems (such as fear) and not specific undesirable behaviors (such as petting-induced aggression). Finally, training is required on the behavioral definitions and rating scales of the behaviors or behavioral indicators being measured, and ideally, interobserver reliability of raters should be assessed. This could be challenging for shelter environments where time is already stretched thin.

15.2.3 *Ad Libitum* Behavioral Observation

This framework involves observing and making inferences about an animal's behavior outside of a structured context. Observations can be made at any time (e.g., intake, medical exam, volunteer interactions). Any notable behaviors (such as those associated with aggression or fear) should be reported and recorded, as should the context in which the behavior(s) took place. For example, a volunteer interacting with a cat may observe that the cat was pushing into her hand while she was petting him, but that he hissed and retreated to his hiding box after five minutes of petting. This observation could contribute to the inference that the cat is exhibiting petting-induced aggression

A major advantage afforded by this framework is that it does not necessarily involve extra staff time. Notable behaviors are already being observed ad libitum by shelter staff and volunteers during their regular activities; all that is required is an organized system for reporting and recording them. Although the behavior exhibited in a shelter is always prone to the impact of stress, ad libitum observation of behavior in a free setting may avoid some of the behavioral abnormalities that may result from an artificial test situation. As a result, this framework is far less likely to result in false positives.

Unfortunately, this framework does not have clear criteria for interpretation, and thus does not lend itself to quick decision-making. Since it is based on observations made opportunistically over time, it may take time for issues to emerge. It also suffers from a lack of standardization, which can make observations difficult to interpret. As these observations can be made by a range of different people, this introduces a lot of variability in terms of the quality of the observations and the context of the interactions. Dawson et al. (2019) found that people vary widely in their ability to interpret feline emotion from cats' faces and that this ability was not related to owning a cat in the past. This study highlights the importance of a thorough training program in feline behavior for staff and volunteers if observations in a free setting can be trusted as a valid source of information. The context of the interaction needs to be considered as well. A cat exhibiting hissing and growling while a volunteer reads to them through their cage bars should be interpreted differently than the same behaviors exhibited while a technician is drawing blood. In shelters that are under resourced and cannot allocate much staff or volunteer time for positive enrichment-based interaction, most of the interaction the cats experience may take place during unpleasant activities such as cleaning and intake exams. This may bias the data to include higher rates of negative behaviors.

Finally, compliance with recording behaviors may not be high. Some people may elect not to record a behavior such as a bite or swat if they fear it may contribute to a euthanasia decision or if they are embarrassed they did not read warning signs and end the interaction earlier.

15.2.4 Trait Rating

Under this framework one or more individuals who have extensive experience with the animal rate them for various traits (e.g., agreeableness, neuroticism) using a Likert or visual analogue scale. Ratings on each trait can be compared between cats to identify differences, or within cats to identify common patterns of traits. This method is used broadly in the study of human individuality (e.g., the five-factor model; McCrae and John 1992), quality of life in farm animals (e.g., Qualitative Behavior Assessment; Wemelsfelder and Lawrence 2001), and within cats specifically (e.g., Feaver et al. 1986).

This framework benefits from the ability to measure the subtle aspects of a cat's behavior that do not fit well within the structures imposed by conventional methods of measuring behavior (Meagher 2009). Trainers familiar with each animal can rate them on traits in moments, and thus little staff time would need to be allocated to testing or data collection. Criteria could then be set for how to proceed based on an individual's score (e.g., if an animal scores ≥4 for "aggressiveness").

However, trait rating requires raters to have extensive experience with the individual animal, so even though the rating itself does not require significant staff time, ratings could not be made until the animal had been in care for enough time for the raters to have spent extensive time with them. Furthermore, the method is subjective and is thus subject to personal bias. Comparison between observer ratings is intended to help assess this problem (Meagher 2009), but this requires at least two observers, which could reduce the feasibility of using this method in shelters.

15.2.5 Qualitative Behavior History

This framework derives inferences about an animal's behavior through free text descriptions provided by someone with extensive experience with the individual. Within animal sheltering, this type of information is often collected through conversations with surrendering parties or intake forms. This structure allows for the description of an animal's temperament that may not be evident in the shelter situation, for anecdotal incidents that may be revealing about individual preferences or responses to specific stimuli, and for combinations of individual quirks.

However, it is easy to imagine how personal bias or emotion may play a role in the quality of information provided in owner reports, or how a lack of expertise in feline behavior may lead the owner to flawed conclusions. Details in intake profiles may be skewed to downplay behavioral issues if an owner thinks an honest description of the animal's behavior may result in euthanasia. Similarly, these descriptions may convey an exaggerated representation of negative qualities, as owners are often very frustrated with their cats when filling out these forms. They also can describe behaviors without the relevant context required to understand the motivation for the behavior. Furthermore, the qualitative behavior histories provided by owners do not lend themselves to clear criteria for acceptability, resulting in less clear-cut outcome decision-making. This increases the time required to debate each case and increases the burden of guilt on shelter staff that is often associated with rejecting an animal.

15.3 Goals of Behavior Assessments

When conducting a behavior assessment, it is imperative that the shelter has a clear understanding of their goal. There are a variety of goals that can be addressed using a behavior assessment, and each goal would be linked to different actions to ensure the well-being of the cat. The following section will describe how behavior assessments can be tailored to each specific goal, including the applicability of the frameworks outlined above.

15.3.1 Identify Propensity for Undesirable Behavior

A common goal of behavior assessments is to determine whether an individual animal is prone to specific undesirable behaviors. The propensity for such behaviors can influence whether a shelter feels equipped to accept an animal, whether an animal is deemed "adoptable," the housing and training/management that might be required for that animal's care while in shelter, and the home or environment deemed appropriate for that animal's placement.

A standardized behavioral test administered shortly after arrival at the shelter can seem an ideal framework for determining a propensity for undesirable behaviors. Predetermined pathway plans associated with the results from such a test can eliminate the necessity to debate the outcomes of animals, and alternative endpoints (e.g., euthanasia, return to colony, working cat programs) can be pursued quickly in appropriate cases. This would reduce the unnecessary suffering associated with a prolonged length of stay resulting from indecision, reduce the burden of guilt often felt by shelter staff, and focus time-consuming behavior modification efforts on individuals with the highest likelihood of being successfully rehomed. Furthermore, van der Borg et al. (1991) found that structured behavioral tests provided a better prediction of problem behavior than did the opinions of the staff based on ad libitum observations. However, there are several problems inherent in relying solely on the results of a standardized behavioral test including the stress of the shelter environment, the speed of assessment after intake, the reliance on the data from a single

assessment, debate about the ability of the test to predict the exhibition of unwanted behavior in subsequent homes, and the relative lack of tests developed for use with shelter cats.

It can be difficult to get an honest representation of how an animal is likely to behave in a home environment based solely on their behavior in a shelter. Despite the best efforts of staff and volunteers, shelters are an inherently stressful place for animals due to exposure to novel stimuli, confinement, reduced enrichment, and an absence of stable positive relationships. As behavior is a key part of the stress response, it is logical that an animal's behavior in a shelter environment would be impacted by the stress inherent in this environment. This is particularly true for cats as, unlike dogs, they are notoriously poorly socialized to novelty. Most cats are kept within the owner's home for the majority of their lives (with the exception of negative experiences, such as veterinary visits). In times of stress, the behavioral response of most animals is fight, flight, or freeze (Skinner et al. 2003). In the traditional shelter cage environment, the option to flee is largely removed or eliminated. This greatly increases the risk of aggression—a behavior that places a cat at increased risk for euthanasia. It is important to note that aggressive behaviors exhibited under these conditions are a normal behavioral response and not indicative of a pathological behavioral condition.

While the shelter environment is likely to be stressful for animals for the duration of their stay, it is experienced most profoundly during the first few days or weeks. Kessler and Turner (1997) found a sequential significant decrease in Cat-Stress-Scores (CSSs) each day a cat was in a boarding facility until day five, and Ellis et al. (2014) found that CSS decreased from week one to week two, and fecal glucocorticoid metabolites decreased from week one to week five in a shelter-like environment. These studies suggest that the average time for cats to habituate to a shelter environment ranges from five days to five weeks. While the ability to make quick decisions about an animal's fate provided by structured behavioral tests is ideal from an efficiency standpoint, the profound stress experienced by a cat immediately following intake has the potential to greatly impact the validity of an assessment conducted during this period.

Many problem behaviors identified by behavior assessments depend on a range of conditions, such as the cat's experience that day, previous experience with handler, hunger, or pain. For example, attempts to pet a cat who has spent all day napping could easily be met with a different outcome than a cat who has spent all day enduring painful medical procedures. Slater et al. (2013b) found that cats needed to be interacted with on multiple occasions in order to capture key behaviors that are indicators of socialization. Standardizing conditions for behavioral tests can be difficult even in a laboratory context, and in a busy shelter environment can be next to impossible. As decisions about animals are often based on the results of a single behavioral test, it is impossible to account for the impact of variables, such as affective state, on test results (Patronek and Bradley 2016).

There is a growing body of research questioning the ability of behavioral tests conducted in shelters to predict behavior in subsequent homes. Within the dog literature, Christensen et al. (2007) found that more than 40% of dogs that passed an in-shelter behavioral test designed to identify a propensity for aggressive behavior exhibited aggressive behaviors in their subsequent home, and Mohan-Gibbons et al. (2012) found that adopters of dogs identified as exhibiting food-guarding behaviors in shelter via a standardized behavioral test reported this behavior as rare or absent in their home during follow-up surveys. The standardized behavioral tests used in both of these studies had been published and subjected to the rigor of the peer review process. However, the incongruency of behavior in the home and shelter environment point to these tests having poor predictive value. See Chapter 9 for more information on assessing the behavior of shelter dogs.

Adding further difficulty to the use of standardized behavioral tests is the relative lack of such tests in the literature for cats as compared to dogs. The Feline Temperament Profile (FTP) may be the only published example of such a test, at least for use with socialized cats. The FTP was originally designed (Lee et al. 1983) to determine the suitability of individual cats for companion animals in nursing homes by identifying "acceptable" and "questionable" behaviors through 10 sequential mini-tests of increasing contact (e.g., calling the cat, petting the cat, holding the cat) with an unfamiliar person. Due to the to the ease of administration, small time commitment, and absence of the need of observers with extensive knowledge of the animal, Siegford et al. (2003) recognized the potential for use of this test in shelter conditions and set about evaluating its validity and predictive value by comparing the test results to behavioral observations in other settings and the test's ability to predict behavior after adoption. Researchers found that FTP scores lined up well with the behavioral observations in other settings, and that the difference in FTP scores was minor between those in the shelter compared to those in the home environment after adoption. The authors contend that FTP scores are valid, consistent, and can be used to determine how applicable a cat would be for particular types of homes. For example, cats with high scores could be placed with families, novices, or people wanting a sociable pet, while cats with low scores would require an experienced cat owner or someone who does not desire a high degree of interaction. However, this test is not designed to identify propensity for *specific* undesirable behaviors, as exist for dogs (e.g., food guarding). Accordingly, many standardized behavioral tests conducted by shelters for this purpose would be developed outside of the peer-review process, where rigorous analysis of the validity or reliability of the test is less likely.

It is often said that the best predictor of future behavior is past behavior. Shelters should focus on collecting the most detailed information possible at intake to identify propensity for undesirable behaviors, as this framework could provide a more honest reflection of the cat's behavior in a home environment. Unfortunately, relying on the information provided on an intake profile has other potential confounders to validity. Most prominently, this relies on accurate reporting by the previous owner. Within shelters, it is commonly suspected that some owners report relinquishing animals due to reasons such as "allergies" to reduce feelings of guilt associated with relinquishing because they are unable to manage unwanted behaviors. It is also supposed that some owners fail to report behavioral concerns out of fear that this will result in immediate euthanasia. Even when previous owners do report previous behavior concerns, these behaviors are communicated through the subjective experience and interpretation of the owner. Cats may be described as "mean" and "attacking out of spite," when an objective retelling of events might reveal that incidents resulting in injury started with cornering and forceful restraint of the cat. The first scenario may lead shelter staff to conclude that the cat is prone to exhibiting redirected aggression (a behavior that is notoriously difficult to predict and has high likelihood of injury), while the second scenario would be interpreted as defensive aggression (a normal behavioral response to frightening conditions, which can be much easier to manage). These profiles often suffer from a non-standardized use of terms. For example, the word "friendly" may be used by one owner to describe a cuddly lap cat, while another may use it to describe a cat that has never exhibited aggression but does not enjoy human interaction. Similarly, the word "feral" may be used to describe a cat that is not socialized to people, or to describe a cat that lives outside but actively solicits interaction with people and enjoys petting. Additionally, a cat's behavior is directly influenced by the conditions in which he was kept, and intake profiles

do not always collect this information. Conditions of the home that could contribute to the cat's behavior include the amount of enrichment provided; the composition of the home (number of other people/pets, etc.); the routine and level of activity within the home; the amount and quality of attention paid to him; and the owner's response to any unwanted behaviors exhibited. Complicating the picture, even if all these details are accurately relayed, shelter staff cannot say with certainty that the cat would exhibit the unwanted behavior under different conditions. Finally, trusting the information on an intake profile presupposes that it requests behavior information in the first place. The questions asked on intake profiles vary widely between shelters, and not all institutions request information about behavior at all. Furthermore, in those that do, the phrasing of questions may be misleading. Any of these factors can result in shelter staff having an incomplete or inaccurate picture of the cat's behavior in a previous home.

Careful design of an intake profile can be one of the most important strategies of any shelter in caring for the behavioral health of the animals in their care. As outlined above, behavioral information should be requested and special attention should be given to the wording of each question. Most shelters develop their own intake profiles, but few shelters have the resources to devote to analyzing which questions provide the most useful responses and which questions should be refined or removed. A tool called Fe-BARQ (Feline Behavior Assessment and Research Questionnaire; Duffy et al. 2017) may serve as a useful supplement to, or replacement for, behavioral questions on intake profiles. The Fe-BARQ was developed as a companion tool to the C-BARQ (Canine Behavior Assessment and Research Questionnaire; Hsu and Serpell 2003), which has been used to investigate specific undesirable behaviors (van den Berg et al. 2010), suitability of young dogs as guide and service dogs (Duffy and Serpell 2012), and the applicability of the test in different geographical regions (Nagasawa et al. 2011; Tamimi et al. 2015; González-Ramírez et al. 2017). The Fe-BARQ was designed to measure feline behavior through indirect behavioral information provided by the cat's owner in a 149-question questionnaire. Questions were selected based on a literature review, and a panel of five experts on cat behavior reviewed and revised them to establish content validity. The authors' construct validity was ensured by (i) comparing results to owner's rating of severity of their cat's behavior problems; (ii) comparison of results with expectations associated with demographic and/or lifestyle characteristics (e.g., playfulness should decline with age); and (iii) whether differences in results from various breeds of cats aligned with previously published findings. The results reveal how the cat scores on 23 different behavioral factors and compares it to the average for all cats that have taken the test. Shelters may then use this standardized information to make inferences about the cat's behavior and potential for rehoming. Additionally, Wilhelmy et al. (2016) modified the Fe-BARQ to screen for six behavioral pathologies (e.g., redirected aggression, separation anxiety, inappropriate elimination/marking). Although the modified Fe-BARQ has potential to reveal a lot about a cat's propensity for undesirable behavior and could be a valuable tool for use in shelters, further work is required to investigate its predictive value.

In some cases (e.g., strays) it is not possible to answer the full range of behavioral questions asked on the Fe-BARQ or most intake profiles. However, even in these cases, there are many questions that can be asked of the Good Samaritan to arm shelter staff with information that could be useful in pathway planning (e.g., How did you get the cat into the carrier? Did the cat approach you? See Appendix 15.A). These basic behavioral histories can be used as a foundation for making some assumptions about the cat's level of socialization to people. Assessment of the

cat's behavior in shelter (either standardized tests or ad libitum observations) can then be used to supplement this information and make conclusions about the propensity for other behavioral concerns. Compared to owner surrendered cats, these observations may be less influenced by the stress of shelter conditions. Dybdall et al. (2007) found that owner surrendered cats showed greater behavioral signs of stress and developed upper respiratory infections more quickly than did stray cats. This may be because stray cats are more accustomed to novelty.

15.3.1.1 Unsocialized Cats

An important subset of these "undesirable behaviors" are those exhibited by cats that have not been properly socialized to humans. Some cats have never been exposed to people and flee at the sight of them, while others have lived their whole lives in loving homes and crave attention from humans. Many cats are somewhere in between. When cats have a lot of positive experiences with humans (especially if these experiences start at an early age), they learn to trust and form close relationships with people. This process is called socialization, and all cats exist somewhere on the socialization spectrum. It is possible for a cat's location on the spectrum to change over time: less socialized cats can become more socialized if exposure to people is paired with positive associations, and more socialized cats can become less socialized if their exposure to humans is reduced and/or paired with negative associations (Slater 2004). With time and effort most cats can become more socialized, but there is often a ceiling effect on these efforts. This means that the "more socialized" version of a previously unsocialized cat may still be poorly suited for a home environment. Moreover, these cats are especially at risk of euthanasia (Lepper et al. 2002; Slater et al. 2010; Tanaka et al. 2012) and experiencing extreme stress in shelters, making them at greater risk of contracting disease (Tanaka et al. 2012). For these reasons, it can be of paramount importance to identify quickly if a cat is truly unsocialized (Slater et al. 2013) and make outcome decisions that would reduce unnecessary suffering in these populations (i.e., euthanasia, trap-neuter-return, return to field, or alternative placement).

Unfortunately, it can be exceedingly difficult to differentiate between unsocialized cats or cats that are fearful due to the shelter conditions. There are limited resources available for shelters to help make these decisions. Slater et al. (2010) found that only 15% of shelters had written guidelines for identifying unsocialized cats. While researching the impact of group housing on shelter cat welfare, Kessler and Turner (1999) identified cats as unsocialized if they scored a mean CSS >4 in eight tests. However, this was never validated by comparing the results of this assessment to known socialization status. Alley Cat Allies has a guide on their website aimed at helping differentiate between unsocialized and stray cats (Alley Cat Allies 2017). However, again no evidence of validation is presented. Furthermore, the criteria presented are not clear enough for shelter staff to differentiate confidently between unsocialized and fearful but socialized cats.

The ASPCA has produced the Feline Spectrum Assessment (FSA) to help shelters identify where a cat falls on the socialization spectrum, based on a series of studies by Slater et al. (2013a, 2013b, 2013c). The authors first developed the Cat Behavior and Background Survey based on personal experience and data published on feline behavior. The results produced a Socialization Score ranging from 0 (extremely unsocialized) to 10 (extremely socialized). After testing and revision, they described the questionnaire as "sufficiently reliable and valid. . .to describe the socialization level of cats to humans when the cats are in a variety of situations in their normal environment" (Slater et al. 2013b). Next, the authors wanted to develop a standardized behavioral test for use in shelters that could determine a cat's level of socialization as accurately, quickly,

and easily as possible. They started with six mini-tests consisting of 46 individual measures, conducted at five time-points. Next, they tested the validity of each test and measure by comparing the results of individual cats to their corresponding Socialization Scores, derived from the questionnaires filled out by their owners or caregivers. After dropping tests and measures with poor predictive value, the authors describe the final test as having adequate validity (Slater et al. 2013a). The publicly available FSA (ASPCA n.d.) consists of four mini-tests (see Figure 15.1), with 25 individual measures, conducted at four time points, over a two- to three-day period. Results are interpreted through process of elimination: (i) if at any point a cat is observed exhibiting a strong indicator, they can be classified as socialized, and no further testing is required; (ii) if a cat is observed exhibiting a weak indicator four or more times across the days, they can be classified as socialized, and no further testing is required; and (iii) during a.m. observations some measures result in point values (determined through statistical modeling)— the points scored can be compared to a matrix to determine the corresponding interpretation of how likely the cat is to be socialized. While more testing is needed to determine the true validity of this test, it remains the best tool available for determining the socialization status of cats for whom no behavior history is available, especially where speedy decision-making is paramount. Nevertheless, the manual encourages shelter staff to supplement the test results with any other available information when making outcome decisions, including ad libitum observations of behavior, behavioral information provided by whomever brought the cat into the shelter (e.g., was the cat trapped or picked up and put into a carrier), heath status, and previous experience (e.g., an unsocialized basement cat may not be suitable for a barn program).

Finally, in cases where the presence of behavioral issues that would preclude the cat from being deemed "adoptable" is suspected, but there is reason to believe that this may be

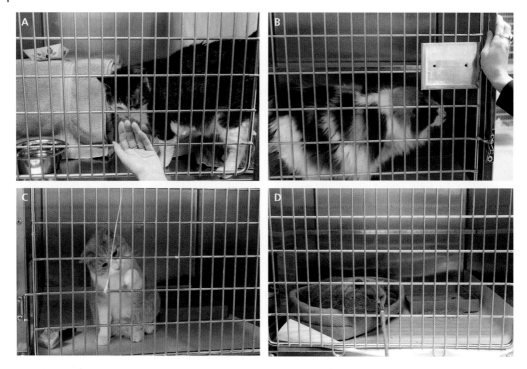

Figure 15.1 The four mini-tests on the ASPCA's Feline Spectrum Assessment: A = greet, B = hand on cage and cracking the cage door, C = interactive toy, and D = touch with wand.

exacerbated by the stress inherent in the shelter conditions, placing the cat in a foster home may provide valuable insight into how the cat might behave in subsequent adoptive homes.

While a standardized behavioral test can be a tempting framework for identifying an individual animal's propensity for undesirable behavior, in practice, a holistic approach using information from all possible frameworks of assessing behavior is likely the best approach.

15.3.2 Behavior Assessment for Matching Cat and Adopter

The terms personality and temperament are often used interchangeably. Several authors have challenged this, but there is currently no consensus across disciplines about the definition or proper usage of either (MacKay and Haskell 2015; Cloninger, 1994). For the purposes of this chapter, the term temperament will be used and will be defined as a tendency

to react or behave in a way that is generally consistent across time and context and is composed of various traits.

Within companion animals, the study of temperament is generating increasing interest. Gartner (2015) reported 51 studies of temperament in the domestic dog and 24 in the domestic cat. Each study has identified various temperament traits in each species and often attempted to categorize individuals on the spectrum of each trait. These studies are composed of a combination of structured behavioral tests and behavior ratings via surveys filled out by owners or caretakers who have extensive experience with the animal. For example, Feaver et al. (1986) investigated the validity of using observer rating to assess the temperament of the cats in their colony. After three months of conducting behavioral observation in a free setting, two observers were asked to rate the cats on 18 behaviorally defined traits (e.g., curious, fearful of people, tense) using a visual analogue scale. Each trait was rated by marking a cross on a 14 cm line, with a cross near the far left of the line representing the minimum expression of that trait and the right side representing the maximum expression of the trait. After dropping the traits with low interobserver reliability (<0.7) the authors examined the scores of the remaining traits for patterns. Three temperament types emerged: (i) active, aggressive, bossy; (ii) timid, nervous; and (iii) sociable, confident, easygoing. The authors declared the ratings to be adequately validated because the ratings correlated significantly with equivalent behaviors measured via the quantitative behavioral observations conducted in a free setting during the first three months.

There is potential value for evaluating the temperament of an animal in a shelter setting. Careful matching of cats and adopters may improve satisfaction, contribute to a better human-animal bond, and reduce the number of returns. Shore (2005) determined that unrealistic expectations were an important risk factor for the return of adopted dogs and that better understanding of the animal's temperament would be a key to successful placement. Cat temperament is the best predictor of owner satisfaction (Elvers and Lawriw 2019; Evans et al. 2019) and humans with certain traits are more likely to be satisfied with cats of certain traits. For example, Evans et al. (2019) found that owner satisfaction was high in dyads in which the owner scored high in the trait "impulsiveness" and the cat scored low in the trait "agreeableness." There is also reason to believe that cats of different temperaments might experience stress differently, be stressed by different stimuli, and/or benefit from different management practices (McCune 1994).

Given the potential benefits of assessing temperament in a shelter environment, it is essential to evaluate the best methods for assessment under these conditions. It has been asserted that trait ratings are more efficient (Gosling 2001) and more reliable than behavior observation (Vazire et al. 2007), assuming

the rater has extensive experience with the animal. Unfortunately, this is not always practical in a shelter environment since staff are unlikely to have sufficient experience with cats—with the possible exception of long stay individuals.

Compared to dogs, there have been relatively few standardized behavioral tests published to assess temperament in cats. As described earlier, the Feline Temperament Profile was designed to assess the suitability of individual cats for companion animals in nursing homes. The name suggests that it is designed to assess temperament, but this test was not designed to identify propensity for *specific* undesirable behaviors, nor does it assess *specific* temperament traits. In practice, it addresses *both* undesirable behaviors (as behaviors in response to each mini-test were classified as either "acceptable" or "questionable") *and* temperament (as many of the mini-tests measured response to an unfamiliar person, and "sociability' is a common temperament trait assessed in cats [Gartner and Weiss 2013]). Furthermore, the author contends that this test could be used by shelter staff to assess a cat's temperament to place the cat in a compatible home.

The ASPCA's Meet Your Match® Felineality™ was specifically designed to assess temperament in shelter cats in order to match them with appropriate adopters (Weiss 2007). It consists of a standardized behavioral test (based largely on the FTP) and a survey for potential adopters to fill out about what they are looking for in a new pet. Data from the behavioral test is used to rate the cat on both a valiance scale and a gregarious scale and the cat is then categorized within one of nine possible cat temperament types (e.g., the "love bug" or the "secret admirer"). Adopter surveys are scored based on the same scales and determine which cat temperament type would best suit the adopter's expectation and lifestyle. Adoption suggestions can then be made based on matching the results. A modified version of the program has since been found to be predictive of cat behavior post-adoption (Weiss et al. 2015) and applicable to cats in a different geographical region (Fukimoto et al. 2019). Individual shelters have also reported a reduction in adoption returns since implementing the program (Weiss 2007). Based on these findings, there is reason to believe that this test could be useful in helping place cats in the best possible homes. While both the FTP and the ASPCA's Meet Your Match Feline-ality are designed to be quick, they may not be practical for shelters with few staff, high feline intake, or short length of stay.

Despite the promising but limited findings of studies using standardized behavioral tests to assess temperament in shelter cats, it is still unclear how shelter conditions impact the expression of associated behaviors. For owner surrendered cats, it is possible that the information that is most reflective of temperament could be collected during the intake process. The Fe-BARQ (described in Section 15.3.1) could be useful in gaining insight in the temperament of a cat in a home environment.

15.3.3 Behavior Assessment to Monitor Well-Being

Perhaps the most underused way to use behavior assessments in a shelter is to inform enclosure design, husbandry, and behavior modification programs, with the goal of improving feline well-being. The growth of the no-kill movement may lead to an increase in emphasizing the importance of behavior assessments for this purpose. This can be done on a group or individual level, and within or between shelters. In these assessments, behavior can be measured in a range of ways.

By far the most common behavioral measure used for assessing well-being in shelter cats is the CSS (Kessler and Turner 1997). In this assessment, a trained observer assigns a cat a score between 1 (fully relaxed) and 7 (terrorized) by comparing that cat's body language and behavior to operationally defined descriptions of body language and behavior within a matrix. The Fear Free certification program (Fear Free Pets n.d.) also offers a similar rating

scale called the Fear, Anxiety, and Stress score for use in cats. The program also has a Fear, Anxiety, and Stress score in dogs and the potential to use a consistent scale with both species could be appealing to shelters. However, as of yet no studies have evaluated the reliability or validity of these scales in shelters, so institutions choosing to use them must keep this in mind.

Well-being has also been assessed behaviorally in shelter cats by measuring the percentage of time spent in various postures, locations, or activities (e.g., Ellis et al. 2014), the presence or absence of behaviors that are associated with positive or negative emotions (e.g., attempting to hide [Kry and Casey 2007]), or behavior in response to a standardized behavioral test (e.g., approach test [Kessler and Turner 1999]).

By assessing behavioral indicators of well-being in the same individual over time, it is possible to make inferences about adaptation to shelter conditions or the success of interventions made by shelter staff to address well-being concerns. For example, CSS could be collected before and after the provision of a social companion (see Figure 15.2), instances of emerging from hiding could be measured in response to socializing kittens, or number of pets tolerated could be measured when desensitizing and counter-conditioning cats to petting. A record of behavioral indicators of well-being over time could also help in making euthanasia decisions when quality of life is in question.

Optimizing shelter conditions is one of the most impactful ways staff and volunteers can improve the well-being of the cats in their care. Shelter design, husbandry, and behavior modification programs have direct impact on the behaviors expressed by the animals. Assessing and comparing these behaviors can give insight into the quality of the environments; animals will exhibit less stress, more desirable behaviors, and fewer undesirable behaviors when their environments are designed to meet their behavioral and

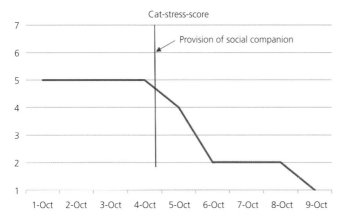

Figure 15.2 Cat-Stress-Score in response to provision of a social companion as an example of using behavioral assessments to monitor the impact of behavioral interventions on the well-being of shelter cats.

psychological needs. To capitalize on this, researchers compare the behaviors assessed by animals in similar environments that differ in one aspect, to make inferences about how that aspect impacts their well-being. The results of these studies allow researchers to make recommendations for optimizing environments that can be adopted by shelters worldwide. For example, several studies have focused on the impact of providing hiding boxes to shelter cats (Kry and Casey 2007; Vinke et al. 2014; van der Leij et al. 2019). Each of these studies showed that the provision of a hiding box facilitated a quicker reduction in stress after arrival in a shelter. Additionally, cats given hiding boxes were more likely to approach the cage front (Kry and Casey 2007) and spent less time behind their litter box (Vinke et al. 2014). The provision of hiding boxes is now considered essential for housing cats in shelter environments (Wagner et al. 2018), likely as a result of the findings of these and other studies.

It is possible to make inferences about the quality of conditions in different shelters by comparing the behaviors assessed in each. McCobb et al. (2005) monitored CSS at four different animal shelters that provided cats with varying degrees of environmental enrichment, housing designs, proximity to canine

housing, and number of caregivers. While the study did not find a difference in CSS between the sites, it introduced the idea of using a standardized behavioral assessment to compare stress levels between sites and making inferences about the quality of the environments provided by each.

15.4 How to Structure A Behavior Assessment Program in Your Shelter

The behavior assessment process can be overwhelming. It is essential that each shelter have a firm grasp on what they are trying to assess and the methods that will contribute to their assessments, have written protocols for the process, and have a clear chain of authority and oversight for the program.

The first step in any behavior assessment program is careful consideration of the behavioral information collected at intake. Ensure that each question is designed to elicit information regarding specific behavior concerns (previous exhibition of specific behaviors, context, temperament, etc.). If creating your own intake form, consider including questions that require people to select from defined categories to ensure a common language, in addition to including room for free text responses. If your shelter decides to use an available resource to collect behavioral information (e.g., Fe-BARQ), ensure that you have a proper understanding of the tool and a plan for interpreting/using results. It is also important to collect behavioral information during intake through non-traditional routes (strays, custodial surrender, transfer from another shelter), and therefore additional intake/behavioral history forms should be created for these purposes. Although less information will be available for animals brought in through these sources, there is almost certainly information available that will prove beneficial.

Aspects of the behavior assessment program designed to be conducted in shelter must be tailored to the resources and needs of each shelter. If you have a dedicated behavior department a more thorough and continual process will be possible, but if behavior assessments must be conducted by animal care workers or volunteers who have other competing responsibilities, your program will likely be less intensive. Think carefully about what information you collect, ensuring the most effective use of these resources. The amount of data you collect may also be limited by the method of recording. If information is recorded directly into an electronic database, this will allow more to be collected, as transferring from paper to a computer program requires more time and is an additional source of human error. If your shelter does not have a dedicated space where tests such as the ASPCA's Meet Your Match Feline-ality can be conducted, this will limit the feasibility of these tests for your institution. Finally, you must consider the characteristics typical of the cats taken in at your shelter and your shelter's average length of stay to determine the appropriateness of each assessment method. For example, the FSA would not be appropriate for facilities that only receive socialized cats, and the ASPCA's Meet Your Match Feline-ality may not be beneficial for shelters with short length of stay.

At minimum, all shelters should have:

- A person (or persons) responsible for the behavior assessment program
- Intake profiles requesting behavioral information
- A repository for keeping behavioral records for individual animals
- A method for flagging animals exhibiting concerning behaviors to be assessed more thoroughly
- A system for addressing these concerns
- And preferably, a daily record of basic behavioral indicators (e.g., food intake, CSS, hiding).

Finally, once you have designed your behavior assessment program, it is important to be open to change. Research is always producing new findings that can help make our assessments more efficient and effective. Keep up to date with developments by attending conferences or setting Google alerts to notify you when new research is published. Reassess your process periodically to see what can be added or to streamline your program by removing cumbersome methods that are not providing actionable information.

15.4.1 Creating Your Own Structured Behavioral Test

Despite the disadvantages of a structured behavioral test, many shelters find them appealing and create their own to assess a range of issues. If for any reason your shelter feels the need to create their own structured behavioral test to aid in your behavior assessment program, there are several factors that need to be considered:

- Validity: the degree to which a test accurately measures the intended concept
- Reliability: the extent to which a test yields consistent results when conducted multiple times
- Feasibility: the potential for the test to be carried out given the resources available (e.g., time, space, skill).

Table 15.2 Types of reliability and validity.

	Subcategory	Definition
Reliability	Inter-observer	Agreement between multiple people independently rating the same observation
	Intra-observer	Agreement between multiple ratings made by one person of the same observation (i.e., via a video recording)
	Test-retest	Agreement between results on the same test conducted at different times
	Internal consistency	Agreement between measures designed to measure the same construct
Validity	Content	The extent to which a research instrument accurately measures all aspects of a construct
	Criterion	Accuracy of the measure in predicting scores of a related measure
	Predictive	Accuracy of the measure in predicting another measure assessed in the future
	Concurrent	Accuracy of the measure in predicting another measure assessed at the same time
	Construct	The extent to which inferences can be drawn based on the measures
	Convergent	The extent to which the measure correlates with others to which it is theoretically related
	Discriminant	The lack of correlation between the measure and others to which it is not conceptually related

Adapted from Meager 2009; Heale and Twycross 2015.

There are several subcategories of both validity and reliability and for a test to be accurate; each type should be satisfied. It is beyond the scope of this chapter to explain the intricacies of each, but Table 15.2 has been included as an overview and starting place for further research.

15.5 Conclusions

Behavioral assessments of cats are key in helping animal shelters achieve a variety of objectives, such as identifying a propensity for undesirable behaviors, matching with appropriate adopters, and monitoring their well-being. However, relying solely on provocative behavioral tests is quickly falling out of fashion for a number of reasons, largely due to questions surrounding their validity. A holistic approach consisting of not only structured behavioral tests but also scan samples of behaviors, ad libitum behavioral observations, trait-rating systems, and qualitative behavioral histories is a more appropriate approach. Setting clear criteria for how to move forward with pathway planning based on the results of specific assessment techniques can facilitate easy decision-making, but ultimately it is important to consider the needs of each cat as an individual, examining all available evidence. Where possible, shelter behavior assessment programs should use techniques that have been validated in the literature, but when the need to create an in-house structured behavioral test is identified, it is essential to consider validity, reliability, and feasibility. Finally, one of the most important components of a shelter's behavior assessment program is that it is organized and focused to the specific needs of the organization.

References

Alley Cat Allies. (2017). Feral and Stray Cats—An Important Difference. https://www.alleycat.org/resources/feral-and-stray-cats-an-important-difference/ (accessed 5 February 2020).

ASPCA. (n.d.). The ASPCA's Feline Spectrum Assessment: A Tool to Identify the Socialization Level in Cats. https://www.aspcapro.org/sites/default/files/ASPCA-FSA-manual-2016.pdf (accessed 5 February 2020).

Christensen, E.L., Scarlett, J., Campagna, M. et al. (2007). Aggressive behavior in adopted dogs that passed a temperament test. *App. Anim. Behav. Sci.* 106 (1–3): 85–95.

Cloninger, C.R. (1994). Temperament and personality. *Curr. Opin. Neurobiol.* 4 (2): 266–273.

Dawson, L., Niel, L., Cheal, J. et al. (2019). Humans can identify cats' affective states from subtle facial expressions. *Anim. Welf.* 28 (4): 519–531.

Duffy, D.L., de Moura, R.T.D., and Serpell, J.A. (2017). Development and evaluation of the Fe-BARQ: A new survey instrument for measuring behavior in domestic cats (*Felis s. catus*). *Behav. Process.* 141: 329–341.

Duffy, D.L. and Serpell, J.A. (2012). Predictive validity of a method for evaluating temperament in young guide and service dogs. *Appl. Anim. Behav. Sci.* 138 (1–2): 99–109.

Dybdall, K., Strasser, R., and Katz, T. (2007). Behavioral differences between owner surrender and stray domestic cats after entering an animal shelter. *Appl. Anim. Behav. Sci.* 104 (1–2): 85–94.

Ellis, J.J., Protopapadaki, V., Stryhn, H. et al. (2014). Behavioural and faecal glucocorticoid metabolite responses of single caging in six cats over 30 days. *Vet. Rec. Open* 1 (1): e000056.

Elvers, G.C. and Lawriw, A.N. (2019). The behavioral style of the cat predicts owner satisfaction. *Anthrozoös* 32 (6): 757–768.

Epstein, M.E., Rodan, I., Griffenhagen, G. et al. (2015). 2015 AAHA/AAFP pain management guidelines for dogs and cats. *J. Fel. Med. Surg.* 17 (3): 251–272.

Evans, R., Lyons, M., Brewer, G. et al. (2019). The purrfect match: The influence of personality on owner satisfaction with their domestic cat (*Felis silvestris catus*). *Pers. Individ. Differ.* 138: 252–256.

Fear Free Pets (n.d.). Fear, Anxiety, and Stress Spectrum. https://fearfreepets.com/fas-spectrum/ (accessed 5 February 2020).

Feaver, J., Mendl, M., and Bateson, P. (1986). A method for rating the individual distinctiveness of domestic cats. *Anim. Behav.* 34 (4): 1016–1025.

Fukimoto, N., Howat-Rodrigues, A.B., and Mendonça-Furtado, O. (2019). Modified Meet Your Match® Feline-ality™ validity assessment: An exploratory factor analysis of a sample of domestic cats in a Brazilian shelter. *Appl. Anim. Behav. Sci.* 215: 61–67.

Gartner, M.C. (2015). Pet personality: A review. *Pers. Individ.* https://doi.org/10.1016/j.paid.2014.10.042.

Gartner, M.C. and Weiss, A. (2013). Personality in felids: A review. *Appl. Anim. Behav. Sci.* 144: 1–13.

González-Ramírez, M.T., Quezada-Berumen, L., and Landero-Hernández, R. (2017). Assessment of canine behaviors using C-BARQ in a sample from northern Mexico. *J. Vet. Behav.* 20: 52–58.

Gosling, S.D. (2001). From mice to men: what can we learn about personality from animal research? *Psychol. Bull.* 127 (1): 45.

Heale, R. and Twycross, A. (2015). Validity and reliability in quantitative studies. *Evid. Based Nurs.* 18 (3): 66–67.

Hsu, Y. and Serpell, J.A. (2003). Development and validation of a questionnaire for measuring behavior and temperament traits in pet dogs. *J. Am. Vet. Med. Assoc.* 223 (9): 1293–1300.

Kessler, M.R. and Turner, D.C. (1997). Stress and adaptation of cats (*Felis silvestris catus*) housed singly, in pairs and in groups in boarding catteries. *Anim. Welf.* 6 (3): 243–254.

Kessler, M.R. and Turner, D.C. (1999). Socialization and stress in cats (*Felis silvestris catus*) housed singly and in groups in animal shelters. *Anim. Welf.* 8 (1): 15–26.

Kry, K. and Casey, R. (2007). The effect of hiding enrichment on stress levels and behaviour of domestic cats (*Felis sylvestris catus*) in a shelter setting and the implications for adoption potential. *Anim. Welf.* 16 (3): 375–383.

Lee, R.L., Zeglen, M.E., Ryan, T., and Hines, L.M. 1983. Guidelines: Animals in nursing homes. *California Vet.* 3: 22a–26a.

Lepper, M., Kass, P.H., and Hart, L.A. (2002). Prediction of adoption versus euthanasia among dogs and cats in a California animal shelter. *J. Appl. Anim. Welf. Sci.* 5 (1): 29–42.

Levy, J.K., Isaza, N.M., and Scott, K.C. (2014). Effect of high-impact targeted trap-neuter-return and adoption of community cats on cat intake to a shelter. *Vet. J.* 201 (3): 269–274.

MacKay, J.R. and Haskell, M.J. (2015). Consistent individual behavioral variation: The difference between temperament, personality and behavioral syndromes. *Animals* 5 (3): 455–478.

McCobb, E.C., Patronek, G.J., Marder, A. et al. (2005). Assessment of stress levels among cats in four animal shelters. *J. Am. Vet. Med. Assoc.* 226 (4): 548–555.

McCrae, R.R. and John, O.P. (1992). An introduction to the five-factor model and its applications. *J. Pers.* 60 (2): 175–215.

McCune, S. (1994). Caged cats: Avoiding problems and providing solutions. *Newsletter Companion Anim. Study Group* 7: 1–9.

Meagher, R.K. (2009). Observer ratings: Validity and value as a tool for animal welfare research. *Appl. Anim. Behav. Sci.* 119 (1–2): 1–14.

Mohan-Gibbons, H., Weiss, E., and Slater, M. (2012). Preliminary investigation of food guarding behavior in shelter dogs in the United States. *Animals* 2 (3): 331–346.

Nagasawa, M., Tsujimura, A., Tateishi, K. et al. (2011). Assessment of the factorial structures of the C-BARQ in Japan. *J. Vet. Sci.* https://doi.org/10.1292/jvms.10-0208.

Newbury, S., Blinn, M.K., Bushby, P.A. et al. (2010). *Guidelines for Standards of Care in Animal Shelters*. Apex, NC: Association of Shelter Veterinarians.

Patronek, G.J. and Bradley, J. (2016). No better than flipping a coin: Reconsidering canine behavior evaluations in animal shelters. *J. Vet. Behav.* 15: 66–77.

Scarlett, J.M., Greenberg, M., and Hoshizaki, T. (2017) *Every Nose Counts: Using Metrics in Animal Shelters*. CreateSpace Independent Publishing Platform.

Shore, E.R. (2005). Returning a recently adopted companion animal: Adopters' reasons for and reactions to the failed adoption experience. *J. Appl. Anim. Welf. Sci.* 8 (3): 187–198.

Siegford, J.M., Walshaw, S.O., Brunner, P. et al. (2003). Validation of a temperament test for domestic cats. *Anthrozoös* 16 (4): 332–351.

Skinner, E.A., Edge, K., Altman, J. et al. (2003). Searching for the structure of coping: A review and critique of category systems for classifying ways of coping. *Psychol. Bull.* 129 (2): 216.

Slater, M. R. (2004). Understanding issues and solutions for unowned, free-roaming cat populations. *J. Am. Vet. Med. Assoc.* 225 (9): 1350–1354.

Slater, M.R., Garrison, L., Miller, K. et al. (2013a). Physical and behavioral measures that predict cats' socialization in an animal shelter environment during a three day period. *Animals* 3 (4): 1215–1228.

Slater, M.R., Garrison, L., Miller, K. et al. (2013b). Reliability and validity of a survey of cat caregivers on their cats' socialization level in the cat's normal environment. *Animals* 3 (4): 1194–1214.

Slater, M.R., Garrison, L., Miller, K. et al. (2013c). Practical physical and behavioral measures to assess the socialization spectrum of cats in a shelter-like setting during a three day period. *Animals* 3 (4): 1162–1193.

Slater, M.R., Miller, K.A., Weiss, E. et al. (2010). A survey of the methods used in shelter and rescue programs to identify feral and frightened pet cats. *J. Fel. Med. Surg.* 12 (8): 592–600.

Stella, J., Croney, C., and Buffington, T. (2013). Effects of stressors on the behavior and physiology of domestic cats. *Appl. Anim. Behav. Sci.* 143 (2–4): 157–163.

Tamimi, N., Jamshidi, S., Serpell, J.A. et al. (2015). Assessment of the C-BARQ for evaluating dog behavior in Iran. *J. Vet. Behav.* 10 (1): 36–40.

Tanaka, A., Wagner, D.C., Kass, P.H. et al. (2012). Associations among weight loss, stress, and upper respiratory tract infection in shelter cats. *J. Am. Vet. Med. Assoc.* 240 (5): 570–576.

UC Davis Koret Shelter Medicine Program. (2019). Developing Intake and Adoption Decision Making Criteria. https://www.sheltermedicine.com/library/resources/?r=developing-intake-and-adoption-decision-making-criteria (accessed 5 February 2020).

van den Berg, S.M., Heuven, H.C., van den Berg, L. et al. (2010). Evaluation of the C-BARQ as a measure of stranger-directed aggression in three common dog breeds. *Appl. Anim. Behav. Sci.* 124 (3–4): 136–141.

van der Borg, J.A., Netto, W.J., and Planta, D. J. (1991). Behavioural testing of dogs in animal shelters to predict problem behaviour. *Appl. Anim. Behav. Sci.* 32 (2–3): 237–251.

van der Leij, W.J.R., Selman, L.D.A.M., Vernooij, J.C.M. et al. (2019). The effect of a hiding box on stress levels and body weight in Dutch shelter cats; a randomized controlled trial. *PLOS ONE* 14 (10): e0223492.

Vazire, S., Gosling, S.D., Dickey, A.S., and Schapiro, S.J. (2007). Measuring personality in nonhuman animals. In: *Handbook of Research Methods in Personality Psychology* (eds. R.W. Robins, R.C. Fraley, and R.F. Krueger), 190–206. New York: Guilford Press.

Vinke, C.M., Godijn, L.M., and Van der Leij, W.J.R. (2014). Will a hiding box provide stress reduction for shelter cats? *Appl. Anim. Behav. Sci.* 160: 86–93.

Wagner, D., Hurley, K., and Stavisky, J. (2018). Shelter housing for cats: Practical aspects of design and construction, and adaptation of existing accommodation. *J. Fel. Med. Surg.* 20 (7): 643–652.

Weiss, E. (2007). *Meet Your Match Feline-ality Manual and Training Guide.* New York: ASPCA.

Weiss, E., Gramann, S., Drain, N. et al. (2015). Modification of the Feline-ality™ assessment and the ability to predict adopted cats' behaviors in their new homes. *Animals* 5 (1): 71–88.

Wemelsfelder, F. and Lawrence, A.B. (2001). Qualitative assessment of animal behaviour as an on-farm welfare-monitoring tool. *Acta Agric. Scand. B* 51 (S30): 21–25.

Wilhelmy, J., Serpell, J., Brown, D. et al. (2016). Behavioral associations with breed, coat type, and eye color in single-breed cats. *J. Vet. Behav.* 13: 80–87.

Appendix 15.A   Stray Cat Intake Profile
Source: Jacklyn J. Ellis and Toronto Humane Society

Stray intake profile

Name: _____ Date: _____

Address: _____

           Unit   Street Number   Street Name   City

Phone: _____ Email: _____

Location where cat was found: _____

                        Street Number   Street Name   City

If address is unknown, provide nearest cross-streets and/or landmarks:

_____   _____

Background information:

1) What is your main reason for bringing in this cat? _____
_____

2) Did you attempt to find the owner? If yes, how? ☐ No, ☐ Yes _____

3) How long have you seen this cat in the area? _____

4) Have you been feeding this cat? If so for how long? ☐ No, ☐ Yes

_____

5) Are you aware of anyone else feeding this cat? ☐ No, ☐ Yes

6) Are there other cats in the area? If so, approximately how many? ☐ No, ☐ Yes _____

7) How did you contain this cat to bring it here?
☐ Picked up cat and put it into a carrier, ☐ Lured cat into a carrier,
☐ Used a trap, ☐ Other: _____

8) How long has the cat been in your home?
☐ < 1 day/not at all, ☐ 1–3 days, ☐ 3–7 days, ☐ > 1 week

9) How does this cat respond when approached?
When outside: ☐ Comes toward you, ☐ Stays in place, ☐ Runs away
In your home: ☐ Not applicable, ☐ Comes toward you, ☐ Stays in place, ☐ Runs away

10) How does the cat respond to your attempts at petting?
☐ Avoid, ☐ Tolerate, ☐ Enjoy, ☐ Have not attempted

11) How does the cat respond to being picked up?
☐ Avoid, ☐ Tolerate, ☐ Enjoy, ☐ Have not attempted

12) Does this cat have any injuries or signs of illness? ☐ No, ☐ Yes _____

13) Is this cat ear tipped? ☐ No, ☐ Yes, ☐ I don't know

16

Feline Housing for Behavioral Well-Being
Chumkee Aziz

16.1 Introduction: Challenges of Feline Housing in Animal Shelters

No matter what the facility or how long the length of stay, the confinement of sheltering affects the day-to-day welfare of cats (Rochlitz 2007, 2000). Imagine what a cat might experience when it enters a shelter: being placed into a cold, hard box with the smell of disinfectants, the sights and sounds of strange animals, the hurried movements of unknown people, the loss of familiar faces and places. Imagine how alien and uncomfortable it must feel to be overwhelmed with such novel sensory stimuli in a new environment with no ability to control or predict what will happen next. Imagine how a shelter's goals of infectious disease control and sanitation and safety standards can worsen these stressors. Then, imagine how critical appropriate housing in the shelter is to a cat. Without appropriate housing, it is unreasonable to expect cats to psychologically and physically cope with the stressors of novel environments (McCune 1994). Good housing can mitigate the infectious disease, sanitation, safety, *and* welfare concerns mentioned above.

Behavioral stress scores of cats are highest early on in confinement and decrease over time based on husbandry and housing, so good

housing must be present from the beginning of a shelter stay to help acclimate cats to new environments as effectively as possible (Kessler and Turner 1997; Stella and Croney 2016). Along with high-quality, low-stress husbandry, housing is the most important feature that can be harnessed in sheltering to provide cats with a sense of choice and control and thereby improve their welfare while in the shelter setting. Enriched, stimulating housing that allows for the expression of a wide range of normal behaviors is a critical aspect in promoting the health and well-being of shelter cats. This chapter provides recommendations on feline housing that optimize feline behavioral well-being in shelters.

16.1.1 Environmental Stressors

Many studies have researched how the structure, complexity, and interactivity of environments have effects on the behavior and health of confined animals (Morgan and Tromborg 2007). Potential environmental stressors for cats in confined settings include:

- Overcrowding
- Sounds, smells, and sights of unfamiliar dogs and cats as well as other foreign smells
- Loud and startling noises
- New experiences

Animal Behavior for Shelter Veterinarians and Staff, Second Edition. Edited by Brian A. DiGangi, Victoria A. Cussen, Pamela J. Reid, and Kristen A. Collins.
Companion website: www.wiley.com/go/digangi/animal

- Diminished control over and intrusion into personal space
- Unfamiliar surroundings
- Unpredictable routines
- Unnatural social situations.

New environments can cause anxiety, fear, and stress in cats. Being confined, particularly in high-density environments, heightens the problem (Arhant et al. 2015; Kessler and Turner 1999b; Ottway and Hawkins 2003). While some animals express stress through defensive or destructive behavior, confined cats with elevated behavioral stress scores show stress through inhibited or withdrawal behavior (Stella and Croney 2016). In this case, inactivity and the inhibition of normal behaviors such as self-maintenance (decreased feeding, grooming, and elimination and increased feigned sleeping, meaning stress-induced, fake sleeping) as well as the inhibition of exploratory and play behaviors are signs of compromised welfare (Carlstead 1993; McCune 1994; Ottway and Hawkins 2003; Rehnberg et al. 2015) (see Box 16.1). Cats with illness may modify their behavior in a similar way (Rochlitz 1999), so in a shelter setting the early recognition of *lack* of activity and normal behavior are critical in the prompt recognition and differentiation of medical and behavioral concerns. In addition, signs of stress such as inactivity may hinder adoptions since studies have shown that adopters view cats that are more active for longer periods of time and more frequently compared to inactive cats, leading to an increased adoption rate (Fantuzzi et al. 2010).

In addition, stress and immunity are closely linked, with chronic stress contributing to immunosuppression, which can lead to the development of infectious diseases such as upper respiratory disease (Gaskel and Povey 1977). Stress can also lead to behavioral concerns such as inappropriate elimination. Accordingly, reducing stress within the shelter environment is crucial to maintaining feline well-being, health, and adoptability.

Box 16.1 Recognizing Stress in Shelter Cats (Griffin and Hume 2006; Rodan and Cannon 2016)

Inhibited or withdrawal behaviors
- Decreased appetite
- Decreased elimination
- Decreased grooming
- Decreased play and exploration
- Decreased sleep (must be distinguished from feigned sleep)

Defensive behaviors
- At front of cage ready to attack if anyone approaches
- Back arched, trying to appear larger
- Ears back
- Dilated pupils
- Vocalizing

Adaptive behaviors
- Destruction of cage contents for the creation of a hiding place

---

16.2 The Connection between Feline Housing and Well-Being

The greater extent to which a cat can control or cope with a stressor can positively impact their welfare (Carlstead 1993; Griffin and Hume 2006). Appropriate housing that is designed to consider the biological, behavioral, and social needs of cats allows for improved coping mechanisms and a wide range of normal behaviors. Appropriate housing, by encouraging good welfare, also facilitates the provision of the Five Freedoms (referred to here on out as the Freedoms) and the Five Pillars of a Healthy Feline Environment (hereafter the Pillars) (Ellis et al. 2013; Manteca et al. n.d.) (see Box 16.2). Upholding these Freedoms and Pillars means that housing allows for cats to express normal behavior, have access to multiple enrichment sources and does not contribute to discomfort, pain, injury, disease, fear, or distress. As an example,

Box 16.2 Freedoms and Pillars

Five Freedoms of Animal Welfare (Manteca et al. n.d.)

1) Freedom from hunger and thirst
2) Freedom from discomfort
3) Freedom from pain, injury, or disease
4) Freedom to express normal behavior
5) Freedom from fear and distress

Five Pillars of a Healthy Feline Environment (Ellis et al. 2013)

1) Provide a safe place
2) Provide multiple and separated key environmental resources
3) Provide opportunity for play and predatory behavior
4) Provide positive, consistent, and predictable human-cat interaction
5) Provide an environment that respects the importance of the cat's sense of smell

account the unique biological needs of cats and the need for cats to cope with unfamiliar environments; it can be tailored to meet the individual needs of cats, ranging from highly socialized housecats that are relatively comfortable in novel settings to cats that may be poorly socialized with people and highly fearful in novel settings; it upholds animal and public safety; it facilitates reduced disease transmission; it does not aesthetically or emotionally distress adopters and, instead, presents animals in favorable ways and allows for increased interaction with potential adopters. Appropriate husbandry is intimately linked to appropriate housing in maintaining feline well-being.

It is also important to note that in some instances it is inappropriate to house cats in the shelter environment. Feral cats, unaccustomed to confinement and handling, are particularly distressed in shelter settings. Kittens under the age of five months, who are not reliably protected by vaccination, are more susceptible to infectious diseases in the shelter. Avoid housing both populations of cats or, at minimum, minimize their length of stay in the shelter through the use of intake diversion programs and foster homes, respectively.

appropriate feline housing has been shown to be one of the primary tools in mitigating the development of upper respiratory disease in cats by reducing behavioral stress, as reflected by lower stress scores (Tanaka et al. 2012; Wagner et al. 2018b). Not only is the cat's well-being positively impacted, but cats that appear more relaxed and friendly are more likely to be adopted (Fantuzzi et al. 2010; Gourkow and Fraser 2006).

Shelters admit and care for a wide-ranging population of cats, differing in source, health, age, and sociability. Each cat is an individual. Stress can induce different behaviors in different cats and each cat copes with stress through different means. Accordingly, providing a variety of housing and enrichment options is critical in helping each cat acclimate to the sheltering environment in its own way. The size, quality, and ability to offer a sense of control and choice are critical when providing appropriate feline housing.

Appropriate housing addresses multiple factors in the sheltering setting: it takes into

16.3 Macro- and Microenvironmental Considerations for Feline Housing

Appropriate aspects of housing that uphold the Freedoms and Pillars ensure that cats have freedom from discomfort, as well as fear and distress, while also allowing cats the freedom to express normal behavior. In short, this means cats are provided a sense of choice in that they are provided the ability to move freely within their enclosure, choose to engage in a range of normal behaviors, and assume a fuller repertoire of normal postures within their enclosures. Focus should be on both the macroenvironment (the environment immediately outside of the primary enclosure) and the microenvironment (the environment within the primary enclosure) as both are important factors in the ability of confined cats to acclimate to an unfamiliar environment (Stella et al. 2014).

It is important to note that all feline housing within a shelter should strive to meet these macro- and microenvironment recommendations. The quality and quantity of housing in isolation areas should match that of adoption and holding areas. Every cat, regardless of where they are in the sheltering process, deserves sufficient space and the choice to perform normal behaviors.

16.3.1 Considerations for the Macroenvironment

Macroenvironmental factors include lighting, sound, odor, temperature and visual stimulation. Managing the area surrounding primary enclosures is just as important in reducing feline stress as is managing the enclosure itself (Stella et al. 2014).

The macroenvironment should allow for natural light. Light and darkness should be provided to support the natural (circadian) rhythms of wakefulness and sleep (Newbury et al. 2010). Views outside of housing areas, toward outdoor views or neutral indoor spaces are recommended. The use of LED lighting is recommended over fluorescent lighting as LEDs do not emit bothersome flickering or buzzing noises that cats can hear but humans may not. LEDs also provide softer lighting, which mimics natural lighting that is better in line with how cats see (Pollard and Shoults 2018a, 2018b).

Cats have a much broader hearing range than humans, meaning they are more sensitive to noise, particularly when they cannot move away from loud noises. Exposure to noise within the macroenvironment should be minimized, including the barking of dogs (McCobb et al. 2005; Stella et al. 2014), loud conversations, music and slamming of cage doors. Housing areas should aim to minimize noise

levels to less than 60 dB, a quiet conversational level (Stella and Buffington 2016). Design housing wards with highly absorptive ceiling materials to reduce reverberant noise (Pollard and Shoults 2018a).

Cats depend on olfactory cues more than humans, so they are also more sensitive to aversive odors. Minimize exposure to odors including strong disinfectants, unfamiliar animals, cigarette smoke and alcohol-based hand sanitizers (Stella and Buffington 2016; Stella and Croney 2016). Try to maintain familiar scents within the environment when possible, such as familiar bedding containing the scent of the cat itself or its former home (Ellis et al. 2013).

Cats prefer a warmer ambient temperature than many other species, so maintain housing areas at 15.5–26.5° C (60–80° F) for temperature and 30–70% for humidity (Newbury et al. 2010; Stella and Buffington 2016). Higher humidity (e.g., 70%) has been correlated with reduced respiratory disease in animals as the increased moisture helps maintain healthier respiratory passages that can more readily resist pathogens (Griffin 2012).

The macroenvironment also means that cage banks are raised and set at least 18 inches off the floor so cats have a "view" (Griffin 2013; McCobb et al. 2005; Wagner et al. 2018a). Elevated cages are less stressful than floor level cages, because cats can better survey their environment from an elevated position (McCobb et al. 2005). This also allows for cats to be both monitored more readily by staff and viewed more readily by adopters at eye level, which in turn can increase feline adoptions (Fantuzzi et al. 2010; Sinn 2016). Fill top cages before using bottom cages and, if needed, elevate cage banks with cage bases (Wagner et al. 2018a) (see Figure 16.1). Avoid triple-stacking cages as this removes cats from the eye-level of caretakers and adopters.

Views of other animals, including dogs and other cats, should be avoided. Cats grow fearful when seeing conspecifics and even cats that are acclimated to living with dogs will become

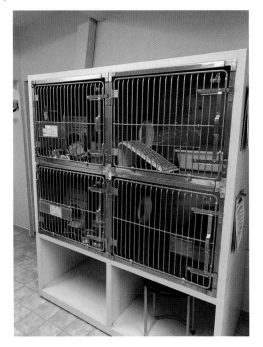

Figure 16.1 Elevated cage bank. *Source:* Courtesy of Dr. Denae Wagner.

frightened when seeing unfamiliar dogs (Rodan and Cannon 2016). Avoid facing housing units toward each other. If this is not possible, try to angle housing units so cats do not directly face one another and ensure there is more than 4 ft. between facing housing units to mitigate droplet transmission of infectious diseases (Gaskell and Povey 1977; Povey and Johnson 1970). Partial cage front coverings can provide an additional way for cats to retreat so they are not forced to see unfamiliar conspecifics.

16.3.2 Considerations for the Microenvironment

Microenvironmental factors include the quality and quantity of space; different functional areas for eliminating, eating, and resting; and size and types of elimination facilities as well as hiding, stretching, and perching opportunities. Traditional, single-compartment cages that provide less than 8–11 ft^2 of floor space per

cat cannot offer these distinct functional areas and limit the expression of species typical behaviors (Stella and Buffington 2016). These smaller cages need to be proactively avoided or adapted, such as through portalization to create double-compartments and overall larger housing areas, to provide improved welfare and well-being.

First and foremost, primary enclosures must be safe for the animal. The Association of Shelter Veterinarians' *Guidelines for Standards of Care in Animal Shelters* states that a "primary enclosure must be structurally sound and maintained in safe, working condition to properly confine animals, prevent injury, keep other animals out, and enable the animals to remain dry and clean. There must not be any sharp edges, gaps or other defects that could cause an injury or trap a limb or other body part. Secure latches or other closing devices must be present. Cage floors should be non-slip and solid. It is unacceptable for primary enclosures to have wire-mesh bottoms or slatted floors" (Newbury et al. 2010).

Primary enclosures should be tall and wide enough to allow cats to move about without touching sides of the cage and to fully stretch and express other common behaviors. The enclosure space should also be sufficient so that there is a minimum of 2 ft. between food and litter (Newbury et al. 2010). Accordingly, 8–11 ft^2 is the minimum amount of floor space required for the healthy housing of cats and to help reduce behavioral and medical concerns, including upper respiratory disease (Newbury et al. 2010; Wagner et al. 2018a, 2018b). Specifically, cats housed in 11 ft^2 of floor space were found to be significantly less stressed than those with only 5.3 ft^2 of space (Kessler and Turner 1999b), while risk of upper respiratory disease was found to be significantly higher in shelters housing cats in cages with less than 8 ft^2 of floor space (Wagner et al. 2018b). This space allotment refers to unobstructed floor space and does not include that provided by perches or other elevated resting areas. Functional separation of food and litter spaces, as well as the ability to move around adequately and change locations, provides a sense of control over the environment, which is necessary for avoiding stress (McMillan 2002). The Freedoms cannot be met without sufficient housing space allotment.

In short, primary enclosures should be large enough to allow for full body length stretching as well as separation of resting and eating areas from elimination areas. Double-compartment enclosures can facilitate this separation by allowing cats to rest and eat in an area away from their elimination area. In addition, during cleaning double-compartments allow for minimized animal handling and therefore less stress. This also leads to reduced likelihood of fomite transmission and increased safety as cats can be secured on one side of the compartment while cleaning occurs on the other side. Double-compartment enclosures, therefore, uphold the tenets expressed in the Freedoms and Pillars.

Single-compartment housing can be retrofitted with a portal to become double-compartmentalized (see Figures 16.2 and 16.3). One common scenario seen is the retrofitting of two side-to-side, 2-ft. wide, single stainless-steel cages with a portal to create a double-compartment configuration, which provides 8 ft^2 of floor space per cat. This modification is an improvement over singled-compartment caging, but shelters purchasing new primary enclosures or entirely replacing older enclosures should consider going beyond this minimum requirement to allow for greater movement and options for cats by providing a minimum of 11 ft^2 of caging floor space per cat. In addition, primary enclosures with multiple portals can allow for additional cage units to be opened up during times of low shelter population, affording cats even more space (Pollard and Shoults 2018a; Wagner et al. 2018a).

New enclosures that are compartmentalized ideally should be configured of two equally sized compartments, as opposed to one large living compartment and one smaller litterbox

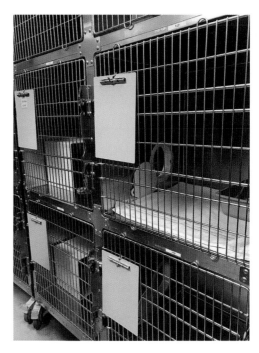

Figure 16.2 Portalized, double-compartment housing. *Source:* Courtesy of Kay Joubert.

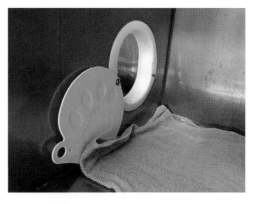

Figure 16.3 Portal installed into existent stainless-steel caging thereby converting this into a double-compartment housing unit. *Source:* Courtesy of Regional Animal Services of King County.

compartment. In unequally sized double-compartment units, fearful cats may seek more secure spaces and choose to rest in their litterboxes within the smaller compartment (Lewis 2017). Instead, the focus should be on providing large, equally sized, enriched spaces on both sides. If this is not possible, the living compartment should be at least 30–36 inches wide and the litterbox compartment should be at least 15 inches wide (Wagner et al. 2018a). Ensure that litterbox compartments do not have shelving that would restrict normal posturing when eliminating. Larger individual units, often manufactured with removable partitions, that meet minimum floor space requirements are alternatives to double-compartment units but are less preferable as they do not allow for distinct separation between resting and elimination spaces.

Walk-in housing that provides adequate space is an alternative to traditional caged housing and has the additional benefit of allowing adopters and caretakers to enter the enclosure and gently interact with cats more readily. If renovating a facility and housing capacity allows for it, dog runs can be converted into walk-in cat housing (see Figure 16.4), while new facilities can create customized walk-in cat living spaces (UC Davis

Koret Shelter Medicine Program 2015) (see Figure 16.5).

Vertical space within primary enclosures, although not included in the minimum floor space requirement, is critical in allowing cats to express normal behaviors. A minimum of 30 inches of vertical height will allow for natural movement and increases the overall functional space and environmental complexity of an enclosure (Lewis 2017), encouraging exploratory behaviors such as climbing and jumping as well as providing space for elevated resting areas that offer a greater sense of security (Rochlitz 2000).

All cats, regardless of their demeanor and where they are housed within the shelter (adoption, isolation, or hold area), must have an opportunity to hide within their enclosure (Newbury et al. 2010). Hiding is a normal, adaptive behavior that reduces stress when cats are exposed to threats or unfamiliar and unpredictable environments (Arhant et al. 2015; Carlstead 1993; Gourkow and

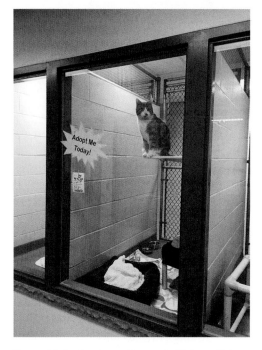

Figure 16.4 Dog kennel converted into walk-in cat housing. *Source:* Courtesy of Dr. Denae Wagner.

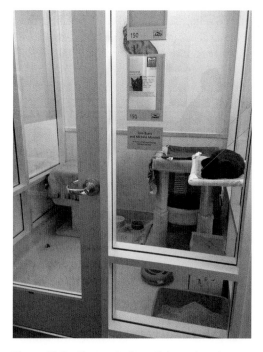

Figure 16.5 Custom-built walk-in cat housing. *Source:* Courtesy of Dr. Denae Wagner.

Fraser 2006; Kry and Casey 2007; McCune 1994; Rehnberg et al. 2015; Stella et al. 2014, 2017; van der Leij et al. 2019; Vinke et al. 2014). Studies show that hiding places are used more by cats with increased stress, indicated by behavioral stress scores (Ottway and Hawkins 2003; Rehnberg et al. 2015; Stella et al. 2014), and that hiding places help reduce stress as indicated by lower behavioral stress scores (Kry and Casey 2007; Vinke et al. 2014). Studies also show that hiding places can increase the behavioral repertoire of confined cats. The sense of security offered by hiding places can at some points increase exploratory behaviors in a cat, while at other points increase resting behavior. In both instances, the provision of hiding places indicates that a cat is more comfortable within its environment (de Oliveira et al. 2015; Kry and Casey 2007). However, attentive recognition of whether a cat is inactive due to comfort or is inactive due to stress is critical to maintaining welfare.

The inability to hide increases stress as it precludes the ability to control aversive stimuli. Persistently stressed cats may not adapt to a new environment and, accordingly, will not display as much active, exploratory play behavior, which may affect their adoption likelihood (Carlstead 1993; Griffin and Hume 2006). Visual concealment can be offered through the provision of hiding places within the primary enclosure or by partially covering the front of an enclosure. Offering the *choice* to hide is equally important, so visual concealment techniques should allow cats the choice to hide if they need to and, conversely, allow them to be exploratory and exposed if they would like to be. Examples of hiding places include cardboard boxes, cat carriers with their doors open, feral dens or beds with high sides. Hiding places should be placed in the back of the cage, turned to the side so cats do not have to look out and, ideally, be enclosed on three sides to maximize the sense of physical protection. In cats that are comfortable in their new environment, hiding boxes can be oriented forward so cats can look out if they

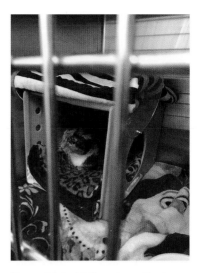

Figure 16.6 Hiding place allowing cat to face outward. *Source:* Courtesy of Kay Joubert.

want to (Rodan and Cannon 2016) (see Figure 16.6). Line hiding places with soft bedding for additional comfort.

If the primary enclosure is not large enough to house a hiding box, then draping a towel over a shelf or an elevated bed (see Figure 16.7) or placing a partial covering on an enclosure's front can also work (see Figure 16.8). Cats that are not given the opportunity to hide have been noted to turn cage furnishings upside down and shred newspaper within their cage at night or crouch behind their bed or litterbox in what seems to be an attempt to conceal themselves (Carlstead 1993; Gourkow and Fraser 2006; Kry and Casey 2007; Vinke et al. 2014). Cats may do this when they are struggling to cope with their environment or when they are sick (Stella and Buffington 2016).

Concerns that hiding opportunities impede adoption rates are unfounded. Studies have shown no negative effect on length of stay or adoption rate when shelters provide cats with hide spots. In addition, no difference in time to adoption has been shown between cats with hiding places versus cats without hiding places (Gourkow and Fraser 2006; Kry and Casey 2007). Studies instead show that providing the option to hide leads to improved

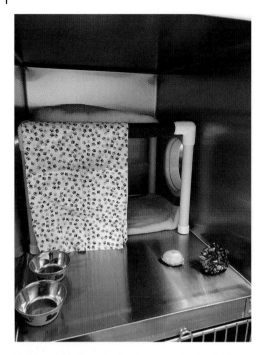

Figure 16.7 Elevated bed creating both a hiding place and a perching spot. *Source:* Courtesy of Dr. Denae Wagner.

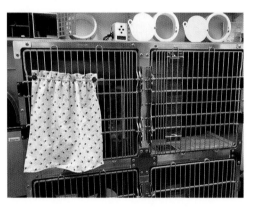

Figure 16.8 Partial cage front covering offering a choice to retreat. *Source:* Courtesy of Dr. Denae Wagner.

welfare and, accordingly, can help cats appear more relaxed and social. These cats are likely to be more affiliative and approach people. Conversely, cats without hiding places have decreased welfare with no adoption advantage.

Bedding not only serves as a source of comfort but as a source of familiarity. Thick soft

bedding should be provided to ensure cats achieve extended periods of normal deep sleep (Griffin 2012). Bedding, which can become a source of a familiar scent, should be laundered only when soiled and/or if a primary enclosure is being prepared for a new cat. Bedding should not cover the entirety of the floor of an enclosure as cats should have the choice to lay on bedding or on a different surface as desired.

Scratching allows cats to exhibit a normal behavior used to mark territory with visual and olfactory signaling. A variety of scratching substrates that can be discarded should be provided as preferred substrates vary between cats. Examples include disposable cardboard scratchers or carpet squares. In addition, while most cats prefer vertical scratch pads, some cats will use horizontal ones, so both types should be provided. Many cats scratch more after resting or sleeping so scratching pads can be strategically placed around resting areas (Rochlitz 2005).

Even color palettes matter when it comes to feline housing. Because cats can see in the ultraviolet B spectrum, avoid manmade materials that appear to fluoresce or reflect such as bright white plastics, which can be visually jarring to cats. Select matte finishes when possible. Cats have superior night vision but cannot see the red end of the human visible spectrum. Reds and oranges appear dull grey and shadowy to cats, making it harder to differentiate surfaces. Accordingly, choose light colors, such as blues, greens, and violets, within and surrounding enclosures so cats can better comprehend the environment around them in low-light situations (Pollard and Shoults 2018b).

Every cat should have a high point to perch on (Newbury et al. 2010). Elevation and the ability to perch are stress reducers as they offer a sense of security from a vantage point and an area to retreat if needed (Ellis et al. 2013; Rochlitz 2007). Cats prefer elevated spaces more than floor areas (Rochlitz et al. 1998). Perches also maximize the functional space of an enclosure and should be both wide and long enough for a cat to fully stretch out (Ellis et al. 2013). At a minimum, perching shelves should be 12 inches wide and raised 13–14 inches off the cage floor to accommodate hiding boxes under them (Wagner et al. 2018a). Ensure ease of access to elevated areas for cats with reduced mobility due to old age, injury, or disease by providing steps and non-slip surfaces. Avoid built-in shelves as they can be hard to clean and limit the configuration of housing (Wagner et al. 2018a). Elevated walkways and hammocks also work well to provide elevation.

16.3.2.1 Specific Design Aspects of Primary Enclosures

Provide quiet cage latches that click instead of slam and quiet hinges to reduce loud noises associated with opening and closing cage doors. Irregular, high amplitude sounds of metal striking metal can be very loud and provoke distress responses in animals (Morgan and Tromborg 2007). For cage fronts, use horizontal bars as they allow for more unobstructed views of the environment and natural ventilation. Having the ability to directly interact with cats is very important to adopters, so avoid the use of completely sealed-in glass cage fronts that prevent adopters from interacting with cats (Sinn 2016). If current enclosure design does not allow for adopter interaction, then ensure that visiting rooms are present within the shelter for adopters to interact and play with potential adoptees and ensure that cats are acclimated to the rooms. Consider transparent backs on cage units to prevent the feeling of claustrophobia for confined cats, while always providing a space to hide if needed (see Box 16.3).

16.3.2.2 Enrichment

The definition of enrichment is an intervention in which changes to environmental structures and husbandry practices result in increasing behavioral choices for animals to promote species-appropriate behaviors and abilities, thus enhancing animal welfare (Young 2003). In

---

Box 16.3   Technical Aspects of the Feline Microenvironment

Specific technical aspects of the feline microenvironment include (Pollard and Shoults 2018; Stella and Buffington 2016; Wagner et al. 2018a):

- Provide quiet cage latches that click instead of slam and quiet hinges to reduce loud noises associated with opening/closing cage doors.
- Use horizontal bars for cage fronts, as they allow for more natural sight.
- Avoid the use of completely sealed-in cage fronts that prevent people from interacting with cats.
- Consider transparent backs on cage units to prevent the feeling of claustrophobia but ensure hiding opportunities are available for cats concurrently.
- Use light color palettes to facilitate sight at night.

Box 16.4   Environmental Enrichment

Goals of environmental enrichment include (Young 2003):

- Increase behavioral diversity
- Reduce the frequency of abnormal behaviors
- Increase the range or number of normal behavior patterns
- Increase positive use of the environment
- Increase the ability to cope with challenges in a more "normal" way.

---

short, environmental enrichment is intended to create and sustain a perception of control and predictability about the surrounding area that permits cats to thrive (Stella and Buffington 2016) (see Box 16.4). Enrichment is required for any duration of confinement and must be appropriate for the length of stay for each animal (Newbury et al. 2010). Enrichment becomes increasingly important as length of stay increases.

Enriched housing provides cats with more choice and control over how to use their environment, potentially improving their welfare and ensuring the provision of the Freedoms and Pillars (Suchak and Lamica 2018). By reducing stress, enrichment can mitigate the development of disease, increase exploratory and a range of species-typical behaviors, and decrease abnormal behaviors that lead to a psychologically and physically healthier animal that can ultimately result in more favorable adoption outcomes (Fantuzzi et al. 2010; Gourkow and Fraser 2006; Uetake et al. 2013). Overall, cats that have been given options to help acclimate to their new environment feel more secure, display more species-appropriate behavior, are less stressed, can appear friendlier and may be of more appeal to adopters.

Each cat's past socialization experience is unique, which influences how it may or may not use enrichment. Some cats require stimulatory enrichment such as toys, while others require enrichment that increases their sense of security such as hiding places (Ellis 2009). The key, then, is to offer different kinds of enrichment that allow cats to adapt to their environment based on their individual behavioral, emotional, physical, and medical needs (Ellis 2009).

In addition to structural enrichment, such as spaces to hide, shelving to allow for stretching, climbing and perching, and abrasive surfaces to allow for scratching, primary enclosures should include visual enrichment that allows for cats to see stimulating environments outside of their enclosure if they wish (Overall and Dyer 2005). Stimulatory enrichment that encourages exploratory and play behavior, such as paper bags, toys that mimic prey, and food toys, is also important. Stimulatory enrichment can improve feline welfare, and, in addition, studies have shown that cats with toys in their cages are viewed more often than cats without toys in their cages, which can in turn positively affect adoptions (Fantuzzi et al. 2010; Sinn 2016). Figure 16.9 demonstrates how to set up a low-stress, double-compartment feline housing enclosure.

Finally, the opportunity for social enrichment with humans or conspecifics is needed.

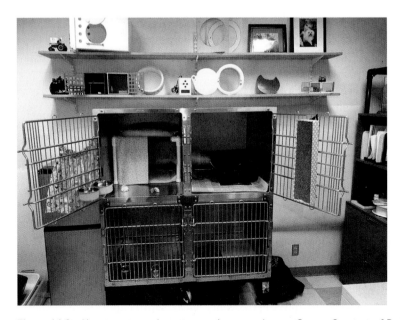

Figure 16.9 How to set up a low-stress primary enclosure. *Source:* Courtesy of Dr. Denae Wagner.

Out-of-cage opportunities are useful for many cats, including those that enjoy socialization with humans outside of their cage but also those that do not enjoy human interaction but just need extra space to be free and move around for a temporary period. Secured outdoor housing, such as catios, that cats can have access to or can temporarily be placed in are also useful for enrichment. Outdoor housing provides increased exposure to natural light as well as natural and often increased ventilation. See Chapter 17 for more information on feline enrichment.

16.3.3 Regarding Ventilation of Macro- and Microenvironments

Because airborne disease transmission is low risk for cats, individually ventilated primary enclosures are not necessary for disease control. Larger cages with barred fronts can allow fresh room air to flow through housing units. In general, because cat housing wards tend to be small, increased ventilation for the ward as a whole should be considered. Some resources state that 10–12 air exchanges per hour are needed (Newbury et al. 2010), while others recommend that 12–20 air exchanges per hour are needed. It should be noted, however, that exchanging air through individually ventilated cages can have the additional benefits of improving air quality and odor control and reducing the overall room air exchange rate needed (Pollard and Shoults 2018a).

16.4 Group-Housing

When designed, used, and monitored appropriately, group-housing can allow for increased welfare of cats, particularly adult cats that are expected to have a relatively longer length of shelter stay (Griffin and Hume 2006; Kessler and Turner 1997). In addition, well-managed group-housing can result in greater exploratory behavior and play in cats, which can help

increase adoption traffic because adopters are attracted to more sociable and playful cats (Fantuzzi et al. 2010; Gourkow and Fraser 2006; Loberg and Lundmark 2016; Uetake et al. 2013; Weiss et al. 2012). The home-like design and aesthetics of group-housing rooms can also increase adoption traffic and allow adopters to interact more comfortably with cats.

The mental and physical benefits of group-housing, including having more space and having conspecifics to interact with, must be carefully weighed against the risks that can arise with group-housing, such as infectious disease exposure, injury, and behavioral stress. Indeed, group-housing can cause intense stress in some cats and negate the benefits of communal enrichment when spaces are crowded and group selection is incompatible (Kessler and Turner 1999b; Ottway and Hawkins 2003). Only cats that are recognized as having been appropriately socialized with other cats and find interacting with conspecifics enriching should be selected for group-housing. Multiple factors contribute to the success of group-housing (see Box 16.5).

Box 16.5   Group-Housing

Factors contributing to the success of group-housing include (based on Arhant et al. 2015):

- Space allowance
- Group size
- The social experience and history of the individual cats
- Careful animal selection
- Stability of the group composition
- Quantity of resources
- Distribution and easy access of resources
- Quality of the space/diversity of enrichment
- Admission procedures
- Disease management
- Monitoring to ensure social compatibility.

16.4.1 Animal Selection

Selecting cats for group-housing should be done carefully with ongoing monitoring and follow-up. It is unacceptable to group animals who fight with one another or to randomly group animals without considering their age, health, and behavioral status. In addition, group-housing should not be used because individual animal housing space is insufficient within a facility (Newbury et al., 2010). Group-housing is ideal for healthy, appropriately socialized adult cats that behave and present well in such settings. Kittens under five months of age should not be randomly co-mingled or co-housed as the infectious disease risk for this population of animals is significant. In addition, adoptable kittens typically have a short shelter length of stay so the risk of infectious disease exposure that is associated with group-housing for kittens outweighs the communal enrichment benefits.

Cats that are shy, as well as cats that are assertive, may increase stress levels for other cats within groups (Kessler and Turner 1999a). Shy cats can struggle to interact with assertive cats, which may result in chronic stress and increased hiding (Bradshaw and Hall 1999; Griffin 2013). Assertive or confident cats may threaten other cats and dominate resources and human interactions. Overly shy or aggressive cats may not present favorably in group-housing and may have better adoption chances in individual housing (Griffin and Hume 2006). Shy cats, specifically, may benefit from co-housing with a socially confident cat.

Criteria for cats that can be considered for group-housing are included in Box 16.6.

16.4.2 Density

Group-housing rooms should maintain a minimum density of 18 ft^2 of floor space per cat (Kessler and Turner 1999a). This is a greater amount of floor space than what is recommended for individually housed cats due to the possibility of inter-cat aggression (Kessler and

---

Box 16.6   Group-Housing Selection and Removal

Animals selected for group-housing should be:

- Healthy
- Predicted to have relatively longer shelter length of stay
- More than five months of age (unless they are littermates)
- Sterilized or of the same sex
- Grouped by age
- Behaviorally compatible
- Seeking out positive interactions with other cats.

Animals that should be removed from group-housing are:

- Consistently hiding or staying in an elevated area
- Not eating during feed time
- Consistently feigning sleeping
- Sitting with their back to the group or hunched in a corner
- Inappropriately eliminating
- Lacking exploratory behavior
- Not showing signs of relaxed body posture
- Guarding resources
- Deliberately trying to restrict the movement of other cats.

Turner 1999b). From an evolutionary standpoint, it is believed that cats lack distinct dominance hierarchies so they cannot truly form stable hierarchies within groups (van den Bos 1998). As such, establishing distances between themselves and avoidance are key mechanisms for conflict resolution within groups of cats. The increased space requirement of group-housing within shelters facilitates avoidance and allows for the maintenance of social distances (Crowell-Davis et al. 2004; van den Bos 1998). Group-housed cats must have this additional space to be able to avoid one another and freely use communal resources without competition and social conflict. If adequate space is not provided, for instance in an overcrowded group-housing scenario, cats will attempt to avoid each other by decreasing their activity (van den Bos 1998).

Outdoor space to which cats have continuous access counts toward this space requirement; however, vertical space, although critical, is not included. Group-housing should not be relied on to artificially increase the holding capacity of a shelter and, as it requires more space per cat, is not a cost-effective solution for capacity expansion (Griffin 2012).

16.4.3   Size

Small groups of three to six individuals or pairs are recommended for group-housing. In general, smaller group-housing rooms with small groups of cats are preferable over large or warehouse-type rooms for reasons related to welfare, stress, and infectious disease exposure. The introduction or removal of individuals results in an adjustment period that can be stressful for group-housed cats (Finka et al. 2014). Small rooms with fewer cats minimize the need for frequent introductions and the reorganization of groups, resulting in more stable group compositions and therefore less stress (Kessler and Turner 1999a; Rochlitz 2007). It should be noted that even more floor space is needed per cat than the recommended minimum noted above if groups are unstable and additions and departures to the group are more frequent (Kessler and Turner 1999b).

Smaller group-housing rooms can also facilitate an "all-in, all-out" approach. In this strategy, cats identified as appropriate candidates for group-housing are placed into a group-housing room simultaneously and no new cats are added until all existent cats are adopted. This strategy reduces the frequency of stress-inducing introductions (Ottway and Hawkins 2003). It also allows for group-housing rooms to be completely cleared out and thoroughly sanitized, thereby breaking any chains of infectious disease that may unknowingly be present before housing a new

cohort of cats in the room. Small rooms with smaller groups allow for more effective group monitoring as well.

16.4.4   Enrichment

The functional space of a group-housing room should be maximized by distributing resources widely and providing quality enrichment. Functional separation of resources provides a sense of control over the environment, which is necessary for avoiding stress (McMillan 2002). The quality and complexity of the environment within group-housing is just as important as the density of group-housing (Griffin 2013; Rochlitz 1999). The environment should offer an abundance of choice and options that meet the physical and behavioral needs of cats. Cats should be allowed to choose their own degree of seclusion and proximity to other cats (McCune 1994). Offering multiple resources and sources of enrichment can prevent social conflict.

Cats must have the ability to hide, perch, stretch, climb, rest, feed, and eliminate without social conflict such as resource guarding. Enrichment such as hiding places and elevated perches can facilitate reduced agonistic behaviors between confined cats and improve behavioral stability within groups (de Oliveira et al. 2015; Desforges et al. 2016). Resources such as resting places, feeding/watering stations, and litterboxes should be abundant, positioned strategically, and made easily accessible. Maximize the distance between resting places so cats can readily avoid one another as desired. Use uncovered litterboxes so cats have a safe vantage point of approaching cats during elimination (Herron and Buffington 2014). Avoid placing resources in corners to allow for access to each resource from multiple sides. Otherwise, stressed cats may avoid such resources as a way of minimizing negative interactions with other cats. Place at least one of each type of resource (litterbox, feeding/watering station, rest spots) per cat, plus one spare, to reduce social

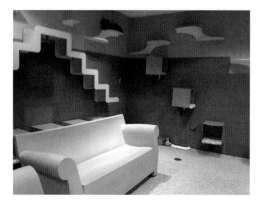

Figure 16.10   Group-housing with environmental enrichment.

conflict (Foreman-Worsley and Farnworth, 2019) (see Figure 16.10).If space is limited, then provide at least one of each type of resource per cat.

Consider certain technical aspects when outfitting a group-housing room. For instance, elevated perches should be sturdy and wide and allow for normal posturing and good footing. Use adhesive-backed, washable cloths on perches to provide soft surfaces. For furnishings, use washable, non-cloth and non-wooden furniture such as patio furniture or toddler play structures. If cloth or wooden furniture are used, ensure these furnishings are readily disinfected or disposable.

16.4.5   Safety

Group-housing rooms should be designed so cats cannot readily escape. A foyer at the room's entrance can provide additional protection and, at a minimum, group-housing doors should not open directly to the outdoors (UC Davis Koret Shelter Medicine Program 2015). In addition, group-housing rooms should have ceilings or covers that cannot be dislodged by cats (Griffin 2012). Windows, which can enrich confined spaces by providing natural daylight and ventilation as well as allow for the observation of the outside environment, should have securely fitted screens. The floors should be non-slip and should be able to withstand chemical disinfectants. Ideally, the floor should be minimally sloped toward a drain to allow for periodic, thorough disinfection of rooms (Geret et al. 2011).

16.4.6   Monitoring

Daily monitoring of individual cats and group dynamics to recognize signs of stress and negative interactions is imperative. Monitoring, especially after a new cat is introduced as well as during feeding time, is critical to ensure that all cats are appropriate for and benefitting from group-housing. Given that weight loss and poor coat condition can be reflective of stress, physical examinations, including weigh-ins and coat/skin condition assessments, should be scheduled monthly for group-housed cats who remain in care for longer than one month (Arhant et al. 2015; Newbury et al. 2010). Volunteers or staff should be trained on how to recognize resource guarding, negative interactions, and other signs of social conflict. Cats that are stressed in group-housing should be removed into individual housing enclosures or placed into a foster home instead of trying to repeatedly move them until a more suitable grouping is found. Criteria for cats that should be removed from group-housing are included in Box 16.6.

16.5   Conclusions

Improved welfare and well-being within a shelter starts with the provision of appropriate housing for cats, especially since cats are particularly susceptible to shelter stressors. Feline housing must meet the safety and biosecurity needs of a shelter while also meeting the physical and psychological needs of cats. The quality (structures and design that encourage behavioral choice) is just as important as the quantity (size) of feline housing. The availability of practical modifications to feline housing means that positive welfare, well-being, and outcomes for cats are possible for any shelter to achieve.

Acknowledgments

Special thanks to Dr. Denae Wager and Dr. Kate Hurley of the University of California, Davis Koret Shelter Medicine Program as well as Dr. Erin Doyle and Dr. Elise Gingrich of the ASPCA for their support on this chapter.

Please visit the companion website for video clips and downloadable resources associated with this chapter.

References

Arhant, C., Wogritsch, R., and Troxler, J. (2015). Assessment of behavior and physical condition of shelter cats as animal-based indicators of welfare. *J. Vet. Behav.* https://doi.org/10.1016/j.jveb.2015.03.006.

Bradshaw, J.W.S. and Hall, S.L. (1999). Affiliative behaviour of related and unrelated pairs of cats in catteries: A preliminary report. *Appl. Anim. Behav. Sci.* https://doi.org/10.1016/S0168-1591(99)00007-6.

Carlstead, K. (1993). Behavioral and physiological correlates of stress in laboratory cats. *Appl. Anim. Behav. Sci.* 38: 143–158.

Crowell-Davis, S.L., Curtis, T.M., and Knowles, R.J. (2004). Social organization in the cat: A modern understanding. *J. Fel. Med. Surg.* https://doi.org/10.1016/j.jfms.2003.09.013.

de Oliveira, A., Terçariol, C., and Genaro, G. (2015). The use of refuges by communally housed cats. *Animals.* https://doi.org/10.3390/ani5020245.

Desforges, E.J., Moesta, A., and Farnworth, M.J. (2016). Effect of a shelf-furnished screen on space utilisation and social behaviour of indoor group-housed cats (*Felis silvestris catus*). *Appl. Anim. Behav. Sci.* https://doi.org/10.1016/j.applanim.2016.03.006.

Ellis, S.L. (2009). Environmental enrichment: Practical strategies for improving feline welfare. *J. Fel. Med. Surg.* https://doi.org/10.1016/j.jfms.2009.09.011.

Ellis, S.L.H., Rodan, I., Carney, H.C. et al. (2013). AAFP and ISFM feline environmental needs guidelines. *J. Fel. Med. Surg.* https://doi.org/10.1177/1098612X13477537.

Fantuzzi, J.M., Miller, K.A., and Weiss, E. (2010). Factors relevant to adoption of cats in an animal shelter. *J. Appl. Anim. Welf. Sci.* https://doi.org/10.1080/10888700903583467.

Finka, L.R., Ellis, S.L., and Stavisky, J. (2014). A critically appraised topic (CAT) to compare the effects of single and multi-cat housing on physiological and behavioural measures of stress in domestic cats in confined environments. *BMC Vet. Res.* https://doi.org/10.1186/1746-6148-10-73.

Foreman-Worsley, R. and Farnworth, M.J. (2019). A systematic review of social and environmental factors and their implications for indoor cat welfare. *Appl. Anim. Behav. Sci.* https://doi.org/10.1016/j.applanim.2019.104841.

Gaskell, R. and Povey, R. (1977). Experimental induction of feline viral rhinotracheitis virus re-excretion in FVR-recovered cats. *Vet. Rec.* https://doi.org/10.1136/vr.100.7.128.

Geret, P.C., Riond, B., Cattori, V. et al. (2011). Housing and care of laboratory cats: From requirements to practice. *Schweiz. Arch. Tierheilkd.* https://doi.org/10.1024/0036-7281/a000175.

Gourkow, N. and Fraser, D. (2006). The effect of housing and handling practices on the welfare, behaviour and selection of domestic cats (*Felis sylvestris catus*) by adopters in an animal shelter. *Anim. Welf.* 15: 371–377.

Griffin, B. (2012). Population wellness: keeping cats physically and behaviorally healthy. In: *The Cat: Clinical Medicine and Management* (ed. S.E. Little), 1312–1356. St. Louis, MO: Elsevier Saunders.

Griffin, B. (2013). Feline care in the animal shelter. In: *Shelter Medicine for Veterinarians and Staff* (eds. L. Miller and S. Zawistowski), 145–184. Hoboken, NJ: Wiley Blackwell

Griffin, B. and Hume, K.R. (2006). Recognition and management of stress in housed cats. In: *Consultations in Feline Internal Medicine*, 5th ed. (ed. J.R. August), 717–734. St. Louis, MO: Saunders Elsevier.

Herron, M.E. and Buffington, C.A.T. (2014). Environmental enrichment for indoor cats. *Compend. Contin. Educ. Vet.* 32: E1–E5.

Kessler, M.R. and Turner, D.C. (1997). Stress and adaptation of cats (*Felis silvestris catus*) housed singly, in pairs and in groups in boarding catteries. *Anim. Welf.* 6: 243–254.

Kessler, M.R. and Turner, D.C. (1999a). Socialization and stress in cats (*Felis sylvestris catus*) housed singly and in groups in animal shelters. *Anim. Welf.* 8: 15–26.

Kessler, M.R. and Turner, D.C. (1999b). Effects of density and cage size on stress in domestic cats (*Felis silvestris catus*) housed in animal shelters and boarding catteries. *Anim. Welf.* 8: 259–267.

Kry, K. and Casey, R. (2007). The effect of hiding enrichment on stress levels and behaviour of domestic cats (*Felis sylvestris catus*) in a shelter setting and the implications for adoption potential. *Anim. Welf.* 16: 375–383.

Lewis, H.E. (2017). *Design of Animal Housing*. Long Beach, CA: PacVet.

Loberg, J.M. and Lundmark, F. (2016). The effect of space on behaviour in large groups of domestic cats kept indoors. *Appl. Anim. Behav. Sci.* https://doi.org/10.1016/j.applanim.2016.05.030.

Manteca, X., Mainau, E., and Temple, D. (n.d.). What Is Animal Welfare? https://www.fawec.org/en/fact-sheets/28-general-welfare/106-what-is-animal-welfare (accessed 29 December 2019).

McCobb, E.C., Patronek, G.J., Marder, A. et al. (2005). Assessment of stress levels among cats in four animal shelters. *J. Am. Vet. Med. Assoc.* https://doi.org/10.2460/javma.2005.226.548.

McCune, S. (1994). Caged cats: Avoiding problems and providing solutions. *Newsletter Companion Animal Study Group* 7: 1–9.

McMillan, F.D. (2002). Development of a mental wellness program for animals. *J. Am. Vet. Med. Assoc.* https://doi.org/10.2460/javma.2002.220.965.

Morgan, K.N. and Tromborg, C.T. (2007). Sources of stress in captivity. *Appl. Anim. Behav. Sci.* https://doi.org/10.1016/j.applanim.2006.05.032.

Newbury, S., Blinn, M.K., Bushby, P.A. et al. (2010). *Guidelines for Standards of Care in Animal Shelters*. Apex, NC: Association of Shelter Veterinarians.

Ottway, D.S. and Hawkins, D.M. (2003). Cat housing in rescue shelters: A welfare comparison between communal and discrete-unit housing. *Anim. Welf.* 12: 173–189.

Overall, K.L. and Dyer, D. (2005). Enrichment strategies for laboratory animals from the viewpoint of clinical veterinary behavioral medicine: Emphasis on cats and dogs. *ILAR J.* https://doi.org/10.1093/ilar.46.2.202

Pollard, V.J. and Shoults, A.M. (2018a). Animal housing. In: *Practical Guide to Veterinary Hospital Design: From Renovations to New Builds*, 212–219. Lakewood, CO: American Animal Hospital Association Press.

Pollard, V.J. and Shoults, A.M. (2018b). The fear free design movement. In: *Practical Guide to Veterinary Hospital Design: From Renovations to New Builds,* 51–55. Lakewood, CO: American Animal Hospital Association Press.

Povey, R.C. and Johnson, R.H. (1970). Observations on the epidemiology and control of viral respiratory disease in cats. *J. Small Anim. Pract.* https://doi.org/10.1111/j.1748-5827.1970.tb05599.x.

Rehnberg, L.K., Robert, K.A., Watson, S.J. et al. (2015). The effects of social interaction and environmental enrichment on the space use, behaviour and stress of owned housecats facing a novel environment. *Appl. Anim. Behav. Sci.* https://doi.org/10.1016/j.applanim.2015.06.002.

Rochlitz, I. (1999). Recommendations for the housing of cats in the home, in catteries and animal shelters, in laboratories and in veterinary surgeries. *J. Fel. Med. Surg.* https://doi.org/10.1016/S1098-612X(99)90207-3

Rochlitz, I. (2000). Recommendations for the housing and care of domestic cats in laboratories. *Lab. Anim.* https://doi.org/10.1258/002367700780577939.

Rochlitz, I. (2005). A review of the housing requirements of domestic cats (*Felis silvestris catus*) kept in the home. *Appl. Anim. Behav. Sci.* https://doi.org/10.1016/j.applanim.2005.01.002.

Rochlitz, I. (2007). Housing and welfare. In:*The Welfare of Cats* (ed. I. Rochlitz), 177–203. Dordrecht, the Netherlands: Springer.

Rochlitz, I., Podberscek, A., and Broom, D. (1998). The welfare of cats in a quarantine cattery. *Vet. Rec.* 143: 35–39.

Rodan, I. and Cannon, M. (2016). Housing cats in veterinary practice. In: *Feline Behavioral Health and Welfare* (eds. I. Rodan and S. Heath), 122–136. St. Louis, MO: Elsevier Health Sciences.

Sinn, L. (2016). Factors affecting the selection of cats by adopters. *J. Vet. Behav.* https://doi.org/10.1016/j.jveb.2016.06.001.

Stella, J.L. and Buffington, C.A.T. (2016). Environmental strategies to promote health and wellness. In: *August's Consultations in Feline Internal Medicine*, vol. 7, 718–736. https://doi.org/10.1016/B978-0-323-22652-3.00073-6.

Stella, J.L., Croney, C.C. (2016). Environmental aspects of domestic cat care and management: Implications for cat welfare. *Sci. World J.* https://doi.org/10.1155/2016/6296315.

Stella, J., Croney, C., and Buffington, T. (2014). Environmental factors that affect the behavior and welfare of domestic cats (*Felis silvestris catus*) housed in cages. *Appl. Anim. Behav. Sci.* https://doi.org/10.1016/j.applanim.2014.08.006.

Stella, J.L., Croney, C.C., and Buffington, C.T. (2017). Behavior and welfare of domestic cats housed in cages larger than U.S. norm. *J. Appl. Anim. Welf. Sci.* https://doi.org/10.1080/10888705.2017.1317252.

Suchak, M. and Lamica, J. (2018). A comparison of cats (*Felis silvestris catus*) housed in groups and single cages at a shelter: A retrospective matched cohort study. *Animals* https://doi.org/10.3390/ani8020029.

Tanaka, A., Wagner, D.C., Kass, P.H. et al. (2012). Associations among weight loss, stress, and upper respiratory tract infection in shelter cats. *J. Am. Vet. Med. Assoc.* 240: 570–576.

UC Davis Koret Shelter Medicine Program. (2015). Facility Design and Animal Housing. https://www.sheltermedicine.com/library/resources/?r=facility-design-and-animal-housing#4 (accessed 30 December 2019).

Uetake, K., Goto, A., Koyama, R. et al. (2013). Effects of single caging and cage size on behavior and stress level of domestic neutered cats housed in an animal shelter: Effect of caging in cats. *Anim. Sci. J.* https://doi.org/10.1111/j.1740-0929.2012.01055.x.

van den Bos, R. (1998). Post-conflict stress-response in confined group-living cats (*Felis silvestris catus*). *Appl. Anim. Behav. Sci.* 59: 323–330.

van der Leij, W.J.R., Selman, L.D.A.M., Vernooij, J.C.M. et al. (2019). The effect of a hiding box on stress levels and body weight in Dutch shelter cats; a randomized controlled trial. *PLOS ONE.* https://doi.org/10.1371/journal.pone.0223492.

Vinke, C.M., Godijn, L.M., and van der Leij, W.J.R. (2014). Will a hiding box provide stress reduction for shelter cats? *Appl. Anim. Behav. Sci.* https://doi.org/10.1016/j.applanim.2014.09.002.

Wagner, D., Hurley, K., and Stavisky, J. (2018a). Shelter housing for cats: Practical aspects of design and construction, and adaptation of existing accommodation. *J. Fel. Med. Surg.* https://doi.org/10.117 7/1098612X18781390.

Wagner, D., Kass, P.H., and Hurley, K.F. (2018b). Cage size, movement in and out of housing during daily care, and other environmental and population health risk factors for feline upper respiratory disease in nine North American animal shelters. *PLOS ONE.* https://doi.org/10.1371/journal.pone.0190140.

Weiss, E., Miller, K., Mohan-Gibbons, H. et al. (2012). Why did you choose this pet?: Adopters and pet selection preferences in five animal shelters in the United States. *Animals.* https://doi.org/10.3390/ani2020144.

Young, R.J. (2003). Environmental cnrichment: An historical perspective. In: *Environmental Enrichment for Captive Animals*, 1–19. Oxford, UK: Blackwell Science.

17

Feline Enrichment
Jacklyn J. Ellis, Katherine Miller, and Katie Watts

17.1   Introduction

Separation from what is familiar coupled with exposure to an unfamiliar environment, especially to a species that is often poorly socialized to novel environments, makes shelters particularly stressful for cats. Although not all stress is bad, prolonged stress without the ability to escape or engage in normal coping mechanisms can have deleterious effects on a cat's health, lead to the development of lasting behavioral problems, and result in a lower likelihood of adoption.

Environmental enrichment can improve a cat's perception of their environment, resulting in a reduced stress response. Space and resources in a shelter can be limited, so careful consideration of how to employ enrichment effectively and efficiently is key to the success of any enrichment program. A standard program of enrichment should be provided for all cats, while a more diverse range of enrichment opportunities may be prioritized to meet the needs of individuals expressing certain behaviors or health concerns or that have longer projected lengths of stay. It is also key to assess the impact of enrichment efforts so as to continually optimize the quality of the program overall and its impact on the well-being of each individual.

17.2   The Value of Environmental Enrichment

The primary role of an animal shelter is to find appropriate outcomes for the animals in their care. However, within that role they have the responsibility to provide for the medical and psychological needs of the animals until outcomes can be finalized. Despite our best efforts, the shelter can be a stressful place. The activation of the stress response largely revolves around the perception of a situation by the individual. The use of enrichment can reduce or eliminate the associated stress by influencing the way the individual appraises its circumstances.

The term *environmental enrichment* can be defined as any addition to an animal's environment resulting in an increase in the environment's quality, and a subsequent improvement to the animal's well-being. Environmental enrichment can influence whether or not an animal perceives a situation as stressful by helping them to habituate to stimuli they do find risky, or by coping with these stimuli by facilitating concealment or escape. It can also reduce boredom by providing stimulation and opportunities for interaction.

Some scholars maintain that the term should be reserved for additions that are made to the environment after the physiological and

Animal Behavior for Shelter Veterinarians and Staff, Second Edition. Edited by Brian A. DiGangi, Victoria A. Cussen, Pamela J. Reid, and Kristen A. Collins.
© 2022 John Wiley & Sons, Inc. Published 2022 by John Wiley & Sons, Inc.
Companion website: www.wiley.com/go/digangi/animal

behavioral needs of the animal are met and should not be used to refer to changes that result in a reduction of stress-related behavior (Duncan and Olsson 2001), but that debate is largely academic. Shelters should—at a minimum—focus on providing whatever is within their means to improve the well-being of the animals in their care, with a priority given to reducing signs of fear and stress, and then providing positive experiences whenever possible.

17.2.1 Value for the Cats

From the moment a cat enters a shelter, it is challenged by a broad range of potential, unavoidable stressors. These include the following (Morgan and Tromborg 2007):

- Confinement in unfamiliar, small, often uncomfortable surroundings
- Change of daily routine
- Disruption of social bonds and isolation
- Reduced positive social contact with people
- Increased negative social contact with people (restraint, medical procedures, etc.)
- Reduced physical and mental exercise
- Aversive, inescapable thermal or sensory stimulation including drafts, loud and sudden noise, and unfamiliar and aversive odors
- Exposure to conspecifics especially if not previously socialized with other cats
- Exposure to unfriendly conspecifics and unfamiliar humans
- Reduced ability to retreat or hide
- Boredom
- Unpredictability
- Lack of choices and control over interactions with the environment.

The cats in shelters tend to have a wide range of socialization histories with people, ranging from former house pets to free-roaming, unsocialized cats (Clancy and Rowan 2003; Levy et al. 2003; Slater 2004). Many pet cats have never left the house before, while many free-roaming cats have never been indoors. Depending on experience, genetics, age, personality, and the shelter environment itself, cats may respond to confinement in a shelter with varying levels of distress. Their stress levels can take more than two weeks to return to baseline (Kessler and Turner 1997, 1999), and some, especially unsocialized cats, will never adapt.

Distress in sheltered cats is often characterized by reduced activity, withdrawal, and motivation to hide (usually in the litterbox or under bedding if no suitable concealment area is available). Stressed cats often feign sleep, which is easily mistaken for relaxation. Distressed cats are tense and so may be hypervigilant, destructive, defensively aggressive, or escape-oriented. Overgrooming, decreased grooming, panting, and excessive drooling may also be signs of distress, as can failure to eat or use the litterbox during daytime hours. Some distressed cats refuse to eat or drink, while others will urinate or defecate where they lie rather than move from their hiding spot or bed to use the litterbox. Even cats who are withdrawn during the day may throw their cage into disarray at night when no people are around, apparently seeking to escape (see Griffin and Hume 2006 for a review of fear and stress behaviors).

Youngsters and active adult cats can quickly find confinement to be understimulating, leading them to make playthings out of any item in their cage. Shelter staff may find them batting playfully at grains of cat litter or the water in their dish, overturning their bowls or litterbox, chewing or tearing bedding, or reaching their paws through the bars of the cage when people pass by. Such boredom behavior can also include biting or scratching caretakers' or visitors' hands or legs as though toys or prey, making it difficult or even dangerous to clean the cage or handle the cat, and potentially result in increased length of stay due to bite quarantine periods or even euthanasia.

Cats displaying fearful, avoidant, defensive, destructive, or aggressive play behaviors are likely to have difficulty attracting adopters (Gourkow and Fraser 2006; Weiss et al. 2012). Furthermore, research indicates that stressed cats are at increased risk of physical illness (Tanaka et al. 2012; Stella et al. 2013) that can further increase their length of stay or increase risk of euthanasia. Also, any animal with a prolonged experience in a chronically barren environment may be subject to lasting detriments to brain structure and function (Rosenzweig and Bennett 1996), a welfare concern both during and after a cat's stay in a shelter.

While research examining the efficacy of environmental enrichment to improve the welfare of shelter cats is still sparse, clearly stress and deprivation can reduce a cat's quality of life (both physically and psychologically) and its chance of successful adoption.

17.2.2 Value for the Staff and Adopters

Stress in shelters is not limited to the animals, however. Shelter staff are likewise regularly exposed to stressors; high turnover and compassion fatigue are common. The creation of an environmental enrichment program is one way to heighten morale by increasing positive interaction between cats and staff, which can reduce stress for both (Carlstead et al. 1993). Interacting with one's own cat has been shown to improve negative moods. Cats have even been found to be sensitive to human depressive moods and are more likely to initiate interactions and rub against owners when they are exhibiting them (Turner 2017). It is reasonable to suggest these benefits could be extended to interacting with shelter cats.

The effects of enrichment can extend to adopters as well, who seem to show a preference for cats that are more active or housed in more interesting environments (Fantuzzi et al. 2010). Enrichment can also facilitate positive interactions between cats and adopters (e.g., through play with interactive toys), helping adopters to bond with a cat while encouraging the cats to approach, important factors in the choice to adopt (Dybdall and Strasser 2011; Weiss et al. 2012).

17.3 Categories of Enrichment

For ease, scientists often think about enrichment in several categories. Different systems of categorization are used in different texts. Ultimately, the idea that every environmental enrichment item falls into one of these categories is false—many items fit into more than one of these categories. However, the purpose of these categories is to help get caregivers thinking about the range of ways they can improve an animal's environment, and to help brainstorm innovative ways to improve the environment's quality.

17.3.1 Structural Enrichment

Structural enrichment is probably the most basic type of enrichment when considering the environment in which an animal lives but can go a long way to helping meet their needs if thoughtfully used. This category refers to all architectural aspects of an animal's environment including space, materials, furnishings, and the organization of these components. See Chapter 16 for further discussion of optimizing feline housing for behavioral well-being.

17.3.1.1 Enclosure Size

Confinement to small spaces can be one of the biggest stressors a cat faces in a shelter, as it limits the cat's ability to flee from perceived threats. Increasing the space available can decrease stress by allowing for the behavioral coping strategy of fleeing. The easiest way to increase the space available to a shelter cat is to house it in a foster home. This is recommended for all cats, unless prohibited by medical (i.e., requires continued ongoing treatment and/or monitoring that cannot be provided by a foster home) or behavioral (e.g., cat is unsocialized to people and unsuitable for a traditional home environment) reasons, or if the cat has a short projected length of stay and can be fast-tracked for adoption. At very least, space requirements should allow for separate functional areas for resting, eating/drinking, elimination, and locomotion. See Chapter 16 for more information on feline housing.

17.3.1.2 Hiding Opportunities

Providing hiding opportunities to shelter cats is crucial. When available, cats engage with them at very high rates. Both Vinke et al. (2014) and Ellis et al. (2021) found that when provided a hiding box, shelter cats will spend approximately 50% of their time inside. Using a preference test, Ellis et al. (2017) found that cats chose to spend significantly more time in the compartment containing a hiding box than in the compartment containing other types of enrichment (a motion-activated toy or an elevated shelf).

The ability to conceal themselves from perceived threats is an important behavioral coping mechanism for stressed cats, and the provision of a hiding box can greatly reduce stress in shelter cats. Vinke et al. (2014), van der Leij et al. (2019), and Kry and Casey (2007) all found that cats who were provided a hiding opportunity had significantly lower Cat-Stress-Scores than the control group, while Kry and Casey also found that cats with a hiding box were significantly more likely to approach a researcher during an approach test and slept restfully significantly more often than the control group. Ellis et al. (2021) found that cats provided with a hiding opportunity had significantly lower fecal glucocorticoid metabolites and greater food intake than cats who were provided with an elevated shelf or the control group.

There are a range of ways that hiding opportunities can be provided for shelter cats, including cardboard boxes (such as the Hide, Perch & Go™ box [British Columbia Society for the Prevention of Cruelty to Animals, Vancouver, British Columbia, Canada], which can also be used as a carrier in which to send the cat home), carriers, or hanging curtains across cage fronts.

17.3.1.3 Elevated Perches

Elevated areas, such as shelves or other platforms, have been described as essential for cats' well-being (Rochlitz 1999). Shelves or perches provide environmental complexity and the opportunity for active behavior as well as vantage points from which cats can monitor their surroundings (Ellis 2009) and could play a key role in exhibiting vigilance to cope with novel circumstances. Podberscek et al. (1991) found that communally housed laboratory cats spent 58% of their resting time on elevated shelves, and Ellis et al. (2014) found that after their initial habituation period, singly housed cats spent 53% of their time on elevated shelves. These findings suggest that elevated perches are a resource of value to confined cats, and that their inclusion in enclosure design may be important.

Many standard shelter cages come equipped with a shelf, but additional shelves can be added by including cardboard boxes (such as the Hide, Perch & Go box) in cages or cat trees and/or shelving units in out-of-cage spaces.

17.3.1.4 Scratching Surfaces

Scratching is a highly motivated behavior in cats; even declawed cats do it. Scratching has a variety of functions, including claw maintenance, stress reduction, stretching, exercising the muscles involved, and communicating a message—both through the visual cues their scratches leave behind and by depositing pheromones from their interdigital glands (DePorter and Elzerman 2019). Destructive scratching is usually easy to redirect if appropriate scratching surfaces are provided (Mengoli et al. 2013). Although it has not been shown to be a common behavioral reason that cats are relinquished to shelters (only 1%; Casey et al. 2009), Wilson et al. (2016) reported that preventing damage to objects in the house was the leading reason that owners elected to declaw their cats.

Providing appropriate scratching surfaces in shelter may help increase the likelihood of recognizing and using these surfaces for scratching in subsequent adoptive homes. The use of appropriate scratching surfaces can be further increased if scratching options are selected that most closely align with the individual's preferences. Zhang and McGlone (2020) found that adult cats prefer to use upright scratchers covered with cardboard or rope, and that adding catnip or silvervine to scratchers can increase its use. Zhang et al. (2019) found that kittens prefer S-shaped cardboard scratchers. In shelters, small, disposable cardboard scratchers (such as the Stretch and Scratch, Encinitas, CA) could be hung vertically on the door for adult cats housed in cages as space is limited, and for cats housed in larger environments scratching surfaces can be provided in the form of scratching posts or as a part of a cat tree. For kittens, where possible, the inclusion of an S-shaped scratcher is advisable.

17.3.1.5 Resting Places with Soft Bedding

Cats in shelters spend the majority of their time inactive (91%; Ellis et al. 2014). Providing comfortable resting places can provide relief from hard surfaces; encourage cats to rest in an area away from their litterbox; permit digging and exploration (e.g., if food is tucked inside or under it); and facilitate hiding. Crouse et al. (1995) found that when provided a cushion, cats demonstrated preference by spending the vast majority of their time in a lying posture on the cushion compared to other surfaces. They also found that the provision of a cushion dramatically decreased the percentage of time they spent lying in the litter pan. Roy (1992, as cited in McCune 1995) found that cats prefer resting on materials that offer a constant temperature, and Hawthorne et al. (1995, as cited in Rochlitz 2002) found cats seem to prefer polyester fleece fabric over less textured fabrics. Importantly, Desforges et al. (2016) found that removal of an enrichment item that provided multiple resting places resulted in an increase in aggression. Thus, co-housed cats require multiple widely spaced beds to reduce the likelihood they will be monopolized or fought over.

17.3.2 Social Enrichment

Contrary to popular opinion, cats are a social species (Macdonald et al. 2000). Providing cats opportunities for social interaction can be an immensely effective form of enrichment, as it provides stimulation, comfort, and may also facilitate social learning.

17.3.2.1 Interaction with Humans

Provided a cat is socialized to humans, most find human interaction very rewarding. Shreve et al. (2017) showed that cats preferred human interaction to a biologically relevant scent, toys, and even food. More than simply an enjoyable experience, human interaction can also help reduce stress and prevent disease development in shelter cats. Rehnberg et al. (2015) found that cats provided extended social interaction (60 minutes/day) with humans had a significant reduction in Cat-Stress-Score from day one to day two, while cats provided standard social interaction (20 minutes/day) did not express a similar reduction. Gourkow et al. (2014) found that cats deemed "anxious" on arrival at the shelter who were "gentled" (gently pet and spoken to softly, 40 minutes/day) were more likely to be rated in a positive mood, had higher S-IgA, and were less likely to develop upper respiratory disease than anxious cats that were not gentled. Gourkow and Phillips (2015) found similar results for cats deemed "contented" on arrival at the shelter. Liu et al. (2020) found that gentled cats were also less likely to spend time at the back of their cage, which may make them more attractive to potential adopters. Moreover, they showed this with only six to nine minutes of gentling daily.

Offering cats opportunities to interact with humans on a regular basis can be time-consuming for staff, but volunteer programs are a helpful resource for meeting the time requirements. All human contact with sheltered cats should be positive, consistent, and avoid excessive restraint. Cats less accustomed to close contact with people may prefer interaction via a toy or treat or for the person to sit nearby and simply read aloud rather than attempt physical interaction (although for well-socialized cats there is evidence that restricting physical interaction may induce frustration; Tuozzi et al. 2021). Incorporating simple training procedures into daily caretaking is a simple way to increase positive human social interaction, desirable animal behaviors, and mental stimulation. Training techniques are discussed in Section 17.3.3.3 and in Chapter 18.

17.3.2.2   Interaction with Other Cats

Cats have a flexible social structure, whereby they can live independently or in groups, depending on availability of food and other resources (Macdonald et al. 2000). Housing cats communally can provide them with social companionship and motivation to move and play. Uetake et al. (2013) found that group housed cats spent more time in locomotion and social/solitary play than singly housed cats and tended to have lower cortisol-to-creatinine ratios. However, when selecting cats to house communally, it is important to consider whether they have been previously socialized to other cats. Kessler and Turner (1999) found that cats without previous socialization to other cats had significantly higher Cat-Stress-Scores in group housing conditions as compared to single housing. Care should also be taken to ensure group housed cats are appropriately matched by age, health, and behavioral compatibility (Newbury et al. 2010). Well-socialized juveniles and kittens may adapt most quickly to new social groupings and can greatly benefit from the socialization and exercise that co-housing provides. While it is advisable to avoid admitting or housing cats that are not socialized toward people in shelters at all due to the inherent stress (Kessler and Turner 1999), invariably this happens from time to time. These cats often come from colonies and therefore are likely to be socialized toward other cats and may find great comfort in communal housing.

The initial introduction of unfamiliar animals is often the time of highest social tension, so integrate several newcomers at once on a weekly or biweekly basis to reduce frequency of stressful introductions (Ottway and Hawkins 2003).

To reduce aggression, the new cat may be housed with food, water, bed, and litterbox in a large wire dog crate inside the communal cage for the first day or more, depending on its and the resident cats' reactions (Griffin and Hume 2006). Use of Feliway® (CEVA Animal Health, Lenexa, KS), may ease the introduction (although see Section 17.3.4.1 on olfactory enrichment regarding evidence of efficacy). Ideally, staff will provide the chance to play and eat treats simultaneously to form initial positive associations. An elevated perch or hiding area with two exits and at least one soft bed should be provided for every socially housed individual. All such resources as well as food bowls, water bowls, and litterboxes should be spatially dispersed to minimize fighting and monopolization (Newbury et al. 2010). Staff should check on newly introduced cats multiple times during the first few hours and days to monitor for signs of bullying, fear, or aggression.

17.3.2.3   Interaction with Other Species

While it is not generally recommended to house cats with other species, there may be circumstances where this could be beneficial to individual cats. For example, if a dog and cat are surrendered together and are reportedly bonded, housing them communally could have obvious benefits to both of their well-being.

17.3.3   Cognitive Enrichment

Cognitive enrichment provides animals with opportunities to solve problems and offers some degree of control over their environment. Control may be the single most important factor in maintaining quality of life, and enrichment is an important means by which it is provided. An animal has control when it can help itself by expressing a behavior that satisfies a need. Animals without control develop unresponsiveness termed learned helplessness (Maier and Seligman 1976). It usually also offers the opportunity for the animal to earn a reward.

17.3.3.1 Feeding Enrichment

The wild relatives of domestic cats spend a large proportion of their day seeking, obtaining, and processing food and other resources, often traveling great distances, remembering and locating past food sources and caches, exploring unfamiliar places, and learning new useful behaviors. Foraging and hunting are means of gaining sustenance as well as gathering information about the environment. Confined animals have few options to occupy themselves in this way, which may result in frustration, lethargy, and weight gain. Foraging enrichment offers opportunities for mental and physical activity and can be part of an enhanced activity program for overweight cats (Clarke et al. 2005).

Reduction in food intake is a common sign of stress in shelter cats (Ellis et al. 2014; Tanaka et al. 2012), so it is advisable to provide food in a bowl until a cat has demonstrated that it is eating an acceptable amount of food. Once acceptable food intake has been established, food can be offered in a puzzle feeder. Ideally, food delivery will mimic cats' natural feeding strategy, which is to hunt, chase, grab, bat, or pounce to obtain multiple small meals (Young 2003). The device should be difficult enough so that the cat is not able to get all the food out at once but not so difficult that they give up. The Aikiou Stimulo Cat Activity Feeding Center (Aïkiou, Quebec, Canada; see Figure 17.1) or Catit® Senses 2.0 Digger (Catit, catit.com) are good options for dry food, because cats are only able to get a few kibbles at a time, tubes of different lengths can be used to increase/decrease the difficulty, and they are easily cleaned. For wet food, ice cube trays can be a quick and easy way to increase the length of a meal and the mental/physical effort required for the cat to access the food. There are also many inexpensive and easy DIY ways to increase the stimulation cats get from meal time, such as scattering food in bedding or shredded paper, hiding it in nooks and crannies, creating a scent trail with tuna juice to a hidden meal, tucking food into wads of paper or empty paper towel rolls, or freezing canned food inside empty plastic bottle caps or halves of plastic Easter eggs to make it a moving, lickable challenge. Making creative forms of foraging enrichment is usually an appealing project to shelter volunteers. Cats vary in their motivation and skill to work for their food, however, so if food is provided solely or primarily through foraging devices, monitor to ensure each cat consumes its daily ration. Clean and disinfect foraging devices before reuse to limit disease transmission.

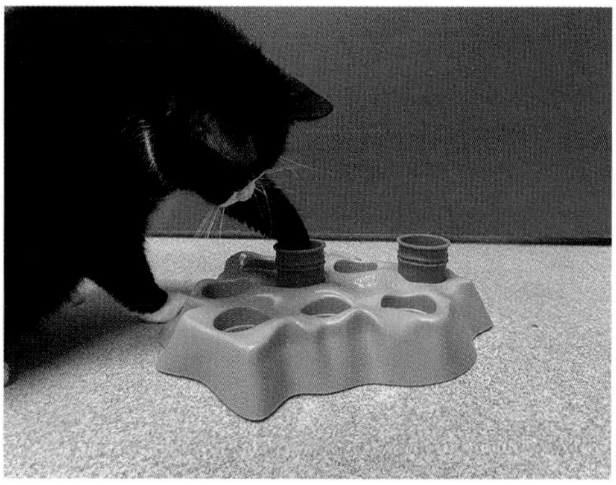

Figure 17.1 Feeding enrichment with the use of a puzzle feeder (Stimulo Cat Activity Feeding Center, Aïkiou, Quebec, Canada). *Source:* Courtesy of Jacklyn J. Ellis and Toronto Humane Society.

17.3.3.2 Toys

Play can be a fantastic way to reduce boredom, increase physical activity, and help a cat gain confidence in its surroundings. The traditional shelter environment does not inherently stimulate play but providing toys can help increase this behavior.

Toys can be separated into two categories: interactive toys that require human participation (such as wand toys), and solo-play toys (such as balls or felt mice). In a toy preference test, Denenberg (2003) found cats played for longer with interactive toys, likely because the movement of the toy generated by the human simulated prey and stimulated a range of natural behaviors (such as pounce, stalk, bat). Interactive toys should be available to people interacting with cats at shelters as they likely confer the most benefit to cats, but these toys should not be left in the cat's enclosures, as they often contain components that could be dangerous for the cat to have access to while unsupervised (e.g., they could consume the string portion of a wand toy). Solo-play toys tend to stimulate less interest from cats but should be available at all times to increase environmental complexity and allow for play from those cats that are interested. Cats seem to prefer small to large toys (de Monte and Le Pape 1997) but solo-play toys should not be so small that ingestion of these items is possible. Cats can habituate to and grow bored of toys surprisingly quickly (Hall et al. 2002) so a daily toy rotation of appropriate toys is recommended to increase interest. Fantuzzi et al. (2010) found that active cats were more likely to be adopted, so if the presence of toys in the cage does stimulate more play this may increase the cat's chances of adoption. However, the authors also found that potential adopters spend more time looking at cats with toys in the cage, regardless of activity levels. So even without the increase in play, the presence of these toys may aid in adoption.

17.3.3.3 Training

Training can provide mental exercise to cats who are eager to work to earn kibble or treats or to play with a toy. Training can also encourage physical exercise, for example, by teaching cats to walk on a harness and leash or perform tricks. Shy animals can be taught to touch their nose or cheek to an outstretched target or approach the front of the cage for a treat. Handling, husbandry, and veterinary procedures can be eased through desensitization and counter-conditioning training to change the animal's perception of these experiences from aversive to positive (see Figure 17.2).

The stress inherent in animal shelters can make learning more difficult, and training can be considered too time-consuming, but Kogan et al. (2017) found that 79% of cats

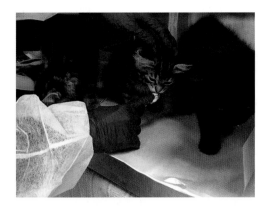

Figure 17.2 Using desensitization and counter-conditioning to socialize a kitten. *Source:* Courtesy of Jacklyn J. Ellis and Toronto Humane Society.

mastered the ability to touch a target in only five 15-minute training sessions. However, they did report that training success was significantly greater for bold as compared to shy cats. Training of shelter cats has also been shown to reduce stress and increase health. Gourkow and Phillips (2016) found that cats deemed "frustrated" on arrival at the shelter who had four 10-minute training sessions/day for 10 days were more likely to be rated in a positive mood, had higher S-IgA, and were less likely to develop upper respiratory disease than frustrated cats that did not experience training sessions. Furthermore, Grant and Warrior (2019) found that after clicker training, cats engaged in more exploratory behavior, spent less time inactive, and spent more time at the front of the cage than they did before. Although this study had no control group and could therefore not rule out the contribution time/habituation had in this behavior change, the behaviors the cats were exhibiting after training suggest they would be more likely to be adopted (Fantuzzi et al. 2010).

The critical aspect is use of positive, reward-based methods of training. Shelter animals will always benefit from more positive interactions with humans, whereas, unless prescribed and applied by a trained, certified behavior professional, punishment can rapidly reduce shelter animals' already fragile quality of life and increase fear and aggression (Herron et al. 2009). To learn more about behavior modification and training for cats, please see Chapter 18.

17.3.3.4 Novelty

Providing predictability for sheltered cats is critical to their quality of life, and most new arrivals likely suffer from an overload of novel experiences and stimuli. However, several weeks or months in a relatively barren shelter environment can engender lethargy, depression, withdrawal, and abnormal repetitive behavior. An intrinsic need for sensory change, exploration, or cognitive "challenge" has been postulated as a requirement for maintaining adequate quality of life for animals in long-term confinement (Hughes 1997; Wemelsfelder and Birke 1997).

While too much or unavoidable novelty can be stress-inducing (Carlstead et al. 1993), optional access to (and the ability to avoid) some novelty is interesting and encourages exploration, helping to satisfy animals' basic need to gain information about their surroundings (Mench 1998). Cats tend to habituate to most environmental enrichments relatively

quickly if they are unchanging and completely predictable. Effective enrichment protocols must therefore balance overall predictability with an appropriate amount of variation (e.g., by alternating or modifying enrichments, adding new enrichments, modifying methods of delivery, teaching new behaviors, and providing opportunities to explore somewhat novel objects and places such as exercise areas, changeable perches or retreats, or a view of the ever-dynamic outdoors). As mentioned above, a daily toy rotation may be a good way to introduce novelty (see Figure 17.3).

17.3.4 Sensory Enrichment

A cat's sense of hearing and smell are significantly sharper than humans, and their vision is finely tuned to detecting movement. Given the loud sounds, strong odors, and inescapable view that cats often experience in shelters, most may benefit more from a reduction of sensory stimulation than an increase. However, for longer-term shelter residents, thoughtful implementation of sensory enrichment can be a means to increase behavioral repertoire and reduce boredom.

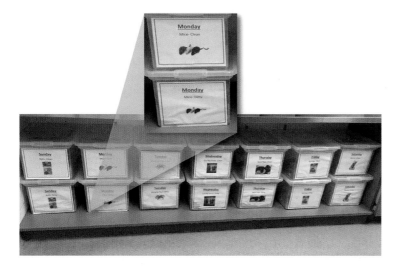

Figure 17.3 Organization of cat enrichment toys to ensure a daily rotation of items. *Source:* Courtesy of Jacklyn J. Ellis and Toronto Humane Society.

17.3.4.1 Olfactory Enrichment

A cat's sense of smell is one of the first senses to develop, and it continues to play an important role throughout their lives in hunting, defining home ranges, and social relationships—including with humans (Shreve and Udell 2015). It is possible for shelters to use olfactory enrichment to both increase stimulation and provide comfort.

To reduce boredom in longer-term shelter residents, bedding or other objects from rodent caging can be placed in small sacks or can be trailed around an exercise area leading to food stashes to provide an outlet for exploration, tracking, and hunting behavior. Catnip has well-known activity-increasing effects on cats, as does the lesser-known silvervine, although not all cats respond to either. Bol et al. (2017) found that 79% of cats responded to silvervine, while only 68% of cats responded to catnip, and that the intensity of the response to silvervine was significantly greater than to catnip. Ellis and Wells (2010) compared the behavioral responses of shelter cats given cloths impregnated with different smells (including prey and catnip) and found that although the interest was relatively low overall, cats with the catnip-impregnated cloth spent more time active and playing than the other treatment groups. Investigating the use of catnip or silvervine in longer-term shelter residents or those exhibiting behaviors indicative of frustration or boredom may reveal an even greater value in these products. These may be mixed into water and sprayed onto small cloths, wads of paper, or plush toys, or toys can also be "marinated" in containers of dried catnip to increase their interest. Silvervine is also often sold in the form of chew sticks.

Synthetic forms of feline facial pheromone (FFP; e.g., Feliway) are marketed to reduce fear, anxiety, and stress-related behaviors including urine marking, as well as to promote calming during stressful episodes such as adjustment to new environments. Reviews of published studies found evidence of efficacy of FFP in reducing urine spraying (Mills et al. 2011), but Chadwin et al. (2017) found the use of FFP in shelters did not reduce Cat-Stress-Scores or incidence of upper respiratory disease. In shelters, the pheromones' effects may be swamped by high levels of other stimulation, plus several weeks of continuous exposure to the pheromones may be necessary to note significant behavior changes (Mills et al. 2011). Because the effects of an FFP diffuser could be reduced by frequent room air exchanges, FFP may be more effective in its spray form, spritzed onto a soft toy or ball of paper inside the cages of cats who seem to benefit from it. Because FFP tends to be relatively expensive, its effects should be monitored to ensure its use is money well spent.

17.3.4.2 Visual Enrichment

Cats' eyes are well designed to detect motion and see well in dim light; however, they cannot appreciate the same spectrum of color that humans do, and they are a bit nearsighted—meaning they cannot focus as acutely on objects at a distance. These factors mean that they are well suited for hunting prey (Beaver 2003). Animal shelters may capitalize on this by using visual enrichment to reduce boredom or to help gain trust from more fearful cats.

Anything involving motion is likely to be most effective. This includes the movement inherent in interactive toys but also video images. Ellis and Wells (2008) found that cats paid more attention to video images that involved linear movement (either animate or inanimate), although their interest in these videos dropped significantly over time. This suggests that constant exposure to videos of movement may not be of much value, but using these videos during human interaction sessions may be a valuable way to add novelty and variety to these visits. There are many commercially available videos marketed for cat enrichment, typically featuring images of wildlife or other moving things, as well as many similar videos available freely on YouTube.

Housing cats in view of windows will also provide visual access to movement. A survey indicated that 98% of pet cats spend some time looking out of windows, with 89% of them spending between one and five hours per day in this activity (Shyan-Norwalt 2005). The vast majority were reported to watch birds and small wildlife outside the window. These findings highlight the importance of a view for cats and of the ability to watch activity and interesting stimuli through windows. The view from shelter windows can be enhanced by strategic placement of bird and squirrel feeders.

17.3.4.3 Auditory Enrichment

Because cats are nocturnal hunters of small, fast-moving prey, their sense of hearing is incredibly sensitive and their rotating ears allow them to pinpoint sounds with great accuracy (Beaver 2003). Shelters can go from very quiet to very loud in an instant (e.g., metal bowls accidentally clattering to the ground), which can be very stressful to cats; particularly to those already experiencing fear. Playing music in cat rooms can be one method of dampening the shock of sudden noises. Some music has further calming effects on cats. Snowden et al. (2015) tested music developed with pitch, pulse rate, and other features ecologically appropriate for cats and found that cats showed more positive responses to music composed for cats than to music composed for humans, and they became calmer after hearing the cat music. Hampton et al. (2020) then tested the effects of the cat music on behavior and physiological stress response of domestic cats in a veterinary clinic and found that cats played the cat music during an examination had significantly lower Cat-Stress-Scores and were significantly easier to handle than cats played either classical music or silence.

This cat music is now commercially available under the name "Music for Cats" and is provided free to veterinary clinics and animals shelters that do not practice declawing: https://www.musicforcats.com/shelters. Playing this music at appropriate volumes during business hours may help reduce stress in shelter cats, but staff should be sure to avoid placing music delivery systems on top of cages to prevent vibrating the cages, which could be stressful to cats given their fine tactile senses. Talk radio may be useful for socializing kittens and cats to the sound of human voices, but this has not been scientifically evaluated.

17.3.5 Husbandry Practices

The contents of this section are geared toward optimizing husbandry practices through reducing negative experiences rather than providing opportunities for positive ones and therefore do not technically qualify as environmental enrichment. However, in order for enrichment interventions to have maximum impact it is important that overall stress reduction is a priority.

Whenever interacting with a cat – but especially a fearful cat –always approach them in a way that will make them feel comfortable; turn your body sideways, avoid towering over them, limit eye contact, verbalize soothingly, and gesture enticingly. It is best if they approach and initiate the interaction. If the cat is showing signs of fear, the intensity of the interaction should be reduced, and their personal space should be respected. This may mean a brief reduction in intensity, but it might require ending the interaction altogether and coming back to try again later. It is particularly important to use a considerate approach during cleaning and medical procedures, as these are interactions that cats may find unpleasant.

Predictable caretaking routines are crucial to reducing anxiety. Carlstead et al. (1993) found that cats subjected to irregular caretaking and feeding schedules exhibited significantly higher concentrations of urinary cortisol, reduced frequency of active exploratory and play behavior, and increased frequency of time awake/alert and attempting to hide. Ensuring cats are fed and cleaned at the same time every day should be standard in any animal shelter husbandry program.

It used to be standard when cleaning cat cages in animal shelters to put the cat in a carrier while everything was taken out to be sanitized, and contents such as bedding were replaced with freshly cleaned items. The industry is now moving to a spot-cleaning model, where the cat is left in the cage while soiled areas are cleaned using a mild cleanser, debris such as litter is shaken out of bedding (but not replaced), and the litterbox is changed. This new model is much less stressful for the cat, as they are not forcibly removed from their environment, and it allows for the retention of familiar odors, which may be comforting to the cat.

As was described in the section on auditory enrichment, cats have very sensitive hearing. Accordingly, the noises of the shelter environment can be very distressing. In one newly built shelter of cinder block construction, noise in holding areas regularly exceeded 100 dB, which is equivalent to a jackhammer, and even when the shelter seemed quiet noise was 50–60 dB (Coppola et al. 2006). Likely results include physiological and behavioral arousal and stress and even hearing damage. It is likely that sound reduction would be more beneficial to cats' quality of life than sound introduction. This can be done by asking staff to refrain from shouting or banging doors/litterboxes, using spray lubricant on squeaky wheels, keeping doors to cat rooms closed, and installing sound baffles (Wagner et al. 2018a). Many cages have very loud latches despite lubrication between inhabitants. In these cases, coating the latches with Plasti Dip® (Plasti Dip International, Inc., Circles Pines, MN) can be an inexpensive way to significantly reduce the noise involved with opening and closing cage doors. Plastic, quiet-close hinges and latches are also available from some enclosure manufacturers. Finally, it is important that shelters house cats far enough away from the dogs that the barking is not audible. McCobb et al. (2005) found that cats with the highest exposure to dogs had the highest urinary cortisol-to-creatinine ratio.

Reducing the frequency of cage moves seems to also have a positive impact on stress and can result in an increase in overall health. Wagner et al. (2018b) found that moving a cat two or more times in their first week in the shelter greatly increased their likelihood of upper respiratory disease.

For additional training on methods for reducing stress in shelters, the Fear Free Shelter Program offers an online training at no cost to all shelter, rescue, and animal welfare employees and volunteers: https://fearfreeshelters.com/ and Chapter 14 is dedicated to low-stress handling techniques for shelter cats.

17.4 Prioritizing Enrichment among Different Types of Cats

In an ideal world, all types of enrichment would be available to every cat they might benefit. In reality, the space and resource limitations of a shelter mean that this is simply not possible. Regardless, a base enrichment program should be available to all cats, which should include at a minimum: 2 ft. of space between food, resting places, and the litterbox; a hiding opportunity (with an opportunity for perching on top); a resting place with soft bedding; regular opportunities for positive interactions with human caregivers; solo-play toys available in their cages; a predictable caretaking routine; and the use of low-stress husbandry practices.

However, when cats present with particular concerns regarding their behavioral or physiological functioning, additional enrichment should be prioritized to meet the specific needs of the individual. Below are some examples of the types of needs that might present, and strategies that might be useful to address these concerns. It is important to note that cats presenting with any of the below concerns (with the exception of unsocialized cats) should be prioritized for appropriate foster placement, as a foster home is inherently more enriching than the shelter environment.

17.4.1 Kittens

For normal neurological and social development, kittens must be raised in a complex, variable, and interactive environment that includes regular social interaction and opportunity to exercise their growing bodies and minds. Kittens with restricted experiences show later deficiencies in social skills, enhanced irritability, fear, and aggression toward unfamiliar people and things, and reduced learning capabilities (Guyot et al 1980; Turner 2000). Kittens should be introduced between two and seven weeks of age to the types of people, animals, environments, handling, and situations they are likely to encounter as adults (Turner 2000). Casey and Bradshaw (2008) reported the lasting behavioral benefits of providing neonates with even just a few minutes of gentle handling and play per day, contact with multiple people, and exposure to recordings of human household sounds. A year later, these kittens were less fearful of people and provided more emotional support to their owners than kittens who experienced only the normal daily shelter caretaking routine.

Therefore, there is no time to lose when it comes to enriching and training kittens and juveniles, including those who are ill or injured. Fortunately, it is usually easy to recruit volunteers for this duty, and the most trustworthy can be instructed in proper precautions when interacting with sick animals. Ideally, kittens will receive at least 20–30 minutes of human interaction and some basic training per day by a variety of people (age, gender, ethnicity, and size) while accompanied by their littermates or similar-aged young ones (Turner 2000). The mother and littermates are crucial to normal social and behavioral development. Therefore, the queen should be housed with the kittens until weaning, then the kittens should be co-housed.

17.4.2 High-Energy Cats

These cats rarely show traditional signs of stress (fear-related behaviors) and are therefore often considered to have good well-being

in the shelter. However, they can suffer from frustration due to understimulation and inability to control their environment. This can lead to loud and persistent meowing, reaching though the bars in an attempt to stimulate interaction from people walking past, pacing or pawing at walls, disrupting their cage contents, excessive grooming, and alternating between a friendly response (rubbing on a handlers' hand) and the delivery of an unexpected bite or swat.

To increase the effectiveness of a base enrichment program for high-energy cats, it is crucial to employ strategies to engage their mind and body. Out-of-cage space, increased climbing opportunities, and scratching surfaces should all be provided. Cognitive enrichment should be a major focus in these cases. Meals should be delivered in feeding puzzles, automated toys may be left in their environments, and these cats are often particularly adept at learning tricks, so training sessions are strongly recommended. Adding novelty or sensory enrichment (particularly stimulating rather than relaxing options) could also be wise.

Chronic frustration can lead to depression, which should be treated as a welfare emergency. Frustration is a common condition in animals living in prolonged captive conditions that do not meet their needs and can result in a long-lasting alteration of the immune and endocrine systems (Sumida et al. 2004). Common signs of depression in cats include high degrees of inactivity, a reduction of grooming, inappetence, and reduction of interest in interaction with humans. Increasing the options for engagement for these cats is essential. If foster placement is unavailable, these cats should be housed in an office with access to human companionship all day or should receive multiple opportunities for human interaction daily.

17.4.3 Cats with Low Tolerance of Petting

Some cats seem to seek out petting, or even actively enjoy it for a time, only to turn around and scratch or bite. Petting for some cats is much like tickling for humans—it may be fun for a while but can turn unpleasant, fast. The threshold for tolerance of petting can vary widely in cats. Moreover, some cats may want to be near humans but do not actually want to be petted. The problem arises when the person's desire for petting is greater than the cat's tolerance. If a cat is showing signs of petting aggression, traditional human-animal interaction can be difficult. Staff and volunteers interacting with cats instinctively want to pet them. If a cat responds to these efforts with a swat or by recoiling, caregivers can be offended and become less likely to want to interact with them in the future. Likewise, adopters can have a hard time picturing a cat exhibiting these behaviors as a part of their lives, and they may have a lower likelihood of adoption.

When dealing with a cat exhibiting these behaviors, the first step is to ensure you are petting them in a "cat-friendly" way. One of the main reasons cats rub against each other and the environment is to deposit pheromones that mark things as familiar and safe, thereby creating a "group scent." When we pet them, this pheromone gets on us and we effectively join their group. When petting your cat, think about this and focus on where they have glands, especially around the face (see Figure 17.4). Research shows that petting at the base of the tail can cause a negative response in cats (Ellis et al. 2015; Soennichsen and Chamove 2002), so it should be avoided unless the cat clearly enjoys it. Most cats prefer to be pet in short bursts, rather than marathon petting sessions. This is likely particularly true in cats with low thresholds for petting.

Cats with low thresholds for petting usually exhibit some warning signs before they lash out. The specific signs vary between cats, but common signs include thrashing tail, enlarging pupils, watching the petter's hand, ears to the side/back, and skin rippling on their back. The easiest way to avoid petting-induced aggression is to learn how much petting a cat enjoys before they start showing these warning signs and ceasing petting them before that. It's important to remember that they are not exhibiting this behavior out of spite but out of discomfort.

Petting is often how people bond with their cats, so asking them to hold back can be hard on this relationship. Interactive play or trick training is a fantastic way to facilitate the human-animal bond without causing the cat discomfort. And knowing a repertoire of

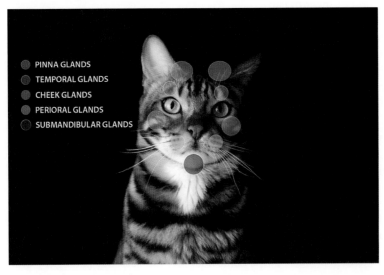

Figure 17.4 Location of scent glands on the feline head. *Source:* Courtesy of Alexander McAvoy and Toronto Humane Society.

tricks may make a cat more appealing to adopters.

It may be possible to increase a cat's tolerance for petting through a process called desensitization and counter-conditioning. This means gradually exposing an animal to something it does not like and pairing this with food. This process can change an animal's perception of something from bad to good. Briefly, as it relates to increasing tolerance for petting:

1) Figure out how long the cat can always be pet before exhibiting warning signs.
2) Pet the cat for that amount of time, and then give a high-value reward.
3) Gradually increase the amount of time the cat can be pet, without pushing the cat past their threshold (i.e., they do not exhibit any warning signs). Continue using the reward.

It is very important that cats are never punished when exhibiting low tolerance to petting. This may reduce the likelihood the cat will exhibit warning signs and may increase the intensity of the reaction in the future.

17.4.4 Overweight Cats

Overweight cats face unique welfare concerns in a shelter environment, including the health concerns inherent in their condition, the limited space contributing to further weight gain, and reduced food consumption (a common sign of stress) leading to feline hepatic lipidosis. Encouraging activity should be prioritized for these cats, including housing them in out-of-cage-space, providing meals in puzzle feeders (once acceptable food intake has been established), and training them to do tricks that require exercise, including target training and agility.

17.4.5 Fearful or Anxious Cats

The reasons why cats find shelter conditions stressful have been well established earlier in this chapter. However, some cats are prone to being more fearful than others. Assuming the cats are socialized to people, this may be due to improper socialization to novelty or a genetic predisposition to a shy temperament (Turner et al. 1986).

Although a base enrichment program should already include hiding and perching aspects, these may be especially important to fearful cats to allow for the coping strategies of concealment and monitoring threats. Routine can also be of particular importance to these cats, reducing anxiety by increasing predictability. Learning to identify body language indicative of fear in cats can help staff and volunteers know when to modify their interaction style by using a more considerate approach. Common signs of fear in cats include large pupils; ears to the side/back; tail tucked or tight to body; hissing, growling, or yowling; hair standing on end; leaning away, crouching, or tense body posture; and rolling on back with feet ready to strike or feet tucked under with paws on the ground, ready to flee.

If possible, identify what things frighten the cat, and do what you can to limit their exposure to them. If these things are nonessential and can be removed from their environment (e.g., human interaction with a specific gender), this is often easiest. For triggers that are unavoidable or frequent, gradually introduce them to these things in combination with something they like (e.g., treats or play). Ensure the introduction is done so slowly that the cat does not go above their threshold (i.e., they do not exhibit fearful behaviors).

Training can be a fantastic way to increase a cat's confidence, although fear can inhibit learning and fearful shelter cats have shown less success in training (Kogan et al. 2017). Learning to touch a target is often the easiest trick to teach a fearful cat. Getting a fearful cat into a carrier can be particularly difficult so carrier training can be especially valuable in this context. This process gives the cat a "safe" place to hide in their enclosure and also ensures that getting the cat into the carrier when necessary will be less stressful for both cat and caregiver.

17.4.6 Unsocialized Cats

As previously stated, it is not advisable to house unsocialized cats in shelters at all due to the inherent stress. Priority should be given to returning these cats to their previous environment through trap-neuter-return or return to field programs, and when that is not possible using alternative placement pathways. While unsocialized cats are awaiting these outcomes in shelters, housing them with a social companion may provide great comfort, as these cats often come from colonies and therefore are likely to be socialized toward other cats. During this time, human contact should be limited, although interactions from a distance using tossed treats and low-key play strategies (such as jiggling the wand of a toy under a towel or gently dragging a string) are acceptable to see if friendly behaviors can be elicited. Chapter 7 includes additional details on managing unsocialized community cats in the shelter.

17.5 Removing Obstacles to Enrichment

Provision of enrichment is not without expenditure of resources and other potential drawbacks, but these can be mitigated if enrichment is thoughtfully implemented and monitored for efficacy. Concerns over disease control can be minimized by focusing on disposable or disinfectable items, sensory enrichment, nonmaterial playthings like bubbles and laser toys, human interaction, and training cats inside their cages.

To reduce staff time required, volunteers can manage the enrichment program, which is usually a very popular assignment. Employing volunteers for tasks outside of human-animal interaction is often overlooked. Tasks such as entering data on human-animal enrichment sessions (or even creation of proprietary software to track human-animal enrichment sessions), automating audio systems to play music at designated times of day, or sewing cage bedding or curtains may all be abilities within the skill set of existing volunteers. If not, advertising for volunteers with these skill sets may expand the capabilities of a shelter enrichment program.

Exploiting corporate partnerships can be a very effective way to supplement an enrichment program. Shelters can host team-building days where members of the corporation come to the shelter and interact with animals or build enrichment devices such as toys or puzzle feeders. Some companies may be willing to donate certain items in exchange for positive press or placement of their company brand and logo on the products within the shelter or on the shelter's website or newsletter. Finally, corporations can be approached with sponsorship opportunities where in exchange for a donation of funds, they can design and install a floor-to-ceiling overhaul of an out-of-cage space environment to meet the enrichment needs of an animal in a way that embodies and advertises their brand (see Figure 17.5). This way, the animals have an enriched environment, the company markets their brand in a way that appeals to the hearts of potential customers, and visitors have a much more engaging experience.

Monetary costs can be minimized by using donated items and recycled materials like cardboard, scrap paper, and bottle caps. More on-going (e.g., towels and bedding) or high-ticket items (e.g., cat trees or audio systems) can be acquired by posting about specific needs on social media or by creating an Amazon Wish List.

17.6 Assessing Efficacy of Enrichment

As was stated in the definition provided in Section 17.2, an item only qualifies as environmental enrichment if it results in an improvement to the animal's well-being. Enrichment efforts will impact individuals differently, and

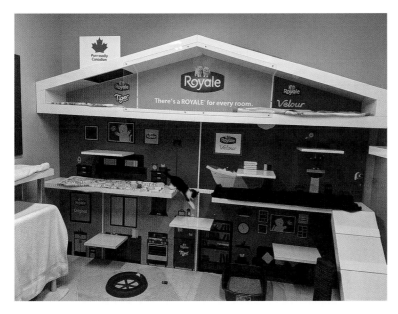

Figure 17.5 An enriched cat housing environment funded by a corporate sponsor. *Source:* Courtesy of Aimee Holmes and Toronto Humane Society.

the relative importance of these efforts will change over time and conditions. While seeing an animal using an enrichment is a good start, it is not sufficient to ensure efficacy in improving quality of life since some animals may require time to figure an enrichment out or will turn to an enrichment only in certain situations, while others' interest may peak quickly and then diminish. Identifying which items might be most effective for different individuals can be accomplished by monitoring their behavior and physiological functioning, then providing items tailored to address what stressor seems negatively impacting them (e.g., fear, boredom, frustration). Improvements to the animal's well-being (and therefore, the efficacy of the item as enrichment) can be assessed by measuring changes in their behavior and physiological functioning after the item is provided.

In order to measure indicators of well-being, the first step is to select a framework. Frameworks that lend themselves best to this purpose in shelters include scan sampling and ad libitum behavioral observations. Scan sampling involves an observer approaching an

animal's enclosure and recording specific behaviors or behavioral indicators at multiple timepoints on a regular schedule (e.g., daily before feeding and cleaning). Ad libitum behavioral observations involve recording an animal's behavior outside of a structured context. Both of these frameworks have the advantage of requiring relatively little extra staff time, as they can be done in combination with tasks that are already being done (e.g., feeding/ cleaning, human-animal interaction, vet exams) (see Chapter 15 for a more thorough discussion of each framework).

Next, select what behaviors to record and how to measure them. The reporting of behavior in shelters often suffers from being qualitative, and thus difficult to compare over time and between individuals reporting it. Instead, it may be more helpful to record the presence or absence of target behaviors that are indicators of positive (e.g., approaches cage front, playing) and negative (e.g., hiding, hissing) emotions. Other indicators linked to well-being could also be recorded, for example food intake (Ellis et al. 2014; Tanaka et al. 2012) or sickness behaviors (Stella et al. 2013; Tanaka et al. 2012). Certain behaviors could also be assessed on a continuum, such as pain (Epstein et al. 2015) or stress (e.g., the Cat-Stress-Score; Kessler and Turner 1997).

If, after monitoring, an individual is identified as having consistently poor well-being indicators despite the base enrichment program provided to all cats in a shelter, this would identify the cat as having additional needs. Staff may consider implementing additional enrichment strategies, such as moving this cat to out-of-cage space, housing them with a social companion, or implementing training techniques. Through continued assessment of the same indicators, it becomes much easier to assess the efficacy of the targeted enrichment intervention(s). For a more thorough discussion of these frameworks, well-being indicators, and tips for implementing a program to monitor these indicators to meet the needs of your shelter, see Chapter 15.

17.7 Conclusions

Environmental enrichment is a key tool available to shelter staff and volunteers to reduce the stress response of the cats in their care by facilitating regular behaviors and coping mechanisms, thereby improving cats' perception of their environment. Shelters should provide a base enrichment program to all cats consisting, at a minimum, of a hiding opportunity; a resting place with soft bedding; regular opportunities for positive interactions with human caregivers; solo-play toys available in their cages; physical space between their food, litter, and resting places; a predictable caretaking routine; and the use of low-stress husbandry practices. Shelters should strive to go above and beyond these basics for all cats, but when cats present with particular needs, additional enrichment should be prioritized to meet the specific needs of the individual. Shelters are still a relatively new frontier in the implementation and study of environmental and behavioral enrichment for cats. It is therefore strongly recommended that shelters track and share their experiences to ensure effective use of valuable resources and to create a more shelter-specific knowledge bank. However, even the most optimal in-shelter enrichment program is unlikely to compare to the enrichment provided in a foster home, so placing as many appropriate cats in foster homes as possible is likely to be the most effective enrichment strategy.

Acknowledgments

The authors would like to acknowledge Nadine Gourkow for contributing an early version of this chapter's manuscript.

Please visit the companion website for video clips and downloadable resources associated with this chapter.

References

Beaver, B.V. (2003). *Feline Behavior: A Guide for Veterinarians*, 2nd ed. Philadelphia, PA: Saunders.

Bol, S., Caspers, J., Buckingham, L. et al. (2017). Responsiveness of cats (Felidae) to silver vine (Actinidia polygama), Tatarian honeysuckle (Lonicera tatarica), valerian (Valeriana officinalis) and catnip (Nepeta cataria). *BMC Vet. Res.* 13 (1): 1–16.

Carlstead, K., Brown, J.L., and Strawn, W. (1993). Behavioural and physiological correlates of stress in laboratory cats. *Appl. Anim. Behav. Sci.* 38: 143–158.

Casey, R.A. and Bradshaw, J.W.S. (2008). The effects of additional socialisation for kittens in a rescue centre on their behaviour and suitability as a pet. *Appl. Anim. Behav. Sci.* 114 (1): 196–205.

Casey, R.A., Vandenbussche, S., Bradshaw, J.W. et al. (2009). Reasons for relinquishment and return of domestic cats (*Felis silvestris catus*) to rescue shelters in the UK. *Anthrozoös* 22 (4): 347–358.

Chadwin, R.M., Bain, M.J., and Kass, P.H. (2017). Effect of a synthetic feline facial pheromone product on stress scores and incidence of upper respiratory tract infection in shelter cats. *J. Am. Vet. Med. Assoc.* 251 (4): 413–420.

Clancy, E.A. and Rowan, A.N. (2003). Companion animal demographics in the United States: A historical perspective. In: *State of the Animals II* (eds. D.J. Salem and A.N. Rowan), 9–26. Washington, DC: Humane Society Press.

Clarke, D.L., Wrigglesworth, D., Holmes, K. et al. (2005). Using environmental and feeding enrichment to facilitate feline weight loss. *J. Anim. Physiol. Anim. Nutr.* 89: 427.

Coppola, C.L., Enns, R.M., and Grandin, T. (2006). Noise in the animal shelter environment: Building design and the effects of daily noise exposure. *J. Appl. Anim. Welf. Sci.* 9 (1): 1–7.

Crouse, S.J., Atwill, E.R., Lagana, M. et al. (1995). Soft surfaces: A factor in feline psychological well-being. *Contemp. Top. Lab. Anim. Sci.* 34 (6): 94–97.

De Monte, M. and Le Pape, G. (1997). Behavioural effects of cage enrichment in single-caged adult cats. *Anim. Welf.* 6 (1): 53–66.

Denenberg, S. (2003). Cat toy play trial: A comparison of different toys. *Annual Scientific Symposium of Animal Behaviour*, Denver, CO.

DePorter, T.L. and Elzerman, A.L. (2019). Common feline problem behaviors: Destructive scratching. *J. Fel. Med. Surg.* 21 (3): 235–243.

Desforges, E.J., Moesta, A., and Farnworth, M.J. (2016). Effect of a shelf-furnished screen on space utilisation and social behaviour of indoor group-housed cats (*Felis silvestris catus*). *Appl. Anim. Behav. Sci.* 178: 60–68.

Duncan, I. and Olsson, I. (2001). Environmental enrichment: From flawed concept to pseudo-science. *Proceedings of the International Congress of the ISAE,* Davis, CA (4–8 August 2001). Davis, CA: Center for Animal Welfare.

Dybdall, K. and Strasser, R. (2011). Measuring attachment behavior and adoption time in shelter cats. *Proceedings of the 20th Congress of the International Society of Anthrozoology,* Indianapolis, IN (4–6 August 2011). Indianapolis, IN: International Society of Anthrozoology.

Ellis, J.J., Protopapadaki, V., Stryhn, H. et al. (2014). Behavioural and faecal glucocorticoid metabolite responses of single caging in six cats over 30 days. *Vet. Rec. Open* 1 (1): e000056.

Ellis, J.J., Stryhn, H., and Cockram, M.S. (2021). Effects of the provision of a hiding box or shelf on the behaviour and faecal glucocorticoid metabolites of bold and shy cats housed in single cages. *Appl. Anim. Behav. Sci.* 236: 105221.

Ellis, J.J., Stryhn, H., Spears, J., and Cockram, M.S. (2017). Environmental enrichment choices of shelter cats. *Behav. Process.* 141: 291–296.

Ellis, S.L.H. (2009). Environmental enrichment: Practical strategies for improving feline welfare. *J. Fel. Med. Surg.* 11 (11): 901–912.

Ellis, S.L.H., Thompson, H., Guijarro, C. et al. (2015). The influence of body region, handler familiarity and order of region handled on the domestic cat's response to being stroked. *Appl. Anim. Behav. Sci.* 173: 60–67.

Ellis, S.L.H. and Wells, D.L. (2008). The influence of visual stimulation on the behaviour of cats housed in a rescue shelter. *Appl. Anim. Behav. Sci.* 113: 166–174.

Ellis, S.L.H. and Wells, D.L. (2010). The influence of olfactory stimulation on the behaviour of cats housed in a rescue shelter. *Appl. Anim. Behav. Sci.* 123 (1–2): 56–62.

Epstein, M.E., Rodan, I., Griffenhagen, G. et al. (2015). 2015 AAHA/AAFP pain management guidelines for dogs and cats. *J. Fel. Med. Surg.* 17 (3): 251–272.

Fantuzzi, J.M., Miller, K.A., and Weiss, E. (2010). Factors relevant to adoption of cats in an animal shelter. *J. Appl. Anim. Welf. Sci.* 13 (2): 174–179.

Gourkow, N. and Fraser, D. (2006). The effect of housing and handling practices on the welfare, behaviour and selection of domestic cats (*Felis sylvestris catus*) by adopters in an animal shelter. *Anim. Welf.* 15: 371–377.

Gourkow, N., Hamon, S.C., and Phillips, C.J. (2014). Effect of gentle stroking and vocalization on behaviour, mucosal immunity and upper respiratory disease in anxious shelter cats. *Prev. Vet. Med.* 117 (1): 266–275.

Gourkow, N. and Phillips, C.J. (2015). Effect of interactions with humans on behaviour, mucosal immunity and upper respiratory disease of shelter cats rated as contented on arrival. *Prev. Vet. Med.* 121 (3–4): 288–296.

Gourkow, N. and Phillips, C.J. (2016). Effect of cognitive enrichment on behavior, mucosal immunity and upper respiratory disease of shelter cats rated as frustrated on arrival. *Prev. Vet. Med.* 131: 103–110.

Grant, R.A. and Warrior, J.R. (2019). Clicker training increases exploratory behaviour and time spent at the front of the enclosure in shelter cats: Implications for welfare and adoption rates. *Appl. Anim. Behav. Sci.* 211: 77–83.

Griffin, B. and Hume, K.R. (2006). Recognition and management of stress in housed cats. In: *Consultations in Feline Internal Medicine*, 5th ed. (ed. J.R. August), 717–734. St. Louis, MO: Saunders.

Guyot, G.W., Bennet, T.L., and Cross, H.A. (1980). The effects of social isolation on the behavior of juvenile domestic cats. *Dev. Psychobiol.* 13 (3): 317–329.

Hall, S.L., Bradshaw, J.W., and Robinson, I.H. (2002). Object play in adult domestic cats: The roles of habituation and disinhibition. *Appl. Anim. Behav. Sci.* 79 (3): 263–271.

Hampton, A., Ford, A., Cox III, R.E. et al. (2020). Effects of music on behavior and physiological stress response of domestic cats in a veterinary clinic. *J. Fel. Med. Surg.* 22 (2): 122–128.

Hawthorne, A.J., Loveridge, G.G., and Horrocks, L.J. (1995). The behaviour of domestic cats in response to a variety of surface textures. *Proceedings of the Second International Conference on Environmental Enrichment,* Copenhagen, Denmark (21–25 August 1995). Copenhagen, Denmark: Copenhagen Zoo.

Herron, M.E., Shofer, F.S., and Reisner, I.R. (2009). Survey of the use and outcome of confrontational and non-confrontational training methods in client-owned dogs showing undesired behaviors. *Appl. Anim. Behav. Sci.* 117: 47–54.

Hughes, R.N. (1997). Intrinsic exploration in animals: Motives and measurement. *Behav. Process.* 41: 213–226.

Kessler, M.R. and Turner, D.C. (1997). Stress and adaptation of cats (*Felis silvestris catus*) housed singly, in pairs and in groups in boarding catteries. *Anim. Welf.* 6: 243–254.

Kessler, M.R. and Turner, D.C. (1999). Socialization and stress in cats (*Felis silvestris catus*) housed singly and in groups in animal shelters. *Anim. Welf.* 8 (1): 15–26.

Kogan, L., Kolus, C., and Schoenfeld-Tacher, R. (2017). Assessment of clicker training for shelter cats. *Animals* 7 (10): 73.

Kry, K. and Casey, R. (2007). The effect of hiding enrichment on stress levels and behaviour of domestic cats (*Felis sylvestris catus*) in a shelter setting and the implications for adoption potential. *Anim. Welf.* 16 (3): 375–383.

Levy, J.K., Woods, J.E., Turick, S.L. et al. (2003). Number of unowned free-roaming cats in a college community in the southern United States and characteristics of community residents who feed them. *J. Am. Vet. Med. Assoc.* 223: 202–205.

Liu, S., Paterson, M., Camarri, S. et al. (2020). The effects of the frequency and method of gentling on the behavior of cats in shelters. *J. Vet. Behav.* 39: 47–56.

Macdonald, D.W., Yamaguchi, N.Y., and Kerby, G. (2000). Group living in the domestic cat: Its sociobiology and epidemiology. In: *The Domestic Cat: The Biology of Its Behaviour* (eds. D.C. Turner and P. Bateson), 194–206. Cambridge, UK: Cambridge University Press.

Maier, S.F. and Seligman, M.E. (1976). Learned helplessness: Theory and evidence. *J. Exp. Psychol. Gen.* 105: 3–46.

McCobb, E.C., Patronek, G.J., Marder, A. et al. (2005). Assessment of stress levels among cats in four animal shelters. *J. Am. Vet. Med. Assoc.* 226 (4): 548–555.

McCune, S. (1995). Enriching the environment of the laboratory cat. In: *Environmental Enrichment Information Resources for Laboratory Animals: 1965–1995: Birds, Cats, Dogs, Farm Animals, Ferrets, Rabbits, and Rodents* (eds. C.P. Smith and V. Taylor), 27–42. Darby, PA: Diane Publishing.

Mench, J.A. (1998). Environmental enrichment and the importance of exploratory behavior. In: *Second Nature: Environmental Enrichment for Captive Animals* (eds. D.J. Shepherdson, J.D. Mellen, and M. Hutchins), 30–46. Washington, DC: Smithsonian Institution.

Mengoli, M., Mariti, C., Cozzi, A. et al. (2013). Scratching behaviour and its features: A questionnaire-based study in an Italian sample of domestic cats. *J. Fel. Med. Surg.* 15 (10): 886–892.

Mills, D.S., Redgate, S.E., and Landsberg, G.M. (2011). A metaanalysis of studies of treatments for feline urine spraying. *PLOS ONE* 6 (4): 1–10.

Morgan, K.N. and Tromborg, C.T. (2007). Sources of stress in captivity. *Appl. Anim. Behav. Sci.* 102: 262–302.

Newbury, S., Blinn, M.K., Bushby, P.A. et al. (2010). *Guidelines for Standards of Care in Animal Shelters*. Apex, NC: Association of Shelter Veterinarians.

Ottway, D.S. and Hawkins, D.M. (2003). Cat housing in rescue shelters: A welfare comparison between communal and discrete-unit housing. *Anim. Welf.* 12: 173–189.

Podberscek, A.L., Blackshaw, J.K., and Beattie, A.W. (1991). The behaviour of laboratory colony cats and their reactions to a familiar and unfamiliar person. *Appl. Anim. Behav. Sci.* 31: 119–130.

Rehnberg, L.K., Robert, K.A., Watson, S.J. et al. (2015). The effects of social interaction and environmental enrichment on the space use, behaviour and stress of owned housecats facing a novel environment. *Appl. Anim. Behav. Sci.* 169: 51–61.

Rochlitz, I. (1999). Recommendations for the housing of cats in the home, in catteries and animal shelters, in laboratories and in veterinary surgeries. *J. Fel. Med. Surg.* 1 (3): 181–191.

Rochlitz, I. (2002). Comfortable quarters for cats in research institutions. In: *Comfortable Quarters for Laboratory Animals*, 9th ed. (eds. V. Reinhardt and A. Reinhardt), 50–55. Cambridge, UK: Animal Welfare Institute.

Rosenzweig, M.R. and Bennett, E.L. (1996). Psychobiology of plasticity: Effects of training and experience on brain and behavior. *Behav. Brain Res.* 78: 57–65.

Roy, D. (1992). Environmental enrichment for cats in rescue centres. B.Sc. thesis. University of Southampton.

Shreve, K.R.V., Mehrkam, L.R., and Udell, M.A. (2017). Social interaction, food, scent or toys? A formal assessment of domestic pet and shelter cat (*Felis silvestris catus*) preferences. *Behav. Process.* 141, 322–328.

Shreve, K.R.V. and Udell, M.A. (2015). What's inside your cat's head? A review of cat (*Felis silvestris catus*) cognition research past, present and future. *Anim. Cogn.* 18 (6): 1195–1206.

Shyan-Norwalt, M. (2005). Caregiver perceptions of what indoor cats do "for fun." *J. Appl. Anim. Welf. Sci.* 8 (3): 199–209.

Slater, M.R. (2004). Understanding issues and solutions for unowned, free-roaming cat populations. *J. Am. Vet. Med. Assoc.* 225: 1350–1354.

Snowdon, C.T., Teie, D., and Savage, M. (2015). Cats prefer species-appropriate music. *Appl. Anim. Behav. Sci.* 166: 106–111.

Soennichsen, S. and Chamove, A.S. (2002). Responses of cats to petting by humans. *Anthrozoös* 15 (3): 258–265.

Stella, J., Croney, C., and Buffington, T. (2013). Effects of stressors on the behavior and physiology of domestic cats. *Appl. Anim. Behav. Sci.* 143 (2–4): 157–163.

Sumida, Y., Kaname, H., Mori, Y. et al. (2004). The effects of a switch-off response accompanied by hypothalamically induced restlessness on immunoendocrinological changes in cats. *Neuroimmunomodulation* 11 (2): 103–112.

Tanaka, A., Wagner, D.C., Kass, P.H. et al. (2012). Associations among weight loss, stress, and upper respiratory tract infection in shelter cats. *J. Am. Vet. Med. Assoc.* 240 (5): 570–576.

Tuozzi, A., Arhant, C., Anderle, K. et al. (2021). Effects of human presence and voice on the behaviour of shelter dogs and cats: A preliminary study. *Animals* 11 (2): 406.

Turner, D.C. (2000) The human-cat relationship. In: *The Domestic Cat: The Biology of Its Behaviour* (eds. D.C. Turner and P. Bateson), 194–206. Cambridge, UK: Cambridge University Press.

Turner, D.C. (2017). A review of over three decades of research on cat-human and human-cat interactions and relationships. *Behav. Process.* 141: 297–304.

Turner, D.C., Feaver, J., Mendl, M. et al. (1986). Variation in domestic cat behaviour towards humans: A paternal effect. *Anim. Behav.* https://doi.org/10.1016/S0003-3472(86)80275-5.

Uetake, K., Goto, A., Koyama, R. et al. (2013). Effects of single caging and cage size on behavior and stress level of domestic neutered cats housed in an animal shelter. *Anim. Sci. J.* 84 (3): 272–274.

van der Leij, W.J.R., Selman, L.D.A.M., Vernooij, J.C.M. et al. (2019). The effect of a hiding box on stress levels and body weight in Dutch shelter cats: A randomized controlled trial. *PLOS ONE* 14 (10): e0223492.

Vinke, C.M., Godijn, L.M., and Van der Leij, W.J.R. (2014). Will a hiding box provide stress reduction for shelter cats? *Appl. Anim. Behav. Sci.* 160: 86–93.

Wagner, D., Hurley, K., and Stavisky, J. (2018a). Shelter housing for cats: Practical aspects of design and construction, and adaptation of existing accommodation. *J. Fel. Med. Surg.* 20 (7): 643–652.

Wagner, D.C., Kass, P.H., and Hurley, K.F. (2018b). Cage size, movement in and out of housing during daily care, and other environmental and population health risk factors for feline upper respiratory disease in nine North American animal shelters. *PLOS ONE* 13 (1): e0190140.

Weiss, E., Miller, K., Mohan-Gibbons, H. et al. (2012). Why did you choose this pet? Adopters and pet selection preferences in five animal shelters in the United States. *Animals* 2 (2): 144–159.

Wemelsfelder, F. and Birke, L. (1997). Environmental challenge. In: *Animal Welfare* (eds. M.C. Appleby and B.O. Hughes), 35–47. Wallingford, UK: CAB International.

Wilson, C., Bain, M., DePorter, T. et al. (2016). Owner observations regarding cat scratching behavior: An internet-based survey. *J. Fel. Med. Surg.* 18 (10): 791–797.

Young, R.J. (2003). *Environmental Enrichment for Captive Animals*. Oxford, UK: Universities Federation for Animal Welfare.

Zhang, L. and McGlone, J.J. (2020). Scratcher preferences of adult in-home cats and effects of olfactory supplements on cat scratching. *Appl. Anim. Behav. Sci.* 227: 104997.

Zhang, L., Plummer, R., and McGlone, J. (2019). Preference of kittens for scratchers. *J. Fel. Med. Surg.* 21 (8): 691–699.

18

Training and Behavior Modification for Shelter Cats

Wailani Sung and Jeannine Berger

18.1 Introduction

In the United States, approximately 3.2 million cats are placed in animal shelters and approximately 860,000 cats are euthanized each year (ASPCA 2018). Factors that contribute to relinquishment include owners' specific expectations about the cats' role in the household, being intact, allowed outdoors, inappropriate elimination, lack of knowledge about cats, changes in lifestyle, allergies, being more work than expected, personal problems, new baby, and behavioral issues (New et al. 2000; Patronek et al. 1996; Salman et al. 1998; Scarlett et al. 1999). Cats with behavioral issues are in danger of being euthanized upon intake or having an increased length of stay in the shelter.

The shelter is a stressful environment for cats due to numerous factors such as exposure to the smell of other people and animals, the noises produced in the shelter by staff and other pets, the unpredictable schedules, and lack of control on the cat's part (Stella et al. 2013). Cats that are relinquished by their owners have higher Cat-Stress-Scores compared to cats classified as strays (Dybdall et al. 2007). This indicates that cats that are used to living in homes are more stressed by the change in their environment. The high level of stress affects the cat's overall welfare. Some stressed cats will hide, whereas some cats will exhibit aggressive behavior (Dybdall et al. 2007). Other signs of stress in shelter cats include decreases in appetite, weight loss, use of litterbox, movement, play, and interactions with people (Tanaka et al. 2012). Stressed cats experience elevated levels of cortisol, which is immunosuppressive. Therefore, stressed cats are more likely to develop medical problems such as feline upper respiratory disease (Dybdall et al. 2007; Tanaka et al. 2012) and stay in the shelter longer. Extended stays in the shelter have a negative effect not only on the cat's physical health but also on their mental well-being. The longer the cat stays in the shelter, the more likely they will engage in stress-induced maladaptive behaviors and be less active (Gouveia et al. 2011).

Environmental enrichment and behavior modification exercises are used by many animal shelters to decrease stress and improve the welfare of cats in the shelter environment. It is crucial that shelters employ all resources to address and reduce stress in cats. Providing hide boxes and elevated perches allows cats to have choices in their environment, which can reduce their level of stress (Vinke et al. 2014).

Animal Behavior for Shelter Veterinarians and Staff, Second Edition. Edited by Brian A. DiGangi, Victoria A. Cussen, Pamela J. Reid, and Kristen A. Collins.
© 2022 John Wiley & Sons, Inc. Published 2022 by John Wiley & Sons, Inc.
Companion website: www.wiley.com/go/digangi/animal

Cats that experience lower levels of stress can better adjust to the shelter environment. They hide less and are more interactive with staff and potential adopters. Potential adopters are more interested in cats that approach the front of the cage, play with toys, and are more interactive with people (Weiss et al. 2012).

The length of stay and stress in cats can be reduced by offering environmental enrichment and interactions with people, which can increase the cats' overall level of comfort in the shelter environment (Gourkow and Fraser 2006; Grant and Warrior 2019). Interactions with staff and volunteers can come in various forms, such as a person simply spending time in the enclosure with the cats or offering treats, food puzzle toys, or other interactive toys and playing with or petting them.

For cats that continue to be withdrawn and exhibit signs of fear, anxiety, and stress or inappropriate behavior such as aggression toward the staff, a training and/or behavior modification protocol needs to be implemented. Training involves teaching the cat to respond to verbal or visual cues to exhibit specific behaviors. Behavior modification involves changing a cat's emotional response to certain triggers and reinforcing alternate behaviors. Through behavior modification exercises, the cat's tolerance of certain triggers is increased, positive associations are created, and more acceptable responses are reinforced. This method reduces stress, provides mental enrichment, and facilitates the adoption of the cats. In this chapter, training techniques and behavior modification exercises to address the more commonly encountered behavior problems cats exhibit in the shelter environment will be reviewed.

18.2 Training Shelter Cats

Training has been shown to improve welfare by reducing fear associated with human interactions and distress during husbandry procedures (Westlund 2014). Training is used to teach animals new behaviors and tasks. Specifically, the use of reward-based training is important because it does not increase fear and anxiety such as with training techniques that rely on aversive incentives. Training is often overlooked in cats due to the misconception that cats can't be trained. In addition, shelter cats often miss out on training opportunities due to the lack of awareness by staff of its benefit, the misconception that a huge time investment is needed, and a lack of skills by staff members or volunteers. Cats with difficulty coping with shelter life can especially benefit from positive reinforcement training.

Training shelter dogs has become a more popular concept that can aid in facilitating dog adoptions (Protopopova and Wynne 2015). Dogs are traditionally the companion animal that has received more training focus by their owners and researchers compared to cats. Although cats, like any animal, can be taught novel behaviors and tasks, there is a dearth of studies on training cats compared to dogs. Nonetheless, we can use and adapt the strategies used to train dogs to our domestic cats.

In 1898, Thorndike placed hungry cats in puzzle boxes and studied their attempts to escape the box to get food placed outside the box (Chance 1999). The cats in puzzle boxes had to figure out through trial and error how to escape the box by manipulating a device, whether it was pushing a lever or pulling a wire to escape. These were some of the early studies that demonstrated that cats can learn through association. The more often the cat was placed in the puzzle box, the quicker the cat learned to escape. This indicated the rate of learning in the cat. In the modern age, initially feline training was more focused on large exotic cats kept in captivity and was considered a form of enrichment. As stated by Melfi (2013), training was seen as a part of their enrichment program if the training fulfilled the following criteria for captive animals:

1) Affords learning opportunities
2) Can achieve the same results as conventional environmental enrichment
3) Increases positive human-animal interactions
4) Provides dynamic change in the animal's day
5) Facilitates the provision of conventional environmental enrichment.

The same principles used on exotic animals can be used to address how captive domestic cat populations are treated in the shelter. Training can have a huge positive impact on any cat's life but is especially important in a shelter cat's life. Cats in shelters undergo a similar experience as some of their exotic feline counterparts; life in captivity changes their natural or normal environment and gives them little or no control over it. To fulfill the criteria listed by Melfi, training not only enriches the shelter cat's life but also provides opportunities for positive human interactions. These positive experiences may encourage cats to be more active in their enclosure, which can be a sign of reduced stress (Tanaka et al. 2012). These cats may also be more interactive with people, spend more time in front of the cage, and are more willing to approach, which increases their chances of being adopted (Weiss et al. 2012). Mellen and Shepherdson (1997) reported that positive reinforcement training for 15–30 minutes per day was required to teach a Siberian tiger to present specific body parts for examination. As a result of training the tiger showed more interest in his environment and attention to the keeper. The trainers determined the duration of the training sessions based on the tiger's decline in frequency of response to stimulus or if they had achieved the training goal for that session (Hare and Sevenich 1999).

Operant training has been used for many decades in the husbandry of zoo animals but not with domestic cats. Recent studies used training to reduce stress in cats for veterinary procedures. Acute stress responses can falsely elevate blood glucose level (Rand et al. 2002) and produce blood abnormalities, such as lymphocytosis, neutrophilia, and hypokalemia (Gooding et al. 2012; Lockhart et al. 2013). Lockhart et al. (2013) used operant conditioning along with systematic desensitization in their cat population. Once a week beginning at three weeks of age, they trained kittens to remain in a technician's lap through the various steps of positioning and blood collection until the veterinary technicians were successful in a jugular blood collection. Then training was reduced to once a month and then once a quarter when they reached one year of age. The trained cats had significantly lower cortisol levels and heart rate. The trained cats also exhibited fewer escape attempts compared to the untrained cats. Another study addressed the issue many owners face before their cats even arrive at the veterinary clinic. Many cat owners struggle with placing their cats into a carrier, preventing them from bringing the cats to regular veterinary visits. The process is stressful for both cats and owners. The cat arrives at the veterinary clinic with an elevated level of stress that often further escalates during the physical examination, preventing the veterinarian from performing a proper physical exam. Pratsch et al. (2018) used positive reinforcement training on 22 cats to train them to voluntarily enter a carrier and endure a car ride. The training protocol was set up for seven phases and six repetitions were needed to move to the next phase. The cats averaged two to six training sessions for completing one phase and were limited to 28 sessions over a period of six weeks. Food was used as the primary reinforcer. Cats that were successfully trained had a significant reduction in their Cat-Stress-Score during the car ride. They also had significant changes in frequency of lip licking and changes in body postures such as sitting. In addition, they were more interested in seeking food than controls. The carrier trained cats also experienced a shorter veterinary examination due to less resistance to handling. Ear temperature recordings also indicated that the trained cats experienced lower stress. This study showed that training can be used to decrease stress in cats trained to enter carriers on their own.

More recently, researchers focused specifically on training shelter cats. Kogan et al. (2017) used clicker training to teach 100 shelter cats four novel behaviors: touch a target, sit, spin, and give a high five. Each cat received 15 five-minute clicker training sessions over two weeks. Success was achieved when the cat was able to perform the four behaviors five times in a row within two seconds after the cue was presented. Both verbal and visual cues were used. There was a significant difference between cats that were more food motivated. These cats were more successful in learning target and high five. The researchers also found that some cats were not food motivated but responded to petting. This group of cats also learned to target with petting as the reinforcer.

Willson et al. (2017) compared the efficacy of three positive reinforcement training methods to train cats to perform a novel task, touch a target. The positive reinforcement methods used were a primary reinforcer (food only), a bridging stimulus (beep + food), and a secondary reinforcer (beep only). In the conditioning phase, the beep sound was associated with the delivery of food and consisted of two sessions on consecutive days with 20 beep-food pairings per session. The primary reinforcer group received rewards from the training device without the beep sound. The cats were trained to touch a red target with their nose. The task was considered successful when the cat's nose touched the red target within five seconds after the trial started for three consecutive presentations. Cats that succeeded in learning within the minimum time and trial requirements took a median of four trials and three seconds to achieve the assessment criteria. The cats in the primary reinforcer group acquired the task quicker than the cats in the bridging stimulus group. Interestingly, the secondary reinforcer group did not acquire the task at all. Furthermore, the authors noted that the treatment condition of using the secondary reinforcer alone was associated with aggression.

Grant and Warrior (2019) sought to use clicker training to increase exploratory behavior in shelter cats as a way of improving the cats' welfare. They engaged the cats in 10-minute sessions of clicker training, three times a week for two weeks. Cats were reinforced for moving toward the front of their enclosure when their names were called. After the training was completed, the researchers noted that the cats spent significantly more time in exploratory behavior and less time being inactive. They also spent more time in the front of their enclosure.

These studies clearly prove that cat can be trained and perform behaviors that increases their activity in their enclosure. The primary reinforcer method also known as response reward method, or the bridging stimulus method via clicker training, are both effective in training shelter cats. Training itself provides the cats with an outlet to cope with shelter stress. In the authors' opinions, when working with animals in the shelter, positive reinforcement is the ideal method to use.

Participation in training is voluntary. Before starting any training sessions, the cat needs to be situated in a quiet environment, relaxed, and interested in food. Interest in food is not crucial but a motivator for the cat needs to be determined. Offer a wide variety of food and treats to determine the cat's preference. It is important to determine the cat's preferred food because research indicates that dogs work harder for their preferred food (Riemer et al. 2018). The preferred food item will then be used as the reward during training. To ensure the cat is hungry, training sessions should occur before mealtimes, or a smaller meal is offered earlier in the day. Each session should be short; about one to five minutes at most. Use a small amount of food as a reward. If the cat is not interested in food rewards, then find another rewarding interaction, such as play, pets, brushing, or verbal praise. In the beginning, offer treats every single time the cat performs the desired behavior. Box 18.1 describes helpful tools for training shelter cats.

Box 18.1 Helpful Tools for Training Shelter Cats

- Pom-pom (long thin wooden dowel with a soft fuzzy fabric ball glued to the end)
- Wand toys
- Target tool or click stick (a long stick with a clicker at one end and target ball at the other)
- Feline pheromones
- Food puzzle toys
- Remote-operated toys
- Nail caps/nail clipper
- Scratching posts
- Spoon wand
- Laser pointer
- Mobiles
- iPad/TV
- Soft brushes
- Noise machine/CD player/radio
- Video camera
- Large, uncovered litterboxes
- Fine, granulated litter
  - Clay-based, not scented
  - Clumping and non-clumping
  - Specialty litter for preference tests (inappropriate urination cats)
- Treats and specialty foods
- Boxes/crates to hide and crate train

This is by no means a complete list. Every organization can be creative with this list, and many donors are happy to have a reference of a shelter's specific needs. It is important that only positive tools are being used. The authors do not support the use of any aversive tools.

18.2.1 Clicker Training

While the basic reward-based technique can be used to train cats, clicker training can also be a helpful technique to train a shelter cat. This is another technique that helps improve the human–animal bond and teaches the cat to perform desired behaviors. The clicker is an "event marker." It marks the cat's behavior, the exact moment the cat performs that particular behavior, so timing is important.

Some researchers have questioned the need for clicker training compared to the traditional reward-based method of training. The foundation of clicker training is based on the principles used in the laboratory studies of animal learning where a signal is given prior to delivery of a reward. The signal becomes the predictor that the reward will soon arrive. The animal engaged in a particular behavior when the signal occurred was reinforced for that specific behavior. Clicker training has been shown to be successful in teaching animals new behavior (Feng et al. 2018; Kogan et al. 2017). Clicker training gained in popularity with positive reinforcement trainers because some animals have difficulty learning when there is any delay in reinforcement (Feng et al. 2017). For exotic animals in enclosures or working with fearful or aggressive animals where it is safer for staff members to keep a distance, there will be a delay in the delivery of the reinforcer. The "click" helps bridge the delay until the reinforcer is delivered (Feng et al. 2018). Smith and Davis (2008) found that the clicker trained dogs were more resistant to extinction.

There is merit in using clicker training for cats with behavioral disorders where the staff may not be able to be close enough to deliver a reward immediately after the appropriate behavior, similar to having to toss treats through a kennel door with dogs. Clicker training is also a training philosophy in which there is no coercion involved with training, only positive reinforcement (Feng et al. 2017). See Chapter 3 for more in-depth discussion regarding training techniques and learning.

If the staff member elects to use clicker training, then the trainer must prime the clicker, which means associating the sound of the clicker with an immediate high-value reward. Use 3 to 15 repetitions until the cat associates the sound of the clicker with a reward. Depending upon the interest of each individual cat, the number of possible repetitions may vary. The cat should look at the trainer expectantly after he hears the click. This indicates that the cat has formed an expectation that he will receive a reward. Once that association is made the cat is ready to be trained new behaviors. If the sound of the clicker is too loud and startling for the cat, a quieter clicker can be used or a softer clicking noise can be made with the tongue. The click of a pen, or a verbal marker such as the word "yes" can provide the same effect. The same principles can be applied using a verbal marker in place of a clicker. Appendix 18.A describes sample clicker training protocols useful for shelter cats.

18.2.2 Crate Training

Although the number of movements within the shelter should be minimized, there will always be a need to move the cat. If a cat is comfortable in a crate, it will reduce the stress of placing the cat in the carrier and transporting them to a new enclosure, to seek medical care, or to the new home. It is a service to the potential adopters if the cat can be easily transported. This also improves the welfare of the cat because many owners cannot get the cat in

the carrier in a low-stress manner in order to seek veterinary care. There are different ways to train a cat to go into a carrier. The easiest way is to lure the behavior by placing food next to the carrier and then, over subsequent days, placing the food farther into the carrier. Use a clicker to capture the behavior when the cat goes in on his own or is lured in with the food or a target. Use whichever techniques are the easiest for the staff to implement or to which the cat responds best. Appendix 18.B describes sample crate training protocols.

18.3 Generic Behavior Modification Protocol for Shelter Cats

Behavior modification is the process by which an animal's current behavioral response to a stimulus is changed. As stated earlier in the chapter, training involves teaching the shelter cat to respond to specific verbal or visual cues to exhibit specific behaviors. Behavior modification involves identifying the triggers that can be changed through management, such as avoiding exposure, and through targeted exercises to change established emotional and behavioral responses (Overall 2013). Both classical and operant conditioning principles can be used. Behavior modification involves changing a shelter cat's emotional response to certain triggers and reinforcing alternate behaviors—the alternate behavior being the more desirable behaviors that people want to see. For example, instead of vocalizing, hiding, chasing or exhibiting aggressive behavior toward a particular stimulus, through behavior modification exercises, the cat's tolerance of certain triggers can be increased, positive associations can be created, and more acceptable responses are reinforced. Therefore, the cat's positive emotional state can be preserved. The cat is more accepting of interactions with people, which increases their chance of being adopted and reduces their overall level of stress.

Behavior modification can be successfully implemented in cats to treat a variety of behavior problems, ranging from fear-based disorders to aggressive behavior within and between species and elimination disorders (Overall 2013). These findings are not only based on anecdotal or case reports from animal and veterinary behaviorists but also based on results from research studies. Gooding et al. (2012) acclimated cats to restriction in a respiratory chamber over an 11-week process. The cats were gradually exposed to the respiratory chamber and study room over several weeks. Then the cats were confined in the respiratory chamber toward the end of the protocol. Positive reinforcement was offered during the cats' stay in the study room and after confinement via petting, talking, or playing with the cats. The results of the study indicated that the Cat-Stress-Scores declined over the duration of the study and exposure to each condition. The experimental cats had lower stress scores compared to naïve cats. Gruen et al. (2013) showed that behavior modification can be used to condition cats to being handled and transported in a carrier. In this study, the training sessions lasted 15–20 minutes per room and occurred once daily on consecutive weekdays. There were three phases in the protocol, once the cat reached the goal for one phase, the cat was moved to the next phase. Phase one involved placing treats in the enclosure and subsequently closer toward the door of the enclosure to condition the cats to move toward the front. Cats took an average of two sessions before moving to phase two. Phase two involved gentle petting and handling of the cat when the cat approached the front of the enclosure to eat the treats. Phase three involved introduction of the carrier and reinforcing the cat for entering the carrier. These are all steps involved in desensitization in which cats are slowly introduced to new stimuli at such a rate that they remain below threshold for anxiety and fear. These studies are a few examples in which a step-by-step protocol that exposes triggers or novel conditions to cats under their threshold can be used to modify cats' behaviors.

A generic behavior modification protocol adheres to a few essential principles. The first and most important step is appropriate management, including safety and avoidance. In this step, any of the situations that caused the problem are avoided so as not to make it worse. Safety is critical for the shelter cat, staff, and volunteers. When promoting safety, stress reduction for the shelter cat is an important factor to focus on too (Stella et al. 2014). For example, if a cat is afraid of noise, then the cat should be placed in the quietest area of the shelter. In certain shelter settings, this could be a very challenging part of the program. Often, creative thinking is needed for this critical step in order for the behavior modification protocol to achieve maximum success.

It needs to be emphasized that stress reduction and elimination of any such trigger is crucial to providing the cat with the best welfare possible (Moberg 2000). Maintaining a consistent daily schedule of when certain activities and exposure to people occur, along with having the same staff and volunteers interact with the cats or limiting exposure to strangers helps reduce stress. Not following this step can impair the welfare of shelter cats and often leads to the development of behavior issues. If the animal does not adapt or habituate to the shelter environment in a few hours or days, and this step cannot be accomplished by successfully managing the environment, then all Five Freedoms may be negatively impacted. The Five Freedoms are all interconnected and, in conjunction with each other, lead to the highest level of well-being for animals in our care (Berger and Ho 2017). Therefore, if shelter staff can perform nothing but the management part of the behavior modification protocol, they have already done a great deal to provide the Five Freedoms to the cats. See Chapter 19 for more information about the Five Freedoms and other welfare assessment paradigms.

18.3.1 Step 1: Management

Appropriate management sets the foundation of the behavior modification program and sets the trainer and cat up for success. Management often includes safety measures, which are of utmost importance for shelter animals, staff, and volunteers alike. It is very important when working with fearful or aggressive cats to avoid any triggers that will cause or escalate fear, anxiety, and aggression. This is achieved by keeping any external stressors such as noise, movement, multiple new people, aversive odors and tools to a minimum. If possible, limit the number of handlers to selected, skilled shelter staff and volunteers. Watch closely for fearful body postures and NEVER directly handle an aggressively aroused cat.

Appropriate management includes giving all shelter cats a hiding spot. Cats behaving aggressively should be left alone for a period of time to give them an opportunity to calm down when aroused (Foreman-Worsley and Farnworth 2019). Intake exams, cleaning the cage, and volunteer visits may have to be delayed. Intake exams can be done with sedation to provide the best care. Bites that result in injuries need to be avoided as they can cause an extended shelter stay. A few hours or days of familiarization can help a cat be less stressed and more acclimated (Moore and Bain 2013). As a result, the cat may be less fearful and easier to handle. If a fearful and/or aggressive cat needs to be moved to a different or quieter location, place a crate as the only hiding place in the enclosure and come back a few hours later. The cat might be in the crate and ready for movement without undue stress to all involved.

18.3.2 Step 2: Behavior Modification

This is the interactive part of a generic behavior modification protocol and includes changing a cat's fear or aggression to a more positive behavior and emotion (Landsberg et al. 2012). To achieve this, we commonly use food, petting, or play. This process is also called desensitization and counter-conditioning. For more information on this process, see Chapter 3 on how animals learn.

In addition, personnel may teach the cat some interactive behaviors such as "look" or target touch. These behaviors help strengthen and reinforce the human–animal bond. It also provides a positive mental outlet for the cat. The performance of alternative behaviors helps alleviates stress (Moberg 2000). The cat also forms a positive conditioned emotional response to the cue and behavior, which can aid in the process of relaxation (Mazur 2013).

Behavior modification starts with a plan and determining what is rewarding to the cat. The authors typically recommend finding a high-value, palatable diet or treat to use as a primary reinforcer. Tasty flavors leave long-lasting, strong, and positive emotional memories that motivate the cat to perform (Riemer et al. 2018). Consider the use of pouch treats, baby food, spray cheese, or any yummy, canned option. It is critical that the cat eats the food. It is helpful to determine the cat's food preference prior to initiating behavior modification. Individual cats have different food preferences (Bradshaw et al. 2000). This can be done by offering a variety of diet or treats (cafeteria style) in the enclosure and observing which food the cat prefers (see Figure 18.1). Once a shelter cat eats from the hand, the progress of behavior modification is usually fast and easy.

Food is obviously important for optimal success; however, some cats may be more motivated by certain toys or play. Even a gentle touch with a pom-pom may be rewarding for some cats. The authors recommend starting with food first and then proceeding to toys should food fail. Verbal praise in a soft, soothing voice should always be used when giving attention to cats. We recommend short (2- to 15-minute) sessions two to three times per day (which may also serve to meet enrichment needs) and to track visits and behavior with an exposure log. Appendix 18.C contains a sample behavior log.

Ensuring cats are calm and relaxed for behavioral modification will help increase the chance of success. Animals exposed to high levels of stress have difficulty learning (Seligman 1972). A more relaxed cat will learn faster and retain the information better.

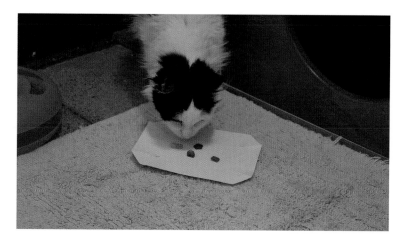

Figure 18.1 Treat selection – offer various treats to determine preference.

In some cases, the first step is to make the cat more comfortable in his enclosure. This can be achieved through enriching the housing environment by offering multiple hiding places, such as perches of various heights. Because an animal eating, and even liking, their food is relied upon, it may also be helpful to place the food and water sources very close to the hiding places at first should the cat be too shy to come toward the food.

It is important that no aggression is displayed during the process of desensitization and counter-conditioning. Should any aggression occur, do NOT use any form of correction as this can only worsen the aggression and increase the risk of injuries. It is critical to avoid the use of physical punishment as these techniques cause pain, fear, increased anxiety, stress, and potentially aggression (Landsberg et al. 2012; Herron et al. 2009). Once triggered to aggression, the cat becomes sensitized by more interaction or handling (Beaver 2004). In these cases, it is best to leave the cat alone and allow him some time to calm down before the next attempt to work with the cat.

A key element in making this part of the behavior modification protocol successful is to proceed in small incremental steps, keeping the cat comfortable at all times (Mazur 2013). That is the very definition of desensitization. It is critical to stay under a cat's threshold, which is the point where a cat escalates their behavior and starts displaying the undesired body language or behaviors. This may mean only a few seconds of interaction per visit are attempted. Whatever it takes to keep the cat relaxed and engaged is important. Simply teaching one small part of a new behavior or touching the cat for one or two strokes to avoid reaching the point where the cat displays any undesired behaviors, including signs of fear or aggression, may still be beneficial.

An important part of a behavior modification protocol is to set a goal and define success for the cat in question. Therefore, it is important to track the sessions, as well as any changes in behavior, in the problem-oriented veterinary behavior record (POVBR); see Box 18.2. To ensure the best process possible, regularly revisiting the predetermined goals, assessing the progress, and adjusting the plan as needed are critical. In the beginning of a new behavior modification plan, daily assessments of progress should be performed, but this will depend on the frequency of sessions. At least once a week, the behavior modification team should meet to assess and discuss any progress or lack thereof and agree on the next steps in the plan. The behavior modification team can include shelter staff (including behavior team personnel), volunteers, local trainers and anyone else with a vested interest in the shelter cats.

Box 18.2   Problem-Oriented Veterinary Behavior Record

The problem-oriented veterinary behavior record (POVBR) is applied for behavioral health. It starts with creating a comprehensive problem list and documenting behavior in a logical manner. This approach to behavior problems allows for a comprehensive treatment plan and should lead to more positive outcomes.

The SOAP

Subjective data	History: Every animal has a story
Objective data	Measurable information and observations
Assessment	Clinical impression of the problem(s)
Plan of action	Outcome options, options and resources for treatment including medications, additional diagnostics, education, and follow-up

---

If progress with the behavior modification plan is not apparent within three to four sessions, consider the following points:

- Check the timing. A reward has to be given immediately after the desired behavior for maximum impact.
- Check the steps. Progression through the exercise may be too fast; the cat may not be ready for the next step. Go back to where the cat was performing well and reinforce those behaviors before moving on to the next step.
- Check the reward. Using an appropriate reward ensures the cat is motivated to learn. Ensure that the reward is meaningful to the cat; for example, try petting instead of food or kibble instead of a soft or moist treat.
- Consider the cat's stress level. If a cat is too stressed to learn, eat, or play, they may need a change in housing, more enrichment, or even psychotropic medications.

Each condition and each individual cat needs a tailored plan to achieve the behavior modification protocol goals. In Section 18.4, the behavior modification protocols designed by the San Francisco SPCA Veterinary Behavior Specialty team, and implemented by shelter staff and volunteers for the most common conditions found in shelter cats as, are outlined. If the behavioral condition of the cat does not improve despite a solid behavior modification plan, or learning cannot be accomplished, then

check if the management is appropriate or can be improved upon, the reward is appropriate, and the timing is accurate. If the animal displays any signs of fear, anxiety, or stress, the use of psychotropic medications may help to alleviate fear and anxiety and improve learning. See Chapter 22 for more information on behavioral pharmacology.

18.4   Behavior Modification Protocols for Common Conditions

18.4.1   The Fearful or Anxious Cat

The goals for treating a fearful or anxious cat are to reduce their response to stressors and help them habituate to the shelter environment. If specific triggers are identified, then desensitization and counter-conditioning exercises can be implemented to increase the cat's tolerance of those triggers and reinforce alternate responses.

Cats are predators to smaller prey. However, they are also prey to larger predators. Therefore, it is important for cats to have a place to hide as this is part of their antipredator strategy when they are threatened. Fearful cats typically stare with dilated pupils or avert their gaze, hold their ears back or sideways, and lower their body into a crouching position. These cats exhibit heightened vigilance and reactivity to stimuli and may display extreme avoidance, withdrawal, or even aggression (Overall 2013). Most fearful cats will use physical attack as a last resort because they are defensive. Fear behaviors are triggered by the "flight or fight" nervous system. These innate responses are within the normal spectrum of cat behavior; however, the severity of the behavior displayed is mostly determined by early positive handling or lack thereof (Collard 1967; McCune 1995). Early socialization improves the animal's coping ability, and environmental factors and genetics will influence the behavior response. Paternal genes determine the friendliness of a cat (McCune 1995). Underlying medical issues, such as pain caused by osteoarthritis, feline resorptive lesions, or interstitial cystitis, need to be ruled out, as they can aggravate the problem. Not being able to hide and avoid the fear-provoking stimulus can, in some cats, increase stress levels and lead to defensive fear aggression (Amat et al. 2016). Because fear is such a universal and basic emotion, all cats, regardless of age, sex, or breed type, are susceptible to fear-related behavior concerns.

Undersocialized cats can undergo the protocol described in Sections 18.4.1.1 and 18.4.1.2; however, if a shelter cat is suspected to be feral, then the shelter team needs to re-assess and determine the best outcome for the cat. The longer a feral cat stays in the shelter, the higher their level of stress and worsening of their physical and mental health and welfare (Stella et al. 2013). Truly feral cats do not make good companions (Slater 2004). This may be a situation where release back to where they were initially trapped or placement in a working situation, such as being a barn cat kept to hunt rodents, is the best way to protect the cat's welfare (see Chapter 7).

18.4.1.1 Management
Cats identified as fearful or anxious should be placed in a quiet area of the shelter, away from busy hallways. They should be offered hide boxes and elevated perches so they can retreat

whenever they need to. The use of a white noise machine can help mask shelter noises. It would be best to minimize any unnecessary handling or movements. Any non-essential interactions with people should be avoided. Take the time to truly assess the NEEDS and WANTS for these cats. Rely on spot cleaning so that these cats can be allowed to remain in their enclosures.

Tool kit: Wand toys, pom-poms, spoon attached to a long stick, remote-type toys, pheromones, soft brushes, and a variety of food and treats; video camera set up in the room; some cats may benefit from the use of nutraceuticals and psychotropic or appetite-simulant medication.

18.4.1.2 Behavior Modification Protocol
Start by determining the appropriate reward to be used for the cat; typically that will be the cat's preferred food. Provide the cat with a few food options, such as canned cat food, moist treats, or baby food. Place these options on the floor and walk a few feet away to observe how much time it takes for the cat to start to eat in the staff member's presence. If the cat will not eat in the staff member's presence, leave the enclosure and come back later to observe which food the cat ate the most. If an obvious preference is not apparent, offer a wider variety. A food scale may be needed to weigh how much the cat actually ate to determine a preference. A 24-hour video surveillance is a useful tool to observe the cat remotely.

Once the highest value reward has been determined, begin the desensitization process. Gradually decrease the distance and get closer to the cat until the cat accepts the handler's presence within 1–3 ft. At this point, used the pom-pom to initiate physical contact (see Figure 18.2). Pheromone spray containing the facial analog can be applied to the pom-pom prior to use to facilitate the cat's tolerance of the pom-pom (Shreve and Udell 2017). Food can be offered in a small tray or on a spoon attached to a long dowel. Always present the pom-pom prior to offering food. Offer the cat

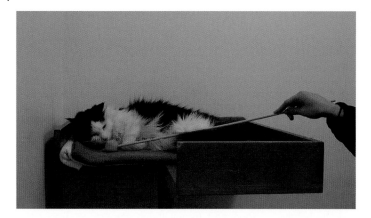

Figure 18.2 Initial approach using pom-pom sprayed with feline facial pheromone.

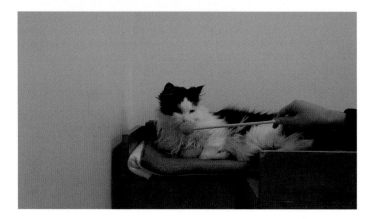

Figure 18.3 Gradual introduction to the hand by moving hand farther down the pom-pom wand.

the high-value food, and while he is eating, place the pom-pom within ½ inch and see if the cat stretches forward for a sniff. Monitor for signs of avoidance, such as moving away, or withdrawal, such as retreating to a farther distance out of reach or to a hide or perch. If there are no signs of avoidance, then use the pom-pom to gently rub the side of the face. Gradually move the pom-pom to rub gently on both sides of the cat's face, on top of the head and under the chin.

For each session, the handler should be stepping 3–6 inches closer. To get the hand closer to the cat, the cat must be desensitized to the hand. With each successful session, the handler should also be holding their hand closer to the pom-pom (see Figure 18.3). The cat should be leaning in, exhibiting soft blinking or closing its eyes and perhaps even purring (see

Figure 18.4). Eventually initiate the rubbing with the pom-pom and slowly replace the pom-pom with your fingers (see Figure 18.5). Observe for signs of withdrawal or stiffening. If there are no signs of stress or fear, then stop the session while the cat appears to be enjoying the interaction or rubbing on the fingers. At subsequent sessions, hold the pom-pom in the hand and slowly reach toward the cat's cheek. Rub both sides of the cat's cheek and lightly rub or scratch under the cat's chin. Then stop the session while the cat appears to be enjoying the interaction. The next session should progress to petting gently and lightly on top of the cat's head. Gradually proceed with gentle petting to the side of the neck and offer light strokes to the side of the body.

After three to four successful sessions, then another handler should follow the same protocol.

Figure 18.4 Desensitization and counter-conditioning to being petted by the pom-pom wand.

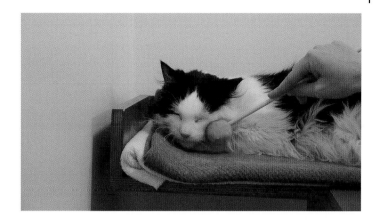

Figure 18.5 Desensitization and counter-conditioning to being petted by the hand.

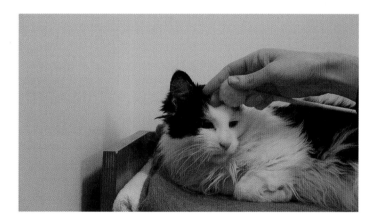

The goal is to generalize to a variety of people. The same concept can also be applied if the cat is not food motivated but shows a toy preference by replacing the food reward with access to the preferred toy.

18.4.2 The Cat That Becomes Easily Overstimulated

The goals for successfully working with cats that become easily overstimulated are to identify their triggers and increase their tolerance of triggers through desensitization and counter-conditioning exercises.

Cats that become easily aroused or excitable by stimuli are commonly referred to as "overstimulated" cats. These cats can solicit attention from people and might accept petting for a short period of time, but they become overstimulated by these interactions and can suddenly escalate to scratching or even biting. Most often, the overstimulation results from people petting the cat in areas of the body that are not commonly touched during social contact with other cats (Crowell-Davis et al. 2004). Some of these cats may be overstimulated by noises or movements. They can hear one octave above human hearing, which means they hear noises we cannot detect (Bradshaw 2018).

There is no age, sex, or breed predilection for overstimulation. These cats appear to have a low tolerance for human interaction or general stimuli, such as noises and quick movements that other cats ignore or even enjoy. Such behavior may be considered normal in some cats, including cats that are undersocialized. This behavior can also be a defense mechanism, where the cat is communicating that they have had enough interaction or, due to high mental arousal, the cat needs an outlet for physical energy. Underlying pain and discomfort have to be ruled out especially for petting-induced aggression (Overall 2013). Too much handling from a person can cause overstimulation or even escalate to aggressive behavior, such as scratches and bites. The distinction needs to be made between overstimulated cats and cats with feline hyperesthesia syndrome. Cats with feline hyperesthesia syndrome will exhibit rippling along their backs, pupil dilation, may lick and/or bite their flank or tail. These signs may or may not be elicited by being stroked along their backs (Overall 2013).

18.4.2.1 Management

For cats that become easily overstimulated, it is important to keep the physical interaction to a minimum. Staff and volunteers should use slow movements within the cat's enclosure. There must be careful handling of items within the cat's enclosure to avoid dropping them and making a loud startling noise and triggering a negative reaction from the cat. Staff and volunteers must avoid playing with the cat using their fingers, hands, and feet. Wand or remote-type toys should be used for play sessions. If staff and volunteers are not able to read the cat's body language, they should not pet the cat with their hands. They can use pom-poms, wand toys or a soft brush to initiate stroking. Use the "1-2-3 rule." This means pet once, pause to assess the body language of the cat, and proceed with another stroke if the cat remains relaxed and receptive. Limit the petting to three strokes maximum. The handler must stop petting when the cat shows any early warning signs, such as tension, vocalization, a hard stare, increased tail movement, pupil dilation, or an aggressive approach.

All behavior modification sessions should include a behavior log. The entries include notes for the next shelter staff member/volunteer, listing the observed body language and human behaviors to avoid, such as petting for prolonged periods. These notes will be used to keep track of progress.

Tool kit: Wand toys, pom-poms, remote-type toys, pheromones, soft brushes, and a variety of food and treats. Some cats may benefit from the use of nutraceuticals or psychotropic medication.

18.4.2.2 Behavior Modification Protocol

Start by determining the reward for the cat (e.g., tasty treats, favorite toy). Then identify the cat's threshold of tolerance for petting. Start with two to three strokes for the initial sessions and stop stroking prior to the cat becoming aroused by the physical attention. Most cats will exhibit signals prior to becoming aggressive, such as a hard stare, skin twitch, tail twitch, or vocalizations. Start petting an area of the body that does not elicit an immediate aggressive reaction, such as under the chin or side of the face. For the first several sessions, limit petting to these areas. Remember to offer food rewards at a constant, steady rate while the hand gently strokes the cat. If the cat vocalizes, stiffens, flattens his ears or gives a hard stare at any point during the exercise, discontinue the session immediately. End the petting sessions by tossing treats or toys to distract the cat. Then slowly stand up and walk away. Over subsequent sessions, gradually increase the amount of time spent stroking the cat. Soft verbal praise should be given along with the food rewards. Gradually increase the amount of petting done away from the head and neck. Focus on the sides of the body because most cats do not enjoy being stroked along their back to the base of their tails (Ellis et al. 2015). Some cats must learn to tolerate this type of petting. Log progress in a journal. Each entry should include the date and duration of the session, the cat's behavior during the session, and progress made.

18.4.3 The Cat That Becomes Overstimulated by Noises

The goal of these exercises is to desensitize and counter-condition the cat to the noises that cause overstimulation. The exercises should progress to a point where the actual sound does not cause a negative or overstimulated response in the cat.

18.4.3.1 Management

Cats that exhibit sensitivity to noises should be placed in the quietest area of the shelter. A white noise machine should be used to mask shelter noises. A soundproof box should be provided for the cat to hide in. Staff members and volunteers should avoid the clanging of any metal items, such as cage doors, food bowls, cleaning equipment, and so on, in the proximity of these cats.

Tool kit: Radio, CD/MP3 player, white noise machines, wand toys, remote-type toys, pheromones, soft brushes, and a variety of dry or canned diets and treats. Some cats may benefit from the use of nutraceuticals or psychotropic medication.

18.4.3.2 Behavior Modification Protocol

First, determine the specific noise the cat reacts to negatively. Play an audio recording of the noise. Start by playing or making the noise at a volume to which the cat does NOT react. Determine whether or not the cat reacts to the recorded noise in the same manner as the actual noise. Watch for early warning signs such as tension, vocalizations, hard stare, piloerection, increased tail movement, pupil dilation, or an aggressive approach. If the cat does not respond to the recorded noise, then attempt to reproduce the actual noise at a controllable volume. High-value food must be offered immediately after the noise is produced. Gradually increase the volume to the next level but avoid eliciting an agitated response. If the cat becomes agitated when the volume is increased, wait for five seconds to see if the cat relaxes. If the cat does not relax, decrease the volume to the previous level. Log progress in a journal. Each entry should include the date and duration of the session, the cat's behavior during the session, the maximum volume reached, and progress made.

18.4.4 The Cat That Becomes Overstimulated by Movements

These exercises are designed to desensitize and counter-condition the cat to the movements that cause overstimulation, such as walking or running past the cat, coming down stairs, or moving hands while speaking or reaching for objects. Ultimately, the goal is to reach a point where the actual movement does not cause a negative or agitated response from the cat.

18.4.4.1 Management

The cat should be housed in a quiet area of the shelter.

The cat should be provided a hide box and a perch. Staff members and volunteers should be informed to minimize any unnecessary handling, foot traffic, and unnecessary interactions with people.

Tool kit: Wand toys, remote-type toys, pheromones, soft brushes, and a variety of food and treats. Some cats may benefit from the use of nutraceuticals or psychotropic medication.

18.4.4.2 Behavior Modification Protocol

Start by determining which movement the cat reacts to by testing the type of movement, speed of movement, direction of movement, and distance from the movement. Watch for early warning signs such as tension, vocalizations, hard stare, piloerection, increased tail movement, pupil dilation, or an aggressive approach. Only work on one factor at a time. For example, focus on the speed of movement. If the cat does not respond to a low level of movement, then increase the speed of the movement. Start by moving at a slow speed to which the cat does NOT react. High-value food must be offered immediately as the movement is produced. Start at a far distance at which the cat does not respond to quick movements, then proceed to work on decreasing the distance. Gradually increase the speed to the next level but avoid eliciting an agitated response. If the cat becomes agitated when the speed of the movement is increased, wait for five seconds to see if the cat relaxes. If the cat does not relax, decrease the speed to the previous level. Log progress in a journal. Each entry should include the date and duration of the session, the cat's behavior during the session, the maximum speed reached, and progress made.

18.4.5 The Confident and Territorial Cat

Status aggression is not clearly defined nor widely accepted. Status aggression refers to a cat with a confident personality who wants to control the situation or resources (Landsberg et al. 2012). Status aggression is rare and usually directed toward other cats but can be directed toward familiar people (Landsberg et al. 2012). The cats exhibit offensive aggression. Territorial aggression includes aggression directed toward an intruder: human or animal. Entering the room or moving objects within the room can cause offensive aggression. Territorial aggression can be directed toward any individual or animal. Cats with either condition display confident body postures and behavior. Therefore, the management and behavior modification protocol will be similar.

A cat of any age, sex, and breed can display status/territorial aggression, but it is more common in socially mature cats (more than one year of age) (DePorter 2018). This behavior can be within the range of normal cat behavior, as the cat might be protective of their vital resources but can be a problem when displayed in the shelter. Cats may show other territorial behaviors such as patrolling the room, cheek and/or urine marking, sham marking, or body rubbing. Cats can exhibit offensive body language and aggressively approach the person entering the enclosure with ears and whiskers forward, direct eye contact, normal size pupils and/or a slow deliberate tail wag. The behavior often escalates (e.g., piloerection, vocalizations, batting, scratching, and biting) until the person moves out of the cat's perceived territory (Landsberg et al. 2012).

18.4.5.1 Management

When managing an aggressive animal in the shelter it is critical to first place them in a quiet location. This may be accomplished by blocking visual access and can be done by covering windows with paper. It also may be helpful to give the animal the largest enclosure available in the shelter as to allow them to retreat and not have to attack. Retreat options, such as a cat tree or even hiding boxes, can also inhibit an aggressive attack. Multiple cats can be co-housed in a larger enclosure unless the aggression is directed at each other. Either way multiple resources should be offered to alleviate the risk of attack, such as multiple hiding places, feed stations, litterboxes, and toys. Limiting social interactions and the number of people coming and going can help the cat feel less threatened in that environment. It is also imperative to always pay close attention to any changes in body language. Early warning signs can include a hard stare, stiffening of the body, and/or certain vocalizations. Increased tail movement with an aggressive approach is a sign of risk to the staff person. Hence a person should never handle an aggressively aroused cat. Using a barrier or shield for increased safety when shelter staff enter the enclosure, such as an x-pen, crate, or a plexiglass shield, can help keep people safe from offensive attacks.

Tool kit: Wand toys, remote-type toys, pheromones, soft brushes, clicker for training, and a variety of food and treats. Some cats may benefit from the use of nutraceuticals or psychotropic medication.

18.4.5.2 Behavior Modification Protocol

Start by determining the favorite reward for the cat (e.g., tasty treats, favorite toy, brushing). Treat showers can then be used upon entry to the room to provide a positive distraction while entering and approaching in the enclosure. Treat showers are four to five small treats tossed into the cat's cage or enclosure as the person approaches. This technique can also be applied to toys. This classically conditions the cat that good things happen when people enter the room. Once this can be accomplished then the cat can be taught various cued behaviors such as "go to mat," "go to perch," "sit," and "target" (see Appendix 18.A). Do NOT use corrections for aggression and it is helpful to keep an exposure log outside the room for next visitors to follow progress.

18.4.6 The Playful Cat

Play and/or predatory-related behavior issues in the shelter are common. Play behavior starts as early as three to eight weeks of age and lasts into adulthood (Overall 2013). Play and predatory-driven behaviors are normal cat behaviors that are intrinsically rewarding to the individual. This means that the cat wants and needs to perform them. Due to this innate drive, play opportunities must be provided for shelter cats as it is one of the Five Freedoms (freedom to perform normal behaviors) and is directly linked to their welfare and well-being. In shelters, cats are commonly confined to small spaces and lack the opportunity to perform these normal behaviors. This is not only a welfare issue for the cat but can quickly become a real safety issue for shelter staff and volunteers.

If cats are not given the opportunity to play appropriately, it can lead to deprivation, frustration, stress, and aggression. All these conditions lower the chance for a positive outcome. Understimulation, or lack of appropriate play and exploratory behavior options, is the main reason for play aggression and often worsens over time in the shelter. A cat's need is so strong that the drive to play or hunt increases and the slightest trigger elicits the behavior (Beaver 2004). Lack of appropriate play can cause a "rebound effect" and cause play behavior to escalate to play aggression. This can lead to behavior problems in a shelter setting. The only time there is any interaction or movement in the cat's enclosure is when humans visit or reach into the confined area for cleaning and feeding. This type of movement then triggers a play or predatory response. This can manifest as unsolicited attacks that range from light scratches to hard, uninhibited, skin-breaking bites. It can be directed toward humans or other animals if the animal is housed in a group setting.

18.4.6.1 Management

To avoid injuries from play aggression is it important to identify the specific triggers and never use human hands or feet to play with the cat. Often the cat is attracted to the movement of hands, feet, or loose clothing, hence it is important to avoid wearing clothing with strings or flowing clothing. Always wear closed-toed shoes and avoid quick hand and feet movements. Consider co-housing cats with similar ages and play behavior. Offer multiple climbing perches and rotate toys frequently to keep it interesting for the cat(s). This can easily be done by providing food in puzzle toys or dividing daily food ration into smaller bowls hidden around the room. A TV or audio stimulation can also help with enrichment in play aggressive cats. It is important that people interacting with the playful cat watch closely for playful arousal and body language such as pupillary dilation, crouching down, treading of the hind legs, pouncing, batting, scratching, and biting.

Tool kit: Food-dispensing toys, toys that make noise, toys that fly/hang, toys that flutter, toys that bounce and move, wand toys, remote-type toys (e.g., laser pointer, crickets), pheromones, soft brushes, a dedicated mat for mat training, clicker for training, and a variety of food and treats. Some cats may benefit from the use of nutraceuticals or psychotropic medication.

18.4.6.2 Behavior Modification Protocol

It is helpful to reward the playful cat for calm and relaxed behavior. Inappropriate play behavior can be interrupted with a mild stimulus that will startle the cat enough to stop the behavior but should not make the cat fearful, such as snapping your fingers or clapping your hands.

Then immediately redirect the cat toward more appropriate behavior, either by throwing toys for the cat, using the wand toys, or engaging in cued behaviors, such as "sit" and "go to mat." Never use physical punishment. It pays to be able to visit the playfully aggressive cat multiple times per day, rather than for one long visit. The behavior should be closely observed and the visit can last as long as the cat enjoys appropriate play. Ideally the cat would at some point start to rest and relax in the presence of the visitor.

A daily log outside the room with notes as to the preferred play style, toys, and any problematic behaviors that occurred is useful for the next visitor. The more specific the notes the better the next visitor can continue to plan, and progress can be tracked. Also, note the duration of the visit and at what time the problem occurred (e.g., "after five minutes of continuous play with the wand toy, the cat's behavior escalated to batting at the hand holding the toy"). Ideally, the next person visiting will know to stop at four minutes and offer multiple bouts of shorter play. It should be stressed that visitors leave the enclosure before the behavior starts to escalate.

18.4.7 The Undersocialized Kitten

Any kitten with a lack of positive human interaction between two and seven weeks of age may be scared of people approaching or handling them (Karsh and Turner 1988). Depending on the kitten's individual temperament, the behavior and genetics of the parents, and any previous experiences, the kitten may show fearful body language or behaviors such as running and hiding, hissing, swatting, scratching, or biting. It is important to understand that most young kittens learn to be comfortable with the presence of humans and human interaction. Even undersocialized kittens can make wonderful companions provided they receive comprehensive behavior modification. The time it takes to grow trust depends

entirely on the individual and can be quick or take months to develop (Bradshaw 2018). These kittens benefit from regular, focused attention; a consistent, quiet routine and a great deal of enrichment. Social facilitation is helpful for establishing affiliative behaviors; hence the presence of a more outgoing cat or kitten can be very beneficial to a fearful kitten.

The process of socialization takes time. In the authors' experience with thousands of kittens, the older the kitten the more difficult it can be to make the change from fearful or not social to social behaviors despite best efforts. It is difficult to place prognosis on age alone. There are multiple factors that play a role for each individual and hence it depends how receptive the kitten is at any given time. For some kittens that are not making progress and have a poor quality of life in the shelter, considerations may include releasing them back to their colony or finding opportunities for them to become working cats (i.e., barn cats). It is important to always remember the Five Freedoms when assessing the cats and their progress. If the kitten does not have a safe place to be released to then it is critical to continue the behavior modification efforts and continuously assess the welfare with ongoing behavior modification and make a quality-of-life decision based on the Five Freedoms.

18.4.7.1 Management
To manage the undersocialized kitten, it is helpful to place them in a small, quiet enclosure for a few weeks until the kitten is fully habituated to humans. This helps avoid having to chase the kitten around in the room to catch them, which obviously would be counterproductive. It is important to provide several safe hiding places, but those should be easily accessed by the person performing the behavior modification. One option for a hiding place could be a cat carrier. When needed the kitten can then be safely removed from the room by closing the carrier door and moving the carrier to another location, such as when the room

needs to be cleaned. Once the kitten is comfortable being in the small space without hiding, the size of the enclosure can gradually increase. It is helpful to provide the fearful kitten with a regular and predictable routine of feeding, cleaning, and handling.

Tool kit: Food-dispensing toys, toys that make noise, toys that fly/hang, toys that flutter, toys that bounce and move, wand toys, remote-type toys (e.g., laser pointer, crickets), pheromones, soft brushes, a dedicated mat for mat training, clicker for training, and a variety of food and treats. Some cats may benefit from the use of nutraceuticals or psychotropic medication.

18.4.7.2 Behavior Modification Protocol

Start with short visits from one or two people at first, so the kitten can bond with them. Feed at set times so the kitten associates visitors with food. Hand-feeding some canned kitten food or kibble at first approach can help make positive associations. Then gradually include more people feeding the kitten. The goal is to work up to multiple, short visits from a minimum of five different people per day to provide gentle handling. Playing with interactive toys is helpful to get the undersocialized kitten used to new people but also not to overwhelm him. It is important to move slowly and talk softly when approaching the kitten. The authors recommend getting down on the ground when in close proximity to the kitten.

Providing an increasing variety of toys for exercise and to build confidence is a fun and good way to bond. The best toys are the interactive kind, like cat dancers or any toys attached to strings. These types of toys, however, should never be left alone with the kitten to avoid ingestion and risk of intestinal blockage. Toys that can be left in the enclosure include ping-pong balls for solitary play or food in a puzzle feeder. To habituate the young animal, handle the kitten often by gently picking him up and holding/cradling him until he is able to relax with handling. When holding, keep the kitten upright. When cradling, keep

the kitten on his back in the handler's arms, like a baby. Some kittens will tolerate both positions and other kittens will resist being cradled. Only hold the kitten in his preferred position at this point. Slow down and briefly pick up the kitten while he is eating a treat and place him back down before any struggling occurs. If the kitten struggles for more than two seconds, the kitten should be released. As the kitten becomes more comfortable with being handled, pet the kitten all over the body as well as get him used to having his paws handled. Only then should the kitten be introduced to nail trims, one nail at a time, paired with a high-value treat.

18.4.8 Feline Inappropriate Elimination

Urination and/or defecation outside the litterbox, often referred to as housesoiling, periuria or, in lay terms, inappropriate elimination, on either horizontal and/or vertical surfaces is one of the most common reasons cats are relinquished to shelters (Casey et al. 2009). Unfortunately, many shelter organizations either refuse to intake or will even euthanize such cats due to the lack of proper treatment protocols that can resolve this problem behavior. The results from a retrospective study conducted at the San Francisco SPCA from 349 cats with a known history of inappropriate urination (IU) over a six-year period provide a compelling argument for managing and adopting these cats (Liu et al. 2019). Not only did the researchers show that their established protocols were successful with cats with urinary house-soiling behavior problems, they also determined that these cats can be successfully adopted with an adoption rate of 94% during the study period. And furthermore, the return rate was similar to the normal cat population. These results support a compelling argument for providing IU cats with opportunities for a positive outcome.

Urination outside the litterbox can be attributed to two different diagnoses: urine marking and house-soiling or toileting. Each diagnosis requires a slightly different treatment approach. Urine marking is when small amounts of urine are deposited on vertical surfaces. It is a form of communication behavior and can be a normal mechanism for cats to express anxiety, territorial behavior, or any agonistic conflict with other animals or humans. Marking behavior may or may not improve when entering a shelter due to the shift in the environment. Cats with urine marking behavior still continue to use the litterbox for both urination and defecation. House-soiling or toileting behavior is characterized by the cat voiding the bladder and/or bowel on horizontal surfaces. In this case, litterbox use needs to be re-established. This type of behavior may be due to preferences for and/or aversions to litterbox locations and/or substrates. This behavior may or may not change due to the availability of the location or substrate in the shelter. In any case of inappropriate elimination, progress within the shelter should be carefully tracked; post-adoption support must be available.

18.4.8.1 Management

To manage behavior problems that include urination or defecation outside the litterbox, it is important to collect as much information as possible from the previous home. Important questions to ask include the following:

- Is the urine deposited on horizontal or vertical surfaces?
- Is the amount of urine small or large?
- Is the posture when eliminating squatting or standing?
- Is the tail straight up in the air or down horizontally by the ground?
- Is the cat digging and covering either in the box or outside the box?
- How often does the cat use the litterbox for urination and defecation?
- How often is the litterbox not used for elimination?

- Are there any specific locations or substrates that the cat uses when going outside the litterbox?

Any cat with a history of IU needs a thorough medical workup. Medical issues are a common reason for IU and should be ruled out before any behavior modification plan is put in place to ensure the highest success and to avoid using shelter resources unnecessarily. A medical workup to rule out any medical causes for the IU could be part of acceptance to the shelter and included in the surrender agreement. A minimum database includes a complete blood count, blood chemistry analysis, thyroid hormone level, urinalysis, and urine culture. Confirm the neuter status of male cats (i.e., identify the presence or absence of penile barbs).

Begin the behavior modification plan immediately after intake. If a cat has a determined preference for bedding, carpeting or any other soft surface, do not provide that surface in the room at first until litterbox use has been re-established (Landsberg et al. 2012).

Tool kit: Elimination tracking sheet, large-size litterboxes, video camera, two different types of granulated clay-based litter, and pheromone therapy. Some cats with marking behavior may need psychotropic medications.

18.4.8.2 Behavior Modification Protocol

When addressing a cat with a history of house-soiling, it is best to house the cat singly until the problem is resolved (unless the cat is part of a bonded pair, and then a video camera needs to be placed for observation and identification of the offender). In general, if space allows, offer two litterboxes side by side, each box containing a different type of granulated, clay-based cat litter. For example, try clumping versus non-clumping, scented versus non-scented, fine versus coarse granulation. The boxes must be the same size and ideally large enough for the cat to enter fully and turn around. Furthermore, it is critical to maintain litterbox hygiene by scooping at least once a day. Never punish a cat for eliminating outside the litterbox as this will not resolve the issue and may cause additional anxiety problems. Then track elimination daily for urine and feces.

In the authors' experience, once a 5-day period of consistent litterbox use has been established, and a preference for a litter type determined, the cat can be made available for adoption. At that point, the lower preference litterbox can be removed and substrates such as bedding, carpets, or towels can be gradually introduced back into a larger enclosure. Prepare adoption counseling and post-adoption support notes with all the pertinent information. These procedures and materials need to address the following:

- Information about the transition to the higher-preference litterbox and substrate reintroduction that happened in the shelter
- Information on the litter preference and instructions around initial confinement to a small area until consistent litterbox use is established in the new home; after reliable litterbox use in the home has been confirmed, the cat can gradually be allowed to roam
- Providing the cat with two litterboxes that are easily accessible in the new home; advise adopters on the use of two different locations, away from food and water, as well as any potentially disturbing household appliances, such as a washer and dryer, or high-traffic areas
- Educating the adopter to maintain litterbox hygiene by scooping at least once a day, thoroughly cleaning the litterbox once per week, and replacing the litterbox entirely once per month
- Counseling the adopter to never punish the cat should there be a relapse.

18.4.9 The Cat Undergoing Ringworm Treatment

Ringworm presents a particularly challenging disease for treatment in the shelter with respect to maintaining behavioral well-being.

The course of therapy is often prolonged, requires intensive handling multiple times per week, and frequently impacts kittens within their sensitive periods of socialization. For these reasons, treatment outside of the shelter setting, such as in a trained foster home, should the first option. The management and behavior modification protocol used for fearful/anxious cats can be applied to cats isolated for ringworm treatment. It is very important that the staff and volunteers continue to visit with these cats several times a day to maintain their sociability. Using low-stress handling techniques with the application of the lime sulfur or other topical therapies should prevent traumatic experiences. Based on the authors' experiences, many of the ringworm-isolated cats can remain very social with concerted efforts from staff and volunteers.

18.5 Conclusions

The shelter is a stressful environment for cats due to numerous factors. The stress can negatively impact the cat's overall welfare. When stressed, some cats will hide, while others will exhibit problem behaviors including aggression. It is important that shelters address and reduce stress in cats. Training and behavior modification exercises can be used to decrease stress and improve the welfare of cats in the shelter. Training involves teaching the cat to respond to verbal or visual cues and perform specific behaviors. Behavior modification involves changing a cat's emotional response to certain triggers and reinforcing alternate behaviors. Through behavior modification exercises, the cat's tolerance of certain triggers can increase, creating positive associations and reinforcing more acceptable responses. This reduces stress, provides mental enrichment, and often facilitates the adoption of the cats, thus reducing length of stay in the shelter.

References

Amat, M., Camps, T., and Manteca, X. (2016). Stress in owned cats: Behavioural changes and welfare implications. *J. Fel. Med. Surg.* https://doi.org/10.1177/1098612X15590867.

ASPCA. (2018). Pet Statistics. https://www.aspca.org/animal-homelessness/shelter-intake-and-surrender/pet-statistics (accessed 30 July 2021).

Beaver, B.V. (2004). Fractious cats and feline aggression. *J. Fel. Med. Surg.* https://doi.org/10.1016/j.jfms.2003.09.011.

Berger, J. and Ho, F. (2017). Introduction to the Five Freedoms. *Animal Care Expo 2017*, Fort Lauderdale, FL.

Bradshaw, J. (2018). Normal feline behaviour. . .and why problem behaviours develop. *J. Fel. Med. Surg.* https://doi.org/10.1177/1098612X18771203.

Bradshaw, J.W.S., Healey, L.M., Thorne, C.J. et al. (2000). Differences in food preferences between individuals and populations of domestic cats *Felis silvestris catus*. *Appl. Anim. Behav. Sci.* https://doi.org/10.1016/S0168-1591(00)00102-7.

Casey, R.A., Vandenbussche, S., Bradshaw, J.W.S. et al. (2009). Reasons for relinquishment and return of cats in the UK. *Anthrozoos.* https://doi.org/10.2752/089279309X12538695316185.

Chance, P. (1999). Thorndike's puzzle boxes and the origins of the experimental analysis of behavior. *J. Exp. Anal. Behav.* https://doi.org/10.1901/jeab.1999.72-433.

Collard, R.R. (1967). Fear of strangers and play behavior in kittens with varied social experience. *Child Dev.* https://doi.org/10.1111/j.1467-8624.1967.tb04608.x.

Crowell-Davis, S.L., Curtis, T.M., and Knowles, R.J. (2004). Social organization in the cat: A modern understanding. *J. Fel. Med. Surg.* https://doi.org/10.1016/j.jfms.2003.09.013.

DePorter, T.L. (2018). Aggression/feline: Territorial. In: *Blackwell's Five Minute Veterinary Consult Clinical Companion: Canine and Feline Behavior*, 2nd ed.

(ed. D.F. Horwitz), 228–240. Hoboken, NJ: Wiley Blackwell.

Dybdall, K., Strasser, R., and Katz, T. (2007). Behavioral differences between owner surrender and stray domestic cats after entering an animal shelter. *Appl. Anim. Behav. Sci.* https://doi.org/10.1016/j.applanim.2006.05.002.

Ellis, S.L.H., Thompson, H., Guijarro, C. et al. (2015). The influence of body region, handler familiarity and order of region handled on the domestic cat's response to being stroked. *Appl. Anim. Behav. Sci.* https://doi.org/10.1016/j.applanim.2014.11.002.

Feng, L.C., Howell, T.J., and Bennett, P.C. (2017). Comparing trainers' reports of clicker use to the use of clickers in applied research studies: Methodological differences may explain conflicting results. *Pet. Behav. Sci.* https://doi.org/10.21071/pbs.v0i3.5786.

Feng, L.C., Howell, T.J., and Bennett, P.C. (2018). Practices and perceptions of clicker use in dog training: A survey-based investigation of dog owners and industry professionals. *J. Vet. Behav.* https://doi.org/10.1016/j.jveb.2017.10.002.

Foreman-Worsley, R. and Farnworth, M.J. (2019). A systematic review of social and environmental factors and their implications for indoor cat welfare. *Appl. Anim. Behav. Sci.* https://doi.org/10.1016/j.applanim.2019.104841.

Gooding, M.A., Duncan, I.J.H., Atkinson, J.L. et al. (2012). Development and validation of a behavioral acclimation protocol for cats to respiration chambers used for indirect calorimetry studies. *J. Appl. Anim. Welf. Sci.* https://doi.org/10.1080/10888705.2012.658332.

Gourkow, N. and Fraser, D. (2006). The effect of housing and handling practices on the welfare, behaviour and selection of domestic cats (*Felis sylvestris catus*) by adopters in an animal shelter. *Anim. Welf.* 15 (4): 371–377.

Gouveia, K., Magalhães, A., and de Sousa, L. (2011). The behaviour of domestic cats in a shelter: Residence time, density and sex ratio. *Appl. Anim. Behav. Sci.* https://doi.org/10.1016/j.applanim.2010.12.009.

Grant, R.A. and Warrior, J.R. (2019). Clicker training increases exploratory behaviour and time spent at the front of the enclosure in shelter cats: Implications for welfare and adoption rates. *Appl. Anim. Behav. Sci.* https://doi.org/10.1016/j.applanim.2018.12.002.

Gruen, M.E., Thomson, A.E., Clary, G.P. et al. (2013). Conditioning laboratory cats to handling and transport. *Lab. Anim.* https://doi.org/10.1038/laban.361.

Hare, V.J. and Sevenich, M. (1999). Is it training or is it enrichment? *The 4th International Conference on Environmental Enrichment*, Edinburgh, UK.

Herron, M.E., Shofer, F.S., and Reisner, I. R. (2009). Survey of the use and outcome of confrontational and non-confrontational training methods in client-owned dogs showing undesired behaviors. *Appl. Anim. Behav. Sci.* https://doi.org/10.1016/j.applanim.2008.12.011.

Karsh, E.B. and Turner, D.C. (1988). The human-cat relationship. In: *The Domestic Cat: The Biology of Its Behaviour* (eds. D.C. Turner and P. Bateson), 159–178. Cambridge, UK: Cambridge University Press

Kogan, L., Kolus, C., and Schoenfeld-Tacher, R. (2017). Assessment of clicker training for shelter cats. *Animals.* https://doi.org/10.3390/ani7100073.

Landsberg, G., Hunthausen, W., and Ackerman, L. (2012). *Behavior Problems of the Dog and Cat*, 3rd ed. Philadelphia, PA: Saunders.

Liu, S., Sung, W., and Berger, J. (2019). Retrospective study of outcomes of cats (*Felis catus*) with house-soiling in a limited intake shelter. *12th International Veterinary Behaviour Meeting*, Washington, DC.

Lockhart, J., Wilson, K., and Lanman, C. (2013). The effects of operant training on blood collection for domestic cats. *Appl. Anim. Behav. Sci.* https://doi.org/10.1016/j.applanim.2012.10.011.

Mazur, J.E. (2013). *Learning and Behavior*, 7th ed. New York: Pearson.

McCune, S. (1995). The impact of paternity and early socialisation on the development of cats' behaviour to people and novel objects. *Appl. Anim. Behav. Sci.* https://doi.org/10.1016/0168-1591(95)00603-P.

Melfi, V. (2013). Is training zoo animals enriching? *Appl. Anim. Behav. Sci.* https://doi.org/10.1016/j.applanim.2013.04.011.

Mellen, J.D. and Shepherdson, D.J. (1997). Environmental enrichment for felids: An integrated approach. *Int. Zoo. Yearb.* 35: 191–197.

Moberg, G.P. (2000). Biological response to stress: Implications for animal welfare. In: *The Biology of Animal Stress: Basic Principles and Implications for Animal Welfare* (eds. G.P. Moberg and J.A. Mench), 1–21. Wallingford, UK: CABI.

Moore, A.M. and Bain, M.J. (2013). Evaluation of the addition of in-cage hiding structures and toys and timing of administration of behavioral assessments with newly relinquished shelter cats. *J. Vet. Behav.* https://doi.org/10.1016/j.jveb.2011.10.003.

New, J.C., Salman, M.D., King, M. et al. (2000). Characteristics of shelter-relinquished animals and their owners compared with animals and their owners in U.S. pet-owning households. *J. Appl. Anim. Welf. Sci.* https://doi.org/10.1207/s15327604jaws0303_1.

Overall, K.L. (2013). *Manual of Clinical Behavioral Medicine for Dogs and Cats.* St. Louis, MO: Elsevier.

Patronek, G.J., Glickman, L.T., Beck, A.M. et al. (1996). Risk factors for relinquishment of cats to an animal shelter. *J. Am. Vet. Med. Assoc.* 209 (3): 582–588.

Pratsch, L., Mohr, N., Palme, R. et al. (2018). Carrier training cats reduces stress on transport to a veterinary practice. *Appl. Anim. Behav. Sci.* https://doi.org/10.1016/j.applanim.2018.05.025.

Protopopova, A. and Wynne, C.D.L. (2015). Improving in-kennel presentation of shelter dogs through response-dependent and response-independent treat delivery. *J. Appl. Behav. Anal.* https://doi.org/10.1002/jaba.217.

Rand, J.S., Kinnaird, E., Baglioni, A. et al. (2002). Acute stress hyperglycemia in cats is associated with struggling and increased concentrations of lactate and norepinephrine. *J. Vet. Intern. Med.* https://doi.org/10.1111/j.1939-1676.2002.tb02343.x.

Riemer, S., Ellis, S.L.H., Thompson, H. et al. (2018). Reinforcer effectiveness in dogs—The influence of quantity and quality. *Appl. Anim. Behav. Sci.* https://doi.org/10.1016/j.applanim.2018.05.016.

Salman, M.D., New, J.G., Scarlett, J.M. et al. (1998). Human and animal factors related to the relinquishment of dogs and cats in 12 selected animal shelters in the United States. *J. Appl. Anim. Welf. Sci.* 3: 207–226.

Scarlett, J.M., Salman, M.D., and Kass, P.H. (1999). Reasons for relinquishment of companion animals US—Selected health and personal issues. *J. Appl. Anim. Welf. Sci.* 2 (1): 41–57.

Seligman, M.E.P. (1972). Learned helplessness. *Annu. Rev. Med.* 23: 407–412.

Shreve, K. R. and Udell, M.A.R. (2017). Stress, security, and scent: The influence of chemical signals on the social lives of domestic cats and implications for applied settings. *Appl. Anim. Behav. Sci.* https://doi.org/10.1016/j.applanim.2016.11.011.

Slater, M.R. (2004). Understanding issues and solutions for unowned, free-roaming cat populations. *J. Am. Vet. Med. Assoc.* https://doi.org/10.2460/javma.2004.225.1350.1.

Smith, S.M. and Davis, E.S. (2008). Clicker increases resistance to extinction but does not decrease training time of a simple operant task in domestic dogs (*Canis familiaris*). *Appl. Anim. Behav. Sci.* https://doi.org/10.1016/j.applanim.2007.04.012.

Stella, J., Croney, C., and Buffington, T. (2013). Effects of stressors on the behavior and physiology of domestic cats. *Appl. Anim. Behav. Sci.* https://doi.org/10.1016/j.applanim.2012.10.014.

Stella, J., Croney, C., and Buffington, T. (2014). Environmental factors that affect the behavior and welfare of domestic cats (*Felis silvestris catus*) housed in cages. *Appl. Anim. Behav. Sci.* https://doi.org/10.1016/j.applanim.2014.08.006.

Tanaka, A., Wagner, D.C., Kass, P.H. et al. (2012). Associations among weight loss, stress, and upper respiratory tract infection in shelter cats. *J. Am. Vet. Med. Assoc.* https://doi.org/10.2460/javma.240.5.570.

Vinke, C.M., Godijn, L.M., amd van der Leij, W.J.R. (2014). Will a hiding box provide stress reduction for shelter cats? *Appl. Anim. Behav. Sci.* https://doi.org/10.1016/j.applanim.2014.09.002.

Weiss, E., Miller, K., Mohan-Gibbons, H. et al. (2012). Why did you choose this pet? Adopters and pet selection preferences in five animal shelters in the United States. *Animals.* https://doi.org/10.3390/ani2020144.

Westlund, K. (2014). Training is enrichment—And beyond. *Appl. Anim. Behav. Sci.* https://doi.org/10.1016/j.applanim.2013.12.009.

Willson, E.K., Stratton, R.B., Bolwell, C.F. et al. (2017). Comparison of positive reinforcement training in cats: A pilot study. *J. Vet. Behav.* https://doi.org/10.1016/j.jveb.2017.07.007.

Appendix 18.A Clicker Training Protocols for Shelter Cats

Goal:

Training is used to teach new behaviors and tasks to shelter cats. Training will help reinforce desired behaviors, reduce fear, allow the cat to form positive associations with people, and improve the cat's overall welfare.

"Sit"

Tools needed: Clicker or some people find it easier to make a clicking noise with their tongue. The cat's preferred reinforcer: treats, toys, or petting.

In this particular exercise, we are capturing the "sit" behavior, which is a normal cat behavior.

- As the cat starts to sit down, click and offer the reward.
- Repeat 5–10 times or more until trainer assesses the cat is ready to progress to the next step.
- When the cat starts to sit, say the verbal cue "sit," click and offer the reward.
- Repeat the verbal cue 5–10 times or more until the cat responds to the "sit" cue.

"Touch"

Tools needed: Target stick with clicker attached. The cat's preferred reinforcer: treats, toys, verbal praise, or petting.

This is a helpful behavior that assists the cat with focus on a target. This exercise will capture the "touch" behavior.

- Hold the tool in the hand with the ball end extended toward the cat.
- When the cat touches his nose to the ball, click, remove the tool with one hand and offer the reward with the other hand.
- Repeat by presenting the ball to the cat again.
- After 2–3 times, move the ball slightly to the left and then slightly to the right to ensure the cat can follow the ball, and perform the nose touch.
- Repeat 5–10 times or more until trainer assesses the cat is ready to progress to the next step.
- Present the ball, say the verbal cue "touch" before the cat moves toward the ball. Once the cat touches the ball, then click and offer the reward.
- Repeat 5–10 times or until the cat has formed an association with the verbal cue.
- To ensure that the cat associates the verbal cue with the behavior, offer the ball without saying the verbal cue. When the cat touches the ball, remove the ball and do not offer a click or treat. Repeat until the cat no longer touches the ball when offered. The cat must learn to only perform the "touch" behavior once the ball is presented and the cat hears the "touch" cue.
- Say the cue, offer the ball, and reward the cat when he performs the behavior.
- Once the cat knows how to "touch," the "touch" cue can be used as a foundation to teach the cat different behaviors. The "touch" cue can be used as a motivator to get the cat to move toward a specific target such as going to a mat or perch. Placing the ball near target/location and cueing the cat to move toward the target/location will speed up the training process.

"Go to mat"

Tools needed: Clicker, small mat (i.e., a fluffy pet mat, yoga mat, bathmat, or towel). The cat's preferred reinforcer: treats, toys, or petting.

This is a helpful behavior that teaches the cat to move to a designated space to provide more space between itself and people. When the cat exhibits fearful or aggressive body language, the person can cue the cat to move away, and the cat learns to move to a specific location when he is uncomfortable. The cat must be left alone when on his mat.

This protocol captures the behavior of the cat stepping onto the mat.

- Start by placing the mat on the floor.
- Wait until the cat steps on the mat, then click and offer the reward.
- Toss a treat or use the target tool to ask the cat to "touch" to get the cat off the mat.
- Wait until the cat steps on the mat, click and offer the reward.
- Repeat 5–10 times or more until trainer assesses the cat is ready to progress to the next step.
- When the cat steps toward the mat, say the verbal cue "mat" before the click and offer the reward.
- Repeat 5–10 times or until cat has formed the association with the verbal cue.
- Once the cat knows the verbal cue, say the cue and the cat will move onto the mat.
- Move the mat around the room so the cat learns to specifically move toward the mat.
- To ensure that the cat associates the verbal cue with the behavior, offer the mat without saying the verbal cue. When the cat moves onto the map, do not offer a click or treat. Repeat until the cat no longer moves onto the mat when offered. The cat must learn to only perform the "mat" behavior once the cat hears the "mat" cue and the mat is presented.

Luring to "mat"

This protocol lures the cat to the mat, then captures the behavior of stepping onto the mat. This is an alternate method of teaching the behavior of going onto the mat.

- Place the mat on the floor.
- Ask the cat to "touch" the tool while the tool is held next to or over the mat.
- When the cat steps on the mat, click, remove the tool and offer the reward.
- The cat does not need to "touch" the tool. The tool is used as a lure to get the cat to move onto the mat.
- Next, toss a treat to get the cat to move off the mat or move the target tool several feet away and ask the cat to "touch" to get him off the mat.
- Initially, the cat may step on the mat with one paw. Click and reward that behavior.
- Next, move the tool a bit farther off to one side of the mat. Click and reward when two paws are on the mat.
- Move the mat around the room so the cat learns to specifically move toward the mat.
- To ensure that the cat associates the verbal cue with the behavior, offer the mat without saying the verbal cue. When the cat moves onto the mat, do not offer a click or treat. Repeat until the cat no longer moves onto the mat when offered. The cat must learn to only perform the "mat" behavior once the cat hears the "mat" cue and the mat is presented.

Shaping to "mat"

This protocol uses shaping to reward the incremental steps toward the final behavior of stepping onto the mat.

- Place the mat on the floor.
- Wait until the cat takes a step in the direction of the mat, click and offer the reward.

- Then wait until the cat takes another step in the direction of the mat, click and offer the reward.
- Repeat 5–10 times or more until trainer assesses the cat is ready to progress to the next step.
- After every 2–3 clicks, wait for the cat to take another step closer to the mat before the next click.
- Click for one paw on the mat.
- Repeat 5–10 times, then click for two paws on the mat.
- Shaping can be used to gradually reward the cat for stepping on the mat with more paws until all four paws are on the mat.
- When the cat steps toward the mat, say the verbal cue "mat" before the click and offer the reward.
- Repeat 5–10 times or until cat has formed the association with the verbal cue.
- Once the cat knows the verbal cue, say the cue and the cat will move onto the mat.
- Move the mat around the room so the cat learns to specifically move toward the mat.
- To ensure that the cat associates the verbal cue with the behavior, offer the mat without saying the verbal cue. When the cat moves onto the mat, do not offer a click or treat. Repeat until the cat no longer moves onto the mat when offered. The cat must learn to only perform the "mat" behavior once the cat hears the "mat" cue and the mat is presented.

"Perch"

This is another helpful behavior that teaches the cat to go to a designated, elevated perching site. This is a helpful behavior that teaches the cat to move to a designated space to provide more space between himself and people. When the cat exhibits fearful or aggressive body language, the person can cue the cat to move to the elevated location. The cat learns that he has the choice to move away when he is uncomfortable. This behavior can be captured or the cat can be lured to the location. Use whichever method works best for the cat. The perch site could be the shelf in the enclosure or the top of a box. It can be any elevated area in the enclosure.

Tools needed: Clicker, perch. The cat's preferred reinforcer: treats, toys, or petting.

Capturing to "perch"
This protocol captures the behavior of the cat stepping onto the perch.

- Whenever the cat gets onto his favorite perch spot, click and offer the reward.
- Repeat the click and reward every time the cat goes onto his perch.
- After 5–10 associations, say the verbal cue "perch" before the click and reward.
- Once the cat learns the verbal cue, say the cue and the cat will move onto the perch.

Luring to "perch"
This protocol lures the cat to the perch, then captures the behavior of stepping onto the perch.

- Use the target tool and place it next to or over the perch.
- Ask the cat to "touch."
- As soon as the cat stands on the perch, click, remove the target tool and offer the reward.
- Next, either toss a treat on the floor or place the target tool close to the floor and ask the cat to "touch." The cat needs to leave the perch so that the behavior can be repeated.
- Repeat 5–10 times, then add in the verbal cue "perch" before you click, remove the tool and offer the reward.
- Once the cat learns the verbal cue, say the cue and the cat will move onto the perch.

Shaping to "perch"

This protocol uses shaping to reward the incremental steps toward the final behavior of stepping onto the perch.

- Wait until the cat takes a step in the direction of the perch, then click and offer the reward.
- Next, wait until the cat steps closer in the direction of the perch, click and offer the reward.
- Repeat 5–10 times or more until trainer assesses the cat is ready to progress to the next step.
- After every 2–3 clicks, wait for the cat to take another step closer to the perch before the click.
- Click for stepping or jumping onto the perch.
- Depending on the location of the perch, it may not be feasible to click for 1–2 paws on the perch, but click when the cat jumps onto the perch.
- Once the cat is on the perch, toss a treat on the floor or move the click tool to the floor and ask him to "touch." The cat needs to leave the perch in order for the behavior to be repeated.
- Say the verbal cue "perch" before the click and offer the reward.
- Repeat 5–10 times or until cat has formed the association with the verbal cue.
- Once the cat knows the verbal cue, say the cue and the cat will move onto the perch

"Scratch"

The clicker can also be used to reinforce appropriate behavior, such as scratching on the scratching post. It can be very helpful for the new adopter if the staff or volunteer can capture the scratching behavior on the scratching post anytime the staff or volunteer is in the enclosure. It is also another way of engaging the cat in a positive manner and using mental enrichment.

Tools needed: Target stick with clicker attached. The cat's preferred reinforcer: treats, toys, or petting. Appropriate scratching surface, with a variety of substrates and angles (horizontal, vertical, or angled).

This protocol captures the behavior of the cat scratching on an object.

- When the cat scratches on the scratching post, click and offer the reward.
- Remember to offer verbal praise while the cat is scratching.
- The cat will be more likely to scratch on the scratching post and be less likely to scratch on the furniture.
- Repeat as often as the cat scratches on the post.
- After 5–10 pairings, as the cat scratches, say the verbal cue "scratch."

Appendix 18.B Crate Training Protocols for Shelter Cats

Goal:

To ease the entry into a crate for shelter cats. By making the crate a positive place, it will be easier to move the cat within the shelter, transport the cat to the new home, and allow the adopter to take the cat to the veterinarian as needed.

Management:

- Do not force the cat into a crate.
- Have a cat carrier available in the enclosure as a hiding place.

Behavior modification:

- Determine the cat's favorite treat or toy.
- Depending on the skills of the handler and the cat, pick one of the following techniques. Continue for a few sessions and switch techniques if that technique seems not to be successful.

Technique 1: Capturing "crate":

- Place the carrier in the cat's enclosure.
- The cat enters the carrier, click and offer the reward.
- Repeat 5–10 times.
- Next, add in the verbal cue "crate" before you click and offer the reward.
- Repeat 5–10 times or until cat has formed the association with the verbal cue.
- Once the cat knows the verbal cue, say the cue and the cat will move into the carrier.
- Next, close the door while the cat is eating the reward.
- He can be kept in the carrier for short periods, starting with a few seconds or minutes, while eating his reward.
- Gradually build up to longer periods of time of the cat being in the carrier, from several seconds to several minutes.

Technique 2: Luring "crate":

- Place the cat's daily meals just outside the open carrier.
- Allow him to eat next to the carrier for 2–3 days.
- Next, place the food just inside the carrier. When the cat moves his head into the opening of the carrier to eat his meal, click before he starts to eat.
- Every 2 days gradually move the food bowl a few inches farther into the carrier.
- Click as he moves into the carrier before he eats.
- After 5–6 days, the cat should be able to walk completely into the carrier. Click as the cat walks in.
- A trail of high-value treats leading in the carrier with a jackpot (a larger portion) of treats for the cat to find inside can also be an effective lure. Click when he enters the carrier.
- When the cat willingly enters the carrier to rest or look for food, say the word "crate" as he enters into the crate, then click.

- Another option if the cat is target trained is to place the target inside the crate and ask the cat to touch the target. The click should occur once the cat enters the crate.
- At this point, the carrier door can be closed during meals.
- He can be kept in the carrier for short periods, starting with a few seconds or minutes, while eating his meals or treats.
- Gradually build up to longer periods of time of the cat being in the carrier, from several seconds to several minutes.

Technique 3: Shaping "crate":

- Place the carrier in the cat's enclosure.
- Click and reward the cat for taking any step in the direction of the crate.
- Repeat 5–10 times.
- After every 2–3 clicks, wait for the cat to take another step closer to the crate before you click.
- Click and offer the reward for placing his head into the crate.
- When the cat takes a step into the carrier, click and offer the reward.
- Repeat 5–10 times.
- After every 2–3 clicks, wait for the cat to take another step farther into the crate before clicking. The goal is to have the entire cat in the crate.
- Next, add in the verbal cue "crate" before you click and offer the reward.
- Repeat 5–10 times or until cat has formed the association with the verbal cue.
- Once the cat knows the verbal cue, say the cue and the cat will move into the carrier.
- Next, close the door while the cat is eating the reward.
- He can be kept in the carrier for short periods, starting with a few seconds or minutes, while eating his reward.
- Gradually build up to longer periods of time of the cat being in the carrier, from several seconds to several minutes.

Appendix 18.C Sample Behavior Log

Behavior diary for: _____   **Start date:** _____

Behavior	Mon	Tues	Wed	Thurs	Fri	Sat	Sun	Notes
Activity level								
Interaction with people								
Anxiety level								
Aggression								

Rating system: 1 = none, 2 = low, 3 = moderate, 4 = high, 5 = very high

In the notes add any specific information that is useful or important to the next visitor.

Training sessions	Mon	Tues	Wed	Thurs	Fri	Sat	Sun	Notes

List the specific behaviors or triggers and threshold worked on. In the top left area, indicate the number of minutes spent on the training session. In the bottom right, indicate the number of sessions. In the notes, add any specific information that is useful or important to the next trainer.

Part V

Special Topics

19

Welfare and Ethical Decision-Making
Victoria A. Cussen and Brian A. DiGangi

19.1   Introduction

The field of companion animal sheltering has undergone major paradigm shifts from its origin in the mid-1800s. Initially intended to provide public safety and protect private property from stray dogs, some societies for the prevention of cruelty to animals (SPCAs) later began providing medical care for unwanted animals and even made them available for adoption. Over the next 150 years, shelter services continued to evolve to include cats more widely and to provide veterinary care for shelter animals. Programs were implemented through which communities could work collaboratively to reduce intake of animals into shelters, increase adoptions, and reduce reliance on shelter euthanasia as a means of population control (Zawistowksi and Morris 2013).

The successes of these developments have been many and far-reaching. Estimates suggest that the number of shelter animals euthanized annually in the United States was as much as 20-fold lower in 2018 compared to the 1960s (representing >10 million fewer animals euthanized yearly), adoptions increase yearly, and improvements in caregiving are widespread (Rowan and Kartal 2018). Along with these successes, however, have come concerns over the increasing complexity of care required for animals remaining in shelters, the duration of time they spend in relative confinement receiving such care, and the impact of those factors on physical and behavioral health. Indeed, increasing length of shelter stay has been associated with increased incidence of upper respiratory infection in cats (Dinnage et al. 2009; Edinboro et al. 1999); increased exposure to canine influenza virus in dogs (Holt et al. 2010); increased frustration behaviors in dogs (Stephen and Ledger 2005); and decreased activity levels, decreased food intake, and increased agonistic behaviors in cats (Gouveia et al. 2011). The link between shelter operational practices, physical health, and behavioral health has never been more apparent.

Fortunately, recent times have also seen growth in the application of animal welfare science to animal sheltering. In 2010, the Association of Shelter Veterinarians published its *Guidelines for Standards of Care in Animal Shelters*, a set of principles guided by scientific evidence and subject matter expertise and founded on the Five Freedoms (Association of Shelter Veterinarians 2010; Farm Animal Welfare Council 2009). Welfare assessment protocols specifically designed for use in animal shelters have also been created (Barnard et al. 2016; Arhant et al. 2014; Kiddie and Collins 2014).

The terms "welfare" and "quality of life" are often used interchangeably, though there are some distinctions that may be useful to

Animal Behavior for Shelter Veterinarians and Staff, Second Edition. Edited by Brian A. DiGangi, Victoria A. Cussen, Pamela J. Reid, and Kristen A. Collins.
© 2022 John Wiley & Sons, Inc. Published 2022 by John Wiley & Sons, Inc.
Companion website: www.wiley.com/go/digangi/animal

consider when applying these concepts to shelter animals. Welfare is the inherent state of an animal, a characteristic that is experienced by the animal itself (Keeling et al. 2011; Bracke et al. 1999; Broom 1996). As an experiential state, it is subjectively determined by the animal, is based on the balance and character of inputs (i.e., the environment and management vs. outputs, which are animal-based welfare indicators), exists on a continuum that is ever-changing, and requires sentience (Mellor and Stafford 2008). Welfare is generally assessed by measurable, objective criteria and should be quantified on a scale from very good to very poor. It may reflect either short-term or long-term states (Broom 2007).

Scientific attempts to assess welfare tend to use one or a balanced combination of three specific viewpoints: biological functioning, affective or emotional state, and natural state. The biological functioning viewpoint holds that when animals are physically healthy, growing, and reproducing, good welfare is present. From an affective state perspective, good welfare is present when animals have positive emotional experiences (e.g., happiness) when interacting with other animals, people, and/or their environment. Alternatively, a positive affective state can also be defined through the absence of pain and suffering. Finally, evaluation of an animal's natural state is dependent upon the degree to which an animal experiences life as compared to the presumed wild state of the species and/or their ability to express normal behavior for their species (Mellor and Stafford 2008; Fraser 2003). Welfare state may also depend on an animal's ability to cope with various stressors and the impact of coping mechanisms on physical or behavioral health (Broom 2007).

It may be best to think of quality of life (QoL) as a component of animal welfare, specifically one that focuses on assessment of an individual animal's affective state over time. QoL measures tend to be subjective and/or assess characteristics that have not been scientifically linked to particular affective states, either physiologically or behaviorally (Lawrence et al. 2019; Mellor and Stafford 2008; Fraser 2003). These measures often involve speculation and focus on the presence of positive experiences and their relative weight as compared to negative experiences (vs. quantification of the absence of negative or detrimental experiences) (Green and Mellor 2011).

As pertains to shelter animals, welfare may best be used to describe, assess, and monitor populations of animals or snapshots of individuals at a given moment in time. QoL may be most appropriate to describe the impact of specific experiences or interventions on an individual animal's emotional state across a specific time frame—past, present, or future (Broom 2007). A simplified description of these concepts contends that states of positive welfare or QoL indicate that "the animal *feels good and enjoys life*" (McMillan 2013). Regardless of the specific terminology used, it is incumbent upon those involved in the care and management of shelter animals to remember that their basic needs remain the same regardless of the mission of the individual sheltering organization or the challenges involved in meeting those needs.

19.2 Animal Welfare Assessment

19.2.1 Frameworks for Welfare Assessment

Animal welfare has moral, ethical, and scientific aspects (Fraser 1995). Assessing welfare involves application of scientific knowledge, while determining what constitutes acceptable welfare is an ethical question guided by the moral standards of the community/society making the determination (Mench 1998). The field of animal welfare science encompasses a wide range of biological disciplines, including behavioral ecology, physiology, zoology, psychology, neuroscience, and ethology (Dawkins 2006). Therefore, a comprehensive review of animal welfare science is beyond the scope of this chapter. The reader is referred to Appleby et al. (2018) or Fraser (2008) for thorough overviews. What follows are brief summaries of several important or influential animal welfare assessment paradigms.

Concern for animal welfare reaches far back in history (Dawkins 2006), though the field of animal welfare science developed following a report by the Brambell Committee (1965), convened by the UK government in response to public concern regarding farm animal welfare. The concern stemmed from practices associated with the intensification of livestock farming and was spurred by the publication of Ruth Harrison's book *Animal Machines* in 1964, which raised awareness of the behavioral restrictions placed on farm animals (Keeling et al. 2011). Most research has concentrated on livestock, including beef and dairy cattle, swine, and poultry. Animal welfare scientists are concerned with the identification and validation of behavioral and physiological welfare indicators, determining how discrete environmental or management factors impact one or a few welfare indicators, and also with the development of assessment protocols that incorporate multiple indicators to determine overall welfare at the individual or facility level (Duncan 2005; Webster et al. 2004). Inferences about how a particular factor influences animal welfare are then made, based on the difference in the behavioral or physiological indicator(s) between treatments or within subjects (in crossover studies). For example, a researcher may assess how space influences the behavior of dogs (Hubrecht et al. 1992).

Welfare research frameworks can be broadly classified as emphasizing biological functioning or subjective feelings (Keeling and Jensen 2002). Commonly used welfare indicators that fall under the "biological function" umbrella include body condition score, gait score, presence of injury and/or illness, production parameters (e.g., milk production in dairy cattle), normal reproduction, and physiological stress as measured by activation of the hypothalamic-pituitary-adrenal (HPA) axis (Mason and Mendl 1993). Indicators used to assess subjective state are mostly behavior and body language based but also include other measures such as spectral analyses of vocalizations (Duncan 2006). Most physiological indicators are not clearly positive or negative, making them of limited use in determining affective state (Polgár et al. 2019). Behavioral indicators include frequency and/or duration of behaviors associated with stress and fear, changes in responsiveness to reward that indicate anhedonia or reward sensitization (Cussen and Reid 2020), choice of and/or latency to acquire resources in preference tests, effort exerted to access resources in motivation tests (Kirkden and Pajor 2006), and the frequency and/or duration of behaviors, such as play, thought to be associated with positive affective state (Boissy et al. 2007).

Historically, animal welfare research focused on pain and physical suffering because their absence indicates minimally acceptable welfare and because they were less contentious concepts among scientists who eschewed the study of internal subjective states in the farm animal production industry (Duncan 2005; Mench 1998). However, animal welfare science has, since its inception, been concerned with the feelings of animals—even the Brambell Report stated that animals' feelings were central to assessing animal welfare (Keeling et al. 2011). While much focus was on negative affective states, or "suffering" (Dawkins 2008), a great deal of research effort concerned what animals wanted (i.e., motivated behaviors; Mason and Burns 2011) and positive affect (Boissy et al. 2007). This was true prior to the advent of "positive welfare." (For a clear discussion of historical context, see Lawrence et al. 2019.) Many welfare scientists, and certainly the general public, have a holistic view in which "animal welfare" means ensuring animals are "healthy and happy" (Keeling 2005). Thus, two questions are fundamental to animal welfare: "Q1: Will it improve animal health? and Q2: Will it give the animals something they want?" (Dawkins 2008).

Most animal welfare assessments evaluate the welfare of individuals but are conducted in production situations that make assessment of every individual impractical. Assessments in these settings must be brief enough to be feasibly completed but thorough enough to determine how well individual animals are coping with their environment. To achieve this, they usually include both input-based and animal-based measures. Input-based measures consider the availability and quality of resources, the condition and safety of the housing environment, and husbandry or management parameters. For example, for group-housed animals, the number of animals per square foot (stocking density) and access to resources determined by the number of drinkers or feeding troughs per animal might be considered. For individually housed animals, input-based measures include access to a clean resting place, air quality, provision of veterinary care, and so forth. The benefit of input-based measures is they are relatively easy to quantify and are objective (e.g., number of kennels with feces, presence or absence of clean drinking water). Animal-based measures can also be objective but are more difficult to measure. For example, physiological parameters like cortisol require blood or saliva samples to be collected and analyzed. Behavioral animal-based measures may also be used and, in general, are rated using a subjective scale or score. This is also true for some health-related animal-based measures like lameness, which is also subjectively determined. While input-based measures are easier and more objective to score, they are less directly tied to welfare than animal-based measures (Berteselli et al. 2019). Because of this, some assessments rely mostly or completely on animal-based measures. The latter approach provides a snapshot of the animal in the moment but fails to provide information about the animal's welfare over any period of time (Webster et al. 2004).

Despite extensive research efforts, welfare indicators are still contentious. There is no "gold standard" measure that definitively indicates good or poor welfare (Mason and Mendl 1993). This is especially true for indicators of positive welfare, which have been more recently developed and less empirically tested than indicators associated with stress (Forkman 2009; Lawrence et al. 2019). With few exceptions, no single measure or indicator is sufficient to assess an animal's overall welfare (Spoolder et al. 2003). An animal may have a disease process, even a painful one, but have adequate or even positive welfare if pain is managed. Additionally, pain itself is subjective, and what may be considered very painful by one animal may be well tolerated by another—so the same injury or illness may have different welfare consequences. Conversely, a healthy animal may have poor welfare if they spend extended periods of time afraid or frustrated by thwarted goal-oriented behavior (Duncan 2006; Jensen and Toates 1993). Further complicating a single-parameter approach, age, sex, breed, and personality may all influence how animals respond to acute and chronic stress, which has implications for how and when they show stress-related behavior(s) (Stephen and Ledger 2005). To assess an animal's overall welfare requires integrating information from indicators of both physical and psychological health (Webster et al. 2004). This can prove difficult for several reasons, including that not all indicators covary, even if they purportedly measure the same thing (e.g., stress) and some indicators vary in the same way in both positive and negative situations (e.g., cortisol may increase with eustress or distress) (Mason and Mendl 1993).

What indicators are included and how they are integrated lies at the heart of animal welfare assessment (Botreau et al. 2007a, 2007b). The Brambell Report laid out minimum criteria for farm animals: the ability to stand up, lie down, turn around, stretch their limbs, and groom their body (Brambell 1965). These original freedoms were later revised by the Farm Animal Welfare Council (FAWC) into the well-known Five Freedoms: freedom from thirst, hunger and malnutrition; freedom from thermal and physical discomfort; freedom from pain, injury, and disease; freedom from fear and distress; and freedom to express normal behavior (Farm Animal Welfare Council 1992). The Five Freedoms framework emphasizes avoiding physical and mental suffering. The freedoms include physical health, behavior, and subjective experience; they are broad categories into which many individual welfare indicators can be placed (Webster 2016; Webster et al. 2004). An early model of animal welfare depicted three interlocked circles representing physical well-being, mental well-being, and natural behavior. Together, these three categories encompass factors associated with each of the Five Freedoms. Each circle overlaps to some degree with each of the others but also includes space unique to that domain (Appleby and Hughes 1997). Natural behavior was initially emphasized because it was thought animals had certain behavioral needs related to performing internally motivated behaviors (see Duncan 1998 for an overview). The concept was later challenged on the grounds that thwarting goal-directed behavior could cause frustration regardless of the loci of motivation (Jensen and Toates 1993) and because "natural" does not necessarily equate with positive as, for example, in the case of aggression. From a practical standpoint, however, the repeated frustration of highly motivated behaviors likely causes animals to suffer (Jensen and Toates 1993), so providing opportunities to express those behaviors is important for animal welfare (Duncan 1998; Mason and Burn 2011). In addition to being intrinsically important to welfare, behavior is relevant to assessing welfare as an indirect indicator of the animal's subjective state—for example, the presence or absence of play behaviors or the frequency and duration of rest.

Unlike the Five Freedoms, which focus on suffering, the criteria included in the Welfare Quality® four principles include the presence of positive physical and mental states. The Welfare Quality (WQ) approach to animal welfare assessment was developed by a multi-year, multi-institution EU-backed research initiative. The project was motivated in part by the need to assess welfare on-site where the animals were housed and to develop relevant, reliable, and practicable indicators of animal welfare (Veissier and Evans 2015). The WQ four principles are good feeding, good housing, good health, and appropriate behavior (Forkman 2009). Twelve criteria were developed, each corresponding to one of the four principles. Multiple welfare measures were included to assess performance on each criterion, with 30 measures in total. For each principle, at least one animal-based measure was included. On-farm assessments use those measures to calculate criteria scores, the criteria scores are then used to calculate a score for each of the four principles, and these principle scores are then used to determine the overall assessment of animal welfare for the facility (Veissier et al. 2009). Welfare assessments are conducted by third-party auditors that are trained in using the WQ assessment, which ensures consistency across facilities and accuracy of implementation.

The Five Domains Model is similar to both the Five Freedoms and the WQ four principles inasmuch as it attempts to group factors relevant to animal welfare under categorical headings to arrive at a picture of overall animal welfare. Similar to the WQ, it includes both the absence of unpleasant states and the presence of pleasant experiences. The domains are nutrition, environment, health, behavior, and mental state. The first four domains are conceived of as inputs to the fifth domain, which represents the affective state of the animal (Mellor 2017). Fraser and Duncan hypothesized that negative affective states underpin "need situations," whereas positive affective states underpin "opportunity situations" (Fraser and Duncan 1998). Similarly, the Five Domains Model segregates survival-related domains from the behavior domain, which is mostly concerned with positive welfare.

But behavior clearly encompasses nutrition (appetitive and consummatory behavior), environment (frustration-related behavior), and health (illness behavior). The model is not an assessment protocol but a framework in which to consider multiple aspects relevant to animal welfare (Mellor 2017). In this respect, it is similar to the Five Freedoms, which Webster (2016) refers to as "guideposts" for considering animal welfare. The Five Freedoms and Five Domains Model differ in the emphasis on absence of suffering versus presence of positive affect, respectively, and the specificity of welfare inputs/outputs. Webster (2016) suggests the Five Domains approach may be more useful in an intellectual than a practical capacity, but it has been widely discussed in the literature.

19.2.2 Assessing Welfare in Animal Shelters

In-shelter welfare assessments share many of the same challenges as on-farm welfare assessments. Typically, large numbers of animals are housed in a facility where the daily schedule cannot be interrupted for extended periods of time. Staff time is needed to perform the assessment in the absence of third-party auditors. This means the welfare assessment must be relatively brief, and animal-based measures should reflect welfare state while also being straightforward to observe within the practical constraints of the assessment. As in production species, welfare indicators include inputs (environment and management) and outputs (animal-based measures).

Welfare inputs include resource-based and management-based measures (Barnard et al. 2016). Examples of relevant input-based measures for dogs and cats in shelters are the *physical environment*, including sound, air quality, temperature and humidity, and housing size and substrate; *resources*, including nutrition, food enrichments, and social resources such as interactions with humans and conspecifics; and *management*, including routine veterinary care,

the facility's operations schedule, opportunities for exercise, grooming, and handling (Timmins et al. 2007). Welfare outputs include health parameters such as body condition score and disease, heart rate, and so on, and physiological and behavioral indicators of affective state. The indicators are generally the same as discussed in the previous section, with species-specific differences (e.g., the preferred social structure or the form of abnormal behaviors exhibited). Recent articles on animal-based welfare indicators in dogs (Polgár et al. 2019) and cats (Arhant et al. 2015) provide valuable resources for practitioners interested in learning more.

Shelter-based welfare studies date back almost 30 years, examining environmental factors such as the effect of space allowance on the behavior of dogs (Hubrecht et al. 1992). Most shelter studies examine how specific interventions influence one or a few behavioral or physiological welfare indicators of dogs or cats housed in the shelter (Protopopova 2016). Less research effort has been applied to developing companion animal welfare assessments, where a series of input- or animal-based measures are used to determine the welfare of animals within a given "typical" shelter environment.

Work from an Italian research group extends WQ indicators (see Section 19.2.1) from on-farm assessment of livestock to in-shelter welfare assessment of dogs. Dubbed "Shelter Quality" after its farm animal counterpart, the assessment protocol includes input- and animal-based metrics that are aggregated to arrive at an overall facility-level welfare determination (Barnard et al. 2014). Shelter Quality maps welfare measures onto the same 12 criteria and four principles developed by the WQ project: good feeding, good housing, good health, and appropriate behavior (Forkman 2009). Measures are a mixture of animal- and input-based; they include continuous (e.g., space dimensions), binary (e.g., presence-absence of disease condition), and ordinal (e.g., emotional state ratings) variables (Berteselli et al. 2019). Measures are split out across the shelter, pen (or kennel), and individual level. A random subsample of pens and individuals are observed for the assessment (Barnard et al. 2014).

Shelter Quality was developed and refined for European shelters, where several countries have legislation prohibiting the euthanasia of physically healthy animals. A surplus of animals led to warehousing dogs, with shelters holding large numbers of animals for long periods—up to the remaining years of the dogs' lives (Barnard et al. 2016). Length of shelter stay is relevant to welfare assessment because the same welfare indicator may be differentially impacted by acute and chronic stress. An example is cortisol, where acute stressors activate the HPA axis, causing an increase in circulating cortisol. Chronic stress, however, can lead to dysregulation of the HPA axis and hypo-secretion of cortisol in response to an acute stressor (Hennessy 2013). Additionally, length of stay can influence the type of welfare threat experienced by the animal. For example, in a large survey study, Stephen and Ledger (2005) assessed the prevalence and onset of 15 behavioral indicators of welfare (positive and negative) in shelter-housed dogs in the UK. They found a higher prevalence of fear-related behaviors (e.g., escape, hiding, inappetence) at the study outset, but these decreased during the six-week period, while frustration-related behaviors (e.g., wall bouncing, pacing) increased. Which behavioral indicators of welfare are relevant may differ between assessments for shorter- or longer-stay facilities. Similarly, it may not be clear that clinical measures pose a long- or short-term welfare threat unless medical records are included in the welfare assessment (Webster et al. 2004). To date, no one has reported implementing the Shelter Quality assessment protocol in a "normal" stay shelter in the United States; for now, it is unclear how directly relevant the Shelter Quality assessment is for shorter-stay facilities.

Shelter Quality has the benefit of using outputs from an extremely large and concerted research initiative as a starting point to validate measures for on-site animal welfare assessment (Veissier et al. 2009). Additionally, because it uses a detailed protocol it can be applied across multiple shelters as a tool to help pinpoint risk factors for poor welfare (Arena et al. 2019). However, because the aim is an "average" facility-level welfare audit, most measures are averaged across the entire shelter or a subset of the shelter's housing units. That means fewer measures recorded at the individual-animal level, including those meant to determine emotional state or abnormal behavior (both measured at "pen" level) (Berteselli et al. 2019). In contrast, an assessment developed by Kiddie and Collins (2014) focused exclusively on animal-based measures of individual dogs in 13 different shelters. Most indicators were aimed at assessing emotional state (positive and negative), with three health-related indicators. An equal number of newly admitted and long-stay animals were included. Dogs within each duration group were assigned to either standard husbandry or additional enrichment (composed of human interaction) treatment groups. Animals' behavior was observed from a distance (i.e., without human disturbance) and during in-kennel interactions. The authors report that the animal-based assessment distinguished between the treatment groups, though most of the variability was explained by the shelter (which was included as a random effect in the statistical analyses) rather than treatment group (Kiddie and Collins 2014). Although a conceptually promising study, the biological relevance of the small difference in scores between the treatment groups is unclear—especially given the large range of scores within groups (see Botreau et al. 2007a). Further, a presence-absence approach to behavioral indicators may not accurately reflect differences in the duration or intensity of emotional states.

An alternative (though compatible) approach to documenting *what* an animal does and/or how frequently they do it is observing *how* an animal expresses behavior. This can be done quantitatively, through kinematic analyses. Kinematic analyses are most familiar in the context of disease or injury assessment (Tashman et al. 2004) but are conceptually linked to an animal's subjective experience and may be useful for assessing welfare (Guesgen and Bench 2017). More research is needed before kinematics is brought to bear on shelter animal behavior assessment.

The most common way to look at the "how" of behavior is an approach called Qualitative Behavior Assessment, or QBA (Wemelsfelder 2007). Unlike typical welfare assessments, QBA does not attempt to measure various welfare parameters and then integrate them (Spoolder et al. 2003). Instead, QBA asks raters to assess the "expressivity of the whole animal" as the animal engages with their environment. The approach is based on the premise that such qualitative assessment better captures the animal's welfare state compared to breaking the whole into parts and then attempting to reassemble them to arrive at a welfare score (Wemelsfelder and Mullan 2014). Multiple raters watch a video clip of the animal in their environment and use their own words to describe the behavior and affect of the animal (a process called "free choice profiling"). Raters then use their own list of descriptors to score other video clips (Wemelsfelder and Lawrence 2001).

QBA was first used as an on-farm tool for assessing welfare of production animals but was subsequently extended to a variety of other farm and companion animal species, including working dogs (Walker et al. 2010) and dogs in animal shelter and home environments (Walker et al. 2016). Qualitative ratings of dogs' overall subjective state were found to generate high agreement between raters (Walker et al. 2010), suggesting QBA may be a useful approach to assess dog welfare. Agreement does not guarantee accuracy; two raters could consistently misinterpret the animals' welfare state and still show high inter-rater agreement. However, a later study comparing dogs in shelters and home environments found a correlation between the QBA ratings and behaviors coded from video using an ethogram, suggesting raters are accurately assessing the dogs' demeanors

(Walker et al. 2016). It is worth noting, however, that the correlations between QBA and quantitative behavior coding appeared to be most robust for relatively straightforward states like "relaxed" and "anxious." How well QBA can parse "depressed" from "bored," and what physiological measures they could be validated against, is still unclear. This question matters because people differ in their interpretation of canine behavior—including experts in animal behavior—regardless of their experience working with dogs (Tami and Gallagher 2009).

19.3 Monitoring Welfare in the Shelter

19.3.1 Methodological Considerations

19.3.1.1 General Considerations

Many behavioral and some physiological welfare indicators can only be interpreted in light of how they change within an individual. This means monitoring animal welfare in the shelter requires an initial assessment followed by recurring, regularly scheduled reassessments (Cussen and Reid 2020). Individuals differ in how a particular environment or event impacts their affective state and behavior (Mason and Mendl 1993), which makes clear "rules" about good or bad welfare metrics difficult, at least as concerns behavioral indicators of mental well-being. For example, opposite changes in behavior—such as less activity and more activity—can both reflect improved welfare, depending on the animal's relative starting point. Decreased activity may be good in the case of a high arousal animal or bad in the case of a normally active animal. Because of this, documenting animal-based welfare measures as soon as possible after acclimation to the new shelter environment is critical for interpreting later results and for detecting and monitoring welfare concerns (Cussen and Reid 2020). Especially for long-stay animals, tracking changes over time is of critical importance for pathway planning and outcome decision-making. Goold and Newberry (2017) reported that predicting shelter-housed dogs' human- and conspecific-directed behavior was improved by longitudinal behavioral monitoring. They also found that dogs showed significant differences in personality and day-to-day variability of behavior—and these differences made group averages and one-off assessments less informative. These findings underscore the need to assess welfare—especially as concerns behavioral indicators—at an individual animal level and over longer periods of time. This need is neglected in "herd health" approaches to welfare assessments (for further discussion see Richter and Hintze 2019).

Variability is a concern not only in the animals but also in the human component of welfare assessment. Assessor training is required to ensure agreement among individual staff members in their understanding of terminology and application of the assessment protocol(s) (Kiddie and Collins 2014). Periodic retraining is necessary to prevent drift in how measures are applied and is also needed when new staff are onboarded. Staff time is also needed to conduct the actual welfare assessment and to review the recorded information. Allocating personnel to document welfare systematically and to synthesize welfare measures from different teams or different time points, can be challenging in the shelter because of constraints on time and staffing. Yet most animal-based measures either require or benefit from longer-duration or more frequent observations, which provide more robust information on the individual's overall patterns of behavior.

Incorporating technology can allow for passive collection of animal-based welfare measures, such as activity counts (Rushen et al. 2012; Whitham and Miller 2016). Passive collection does not require staff time and can help increase the amount of information gathered without disrupting operations or diverting staff (Cussen 2019). Heart rate variability is a promising physiological indicator that provides information on the relative activation of the sympathetic and parasympathetic nervous systems, so it may be informative of positive affective state (Zupan et al. 2016). Some consumer-grade heart rate monitoring products have been validated against EKG for use in dogs (Essner et al. 2015), making this a potentially useful, noninvasive parameter amenable to passive collection. More research is needed, however, before clear heart rate variability welfare indicators are developed (Polgár et al. 2019). Cost can limit the number of units available in a facility, but even a limited number of units can be helpful to monitor focal animal(s) where welfare concerns already exist. For example, activity data from accelerometers can provide information on recovery from a medical procedure or the efficacy of behavior interventions Round-the-clock activity monitoring of shelter dogs found differences in patterns of behavior over longer periods of time that would not have been apparent from short-duration observations (Hoffman et al. 2019).

Not only can more information be captured for each animal with passive collection techniques, thereby facilitating welfare monitoring, *better* information can be captured because it is not influenced by the "observer effect," where human presence changes how animals behave (Martin and Bateson 1993). In a kennel of working German shepherds, for example, human activity elicited significant increases in repetitive behaviors; this was discovered by comparing the dogs' activity during live observations against their activity when no humans were present (Denham et al. 2014). That finding is one example of the usefulness of video monitoring, using camcorders or closed-circuit systems, for observing behavioral indicators of mental well-being. Technology helps avoid overestimating uncommon behaviors and underestimating common behaviors, especially when a behavior is triggered or suppressed by human activity (Normando et al. 2019).

Welfare monitoring requires not just collecting information, but distilling that information in ways that help decision makers better manage their population of animals. After animal-based measures are collected, technology can also facilitate integrating welfare indicators from different teams (e.g., medical and behavior teams) or tracking welfare measures from repeated assessments over time. Creating a cloud-based assessment or allocating space for a dedicated data-entry terminal allows staff to easily and directly enter information, which eliminates a step compared to recording observations on paper and later aggregating. Information "dashboards" are easily created by common spreadsheet software or purpose-made programs. Dashboards provide a high-level overview of current welfare state and changes over time—for the population, the individual, or both.

19.3.1.2 Welfare Indicator Considerations

When assessing welfare in the shelter, it is important to include measures that reflect positive welfare state to ensure positive affect, not just the absence of suffering (Mellor 2017); examples include play (Polgár et al. 2019) and anticipatory behaviors (Cussen and Reid 2020). Furthermore, debate still exists around established measures of negative welfare—such as cortisol or stereotypies—and positive indicators have been studied less rigorously (Lawrence et al. 2019).

Cortisol is one of the most commonly used physiological parameters in shelter-based welfare research. Despite its popularity and long history of use in welfare research generally, there are many difficulties in the interpretation of cortisol level as regards an individual's welfare. Individual differences in baseline levels and temporal fluctuations, the generalized role cortisol plays in the body, and the potential for up- or down-regulation due to chronic HPA axis stimulation (Mason and Mendl 1993; Hennessy 2013) can all muddy the waters. The use of cortisol as a measure is also limited in shelters because of the cost of running assays and the difficulties in collecting samples from fearful or aggressive animals, which leads to sampling bias at the group level and missing information at the individual level. Extracting cortisol from hair or fecal samples may mitigate some, but not all, of these difficulties (Packer et al. 2019).

The use of repetitive or stereotypic behavior as an indicator of negative affect—a common practice in shelter-based welfare assessments—is problematic for two reasons. First, the wide range of definitions used in the shelter research literature for what constitutes repetitive or stereotypic behavior retards progress in understanding causes and/or consequences because findings cannot be readily compared among studies or shelter professionals (Cussen and Reid 2020). Second, the premise that individuals who exhibit stereotypic behavior have poor welfare compared to animals who don't may not always be true. Mason and Latham (2004) synthesized literature across a range of species, where comparisons were made among different types of environments or among individuals in one environment. They arrived at a counterintuitive conclusion: while stereotypic behavior is more common in suboptimal environments (indicating inadequate housing/husbandry at a facility level), within a given environment, animals performing stereotypic behaviors appear to have better welfare than their counterparts who do not (Mason and Latham 2004). In some cases, therefore, stereotypies may help animals cope with the environment and improve their welfare (Rushen and Mason 2006). This means that a high proportion of animals exhibiting repetitive behaviors may be a red flag indicating the housing and husbandry practices of a given facility warrant careful assessment. At the same time, resources should be divided across all the animals in that environment rather than concentrated on the stereotypic individuals. In other words, they may be the canary in the coal mine, but the other animals are breathing the same "air." Finally, using stereotypic behavior as a welfare indicator is also problematic because such behavior may persist as a behavioral "scar" from time spent in a suboptimal environment, even after the animal is moved to an adequate or even above average environment (Swaisgood and Shepherdson 2005).

QBA is an intuitively appealing approach for assessing the welfare of shelter animals. It does not require the recording of behavior frequencies/durations, prevalence of health-related indicators, or measurement of input-based measures (such as space per animal), nor does it require their integration. While this approach may seem more efficient and intuitive, the interpretation of QBA requires a multi-step process to train raters on the free choice profiling method and to develop their individual free-choice descriptors prior to rating individual animals, followed by statistical analyses after rating. The alternative is a simple "gut" description of behavior, which may be inaccurate despite significant hands-on experience with animals (Tami and Gallagher 2009). These considerations may limit QBA's practical usefulness as a stand-alone welfare assessment.

Regardless of the assessment approach used, clear protocols are essential. Protocols for assessing welfare also need to be comprehensive, addressing how and when staff are trained, how and when an animal's welfare is assessed, how records are kept, when they are reviewed, and by whom (see Section 19.3.3). Clear, comprehensive protocols ensure consistent welfare assessments for all animals, facilitate decisions regarding necessary actions to be taken and the monitoring of intervention outcomes, and—when needed—provide a piece of information to inform QoL euthanasia decisions.

19.3.2 Daily Rounds

Daily rounds can serve as an informal and practical means of judging welfare and addressing welfare concerns in a shelter environment and can enhance collaborative care among different teams (medical, behavior, operations). A well-known population management tool, daily rounds have been defined as "a systematic monitoring process to promptly identify any health or welfare problems and help keep the population management plan on track" (Newbury and Hurley 2013); however, they may best be used as a proactive approach to in-shelter care that helps identify animal needs *prior* to problem development. When properly and regularly conducted, daily rounds can help create a sense of urgency in meeting animals' needs and moving them through the shelter system, decrease length of stay, prevent crowding, maintain the population within the available housing capacity, and maintain operations within the available resources of staffing, time, and money. In this way, daily rounds are one of the most effective tools available to protect and promote good welfare in the shelter environment. Daily rounds are functionally distinct from clinical case rounds (i.e., assessing status of clinical conditions and effectiveness of treatment plans) or facility rounds (i.e., addressing maintenance, safety, and cleanliness), although it may be most efficient to conduct each of these processes simultaneously given the overlap of personnel involved.

For each animal in the shelter population, the specific goals of daily rounds are to (i) identify their unique physical and behavioral needs; (ii) create, enact, update, or confirm their anticipated disposition pathway as needed; and (iii) ensure accountability of personnel in addressing goals one and two. It is recommended that daily rounds be conducted by a team of staff members with decision-making authority. Minimally, this team should include individuals to represent shelter operations, medical, and behavior perspectives, and attendees should have direct knowledge of the animals in the current shelter population. A population manager should be appointed to lead the daily rounds team and initiate the action steps identified during the process; this role may be designated to an existing member of the daily rounds team. Perspectives from adoption or animal placement staff as well as executive management team members should also be periodically included.

Active participation in daily rounds should be expected from those assigned to the daily rounds team, and time to engage in the process must be protected. Although there may be a benefit to occasionally conducting rounds at different times of the day, establishing and adhering to a consistent schedule will ensure it is a regular part of daily tasks and may facilitate detection of changes in physical or behavioral health. Conducting daily rounds prior to cleaning and feeding can aid in the identification of animals that are inappetant or otherwise cannot access food or water and can allow for the assessment of physical (e.g., diarrhea, increased urination) and behavioral (e.g., prior housetraining) habits. For group-housed animals, consideration should be given to conducting rounds during feeding on a regular basis to ensure ready access to fresh food and water. Once an efficient system is established, daily rounds can generally be conducted within an hour, even in shelters with large animal populations.

With limited exceptions (e.g., animals in foster homes or infectious disease isolation), the rounds team should physically approach each animal's enclosure to evaluate their status and have real-time access to current animal records. Typically, variations on the following questions should be asked and answered for each animal during each rounds session:

1) Who are you? Do physical, cage-front, and animal record identifiers match?
2) How are you—physically and behaviorally?
3) Are you where you should be? Is your housing location appropriate to meet your needs while also being suitable for the health and well-being of the larger population? Does it match the location indicated in the animal inventory?
4) What resources or services can we provide today to better meet your physical and/or behavioral needs?

5) Where are you going (i.e., What is your anticipated outcome pathway?), and what resources or services can we prepare or schedule in advance to ensure you get there as efficiently as possible?

Discussing the answers to these questions also allows for assessment of the anticipated outcome pathway and the opportunity to follow-up on action steps from the previous day's assessment. Knowledge of the animal's intake date/length of stay and stage in care is also critical context to inform decision-making during daily rounds. Ensuring that these discussions are founded on a welfare-based framework, such as the Five Freedoms, the Five Domains, or the four principles, can help guide decision-making and prioritization of animal needs.

The daily rounds process, decisions made, and action steps identified should be recorded in real-time on an animal inventory log or purpose-made action list to document findings, aid in animal care task assignments, and allow for accountability and follow-up. (A variety of sample logs are available online.) A key component of the daily rounds process also includes regular analysis of such documentation to identify population-level trends and persistent bottlenecks to animal flow. Not only does an effective approach to daily rounds protect and promote animal welfare by optimizing the use of resources and preempting delays in animal care or flow-through; it also ultimately results in increased numbers of animals served.

19.3.3 Monitoring Welfare in a Population of Dogs with Extreme Fear or Anxiety

The ASPCA Behavioral Rehabilitation Center (BRC) is a purpose-built facility dedicated to providing behavioral rehabilitation for extremely fearful dogs and operates on the philosophy that "Everyone is on the Behavior Team." This approach recognizes that, as they do when it comes to animals' physical health, all staff have important insights on the behavior and psychological welfare of animals in the facility, not just the behavior experts on staff. Successful care and rehabilitation require all teams working as a single unit to continually monitor, document, and assess each animal's progress and QoL (see Box 19.1). This collaboration can result in increased recognition of welfare threats and enhanced delivery of care, ultimately hastening the animal's recovery and improving their chances for long-term success. It can also result in timely outcome decision-making when rehabilitative interventions are ineffective and humane euthanasia is appropriate.

Box 19.1 "Everyone is on the Behavior Team" Approach to Monitoring Welfare in a Population of Dogs with Extreme Fear or Anxiety

Monitor

- Behavior staff observe animals during their scheduled behavior modification treatments five days a week, with two rest days each week.
- Daily care and enrichment staff observe animals multiple times a day during their feeding and cleaning duties and when enrichment items are distributed to the animals (twice a day).
- Medical staff observe the animals on a regular schedule.
- Each dog receives a standardized behavior evaluation every three weeks, conducted by the behavior rehabilitation team.
- Quality of life assessments are completed on a regular schedule by multiple members of staff, across teams.

Document

- A central database where animals' treatment records are stored is maintained. Treatment documentation includes the dog's behavior during the day's treatment as well as any extenuating circumstances that may have influenced their behavior (e.g., facilities work, storms).
- Ratings are recorded for fear level, social behavior, and aggressive behavior. Ratings are documented for both treatment sessions and behavior evaluations.
- Data entry rooms are situated in each animal housing area to facilitate documentation by behavior staff, and tablets are used for direct data entry during evaluations. Additional computer kiosks are located by the administrative offices to enable daily care and enrichment staff to document their observations, which are also entered in the central behavior database. Medical records are maintained in a separate database.
- Quality of life assessments are entered via a cloud-based survey platform, allowing any staff to access and complete the survey from a smartphone.

Assess

- Weekly behavior staff treatment meetings are used to review each animal's progress during the preceding week, troubleshoot areas of concern and/or create benchmarks for the next week's progress, and develop treatment plans for each dog.
- An outcome decisions panel meets once a week to review cases. This panel includes staff from all branches (behavior, medical, and operations) and reviews cases selected by the senior director of behavior rehabilitation. The panel determines if the dog should be kept in treatment, advanced to pre-graduation, medicated, sent to foster, considered graduated and ready for placement, or euthanized (see Section 19.5.2).

This philosophy that everyone is responsible for both physical *and* behavioral health is applicable outside a specialized rehabilitation facility, even when staffing structure, roles, and responsibilities vary. To be useful, observations must be recorded and indexed in such a way they can be retrieved and reviewed. Records need to be reviewed on a regular schedule and more frequently for any animal with a welfare concern. Encouraging staff to record and share observations can greatly increase the "eyes" on an animal, thereby improving monitoring capacity. For this approach to work, staff need to speak the same language: training all staff on the use of objective language to describe behavior observations is essential.

19.4 Preventing and Responding to Welfare Threats

Preventing or responding to poor welfare should address the fundamental cause(s) of the problem, rather than relying on ad-hoc treatment of behavioral signs related to the issue. For example, stereotypic behavior is associated with suboptimal housing environments (Mason and Latham 2004) and behavioral restriction (Mason and Burn 2011). Mills and Luescher (2006) emphasize the importance of working to change the environment to reduce the stressor(s) causing stereotypic behavior and emphasize that pharmacologic interventions should not be used in lieu of changing the animal's environment. This is especially important in light of an unpublished interview study with a panel of 32 veterinary behaviorists, where only 50% identified "environmental manipulation/enrichment" as one of the top five treatments for stereotypies (Mills and Leuscher 2006). As discussed in Section 19.3.1.2, it is possible the behavior is a "scar" from previous experiences, but this should be deduced based on the animal's response (or lack of response) to environmental interventions, not assumed to be the case.

Addressing causal factors is straightforward in the case of the physical component of welfare (i.e., injuries and illnesses). Although there are certainly difficulties in protecting basic physical welfare in some facilities, most are constructed and operated to minimize these welfare risks, for example, through the use of impervious surfaces and frequent sanitation. The same facilities and operations, however, may increase risks to the mental component of welfare. For example, restricting social interactions can reduce opportunities for disease transmission and prevent injuries from aggressive interactions but can also increase psychological stress from frustration and boredom. Likewise, frequent cleaning promotes healthy living conditions, but the noise and odors associated with cleaning can be unpleasant or even frightening to some animals. Taylor and Mills (2007) captured this when they extended welfare inputs to the "psychological environment"—an important, and often overlooked, aspect of environmental enrichment and facility design.

Psychological stressors are any stimuli that activate the animal's physiological stress response. What constitutes a stressor varies among individuals and hinges on how an animal perceives a particular stimulus (Jensen 2017). That said, behavioral restriction is a powerful psychological stressor that causes frustration and boredom for many, if not all, animals (Mason and Burn 2011). Increasing animals' ability to predict and control their environment, affording them agency to perform motivated behaviors and avoid aversive situations and/or tasks, can improve the psychological environment and protect psychological well-being in the shelter (Cussen and Reid 2020).

Perhaps the most important aspect of preventing and responding to poor animal welfare is remembering that welfare "is multidimensional and one dimension probably cannot fully compensate for another one (e.g., good health cannot fully compensate for behavioural deprivation)" (Botreau et al. 2007b). Compromises and trade-offs are necessary across domains to maximize welfare. Therefore, best practices for facility design and operations to prevent welfare problems must include management factors as well as both the physical and psychological environment. Additional species-specific aspects are covered extensively in other chapters in this volume, including the physical environment (Chapters 10 and 16), the psychological environment (Chapters 11 and 17), and training and behavior modification (Chapters 12 and 18).

19.5   Ethical Decision-Making

19.5.1   Ethical Frameworks and Structured Decision-Making

Whether formally or informally, assessing and responding to animal welfare needs occurs daily in animal care professions. While there is a robust and growing evidence base on which to determine how operational decisions are likely to impact an individual's welfare status, the importance of that impact and its weight compared to other factors is much more subjective. For example, animal

welfare science might tell us that providing a hiding box for a shelter cat will reduce their stress scores and thereby improve their welfare (Vinke et al. 2014). Whether or not that improvement is "acceptable" or whether the cat should be admitted to the shelter in the first place are ethical determinations. As this example demonstrates, animal welfare and ethics are inextricably intertwined.

Ethics refers to a set of beliefs about what is right or wrong, good or bad, just or unjust (Tannenbaum 1995). As pertains to animals and their care, a variety of ethical frameworks, often used in various combinations, have been used to determine exactly what is "right" or "wrong" (see Table 19.1). The application of these frameworks to everyday scenarios, answering the question of what one *should* do, is the study of applied normative ethics (Mullan and Fawcett 2017b).

Embracing a structured approach to ethical decisions can help legitimize decisions to those with opposing views and allows for the ability to justify one's position in a consistent manner (Palmer and Sandøe 2011); it ensures that decision-making is inclusive, transparent, and evidence-based, thus minimizing challenges based on gaps in information (Kaiser et al. 2007). Tools to facilitate ethical decision-making can

Table 19.1   Common ethical decision-making frameworks (Mullan and Fawcett 2017a; Palmer and Sandøe 2011).

Framework	Decisions based on
Animal rights	Protection of animal life, liberty, and respectful treatment
Contextual	Animal capacities and relationship to humans
Contractarianism	Degree of benefit to humans
Deontology	Rights, freedom, and choices of individuals; conformation to moral norms
Ethics of care	Obligations to and relationships with recipients
Justice as fairness	A social contract of basic rights, void of discrimination by natural assets
Respect for nature	Protection of species and natural processes
Utilitarianism	Best balance of good over bad
Virtue ethics	Expected character traits of the decision-maker

be applied to individual scenarios as well as in policy development. The development and application of a clinical ethics committee in a veterinary environment has also been described (Mepham et al. 2006; Mepham 2010; Adin 2019).

Another potential benefit to structured decision-making in complicated scenarios such as those encountered in animal sheltering is the mitigation of moral stress and associated errors in caregiving. Moral stress has been described as stress arising from the inability to do what one believes is "right" due to external (e.g., legal, institutional) constraints—in other words, stress related to ethical dilemmas (Raines 2000; Kälvemark et al. 2004). Pervasive throughout a variety of caregiving professions, moral stress has been associated with medication errors and lack of reporting of those errors in one national study of critical care nurses (Maiden et al. 2011). Health care professionals with related syndromes of compassion fatigue, secondary traumatic stress, and burnout are at greater risk for breaching the ethical codes of their professions than their colleagues who are not suffering from those conditions (Everall and Paulson 2004; Gentry 2005). Moral stress can compound other types of stress, compel affected individuals to question their choices, and contribute to agonizing over potential mistakes. It is unique in that individualized stress management and resiliency-building techniques are unlikely to have a significant impact on one's ability to cope (Rollin 2011). Rather, organizational resources and structures—including mechanisms for formally facilitated discussion of ethical dilemmas—are needed (Kälvemark et al. 2004; Adin et al. 2019).

There are four basic components of a formal ethical decision-making process. These include: (i) identifying and characterizing the ethical concerns, (ii) identifying the stakeholders and their interests, (iii) determining and obtaining the data needed to inform the decision, and (iv) applying an ethical framework to ensure that the decision-makers have the relevant and same information by which to arrive at a defensible judgment on the question at hand (Mepham et al. 2006; Mullan and Fawcett 2017a). Before subjecting an ethical question to such a process, it is important to define who carries the decision-making authority and when and what sort of questions are subject to review (Tannenbaum 1995). In most sheltering organizations, the "who" should, at minimum, include those in leadership positions and relevant subject matter experts representing the areas of physical health, behavioral health, and shelter operations. Defining the scenarios and types of questions that should undergo an ethical decision-making process will vary by each organization according to their community's expectations, operational model, philosophy, and resources. Some common situations that may benefit from formalized ethical review at both individual animal and policy levels are listed in Box 19.2.

The ethical matrix is a widely used framework for a variety of scenarios in and outside of animal welfare fields. This tool combines the ethical frameworks of utilitarianism, deontology, and justice as fairness to help decision-makers arrive at sound judgments for existing or prospective scenarios (Mepham et al. 2006). Each stakeholder in the scenario at hand is identified, and their interests are compared in relation to the scenario's impact on their well-being (i.e., maximizing the good, utilitarianism), autonomy (i.e., individual rights and freedoms, deontology), and fairness (i.e., equality in treatment, justice as fairness). In most shelter applications, a variety of stakeholders could be considered (e.g., individual animals, animal populations, staff and volunteers, donors, governing bodies, adopters, the general public); however, to overcome practical constraints, limiting the analysis to the interests of four groups of stakeholders is recommended. Groups should be considered for inclusion if they are subjects of ethical consideration in their own right and are affected in a systematically different way by the decision at hand compared to the others (Mepham et al. 2006). The individual cells within this

---

Box 19.2   Common Sheltering Situations That Might Benefit from a Formal Ethical Decision-Making Process

Individual Animal Level

- Medical or behavioral treatment end points
- Medical or behavioral treatment plans requiring an unusually high level of resources, experimental or unproven treatments, or transfer of custody to a third party
- Denial of adoption to an individual person
- Non-medical euthanasia decisions
- Euthanasia of privately owned pets or those relinquished for euthanasia

Policy Level

- Type of physical health conditions that will be treated
- Type of behavioral health conditions that will be managed
- Provision of free or low-cost animal care services
- Adoption procedures for individuals who have previously returned multiple animals
- Situations that warrant filing of criminal charges for cruelty, abuse, or neglect
- Handling of pregnant animals: spay-abortion procedures, housing and care during parturition
- The use of animals and/or their bodies for educational purposes
- Community cat admission, management, and disposition
- Management of animals with a history of bites to humans
- Management of animals with a history of injuring or killing other animals

---

matrix are filled with facts (where available and reliable) or values as appropriate and are weighed in relation to the status quo. Tables 19.2 and 19.3 demonstrate a generic ethical matrix adapted for animal sheltering scenarios and an example of a completed ethical matrix to inform a decision about making a dog available for adoption (i.e., to answer the question, "Should this dog be made available for adoption?").

The International Companion Animal Management Coalition describes two tools that can be adapted to a variety of decision-making scenarios specific to animal sheltering operations. The first, a three-part decision-making algorithm, assists the user in evaluating physical and psychological health and the impact of environment on both of those factors to inform a course of action. (The complete algorithm is available online at www.icam-coalition.org.) The second lays out an objectively scored decision table that can be tailored to assess the needs of a given animal

or situation through the filters of overall need, likelihood of success, and resource requirements. The table can also be adjusted to compare different courses of action for the same scenario. (Appendix 19.A contains a sample decision table based on this tool.) These tools are most appropriately used to reflect the considerations important to each individual organization and as a guide for informed conversation rather than to definitively determine a specific decision.

19.5.2   Behavioral Euthanasia Decisions

Animal welfare assessment, which provides a "snapshot" of an animal at a given point in time (Webster 2016) differs from euthanasia decisions to alleviate an animal's suffering, which are made in the framework of QoL (see Section 19.1). Veterinarians are familiar with clinical QoL assessments for pet animals, such as the HHHHHMM (H5M2) scale. The acronym stands for: hurt; hunger; hydration; hygiene;

Table 19.2 Generic ethical matrix for animal shelters* (adapted from Food Ethics Council 2019).

Respect for:	Well-being (health and welfare)	Autonomy (freedom and choice)	Fairness (justice)
Animals	Animal welfare	Behavioral freedom	Intrinsic value
Shelter staff and volunteers	Good income and working conditions	Freedom of action	Fair laws and operational practices
Members of the community	Safety and quality of life	Democratic, informed choice	Availability and access to animals/animal care

* Each cell describes the main criterion that would be met if the principle was respected for the indicated group of stakeholders.

Table 19.3 Example ethical matrix for making a dog available for adoption.

Respect for:*	Well-being (health and welfare)	Autonomy (freedom and choice)	Fairness (justice)
Individual animal	High degree of physical and behavioral health; minimization of fear, anxiety, stress, and frustration	Ability to express normal patterns of behavior	Treated with respect and compassion as an individual sentient being
Shelter dog population	High degree of physical and behavioral health; minimization of fear, anxiety, stress, and frustration	Ability to express normal patterns of behavior, including intra- and interspecies socialization	Equitable distribution of resources throughout population
Shelter staff	Personal safety, positive outcomes for animals, sufficient resources to perform duties	Allowed to use their skill and judgment in providing animal care; have appropriate input on operational policies and practices	Equitable distribution of shifts, duties, and resources across staff members
Adopters	Safe, friendly pet that meets care expectations and fits within lifestyle	Choice of adoptable animals, sufficient and accurate information regarding medical and behavioral history	Equal consideration, provision of information, and access to resources as other adopters

* Additional interest groups that could be considered include volunteers, donors, governing bodies, and the general public.

happiness; mobility; and more good days than bad. This framework was developed for animals with terminal disease processes such as cancer (Villalobos 2007). Given its application, it is unsurprising that most components focus on physiological functioning. Decisions regarding euthanasia for mental suffering are complicated because, unlike eating, drinking, and so forth, mental suffering cannot be directly observed.

However, behavioral proxies can be used to infer mental state—as they are to assess pain, which is also an internal subjective phenomenon not accessible to direct observation. This raises an important question is: how does one determine a level of mental suffering that justifies euthanasia?

Consultation with a credentialed, well-qualified behaviorist, either a board-certified veterinary behaviorist (Diplomate of the American College of Veterinary Behavior [DACVB]) or an applied animal behaviorist (Animal Behavior Society Certified Applied Animal Behaviorist or Associate Certified Applied Animal Behaviorist [CAAB or ACAAB]), can be helpful in identifying mental suffering and is recommended when establishing policies and protocols or when encountering individual cases that are particularly challenging or controversial. The behaviorist provides their determination based on the animal's history and current behavior, coupled with the probability of improvement or decline. Prognosis for improvement is based upon the animal's response (or lack thereof) to environmental interventions (changes in housing and/or husbandry) and standard behavioral therapies, including systematic desensitization, counter-conditioning, and psychopharmacology (prescribed and supervised by a veterinarian). The behaviorist's expert opinion is based on both their scientific training, including evidence from animal models of psychopathology, and their professional experience working with animals of the same species with a similar degree of psychological trauma. In cases where the animal spends the majority of their time experiencing aversive mental states that do not improve despite interventions *and* where professional experience and the scientific literature indicate a poor prognosis for improvement, *then,* to avoid a lifetime of fear ("mental suffering"), a recommendation would be made for euthanasia. The shelter veterinarian, in conjunction with the appropriate shelter leadership, has final discretion over whether or not to act on that recommendation.

In practice, many euthanasia decisions do not fall neatly into the categories of medical/physical health or behavioral euthanasia, as many shelter animals face multiple types of health and welfare threats simultaneously. In some cases, the disease treatment or behavioral management plan may contribute to mental suffering or inadvertently induce behaviors that pose safety concerns for shelter personnel or future adopters. For these reasons, it is important that policies and decision-making criteria are developed using an integrative approach, involving stakeholders and subject matter experts in shelter operations, veterinary medicine, and animal behavior. Specifically, thought should be given to developing policies and protocols for handling cases where the individual medical or behavioral health concerns may not, on their own, warrant a euthanasia decision but, when taken in congregate, QoL concerns (either in the shelter or post-placement) become apparent. The resources presented in Section 19.5.1 and Appendix 19.A can assist shelter leaders in structuring these discussions and ensure they are founded on a realistic assessment of currently available animal care and programmatic resources. There is currently no universal system for categorizing such euthanasia decisions for the purposes of data analysis; shelters are encouraged to create clear and consistent definitions for their own organization to facilitate analyses of program effectiveness and identify opportunities for future programming. For this reason, it may also be useful to distinguish euthanasia as a result of inherent behavior concerns that prevent safe placement (e.g., aggression) from those of behavior indicators of physical illness or behavioral diagnoses (e.g., inappetence, inactivity).

Euthanasia decision-making should also consider not only the frequency but also the intensity of behavioral indicators of suffering, as well as available management options— both in the shelter and post-placement. Outcomes may differ for two animals showing similar behaviors if one animal shows those behaviors in discrete circumstances that can be reasonably minimized or managed and the other animal shows the behaviors consistently, across a range of circumstances such that it is difficult or impossible to mitigate suffering. Similarly, two animals exhibiting similar frequencies and intensities of behavioral indicators of suffering may have different outcomes if one is responding to behavior modification and the other is not.

It is important to recognize that individual staff members may have different philosophies regarding euthanasia (Sandøe and Christiansen 2007); here again, transparent policies will mitigate conflict associated with ad-hoc decision-making. Where QoL concerns do exist, having multiple staff members assess the same animal ensures consensus or highlights differences of opinion regarding the animal's QoL. This helps staff make difficult decisions especially about the euthanasia of medically sound but psychologically compromised animals. These decisions are made within the framework of protocols, which determine how and when certain things happen, but each case is considered on its own unique combination of circumstances.

19.6 Conclusions

Animal welfare science provides objective, evidence-based approaches to the assessment of animals' experiences, both in and outside of the shelter setting, as well as means by which to guide QoL judgments made by animal caregivers. Ensuring adequate resources for regularly assessing animal welfare is an important part of maintaining a shelter's operations within its capacity for care and providing humane conditions. Because individuals differ, the physical and behavioral impact of a given facility will also differ among individuals. Determining how an individual is coping with that environment throughout the course of their stay is fundamental to pathway planning and outcome decision-making. Welfare assessment protocols provide one piece of information but should not be considered definitive, nor should hard cutoff criteria be used due to the nature of welfare indicators and individual differences among animals.

A variety of decision-making frameworks can be used to guide shelter leadership in formulating policies and protocols, including those involving euthanasia. Employing a structured process can help ensure inclusivity, transparency, and objectivity in operations and prioritize the best interests of the animal populations being served. Above all, animal care professionals must remember that basic animal needs remain the same regardless of the mission of the individual sheltering organization or the challenges involved in meeting those needs.

Please visit the companion website for video clips and downloadable resources associated with this chapter.

References

Adin, C.A., Moga, J.L., Keene, B.W. et al. (2019). Clinical ethics consultation in a tertiary care veterinary teaching hospital. *J. Am. Vet. Med. Assoc.* 254 (1): 52–60.

Appleby, M.C. and Hughes, B.O., eds. (1997). *Animal Welfare*. Boston, MA: CABI.

Appleby, M.C., Olsson, A.S., and Galindo, F. eds. (2018). *Animal Welfare*, 3rd ed. Boston, MA: CABI.

Arena, L., Berteselli, G.V., Lombardo, F. et al. (2019). Application of a welfare assessment tool (Shelter Quality protocol) in 64 Italian long-term dogs' shelters: Welfare hazard analysis. *Anim. Welf.* 28: 353–363.

Arhant, C., Wogritsch, R., and Troxler, J. (2014). Assessment of behavior and physical condition of shelter cats as animal-based indicators of welfare. *J. Vet. Behav.* 10: 399–406.

Association of Shelter Veterinarians. (2010). Guidelines for Standards of Care in Animal Shelters. https://www.sheltervet.org/assets/docs/shelter-standards-oct2011-wforward.pdf (accessed 20 May 2020).

Barnard, S., Pedermera, C., Candeloro, L. et al. (2016). Development of a new welfare assessment protocol for practical application in long-term dog shelters. *Vet. Rec.* https://doi:10.1136/vr.103336.

Barnard, S., Pedernera, C., Velarde, A. et al. (2014). *Shelter Quality Welfare Assessment Protocol for Shelter Dogs*. Teramo, Italy: Istituto Zooprofilattico Sperimentale dell'Abruzzo e del Molise.

Berteselli, G.V., Arena, L., Candeloro, L. et al. (2019). Interobserver agreement and sensitivity to climatic conditions in sheltered dogs' welfare evaluation performed with welfare assessment protocol (Shelter Quality protocol). *J. Vet. Beh.* 29: 45–52.

Boissy, A., Manteuffel, G., Jensen, M.B. et al. (2007). Assessment of positive emotions in animals to improve their welfare. *Phys. Behav.* 92: 375–397.

Botreau, R., Bonde, M., Butterworth, A. et al. (2007a). Aggregation of measures to produce an overall assessment of animal welfare. Part 1: A review of existing methods. *Animal* 1: 1179–1187.

Botreau, R., Bracke, M.B.M., Perny, P. et al. (2007b). Aggregation of measures to produce an overall assessment of animal welfare. Part 2: Analysis of constraints. *Animal* 1:1188–1197.

Bracke, M.B.M., Spruijt, B.M., and Metz, J.H.M. (1999). Overall animal welfare assessment reviewed. Part 1: Is it possible? *Neth. J. Agri. Sci.* 47: 279–291.

Brambell, F.W.R. (1965). *Report of the Technical Committee to Enquire into the Welfare of Livestock Kept under Intensive Conditions*. Command Paper 2836. London, UK: HMSO.

Broom, D.M. (1996). Animal welfare defined in terms of attempts to cope with the environment. *Acta Agric. Scand. Sec. A. Anim. Sci. Suppl.* 27: 22–28.

Broom, D.M. (2007). Quality of life means welfare: How is it related to other concepts and assessed? *Anim. Welf.* 16s: 45–53.

Cussen, V.A. (2019). Beyond coping: Using technology to assess canine quality of life in the animal shelter. *Proceedings of the Interdisciplinary Forum for Applied Animal Behavior Conference 2019*, Tempe, AZ (8–10 February 2019).

Cussen, V.A. and Reid, P.J. (2020). The mental well-being of animals in shelters. In: *Mental Health and Well-Being in Animals*, 2nd ed. (ed. F. McMillan), 257–276. Boston, MA: CABI.

Dawkins, M.S. (2006). A user's guide to animal welfare science. *TREE* 21: 77–82.

Dawkins, M.S. (2008). The science of animal suffering. *Ethology* 114: 937–945.

Denham, H.D., Bradshaw, J.W., and Rooney, N.J. (2014). Repetitive behaviour in kennelled domestic dog: Stereotypical or not? *Physiol. Behav.* 128: 288–294.

Dinnage, J.D., Scarlett, J.M., Richards, J.R. (2009). Descriptive epidemiology of feline upper respiratory tract disease in an animal shelter. *J. Fel. Med. Surg.* https://doi.org/10.1016/j.jfms.2009.03.001.

Duncan, I.J.H. (1998). Behavior and behavioral needs. *Poultry Sci.* 77: 1766–1772.

Duncan, I.J.H. (2005). Science based assessment of animal welfare: Farm animals. *Rev. Sci. Tech.* 24: 483–492.

Duncan, I.J.H. (2006). The changing concept of animal sentience. *Appl. Anim. Behav. Sci.* 100: 11–19.

Edinboro, C.H., Janowitz, L.K., Guptill-Yoran, L. et al. (1999). A clinical trial of intranasal and subcutaneous vaccines to prevent upper respiratory infection in cats at an animal shelter. *Feline Pract.* 26 (7): 7–11, 13.

Essner, A., Sjöström, R., Ahlgren, E. et al. (2015). Comparison of Polar® RS800CX heart rate monitor and electrocardiogram for measuring inter-beat intervals in healthy dogs. *Physiol. Behav.* 138: 247–253.

Everall, R.D. and Paulson, B.L. (2004). Burnout and secondary traumatic stress: Impact on ethical behaviour. *Can. J. Couns.* 38 (1): 25–35.

Farm Animal Welfare Council. (2009). Five Freedoms. https://webarchive.nationalarchives.gov.uk/20121010012427/

http://www.fawc.org.uk/freedoms.htm (accessed 20 May 2020).

Food Ethics Council. (2019). Ethical Matrix. https://www.foodethicscouncil.org/app/uploads/2019/02/Ethical_Matrix_1.pdf (accessed 29 May 2020).

Forkman, B. (2009). Investigating possible measures to include in the assessment systems. In: *Welfare Quality Reports No. 12: Overview of the Development of the Welfare Quality® Project Assessment System* (ed. L. Keeling). Uppsala, Sweden: SLU Services.

Fraser, D. (1995). Science, values and animal welfare: Exploring the "inextricable connection." *Anim. Welf.* 4: 103–117.

Fraser, D. (2003). Assessing animal welfare at the farm and group level: The interplay of science and values. *Anim. Welf.* 12 (4): 433–443.

Fraser, D. (2008). *Understanding Animal Welfare: The Science in Its Cultural Context*. Ames, IA: Wiley Blackwell.

Fraser, D. and Duncan, I.J.H. (1998). "Pleasures," "pains" and animal welfare: Toward a natural history of affect. *Anim. Welf.* 7: 383–396.

Gentry, J.E. (2005). The effects of caregiver stress upon ethics-at-risk behavior among Florida licensed marriage and family therapists. PhD dissertation. Florida State University.

Goold, C. and R.C. Newberry (2017). Modelling personality, plasticity and predictability in shelter dogs. *R. Soc. Open Sci.* 4 (9): 170618.

Gouveia, K., Magalhães, A., and de Sousa, L. (2011). The behaviour of domestic cats in a shelter: Residence time, density and sex ratio. *Appl. Anim. Behav. Sci.* 130 (1–2): 53–59.

Green, T.C. and Mellor, D.J. (2011). Extending ideas about animal welfare assessment to include "quality of life" and related concepts. *New Zeal. Vet. J.* 59 (6): 263–271.

Guesgen, M.J. and Bench, C.J. (2017). What can kinematics tell us about the affective states of animals? *Anim. Welf.* 26: 383–397.

Hennessy, M.B. (2013). Using hypothalamic–pituitary–adrenal measures for assessing and reducing the stress of dogs in shelters: A review. *Appl. Anim. Behav. Sci.* 149: 1–12.

Hoffman, C.L., Ladha, C., and Wilcox, S. (2019). An actigraphy-based comparison of shelter dog and owned dog activity patterns. *J. Vet. Behav.* 34: 30–36.

Holt, D.E., Mover, M.R., and Cimino Brown, D. (2010). Serologic prevalence of antibodies against canine influenza virus (H3N8) in dogs in a metropolitan animal shelter. *J. Am. Vet. Med. Assoc.* 237 (1): 71–73.

Hubrecht, R.C., Serpell, J.A., and Pool, T.B. (1992). Correlates of pen size and housing conditions on the behavior of kenneled dogs. *Appl. Anim. Behav. Sci.* 37: 345–361.

International Companion Animal Management Coalition. (n.d.). The Welfare Basis for Euthanasia of Dogs and Cats and Policy Development. https://www.icam-coalition.org/wp-content/uploads/2017/03/The-welfare-basis-for-euthanasia-of-dogs-and-cats-and-policy-development.pdf (accessed 29 May 2020).

Jensen, P. (2017). *The Ethology of Domestic Animals: An Introductory Text*, 3rd ed. Boston, MA: CABI.

Jensen, P. and Toates, F.M. (1993). Who needs "behavioural needs"? Motivational aspects of the needs of animals. *Appl. Anim. Behav. Sci.* 37: 161–181.

Kaiser, M., Millar, K., Thorstensen, E. et al. (2007). Developing the ethical matrix as a decision support framework: GM fish as a case study. *J. Agr. Environ. Ethic* 20: 65–80.

Kälvemark, S., Höglund, A.T., Hansson, M.G. et al. (2004). Living with conflicts—Ethical dilemmas and moral distress in the health care system. *Soc. Sci. Med.* 58 (6): 1075–1084.

Keeling, L. (2005). Healthy and happy: Animal welfare as an integral part of sustainable agriculture. *Ambio.* 34: 316–319.

Keeling, L. and Jensen, P. (2002). Abnormal behaviour, stress and welfare. In: *The Ethology of Domestic Animals: An Introductory Text.* (ed. P. Jensen), 119–134. Boston, MA: CABI.

Keeling, L.J., Rushen, J., and Duncan, I.J.H. (2011). Understanding animal welfare. In: *Animal Welfare*, 2nd ed. (eds.

M.C. Appleby, J.A. Mench, I.A.S. Olsson, et al.), 13–26. Oxfordshire, UK: CABI.

Kiddie, J.L. and Collins, L.M. (2014). Development and validation of a quality of life assessment tool for use in kenneled dogs *(Canis familiaris)*. *Appl. Anim. Behav. Sci.* 158: 57–68.

Kirkden, R.D. and Pajor, E.A. (2006). Using preference, motivation and aversion tests to ask scientific questions about animals' feelings. *Appl. Anim. Behav. Sci.* 100: 29–47.

Lawrence, A.B., Vigors, B., and Sandøe, P. (2019). What is so positive about positive animal welfare? A critical review of the literature. *Animals* 9. https://doi.10.3390/ani9100783.

Maiden, J., Georges, J., and Connelly, C.D. (2011). Moral distress, compassion fatigue, and perceptions about medication errors in certified critical care nurses. *Dimens. Crit. Care Nurs.* 30 (6): 339–345.

Martin, P. and Bateson, P.P.G. (1993). *Measuring Behaviour: An Introductory Guide*, 2nd ed. Cambridge, UK: Cambridge University Press.

Mason, G.J. and Burn, C.C. (2011). Behavioural restriction. In: *Animal Welfare*, 2nd ed. (eds. M.C. Appleby, J.A. Mench, A.S. Olsson et al.), 98–119. Boston, MA: CABI.

Mason, G.J. and Latham, N.R. (2004). Can't stop, won't stop: Is stereotypy a reliable animal welfare indicator? *Anim. Welf.* 13: 57–69.

Mason, G. J. and Mendl, M. (1993). Why is there no simple way of measuring animal welfare? *Anim. Welf.* 2: 301–319.

McMillan, F.D. (2013). Quality of life, stress, and emotional pain in shelter animals. In: *Shelter Medicine for Veterinarians and Staff*, 2nd ed. (eds. L. Miller and S. Zawistowski), 83–92. Hoboken, NJ: Wiley Blackwell.

Mellor, D.J. (2017). Operational details of the Five Domains model and its key applications to the assessment and management of animal welfare. *Animals* 7. https://doi.10.3390/ani7080060.

Mellor, D.J. and Stafford, K.J. (2008). Quality of life: A valuable concept or an unnecessary embellishment when considering animal welfare? *Australian Animal Welfare Strategy International Conference*, Queensland.

Mench, J.A. (1998). Thirty years after Brambell: Whither animal welfare science? *J. Appl. Anim. Welf. Sci.* 1: 91–102.

Mepham, M. (2010). The ethical matrix as a tool in policy interventions: The obesity crisis. In: *Food Ethics* (eds. F.T. Gottwald, H.W. Ingensiep, and M. Meinhardt). New York: Springer.

Mepham, N., Kaiser, M., Thorstensen, E. et al. (2006). *Ethical Matrix Manual*. The Hague: LEI.

Mills, D. and Luescher, A. (2006). Veterinary and pharmacological approaches to abnormal and repetitive behaviour. In: *Stereotypic Animal Behaviour: Fundamentals and Applications to Animal Welfare*, 2nd ed. (eds. G. Mason and J. and Rushen), 286–324. Cambridge, MA: CABI.

Mullan, S. and Fawcett, S. (2017a). Making ethical decisions. In: *Veterinary Ethics: Navigating Tough Cases*, 37–68. Sheffield, UK: 5M Publishing Ltd.

Mullan, S. and Fawcett, S. (2017b). What is veterinary ethics and why does it matter? In: *Veterinary Ethics: Navigating Tough Cases*, 1–34. Sheffield, UK: 5M Publishing Ltd.

Newbury, S. and Hurley, K. (2013). Population management. In: *Shelter Medicine for Veterinarians and Staff*, 2nd ed. (eds. L. Miller and S. Zawistowski), 93–113. Hoboken, NJ: Wiley Blackwell.

Normando, S., Di Raimondo, G., and Bellaio, E. (2019). An investigation using different data gathering methods into the prevalence of behavioral problems in shelter dogs—A pilot study. *J. Vet. Behav.* 30: 1–8.

Packer, R.M.A., Davies, A.M., Colk, H.A. et al. (2019). What can we learn from the hair of the dog? Complex effects of endogenous and exogenous stressors on canine hair cortisol. *PLOS ONE* 14: e0216000.

Palmer, C. and Sandøe, P. (2011). Animal ethics. In: *Animal Welfare*, 2nd ed. (eds. M.C. Appleby, J.A. Mench, I.A.S. Olsson, et al.), 1–12. Oxfordshire, UK: CABI.

Polgár, Z., Blackwell, E.J., and Rooney, N.J. (2019). Assessing the welfare of kenneled dogs—A review of animal-based measures. *Appl. Anim. Behav. Sci.* 213: 1–13.

Protopopova, A. (2016). Effects of sheltering on physiology, immune function, behavior, and the welfare of dogs. *Physiol. Behav.* 159: 95–103.

Raines, M.L. (2000). Ethical decision making in nurses: Relationships among moral reasoning, coping style, and ethics stress. *JONAS Healthc. Law Ethics Regul.* 2 (1): 29–41.

Richter, S.H. and Hintze, S. (2019). From the individual to the population—And back again? Emphasizing the role of the individual in animal welfare science. *Appl. Anim. Behav. Sci.* 212: 1–8.

Rollin, B.E. (2011). Euthanasia, moral stress, and chronic illness in veterinary medicine. *Vet. Clin. Small Anim.* 41: 651–659.

Rowan, A. and Kartal, T. (2018). Dog population & dog sheltering trends in the United States of America. *Animals.* https://doi:10.3390/ani8050068.

Rushen, J., Chapinal, N., and de Passillé, A.M. (2012). Automated monitoring of behavioural-based animal welfare indicators. *Anim. Welf.* 21: 339–350.

Rushen, J. and Mason, G. (2006). A decade-or-more's progress in understanding stereotypic behaviour. In: *Stereotypic Animal Behaviour Fundamentals and Applications to Welfare*, 2nd ed. (eds. J. Mason and G. Rushen), 1–18, Cambridge, MA: CABI.

Sandøe, P. and Christiansen, S.B. (2007). The value of animal life: how should we balance quality against quantity? *Anim. Welf.* 16 (S): 109–115.

Spoolder, H., De Rosa, G., Horning, B., Waiblinger, S., and Wemelsfelder, F. (2003). Integrating parameters to assess on-farm welfare. *Anim. Welf.* 12: 529–534.

Stephen, J.M. and Ledger, R.A. (2005). An audit of behavioral indicators of poor welfare in kenneled dogs in the United Kingdom. *J. Appl. Anim. Welf. Sci.* 8 (2): 79–96.

Swaisgood, R.R. and Shepherdson, D.J. (2005). Scientific approaches to enrichment and stereotypies in zoo animals: What's been done and where should we go next? *Zoo Biol.* 24: 499–518.

Tami, G. and Gallagher, A. (2009). Description of the behavior of domestic dog (*Canis familiaris*) by experienced and inexperienced people. *Appl. Anim. Behav. Sci.* 120: 159–169.

Tannenbaum, J. (1995). The four branches of veterinary ethics. In: *Veterinary Ethics: Animal Welfare, Client Relations, Competition and Collegiality*, 2nd ed., 14–18. St. Louis, MO: Mosby-Yearbook, Inc.

Tashman, S., Anderst, W., Kolowich, P. et al. (2004). Kinematics of the ACL-deficient canine knee during gait: Serial changes over two years. *J. Orthop.* 22: 931–941.

Taylor, K.D. and Mills, D.S. (2007). The effect of the kennel environment on canine welfare: A critical review of experimental studies. *Anim. Welf.* 16: 435–447.

Timmins, R.P., Cliff, K.D., Day, C.T., et al. (2007). Enhancing quality of life for dogs and cats in confined situations. *Anim. Welf.* 16 (S): 83–87.

Veissier, I., Botreau, R., and Perny, P. (2009). Scoring animal welfare: Difficulties and Welfare Quality® solutions. In: *Welfare Quality Reports No. 12: Overview of the Development of the Welfare Quality® Project Assessment System* (ed. L. Keeling). Uppsala, Sweden: SLU Services.

Veissier, I. and Evans, A. (2015). Principles and criteria of good animal welfare. Welfare Quality®. http://www.welfarequality.net (accessed 29 June 2020).

Villalobos, A.E. (2007). Palliative eare: End of life "pawspice" care. In: *Canine and Feline Geriatric Oncology: Honoring the Human-Animal Bond*. Oxford, UK: Blackwell.

Vinke, C.M., Godijn, L.M., and van der Liej, W.J.R. (2014). Will a hiding box provide stress reduction for shelter cats? *Appl. Anim. Behav. Sci.* 160: 86–93.

Walker, J.K., Dale, A.R., D'Eath, R.B. et al. (2016). Qualitative behavior assessment of dogs in the shelter and home environment and relationship with quantitative behavior assessment and physiological responses. *Appl. Anim. Behav. Sci.* 184: 97–108.

Walker, J., Dale, A., Waran, N. et al. (2010). The assessment of emotional expression in dogs using a free choice profiling methodology. *Anim. Welf.* 19: 75–84.

Webster, A.J.F., Main, D.C.J., and Whay, H.R. (2004). Welfare assessments: Indices from clinical observations. *Anim. Welf.* 13: 93–98.

Webster, J. (2016). Animal welfare: Freedoms, dominions and "a life worth living." *Animals* 35. https://doi.10.3390/ani6060035.

Wemelsfelder, F. (2007). How animals communicate quality of life: The qualitative assessment of animal behavior. *Anim. Welf.* 16 (S): 25–31.

Wemelsfelder, F. and Lawrence, A.B. (2001). Qualitative assessment of animal behavior as an on-farm welfare-monitoring tool. *Acta Agri. Scand.* 51: 21–25.

Wemelsfelder, F. and Mullan, S. (2014). Applying ethological and health indicators to practical animal welfare assessment. *Rev. Off. Int. Epizoot.* 33: 111–120.

Whitham, J.C. and Miller, L.J. (2016). Using technology to monitor and improve zoo animal welfare. *Anim. Welf.* 25: 395–409.

Zawistowski, S. and Morris, J. (2013). Introduction to animal sheltering. In: *Shelter Medicine for Veterinarians and Staff*, 2nd ed. (eds. L. Miller and S. Zawistowski), 3–12. Hoboken, NJ: Wiley Blackwell.

Zupan, M., Buskas, J., Altimiras, J. et al. (2016). Assessing positive emotional states in dogs using heart rate and heart rate variability. *Physiol. Behav.* 155: 102–111.

Please visit the companion website for video clips and downloadable resources associated with this chapter.

Appendix 19.A Sample Decision Table for Animal Care (Adapted from International Companion Animal Management Coalition n.d.)

1) Identify the care, treatment, or condition under consideration.
2) Identify additional factors to be considered in the first column.
3) Enter scores as indicated for level of need, likelihood of success, and resource costs for each factor identified.
4) Tally scores within each row and column.
5) Repeat exercise for each intervention under consideration.
6) Use scores to inform discussion. A high score suggests high need and high cost but little chance of success. A low score suggests low need and low cost but high chance of success.

Question or scenario: _____

	What is the level of need? (1 = low, 10 = high)	What is the likelihood of success? (1 = high, 10 = low)	What is the resource cost of this option? (1 = low, 10 = high)	Total
Physical health treatments				
Behavior modification				
Special housing and husbandry needs				
Total				

20

Behavioral Care during Transportation and Relocation
Brian A. DiGangi and Karen S. Walsh

20.1 Introduction

20.1.1 History of Animal Relocation

Animal relocation for adoption started with small-scale, individual breed rescue in the last two decades of the twentieth century. Shortly thereafter, some animal welfare organizations in the northeastern United States participated in regular high-volume transports of mostly small dogs and puppies to meet an increasing demand for adoptable dogs (Zawistowski and Morris 2013). It was not until 2005 during the response efforts following Hurricane Katrina that the use of large-scale companion animal relocation began to take shape more broadly. The challenges and successes that were a part of the evacuation and rescue during Katrina paved the way for major milestones and shifts in animal welfare, including the large-scale use of relocation to address companion animal homelessness as well as the development of best practice documents to guide relocation programs using a variety of transport methods (see Figure 20.1). This massive undertaking, the public response, and the number of animals placed in homes through relocation led to a new way to manage the regional imbalance of animals needing shelter and people seeking pets.

As used in this chapter, "animal relocation" refers to the long-distance movement of a group of healthy companion animals from one geographic region to another for the purposes of adoption. "Transport" and "transportation" are used to refer to an individual route, regardless of distance, or the logistics and process of animal movement itself. Animals are also commonly relocated as part of a natural or man-made emergency response effort and to provide access to otherwise unavailable services. Specific transport accommodations and considerations that relate to these scenarios will be addressed briefly, though, as described below, an animal's physical and behavioral needs during transport remain the same regardless of the distance or rationale for relocation.

20.1.2 Purpose and Indications

Animal relocation programs are used as a tool to address companion animal homelessness. Through the creation of effective partnerships, they aim to balance population discrepancies between areas where the homeless pet population exceeds adoption demand (known as sources) and organizations located where there is a higher demand for animal adoption than

Animal Behavior for Shelter Veterinarians and Staff, Second Edition. Edited by Brian A. DiGangi, Victoria A. Cussen, Pamela J. Reid, and Kristen A. Collins.
© 2022 John Wiley & Sons, Inc. Published 2022 by John Wiley & Sons, Inc.
Companion website: www.wiley.com/go/digangi/animal

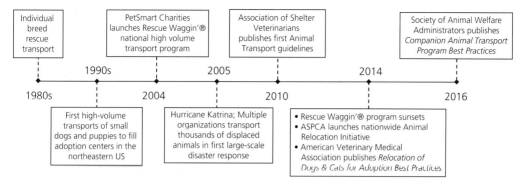

Figure 20.1 Timeline of large-scale companion animal relocation in the United States.

can be met locally (known as destinations). In doing so, over-burdened source shelters can divert resources that would have been needed for basic animal care toward operational enhancements and the development of new programs that offer sustainable, local solutions to animal welfare problems. Similarly, animal relocation programs allow destination shelters to capitalize on their successes in medical and behavioral care, increasing opportunities for positive outcomes for animals and, in many cases, generating resources that can be used to support the source shelter. Well-designed animal relocation programs are a win-win-win scenario that support improved welfare for individual animals as well as the animal (and human) populations in both communities.

Source shelters must have the ability and resources to effectively select and prepare relocation candidates. The benefits of relocation should outweigh the risks for the individual animals involved and the animals selected should meet the needs of the destination shelter's community. Animal relocation is only one of the tools source communities may use to manage their populations. Well-rounded sheltering programs will focus on local, long-term solutions and must not consider relocation a substitute for local community action or a key budget item to maintain financial viability. Some examples of programs that should be used in conjunction with relocation are those that: reduce or divert intake, proactively manage community cat populations, remove

barriers to adoption or foster care, enlist foster homes to serve as adoption ambassadors, work with the local government to create animal-friendly regulations that support community animal and public-health, and focus on creative and innovative ways to decrease length of stay and place animals in homes.

Indications for relocation in a destination community can be numerous and compelling. A community imbalance of available and desirable pets for adoption is often the catalyst to explore a relocation partnership. While the demand for adoptable pets has increased over the past few decades (Rowan and Kartal 2018), in many communities the increasing complexity of medically and behaviorally challenged animals in the shelter may decrease adoptions. When the public is unable to find animals with the characteristics they expect or desire, they may become disillusioned with the lack of variety and seek pets from other sources. Although the shelter may be beloved in the community and have established themselves as the go-to place for information and services for animals, a lack of available animals can jeopardize that hard-won relationship. Animal relocation programs can provide solutions to each of these concerns. In addition, community excitement and the desire for animals that may now be unusual in the region often further increase local demand, driving shelters to increase the number of animals they can accept into their program.

Animal relocation is not without risk to physical or behavioral health and welfare; it is key to remember that the destination often drives the level of risk and its impact on animal welfare during transportation to their community. As such, the responsibility to select appropriate source partners and transporters falls primarily on the destination. It is the responsibility of the destination to ask questions not only about the behavioral and medical history of the animals that will be coming to their facility, but the appropriateness of the transport vehicle and the practices that will be used to move animals. Ensuring humane conditions must be the guiding principle of each transport from start to finish; if essential provisions for safety of both the animals and the drivers cannot be met, the transport should not proceed. The animals' needs are the same regardless of a partner's immediate ability or aspiration to meet them. Once substandard care has been accepted, it becomes more challenging to seek higher ground. A positive outcome does not negate the need to meet minimal standards for both drivers and animals and continually strive toward better practices. Simply surviving a transport is not enough, the conditions should be such that the animals in our care can thrive

20.1.3 Guidelines and Regulations

A number of professional animal welfare organizations have published recommendations, guidelines, and best practices for the responsible relocation of dogs and cats for adoption (see Box 20.1). The Association of Shelter Veterinarians' (ASV's) *Guidelines for Standards of Care in Animal Shelters* was the first such document with a designated Animal Transport section (ASV 2010). This report, founded in the Five Freedoms, addresses responsibilities of individuals and organizations participating in animal relocation programs from the point of origin, through the transportation itself, to the destination. The Association for Animal Welfare Advancement (AAWA) created *Companion Animal Transport Programs Best Practices* that "are generally accepted as those that will produce the best results for animals" and that focus on the operational aspects of such programs (AAWA 2019). In addition, the AAWA's document

---

Box 20.1 Published Guidelines and Best Practices in Companion Animal Relocation

American Veterinary Medical Association
Non-emergency Relocation of Dogs and Cats for Adoption within the United States
https://www.avma.org/sites/default/files/2020-03/AWF-TransportAdoptionBestPractices.pdf

The Association for Animal Welfare Advancement
Companion Animal Transport Best Practices
https://theaawa.org/page/Bestpractice

Association of Shelter Veterinarians
Guidelines for Standards of Care in Animal Shelters
https://www.sheltervet.org/shelter-guidelines

International Air Transport Association
Live Animal Regulations
https://www.iata.org/en/publications/store/live-animals-regulations/

National Alliance of State Animal and Agricultural Emergency Programs
Animal Evacuation and Transportation Best Practices
https://www.thenasaaep.com/workshp-resources

discusses considerations of the role of animal transport programs and their impact on organizations and communities. Recommendations specific to both ground and air transport are described as are limited considerations specific to the transportation of animals in emergency response scenarios. The American Veterinary Medical Association (AVMA) and Association of Shelter Veterinarians offer best practices for *Non-Emergency Relocation of Dogs and Cats for Adoption* that focus on aspects of program design and operation that have direct impacts on animal health and welfare (AVMA 2020a). Special precautions for the responsible handling of vulnerable populations of animals (e.g., young animals, brachycephalic dogs, cats, pregnant animals, seniors) are enumerated. Additional publications of note include the National Alliance of State Animal and Agricultural Emergency Programs' *Animal Evacuation and Transportation Best Practices* and the International Air Transport Association's *Live Animals Regulations.* The former focuses on disaster response planning and the pros and cons of different types of vehicles used to transport animals, while the latter focuses on commercial airline requirements and governmental regulations.

The guidelines and best practices described above should be followed to ensure relocation programs operate in a manner that minimizes risks and maximizes benefits to all stakeholders, including:

- Animals involved in the relocation program
- Animals not involved in the relocation program (source and destination shelters and their communities)
- Drivers, animal handlers, animal care staff
- Veterinarians (shelter, USDA-accredited, and community)
- Shelter leadership and specialty staff (behavior, public relations, development, etc.)
- Adopters.

Adhering to these practices, even when they may seem challenging, is critical for ensuring the long-term success and viability of animal relocation programs nationwide. Following

voluntary guidelines mitigates the need for regulatory interventions that may limit or eliminate this lifesaving tool from the animal welfare playbook.

While essential for both short and long-term success, industry guidelines largely remain just that—guidelines—and not legal requirements. (Note that the Animal Welfare Act sets federal law regulating minimum standards of care and treatment for certain animals bred for commercial sale, used in research, transported commercially, or exhibited to the public. See https://www.nal.usda.gov/animal-health-and-welfare/animal-welfare-act for more information.) Legal requirements for animal relocation programs vary widely by state and may include everything from animal vaccination protocols to housing requirements to minimum holding periods. Some transporters and importing agencies may be required to register with various regulatory bodies prior to participating.

It is important that organizations familiarize themselves with the specific requirements of both the source and destination states. However, while some states may require documentation of companion animals being exported from their state, it is principally the destination state's regulations for importation of companion animals that must be adhered to. Such importation is regulated by the United States Department of Agriculture Animal and Plant Health Inspection Service (USDA-APHIS) and the state veterinarian in the destination state. The USDA-APHIS's Pet Travel webpage (https://www.aphis.usda.gov/aphis/pet-travel) directs users to each state's individual importation and exportation requirements. As requirements can and do change without notice, they should be checked regularly.

Written confirmation of an animal's health and fitness for travel along with a statement indicating the animal is free from contagious disease must accompany each animal. Such documentation is referred to as a Certificate of Veterinary Inspection (CVI) (i.e., health certificate) and in most, but not all, jurisdictions must be signed by a veterinarian accredited by the USDA to perform such inspections as a representative of the federal government. It is the signing veterinarian's obligation to familiarize themselves with the requirements for entry into the destination state and ensure that each animal certified for importation meets those requirements. CVIs typically must be completed within a maximum of 30 days from the date of entry (although many jurisdictions require shorter time periods) and must be submitted to the destination state veterinarian's office. A variety of electronic CVI services are available and can assist with proper completion and submission of the required information. See Box 20.2.

International transports are subject to additional regulations and standards that should be researched thoroughly. Careful consideration should be taken before importing animals from other countries; in many cases prolonged quarantine periods and importation permits are required to minimize the risk of introducing a foreign animal disease to the destination locale (Polak 2019). Long journeys can be arduous for animals that are unfamiliar with confinement and a lack of appropriate safeguards can result in severe and devastating consequences.

The authors are unaware of any import requirements, CVI declarations, or local regulations that address behavioral health. Therefore, it is the responsibility of partnering organizations to ensure the behavioral suitability of animals selected for transport (see Section 20.4.3).

Box 20.2 Electronic Certificate of Veterinary Inspection (CVI) Services

AgMoveCVI
https://agmovecvi.com/

Global VetLINK, LLC (GVL®)
https://www.globalvetlink.com/

Veterinary Services Process Streamlining (VSPS)
https://vsapps.aphis.usda.gov/vsps/
(Livestock species, including equines, only)

20.1.4 Program Models

Companion animal relocation programs can operate under a variety of models that vary based on resource requirements, risk for disease transmission, financial costs, and number of animals served. Core considerations for any model include the distance between source communities and destination communities, the shelter population targeted for relocation, and the mode of transportation (see Figure 20.2).

Local, regional, national, and international transport are all common models used by agencies seeking to relocate populations of animals in need. In general, operating costs and risk for disease transmission increase with distance travelled, so local transport should be considered first. Choosing a partner that is located within the same community, state, or region is more cost-effective and efficient than national or international options and builds connections that can improve animal welfare in the surrounding area. Proactively monitoring animal welfare trends in the region and engaging in outreach within the source or destination state can enhance existing partnerships and identify new ones.

International transport is also pursued by some organizations. Such programs carry the greatest costs and have been repeatedly associated with the introduction of novel diseases (Polak 2019). Prior to accepting transport from an international source, organizations should carefully consider the needs of partners that are closer to home and the impact of international partnerships on their own mission. Criteria for animal selection must take into account suitability for adoption, disease management, long-term quality of life, and the effects of extensive travel on the animals. Shelters that are accepting international transports may find it useful to have a written policy statement regarding the reasons behind the decision to accept these animals.

Regardless of the geographic model selected there are an array of transport options

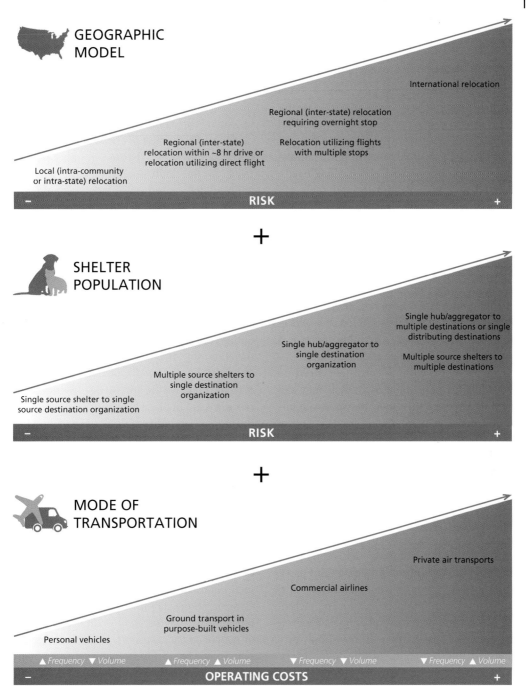

Figure 20.2 Companion animal relocation program models—and the associated risks and costs—vary based on the geographic region and shelter populations intended to be served, as well as the mode of transportation employed. *Source:* Illustration by Laura Nelson.

available. The type of transportation will depend on the population being moved, the numbers of animals that will be relocated at one time, and the distance the animals will be travelling. Organizations that have a small number of animals to move may use volunteers driving personal vehicles or a small rented van. This option is well suited for animals that are part of a harder-to-place population with specific medical or behavioral needs. Nursing or pregnant animals and their offspring or exotic pets can also benefit greatly from this quiet, focused mode of transport. It is important to consider the implications to the organization when using vehicles that are not owned by the organization. Insurance, liability waivers, safety protocols, and a written Memorandum of Understanding (MOU) should all be a part of the creation of a relocation program, even one that only involves a small number of volunteers and animals.

Organizations with a consistent need to move a larger population of animals may still choose to operate their own transport vehicle. In this model an appropriately sized cargo van, cargo trailer, or specialty vehicle should be specifically outfitted for animal transport. The agency may select trained volunteers or staff to drive the animals that are identified and accepted for transport. Transports under this model usually travel regionally or across several states to partner with an appropriate destination. Another common model is facilitated transport through a paid or unpaid third party. The transport company or organization may manage the entire relocation process, including contact and placement of animals between the source and destination, or may simply provide the transportation. Multi-shelter transports between more than one source and/or destination may also participate in this model. Transports that involve a hub or aggregator shelter that gathers animals regionally from smaller partners are often a part of the third-party model. It is important to be sure that the third-party transporter is reputable, insured, and that the transport vehicle is outfitted in

such a manner to ensure a safe and comfortable ride for the animals entrusted to their care. Meeting with the transporter, asking for references, visually reviewing the vehicle(s) to be used, requiring copies of any licenses and insurance policies, and watching loading or unloading at another facility can help to develop a full picture of the service the transporter is providing. The total number of animals on the individual transport, whether appropriately sized and safe kennels are required, the required pre-transfer medical preparation, and the number of partners that are allowed to place animals in one vehicle should all be known and considered before deciding that this transporter is an appropriate choice.

Regardless of the specific program model employed, standing operating procedures must outline the type of vehicle the animals will be travelling in, the distance the drivers will be travelling, the road types and route to be driven, standards for low-stress driving, what resources are in place to ensure safety for both the animals and drivers along the way, and the plans for emergency situations such as adverse weather or vehicle breakdown, including mechanisms for emergency animal removal. The creation of an emergency plan should happen prior to starting a relocation program. Drivers should receive training in basic first aid, management of safety equipment such as a fire extinguisher, and have a rehearsed evacuation plan for every animal on board, incorporating stress reduction techniques. Consideration should be given to vehicle breakdowns, accidents, ill or injured animals or people on the transport, and a contingency plan should be readily available for each potential transport issue. Contingency plans can include the location of partner organizations, including veterinary hospitals, along the travelled route that are willing to be on stand-by and offer assistance. Securing a contract with a national towing service that can support vehicle needs regardless of location is imperative. Some resourceful organizations have added a shuttle vehicle that follows the primary transport vehicle so that resources and assistance are readily available in case of emergency.

To ensure a relocation partnership is built on a strong foundation and expectations are in alignment, organizations should prepare and sign an MOU that sets realistic expectations and spells out the responsibilities of each party. Agreements codified in an MOU are a less formal way of building a relationship that does not imply a legal commitment but creates a place to document and follow up on expectations.

In the authors' opinion, distance is a key component of transport stress for both the drivers and the animals on a transport. Mapping out routes and using United States Department of Transportation (DOT) guidelines as a rule of thumb will keep staff, volunteers, and pets safer. Having two drivers on the transport provides an excellent layer of protection if there is an accident or breakdown that requires removal of all animals on board but does not eliminate the chances of sleep-deprived driving. Transports that cover thousands of miles, involve travel at odd hours, or have prolonged durations with sporadic or no rest put all vehicle occupants, as well as others traveling on the same roadways, at unnecessary risk (Hoffman 2020; Dillane 2020). As little as one to two fewer hours of sleep can result in 2–10 times the crash rate—a rate equivalent to that of driving under the influence (Tefft 2016).

20.2 Moving Animals

20.2.1 Vehicle Selection and Upfitting

20.2.1.1 Ground Transport
The selection of a vehicle is an exciting and daunting part of a program's evolution. There are many companies that design and provide a variety of vehicles specific for animal movement. Most of those contain specialized stainless-steel units originally designed for animal control functions rather than long-distance relocation. Customization and features are usually available and require knowledge on the part of the organization in order to select all options that best meet the needs of the organization and fit the program model. Costs beyond the vehicle purchase should be a part of the initial and ongoing funding plan so that the program created is a sustainable model.

The first consideration is the vehicle type and size that is appropriate for the program. The number of animals the organization would like to relocate, the available resources needed to safely accomplish that task, and the location of the destinations should all be taken into account. A smaller vehicle is often nimbler, and the movement of fewer animals more frequently allows for improved conditions during transport as well as faster placement of animals at the destination. Although it is appealing to consider loading a bus or a tractor trailer full of animals, it is nearly impossible to maintain safe and humane conditions in such a scenario. In the authors' experience, as the number of animals on a transport increases so does the stress level and the possibility of disease exposure and spread.

The factory-installed cargo climate control unit should be avoided when ordering a vehicle. The location, airflow, distribution of heat and cold, and power of pre-installed units are not sufficient to combat the increased internal heat that comes from the body temperatures of the occupants and the amount of space that needs to be cooled or heated. Such systems are designed to perform functions for static items (like flowers) and do not provide for live animal comfort and safety. These units often "pool" cool or warm air in just one area of the vehicle rather than creating an even airflow throughout the vehicle so that animals at the top of the vehicle experience a similar temperature to animals at the bottom of the vehicle. The additional attachment kits that come with many of these units contain corrugated tubes or PVC pipes that create additional hard-to-reach surfaces that are difficult to sanitize. For these reasons, an appropriate low-profile roof-mounted climate control unit is recommended for animal transport vehicles. An evaluation should be completed to determine the cooling capacity of the proposed unit; consideration must be given to the fact that the changing exterior temperature and the heat output of animals are not constant and will directly impact the ability of the unit to maintain the internal temperature. The size of the unit should be approximately twice that of what might be expected if only considering the amount of space that needs to be cooled. Selecting and maintaining a unit that can easily manage the anticipated load will extend the life of the unit and create peace of mind that a comfortable and safe environment is being created for the animals on the transport.

Insulation is an important consideration for a transport vehicle. Both trailers and vans require proper insulation on the sides, roof, and floor of the interior of the vehicle. The layer of insulation must be completely covered and sealed with a non-permeable surface so that there is no possibility of moisture leaching into the insulation when the vehicle interior is cleaned and disinfected. An insulated floor mat covered with bedliner or diamond plate flooring (or a combination of the two) will greatly reduce road heat that affects the comfort of animals housed on the lowest level of the vehicle housing units. Meeting with contractors and upfitters prior to ordering the vehicle will help to expedite the process and ensure the desired result.

Once a type of vehicle has been selected, the type, size, and number of kennels can be considered and are a crucial component of animal safety and comfort. Kennels should be structurally sound, appropriately sized for the animal and length of transport, unable to collapse, designed to minimize the possibility of injury or escape, easy to clean and disinfect, and durable enough for repeated use. When kennels will be placed on both sides of the vehicle animals will need to be provided with a

disinfectable barrier to reduce visual stimulation and act as a physical barrier to respiratory droplets. Roll-down outdoor solar shades can serve this purpose without restricting climate control (see Figure 20.3). Although stainless-steel built-in kennels are easy to clean and attractive, there are drawbacks to having kennels that cannot be removed in an animal relocation vehicle. When faced with a breakdown or an accident, safe and expedient removal of the animals can be impossible for the driver and assistant in such a vehicle. Selecting kennels that can be securely attached to the walls of the vehicle and easily removed without removing the animals from the safety of the

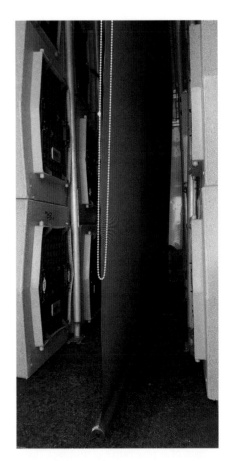

Figure 20.3 A roll-down, outdoor, solar shade provides a visual and physical barrier between opposing kennels without compromising climate control. *Source:* Courtesy of J. Birkenmeier and C. Estrada.

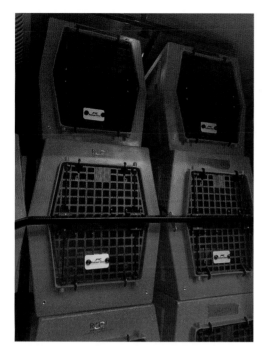

Figure 20.4 Custom cargo control bars allow ease of access during loading/unloading and secure crates to the vehicle during transit. In this image, the bars for the upper row of kennels have been raised to access the kennels for loading/unloading. *Source:* Brian A. DiGangi.

kennel is crucial. In some vehicles, custom-built cargo control bars can be installed to accomplish these goals (see Figure 20.4). When writing protocols and selecting equipment, all of these criteria must be a part of the initial plan for success.

The importance of monitoring and safety in an animal relocation vehicle cannot be stressed enough. Whether using a trailer, a bus, or a van cargo space, monitors and alarms for carbon monoxide, temperature, and humidity and the ability to visualize and hear the animals in the cargo area should be a part of every vehicle design. When driving a van, a bulkhead unit that separates the driver cab from the animal area is essential for driver safety. Items in the cargo area, even when well fastened, can become projectiles in an accident. While allowing the drivers in the cab to have open access to the animals creates an additional monitoring

opportunity, that should not be a substitute for driver safety and must be carefully thought out: a bulkhead with a door or opening is a better option than an open vehicle if constant access is desired for care and monitoring of the animals.

Regulations and proper licensing of a vehicle and the drivers is another programmatic consideration related to vehicle selection. Department of Transportation regulations that require a commercial driver's license (CDL) or Medical Examiner's Certificate must be considered when planning a program and operating a large vehicle. Drivers that obtain a CDL are in high demand and can qualify for a rate of pay much higher than most shelter personnel; finding and retaining a CDL driver can be challenging, and the need for one can drive up the cost of the program. Designing a program that includes, at a minimum, two drivers that can manage the selected vehicle while understanding and complying with all state and federal regulations is crucial.

20.2.1.2 Air Transport

Air transport, through commercial or privately chartered aircraft, is the most expensive method of animal relocation and generally carries the greatest degree of risk. Where animals travel as cargo on a commercial aircraft, animal care and monitoring are absent and/or relegated to airline staff. Generally, this method can only accommodate individuals or small groups of animals at a time and commercial airlines often have breed, species, or conformational restrictions (e.g., brachycephalic, bully breeds) for both dogs and cats due to concerns about liability and animal safety. In the case of chartered aircraft, a large number of animals can be accommodated; however, to fill the charter and improve cost efficiency, multiple populations of animals are often intermingled, which increases the risk for disease transmission. When deciding to use a private carrier for transport, always check references to be sure the organization is reputable and does not violate regulations (see https://aphis-efile.force.com/PublicSearchTool/s/inspection-reports for USDA APHIS Animal Care inspection reports).

One advantage of air over ground transport may be found in the duration of the trip. When appropriately managed, flying animals can result in a shorter travel time, which may be less stressful, reducing illness, resulting in the potential for improved outcomes and shorter length of stay at the destination. Confinement and travel time to and from the airport must also be taken into account when comparing duration of different modes of transport.

20.2.2 Transportation Requirements

20.2.2.1 Ground Transport

Animal comfort and stress reduction should be the primary consideration for each transport. While the temperature, humidity, and concentration of exhaled gases (carbon dioxide) in the vehicle may be acceptable, that in the kennel may be different and lead to an uncomfortable or dangerous environment for the individual animal. Transporting or housing an animal in an unsuitable environment can induce changes in physiology including alterations in disease susceptibility (National Research Council 1996). Thoughtful planning

for animal handling, loading, housing, monitoring, and safety is critical.

Limiting the number, size, and type of animals that can ride in a vehicle are important parts of creating a humane transport. It is also important to consider the species-specific behaviors and the ability to express normal behaviors such as standing, sitting, and laying down without contacting the sides of the enclosure. Just as it is inappropriate to mix species within a housing area in a sheltering facility, the same holds for animal transport. The increased stress for a prey animal being housed in proximity to a predator make this practice unacceptable. In an emergency, when there are no other options, both physical and visual barriers that provide auditory protection should be in place. Stress reduction techniques such as these are important for every transport.

Maintaining the proper temperature, humidity, and ventilation (or airflow) in the animal housing areas is vital to ensure animal safety. Temperature should not be confused with ventilation as they are very different parameters that meet different physiological needs (see Box 20.3). When considering the difference,

---

Box 20.3   Definition and Clinical Implications of Temperature, Humidity, and Ventilation (Blood and Studdert 1999; National Research Council 1996; Hales and Bligh 1969)

Temperature
- A qualitative state of a living being or environment; a measurement of the degree of sensible heat or cold
- Self-regulation, within normal species variation, is necessary for well-being; exposure of unadapted animals to extremes can produce life-threatening clinical effects

Humidity
- The degree of moisture in the air
- Ability to thermoregulate and degree of clinical effects are associated with changes in humidity

Ventilation
- Renewal or exchange of gas in an enclosed space; also referred to as airflow
- Serves to supply adequate oxygen; remove thermal loads caused by respiration, lights, equipment; dilute aerosolized contaminants; adjust moisture content of air

Note that ensuring adequacy of temperature, humidity, or ventilation within a vehicle cargo space does not ensure adequacy within an individual animal enclosure.

picture riding on a school bus with all the windows open on a temperate day. The surrounding temperature may be a balmy 75° F (23.9° C), but it is comfortable due to the flow of air through the open windows of the vehicle. However, riding in the same school bus with the windows closed, the flow of air would be blocked and the environment would quickly become stifling. In a similar way, spacing kennels so that every animal in the vehicle can be visualized and limiting the number of animals in the vehicle helps to allow for adequate ventilation through each kennel and to each individual occupant. Even in an appropriately loaded vehicle, active airflow is needed to maintain sufficient ventilation.

Temperature extremes within the vehicle should never be less than 50° F (10° C) or above 85° F (29.5° C) and humidity should be maintained between 30 and 70% (Animals and Animal Products 2016); maintaining temperatures between 60 and 80° F is preferable (ASV 2019; AAWA 2019). Depending on vehicle size and loading capacity, multiple digital sensors that send a signal to remote battery-operated thermometers and hygrometers should be used. Sensors should be placed at the animal level where the kennels are located, at the air return for vehicles with rooftop units, and the corresponding gauges should be easily visible in the cab of the vehicle. Sensor placement is important because the temperature reading on the factory-installed driver control panel displays the temperature of air leaving the unit, while the sensor placed on the air return will measure the temperature of the air coming back into the unit; the latter may better represent the most extreme temperature experienced by some of the animals in the cargo space. Using this dual-control, remote monitoring system and units that allow for programmed alarms at pre-determined set points can add additional layers of security. In addition, battery operated carbon monoxide detectors must be placed in the animal cargo area to alert the driver in case of an undetected leak so that all vehicle occupants are protected from CO poisoning. All monitors need to be able to be read and/or heard by the driver or passenger while the vehicle is in use, and protocols should be established to provide for continuous monitoring and documentation of these environmental parameters.

Additionally, the use of pheromone sprays; music that may calm the species being transported, played at an appropriate volume and duration of time; and safe, edible enrichment (when animals are housed alone) to occupy the time and mind of the animal should all be common practice in a relocation program (Ellis et al. 2013; Lindig et al. 2020). Scented air-freshener sprays and essential oils, including those that may be useful enrichment tools in animal shelters, are not recommended for use within individual enclosures or the vehicle itself. Such use does not allow an animal adversely affected to escape from the scent and may increase stress. See Chapters 11 and 17 for more considerations regarding canine and feline enrichment strategies.

Transport vehicles, equipment, and enclosures should be well maintained and replaced when damaged, so that they can be adequately cleaned and disinfected prior to and during transport. Meticulous sanitation plays a key role in ensuring the safety and health of groups of animals housed in a confined area. Animals must be provided with solid hard-surfaced kennels that cannot accidently collapse and can be completely sanitized. There should be no rust or corrosion present on any kennel. Animals must be able to comfortably stand up without having to duck their head, lie down, and turn around.

Kennels selected for use should be built to withstand the challenges of volume animal relocation by ground. In the authors' experience, kennels designed as a seamless, one-piece, molded, high-density, polyethylene unit that is durable and easy to clean best meet these requirements (Ruff Land Kennels, Tea, SD). Kennel design must allow for access to fresh water for every animal during breaks. This can be accomplished by filling attached

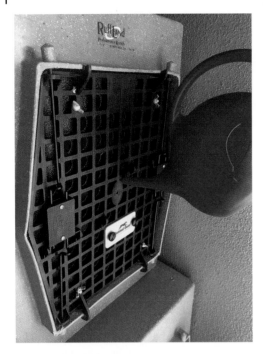

Figure 20.5 A thin-spouted watering can allows drivers to refill water bowls attached to kennel doors without opening them. *Source:* Brian A. DiGangi.

bowls with a thin-spouted watering can. This technique allows for water to be provided without opening the door, which helps minimize arousal during rest stops and reduces chance of escape (see Figure 20.5). In warmer months, crushed ice can be offered as a substitute for water and should be provided in a pet-safe durable container attached to the kennel.

When staffing an animal transport, the following points should be considered. Drivers must travel with cell phones, GPS mapping, a tracking or locating app, and equipment that will help address most common emergencies. If the transport will contain more than two animals and/or take more than two hours, there should be two drivers. At a minimum, the drivers should stop every four hours to check on the animals. The size of the vehicle can make observing and managing the transported population challenging or impossible for one driver. The species and the temperament of the animals being transported (dog, cat, or other) may change decisions regarding

the number of animals transported or the number of personnel that accompany them. Animals that are medically unsound or have behavior concerns may have specific needs. The time of day and year that transport is happening and the expected (or unexpected) weather that can be encountered must be also be considered.

Organizations that are performing animal transport must meet state regulations and DOT rules and regulations (https://www.fmcsa.dot.gov/regulations) in order to provide a safe environment for both the animals and the driver team, regardless of whether they are legally required to comply. These regulations exist to ensure that drivers are well rested when they are behind the wheel and to reduce the risk of fatigue-related accidents. The regulations set a standard limit on hours of drive time in a day, including off-duty time requirements; having two drivers does not increase the amount of drive time available.

Effective training is critical for transport personnel. Before entrusting this important task to any volunteer or staff member they must demonstrate the necessary skill and aptitude for this lifesaving work. In addition to basic animal handling and care skills, drivers should be adept at driving techniques that can mitigate fear, anxiety, and stress during travel in the specific vehicle in use. Aspects of particular relevance to animal stress include minimizing g-forces by avoiding hard-braking, reducing speed before entering curves, making smooth turn and gear-shift transitions, awareness of road surface and its impacts (e.g., vibrations or bumping), and ensuring careful handling in inclement weather. A comprehensive training program (https://www.drivedifferent.com/) must be available that requires trainees to demonstrate skills and sign off on a checklist as each skill is proficiently demonstrated. Training should be written and learned through hands-on work. Drivers should be trained on basic health examination, appropriate loading technique, vehicle set up, first aid, basic vehicle maintenance and troubleshooting, emergency protocols, and safe driving. Familiarizing the team with best practices and establishing transports that follow the recommended processes and guidelines will enable the organization to run a safe and successful program.

20.2.2.2 Air Transport

Planes that are not specifically designed to move animals may present unique challenges. In general, the same handling, loading, monitoring, safety, and environmental accommodations presented for ground transport also apply to air transport (see Section 20.2.2.1). Although there will be limitations based on aircraft model, some basic practices and accommodations should be in place to protect the health and welfare of animals during air transport.

The number of animals that a plane can carry and how they are arranged is dependent on balancing the center of gravity as appropriate for the specific aircraft model. In some cases, weight will need to be shifted or a temporary or permanent ballast installed to ensure stability during flight. Crates should have space between them to allow for free flow of air, and the kennels should be fastened to the body of the aircraft using restraint devices within the cargo hold. The pilot is ultimately responsible for all flight management including the weight and balance of the cargo and should be relied on for aircraft safety. However, the pilot should not be relied on for animal care needs; it is the responsibility of partnering organizations to select appropriate candidates for air transports within the given constraints.

Small and medium-sized planes may need to stop for refueling, which can extend the flight time. The entire travel time should be considered when selecting appropriate candidates for this mode of transport including loading at the source; traveling to the airport; unloading at the airport; organizing and loading onto the aircraft; flight time (including taxiing, tarmac delays, and layovers); unloading at the destination airport; loading destination transport vehicles; traveling to the destination; and unloading at the destination shelter.

All commercial airlines observe seasonal restrictions on pet travel and will not carry animals during extreme weather. In general, this includes temperatures above 80° F (27° C) or below 20° F (−7° C) at any point during routing that the animal is on the ground. For private flights, flight schedules may be more easily adjusted to avoid temperature extremes (e.g., early morning flights). Loading time should not exceed 45 minutes, and climate control machinery should be used, if available. Airport staff should be alerted in advance that live animals will be loaded on the tarmac and request assistance, such as an air conditioning unit for the loading time or access to a shady area for waiting animals, as needed. If the temperature is at or exceeds 85° F (29° C) inside the plane, the plane must not be loaded. Animals should not sit on a loaded plane for more than 30 minutes without take-off if ground temperatures are above 75° F (23.9° C) (AAWA 2019); communication must take place between the flight crew and air traffic control to ensure these safety goals are met.

20.3 The Impact of Transportation on Physiology and Behavior

There is little objective information regarding the physiological and behavioral impact of transportation on companion animals. A study in adult male beagles reported increased serum cortisol and total bilirubin in dogs after long-distance (22-hour) ground transportation that took two weeks to return to baseline levels (Ochi et al. 2016). In another report, beagle dogs transported for 9.5 hours had elevated levels of cortisol and corticosterone during ground transportation that returned to baseline values overnight; red blood cell parameters increased moderately (Kuhn et al. 1991). Increased plasma cortisol was also demonstrated in a group of beagles that underwent a 1-hour ground transport (Frank et al. 2006).

Scan sampling of video recordings during this transport showed dogs spent most of the time in a sitting position and the most frequently observed activity was lip-licking. A survey of dog owners found travel-related problems in 44% of dogs consistent with anxiety, fear, and motion sickness; as much as 29% of those dogs vomited during car travel (Cannas et al. 2010). Behavioral responses consistent with nausea (vomiting, salivation, hiding, and cowering) were ameliorated with the application of a dog-appeasing pheromone collar in another report, with the greatest perceived improvement in the reduction of nausea as compared to excitability and tenseness (Gandia Estellés and Mills 2006). To the authors' knowledge, similar studies have not been conducted in cats.

As with ground travel, the impact of air travel on physiology and behavior of dogs has been evaluated in a limited number of studies. Physiological and behavioral reactions to air transport were measured in a group of beagles that traveled by air to an intermediate destination, were unloaded, then re-loaded and returned to the airport of origin. The experience included an approximately 180-mile road journey each way to and from the airport, being loaded and unloaded into the aircraft cargo hold (about 70 minutes turnaround) and an approximately 43- to 48-minute flight (Bergeron et al. 2002). Study data demonstrated an increase in plasma cortisol concentration after ground transport, an increase in salivary cortisol concentration after both ground and air transport, and higher neutrophil and lower lymphocyte counts after both ground and air transport. Heart rate was significantly higher during loading (and no different from waiting and unloading periods) than during take-off, flying, landing, or turnaround; the largest increase in heart rate was detected during loading and unloading. In-flight video monitoring found the dogs spent more than 50% of the time lying down and the remainder of the time sitting; they remained inactive for 75% of the time. Study authors concluded that

the air travel experience included multiple acute stressors—the loading and unloading processes being the most stressful components. A small study of Greyhounds traveling short distances by air found no significant differences in stress response (as measured by plasma ACTH, cortisol, lactate, and fatty acid concentrations) based on differences in kennel size and construction (Leadon and Muyllins 1991). Presumably due to differences in temperature control and lighting, the data did suggest that dogs travelling in the belly hold of a commercial passenger aircraft had a greater stress response than those traveling in the main cargo hold of a cargo aircraft.

A study of working dogs compared changes in fecal score and microbial composition as a result of airline stress (Venable et al. 2016). Dogs that travelled for 2.5 hours in the cabin of a commercial airline had significantly higher fecal scores (i.e., softer feces) and statistically—but not clinically—significant differences in various blood chemistry values immediately after travelling. On working days (days one to three after travel), scores for completing previously trained behaviors were no different between dogs that travelled and those that did not. Again, statistically—but not clinically—significant differences in various blood chemistry values were observed in the days post-transport along with differences in both the type and abundance of bacterial communities present in fecal samples.

Although crude and non-specific, one other objective measure of the impact of transportation on physical health of companion animals can be found in the monthly animal incident reports published by the US DOT (https://www.transportation.gov/individuals/aviation-consumer-protection/air-travel-consumer-reports). In 2010, the DOT released an analysis of pet deaths during air transport, including a breed analysis, which indicated that approximately half of the deaths were brachycephalic dogs (DOT 2010). It is thought that dogs and cats with such conformation are more vulnerable to changes in air quality and temperature and such animals may be prohibited by individual carriers from flying in the cargo hold (AVMA 2020b).

Although the literature is sparse and targets populations other than healthy companion animals undergoing relocation for adoption, findings consistently identify alterations in both physiology and behavior during transport. For this reason, it is incumbent upon organizations engaging in animal relocation to strategically assess their participation as an organization, establish rigorous animal selection protocols, and maintain recognition that animal relocation is but one of many tools available to protect and promote the welfare of the animals and communities they serve. Program models and operational protocols should be designed to minimize both known and anticipated negative effects on animal health and welfare.

20.4 Animal Selection and Population Considerations

20.4.1 Source and Destination Partners

Creation of animal selection criteria starts with selecting the source and destination partners themselves; it is important to evaluate each individual organization's purpose for participation in a relocation program. Balance is a key consideration when deciding which animals are eligible for transport and what portion of the eligible animals should be sent. As community resources change and grow and the resulting programs available to a source shelter change, the criteria for relocation candidates should change as well. Sending locally desired animals on transport while local adopters have no options for adoption at their community shelter is ill-advised. Losing the support and relationship with the surrounding community while sending animals to "a better place than here" is detrimental to the long-term viability of the organization. Local relationships are equally or more important than long-distance ones. Although relocation is a

valuable tool where needed, the ongoing impact should be evaluated periodically to determine when other tools and programs might benefit the local population more. It is the role of the local shelter to assist the community evolution in animal welfare. Communities that stagnate or are completely dependent on relocation should carefully consider their long-term viability and evaluate program diversification.

The destination community must also evaluate existing resources and local populations prior to making the decision to become a relocation partner. It is important to consider the purpose of the organization, the impact that relocation will have, the parameters for accepting animals, and if those parameters allow the destination shelter to be a supportive entity for the source partner. If the relationship is not mutually beneficial and the source struggles throughout the partnership, the long-term benefit to the welfare of the animals in the source community is lost. Local animals in need of sheltering should have priority over animals that are coming in from other communities. A destination must be able to meet all local, state, and federal laws for animals that are coming to the facility. They should create parameters around acceptance that align with available resources, have systems that allow for appropriate length of stay and throughput of animals, have the capacity to provide timely spay-neuter, and have the medical and behavioral care capacity to isolate and separate incoming populations to avoid disease outbreaks and provide for behavioral health needs. When deciding to become a destination community, ongoing evaluation and a risk-benefit analysis will play an important role in long-term planning. Ensuring consistent positive messaging to the public and the media when discussing the communities and the programs on both ends of the transport is a key consideration in maintaining support for the relocation program and its partners.

It is vital for source and destination shelter partners to sustain change in their communities and always focus on the future of their programs, services, organization, and community. To be a viable source community, the types, variety, and number of available animals must provide for the partnership with the destination community without overwhelming the throughput at the destination end. Sending multiple hard-to-place or medically challenged animals without first discussing the available resources at the destination is inappropriate. Animal selection for relocation requires close collaboration and communication between partners to balance the needs of both organizations and communities. Planning and consistency are important in supporting a sustainable program but equally important is frequent reevaluation and adjustment based on changing needs. Open dialogue is critical to mitigate concerns and to troubleshoot and learn from mistakes.

20.4.2 Physical Health

Once source and destination partners and the general program parameters have been established, consideration should be given to the individual animal relocation candidates and their preparation for transit. Physical and behavioral health are inextricably intertwined and dependent upon one another (see Chapter 4). As it relates to transportation and relocation of animals, physical healthcare should focus on broad spectrum preventive measures to minimize pain and suffering that can result from physical diseases and/or their treatment. Careful animal selection should also occur with the intent of identifying physical conditions that may intensify fear, anxiety, stress, or frustration during the transportation and relocation process.

Animals selected for relocation should receive prophylactic broad spectrum anthelmintics with efficacy against roundworms and hookworms. Infestation with fleas or ticks can cause considerable welfare concerns and must be addressed for all animals prior to boarding a transport vehicle.

Vaccination with modified-live virus products at the time of shelter intake is also essential and should include all core vaccines administered on a schedule appropriate for shelter animals. Rabies vaccination is also typically required prior to importation. The timing of vaccination in relation to transportation should be carefully considered. While core vaccines may take effect three to five days after primary immunization (Brun et al. 1979; Carmichael et al. 1983; Larson and Schultz 2006), delaying transport until full vaccine effect may require animals to remain at the source shelter longer than anticipated. On the other hand, vaccination on the day of transport may result in delayed recognition or treatment in the event of an anaphylactic reaction. The precise timing for vaccine administration in relation to relocation should be determined based on a risk assessment that includes the age of the animal; their vaccination history; the protocols and conditions during transportation; the operational practices, facility design, and access to veterinary care at both the source and destination shelters; the impact of the timing of vaccine administration on animals in place in the source and destination shelters; and endemic disease levels in the source and destination shelters and communities. Evaluation of canine parvovirus cases diagnosed after relocation by one program found that the number of vaccinations, timing of vaccination relative to transport, and timing from intake to transport were not related to the frequency of post-transport canine parvovirus diagnoses. Based on these findings, as long as a minimum of one modified-live virus canine parvovirus vaccination is appropriately administered, the authors believe there is no benefit to maintaining puppies selected for relocation at the source shelter for the purpose of additional vaccinations; completion of the primary vaccination series should continue after arrival at the final destination and/or adoption (DiGangi et al. 2021). Given these findings, in most relocation scenarios transport should not be delayed to wait for vaccine efficacy, but boosters due on the day of transport should be postponed. Expediting transport outweighs the risks associated with remaining at the source for a prolonged period of time where the level of pathogen exposure is likely to be much greater than on the transport vehicle or at the destination.

Some diagnostic screening tests may also be considered as a component of the preventive healthcare plan depending on the individual populations under consideration for relocation and any regulatory requirements imposed by the destination state. Common diagnostic screening tests that might be considered include Wood's lamp examination for dermatophytosis, heartworm antigen and/or microfilarial testing for dogs greater than six months of age, and retroviral screening of high-risk cats.

On occasion it may be desirable to relocate an animal with a non-contagious physical disease or altered physiological state. The appropriateness of relocating such animals should be carefully scrutinized on a case-by-case basis. Consideration should be paid to the impact of the physical condition on the animal's physiological functioning; development of and ability to cope with fear, anxiety, stress, and frustration; reduced mobility and prolonged confinement; and minimal access to food and water that will be encountered during the relocation process. Table 20.1 describes common physical conditions and their potential impacts on health and welfare that may be encountered during relocation. Prior to relocating such animals, relocation personnel should be alerted to the individual animal conditions, trained on recognition of problem development, and know how to address these needs en route. In general, animals with non-contagious physical disease or altered physiological states should not be considered for

Table 20.1 Common physical conditions and potential impacts during relocation.

Physical condition	Potential impact
Cardiopulmonary *Examples: Heart disease, heartworm disease, asthma, brachycephalic conformation*	• Decreased tolerance of heat and humidity • Decreased tolerance of alterations in air flow and ventilation • Stress-induced arrythmias (heart disease) or pulmonary thromboembolism (heartworm disease)
Metabolic *Examples: Diabetes, chronic renal disease*	• Increased access to water and ability to urinate
Musculoskeletal *Examples: Osteoarthritis, chronic bone fracture*	• May need increased and/or altered (i.e., enhanced bedding) kennel space • Confinement may exacerbate pain or cause further injury • Pain management may need to be provided during transportation
Reproductive *Examples: Pregnant, nursing, in-heat*	• Premature parturition • May need increased kennel space during transportation • Decreased ability or desire to nurse or care for young • Increased frustration around other intact animals (in-heat)
Other *Examples: Pediatrics, post-operative*	• Increased access to food and water • Decreased ability to thermoregulate • Post-operative pain and discomfort

relocation unless their safety can be ensured during the journey and their best opportunity for continued management and improved health and welfare lies at the destination.

20.4.3 Behavioral Health

Aside from excluding animals with signs of contagious diseases or those likely to suffer decompensation of existing physical conditions during relocation, physical health considerations tend to emphasize *preparing* animals for relocation. While behavioral health considerations should also include an element of individual animal preparation (e.g., acclimating animals to the transport enclosure, low-stress handling), a focus on *selection* of behaviorally appropriate candidates for relocation is critical. In addition, transportation conditions should be set up so as not to result in the development of new fears or anxieties while also mitigating the effects of potentially stressful experiences. For animals with known behavior concerns, the degree of stress associated with relocation should be balanced against the potential benefits provided at the destination.

At minimum, animals considered for relocation should be easily handled by a variety of people, able to cope with prolonged periods of confinement, and not exhibit overt aggression toward any species of animal that may also be participating in their individual transport. As with physical health conditions, it may be desirable to relocate animals with known behavioral health concerns in order to provide access to behavioral services or otherwise improve their opportunity for adoption (e.g., a city dog with fear of loud noises may best be served by relocation to an adoption center in a rural location, a dog in the southeastern United States with severe thunderstorm phobia may best be served by relocation to an adoption center in a more temperate climate). In such cases, it is incumbent upon the source shelter to disclose any and all behavioral history and observations it has obtained to the destination; given that information, the destination should make a realistic assessment of its ability to meet the needs of that individual animal prior to relocation. Again, relocation personnel should be alerted to the individual animal conditions and trained on how to recognize exacerbation of behavioral health concerns during transport and initial steps needed to address urgent needs. Animals with known behavioral health concerns should not be considered for relocation unless their safety and that of human personnel can be ensured during the journey and their best opportunity for continued management and improved health and welfare lies at the destination; those with known history of aggression toward people may be deemed ineligible.

Protocols that respect behavioral healthcare needs and mitigate the stressors encountered during the relocation process should address the following areas: animal handling, the individual animal enclosures, and vehicle construction and operation. While humane, low-stress animal handling skills should always be practiced (see Chapters 8 and 14), animal handling concerns unique to animal relocation include moving animals contained in crates, manipulating leashed dogs in close quarters, and vehicle loading and unloading practices. The micro-environmental conditions the animal experiences during relocation must also be considered. These include the characteristics of the individual animal enclosure; the presence or absence of co-occupants; and provisions such as bedding, food, water, toys, hiding spaces, and litter boxes. Finally, macro-environmental conditions that can directly impact the emotional experience of animals during relocation include the number and arrangement of animal housing units within the cargo area; the presence or absence of visual, auditory, and olfactory stimulants and/or barriers; mechanisms used for species segregation; vehicle design including HVAC capacity and means of securing animal enclosures; and driver skill and technique. Table 20.2 describes specific behavioral health considerations unique to relocation programs.

Table 20.2 Behavioral health considerations for animal relocation programs and steps to mitigate fear, anxiety, stress, and frustration.

Category	Consideration	Potential mitigation steps
Animal handling	Minimize movement and manipulation of crated animals	Carry crates from the bottom; use two people when necessary
		Place crates on rolling cart for movement
		Load cats into crates the day prior to departure
	Prepare leashed dogs for handling and confinement in close quarters	Load leashed dogs first
		Load vehicle in such a manner to minimize visual contact with other animals (e.g., front to back for a rear-loading vehicle)
		Habituate dogs to entering crates prior to relocation
	Ensure an orderly and efficient loading process	Ensure logistical considerations are completed ahead of time to minimize loading time
		Allow house-trained animals to eliminate prior to loading
	Ensure an orderly and efficient unloading process	Ensure personnel at unloading site are prepared and notified ahead of arrival to minimize unloading time
		Unload house-trained animals first and allow to eliminate prior to re-kenneling
Animal enclosure	Ensure comfort and safety during confinement	Ensure enclosures are large enough for each animal to stand up, sit, and lie down in a normal position
		Ensure enclosures contain a non-slip surface
		Provide bedding of a type and quality appropriate for the individual animal(s)
		For animals that are not house-trained, provide absorbent material to maintain sanitary conditions
	Use co-housing strategically	Reserve co-housing for littermates or bonded pairs
		Limit the number of animals co-housed as appropriate for the size of the enclosure (see above)
	Ensure adequate hydration and caloric intake	Offer treats, and refill water or provide ice chips at each observation stop
		Feed puppies and kittens <20 weeks of age a maximum of four hours prior to transport
	Minimize boredom and frustration	Provide toys of an appropriate type and quality for the individual animal(s)
		For co-housed animals, ensure sufficient toys for each individual

(Continued)

Table 20.2 (Continued)

Category	Consideration	Potential mitigation steps
	Minimize visual stressors	Provide a visual barrier that does not interfere with ventilation or ability to observe occupant
Vehicle construction and operation	Operate within physical capacity of vehicle while maintaining humane conditions	Ensure enclosures are arranged to allow direct visual observation of each animal without moving crates
		Ensure the HVAC system has the capacity to heat, cool, and ventilate the animal cargo area when loaded to full capacity
		Ensure the number of animals contained within the vehicle does not exceed that for which the HVAC can maintain appropriate environmental conditions nor that which exceeds the ability of the drivers to safely and quickly evacuate the vehicle during an emergency
	Provide calming stimuli	Intermittently play calming music at an appropriate volume within the animal cargo area
		Apply species-appropriate pheromones to bedding prior to loading animals
	Reduce stressful stimuli	Install visual barriers between opposing rows of kennels in such a way as to not interfere with ventilation or ability to observe occupant
	Ensure species separation	Avoid mixed-species transports
		When transporting multiple species in the same vehicle, ensure physical, visual, and auditory separation
	Ensure animal safety	Ensure a means of securing each individual enclosure to the body of the vehicle; restraints should be sufficient to prevent dislodging of crates during a rollover and allow for containment of animals in the event of evacuation or vehicle breakdown
	Ensure animal and human safety on the road	Ensure drivers are trained to operate the specific vehicle they will drive in such a manner as to avoid sudden starts, stops, turns, etc.
		Enforce maximum driving time and minimum resting time periods as required by the Department of Transportation for commercial drivers
		Require two drivers to participate in each transport in the event of a human or animal emergency

20.4.3.1 Sedatives and Anxiolytics

Although the efficacy of psychopharmaceutical therapy in companion animals is well established, no data have been evaluated regarding their use in companion animals undergoing relocation for adoption. There is no doubt that, although there are individual differences, the transportation process can result in a measurable stress response. While it is reasonable to assume that psychopharmaceuticals would have similar effects in this population, the transportation experience clearly impacts normal physiology and the environment varies greatly from that of a home, a veterinary clinic, or a shelter. For these reasons, the use of sedatives or anxiolytics in animals undergoing relocation for adoption must be carefully considered and must include assessment of factors unique to such programs (see Box 20.4). Psychopharmaceuticals must only be used under veterinary direction (see Chapter 22).

A placebo-controlled, double-blind study of beagles undergoing a one-hour ground transport evaluated the impact of clomipramine on signs of anxiety or fear (Frank et al. 2006). Dogs treated with twice daily clomipramine starting three days prior to transport had a significantly lower increase in plasma cortisol, lower neutrophil:lymphocyte ratio and lower increase in neutrophil:lymphocyte ratio, and lower average heart rate during transport compared to placebo. These dogs also drooled less frequently as those on placebo as seen by video scan sampling. The authors concluded that pre-treatment with clomipramine led to decreases in physiological responses associated with stress as well as the frequency and duration of behaviors associated with anxiety in the study population.

Although designed to assess impact of treatment on handling during veterinary examination, two studies evaluated cats transported locally via ground (i.e., to a veterinary appointment) after treatment with gabapentin and trazodone. When pre-treated with gabapentin,

> **Box 20.4 Considerations for Use of Psychopharmaceuticals in Animal Relocation Programs**
>
> - Does the animal meet the behavioral health criteria established for the relocation program (i.e., Is this animal a good adoption candidate; should they be relocated?)?
> - Has this medication been administered to the animal previously, and is their response predictable with a minimum of side effects?
> - How long after administration will the medication have the desired effect?
> - Is the veterinary staff at the destination aware of the animal's medication administration history? Are they willing and able to complete the course of therapy?
> - Will the animal require re-dosing along the route to maintain the desired effect?
> - Are drivers and other personnel trained to administer medications, record the appropriate information in the medical record, and monitor for and respond appropriately to side effects?
> - How will medications be stored and handled en route, including any overnight stops?
> - What mechanisms are in place to prevent diversion of medications with human abuse potential?

cats with a history of aggressive behavior during veterinary examination demonstrated significantly reduced stress scores, aggression scores, and heart rates with treatment, while sedation scores increased (van Haaften et al. 2017). Thirty percent of cats treated with gabapentin experienced side effects shortly after administration (e.g., sedation, ataxia, hypersalivation, vomiting), and 90% experienced side effects after returning home. Cats with a history of anxiety associated with transport or veterinary examination pre-treated with trazodone showed improvement in transport-associated anxiety and ease of handling; one cat experienced transient sleepiness after the visit (Stevens et al. 2016). A protocol for successfully conditioning cats to handling, entering, and exiting a transport carrier has been described for cats in laboratory settings (Gruen et al. 2013); adapting these principles to acclimate cats to their carriers the night before transport may mitigate the need for pharmaceuticals.

The use of sedatives for animals while travelling is banned by all commercial airlines. It is likely that the physiological effects of some medications are exacerbated at altitude, as oversedation accounted for half of all canine deaths during air transport in one report (Tennyson 1995). Additional studies on the physiological effects of air transport and the pharmacokinetics of sedatives and anxiolytics under these conditions are needed; it is the authors' opinion that alternative avenues for adoption should be considered for animals requiring psychopharmaceuticals to ensure good welfare during air transport.

20.4.4 Special Populations

At their outset, large-scale relocation programs focused on highly desirable small- to medium-sized dogs and puppies. As the populations of animal welfare organizations have evolved, so have the animals being relocated. Local populations of animals that may previously have been euthanasia candidates, such as community cats or dogs with severe anxiety, are now relocated to specialized programs to help meet their specific needs. Animals are also commonly transported as a component of spay-neuter clinic services or part of large-scale animal cruelty investigations. As these programs expand it is crucial that they are well managed and monitored to ensure the welfare of the individual animal and the adopter remain key indicators of program success. Animals should not be sent without

reasonable expectation of available resources at the destination to meet their specialized needs and opportunities for adoption.

20.4.4.1 Pediatrics

Puppies and kittens 8–20 weeks of age often represent a large component of animal relocation programs. This age range is associated with key behavioral development processes as well as the development of reactivity, fears, and phobias (Overall 2013). For these reasons, particular care should be paid to the accommodations and protocols for the handling, care, and observation of pediatric animals. Specific recommendations include housing un-weaned animals with their mother in appropriately sized enclosures to accommodate nursing; co-housing with weaned littermates in an appropriately sized enclosure to reduce stress associated with social isolation; offering food and water frequently (approximately every four to six hours) to prevent hypoglycemia or ensuring that food and water dishes are attached in such a manner as to allow continual access without soiling; and providing an appropriate amount and type of bedding to ensure adequate thermoregulation and serve as a means to absorb waste.

20.4.4.2 Community Cats

Feral and community cats are one special population that frequently require transport. Such transports are generally short in distance to bring cats to and from surgical clinics or to return them to their community homes. The safe transport of community cats requires additional equipment, time, and patience to achieve minimal human contact and the least amount of stress. Whenever possible, these cats should be moved in a covered trap, transfer cage, or feral cat den. Although a cover decreases the ability to monitor the cat, the stress reduction that comes with the ability to hide and the short duration of these transports often outweigh the need to continuously visualize each cat. Considering the spay-neuter service's specific protocols will guide trappers and transporters in the selection of an appropriate enclosure type, help create a smooth transition for the cats, and foster a positive working relationship with caretakers. For example, some clinics may require that the cats remain in a trap to facilitate handling and drug dosing based on known trap sizes and weights. Transfer cages also offer consistency in enclosure dimensions that may facilitate transport or handling throughout the clinic. However, their small size renders them inappropriate for recovery and care longer than a few hours in duration. Another option that may be discussed is the use of a feral cat den (Animal Care Equipment Services, Broomfield, CO). Also appropriate for short durations (i.e., a few hours) only, this type of enclosure may be preferred over a carrier as they are designed specifically for containing a fearful or fractious cat and the guillotine door creates a layer of safety should handling prior to sedation be required. Compliance with the requests of the clinic will ensure a safe and successful partnership.

Once the type of enclosure is selected, carefully carrying covered enclosures to the vehicle while providing slow and deliberate movement that avoids sudden drops or swinging of the trap will help mitigate stress. As with any transport, enclosures should be secured in the transport vehicle in such a way as to prevent lateral movement and to ensure stability in the event of a rollover. If a personal vehicle is used, a small tarp placed in the vehicle to provide a clean barrier that can be sanitized is recommended. Enclosures should be arranged in a single layer—never stacked—and each individual enclosure should be completely covered so that the cats are not able to see or come in contact with other cats or human handlers. Securing animal enclosures in a personal vehicle can be challenging, though a combination of seatbelts and rubber bungee tarp straps affixed to the vehicle itself may be effective. Purpose-built transport vehicles may contain shelving to increase carrying capacity as well as D-rings and/or E-track rails to facilitate

securing of enclosures to the vehicle. Although not evaluated specifically in community cats during transport, pheromone sprays and feline-specific music may help reduce anxiety (Shu and Xianhong 2021; Hampton et al. 2020; Kronen et al. 2006).

20.4.4.3 Shy, Fearful, or Undersocialized Dogs
Programs that meet the needs of dogs that are shy, fearful, or undersocialized are becoming more common. Well-thought-out processes that help these dogs maintain behavioral health and actively work to prevent transport-induced decline are essential. When loading dogs that are undersocialized and have severe fear or anxiety, use extra caution to prevent bites and escape while employing low-stress handling to minimize stress. The authors recommend using both a Martingale collar with a leash and a slip lead during loading/unloading to limit the chance of escape. Dogs that are not a bite risk can still be an extreme flight risk. GPS trackers for extreme flight risk dogs provide an additional layer of safety, if resources are available. Creating protocols and providing training to staff so that these transports run smoothly is important to minimizing stress for both the drivers and the dogs.

20.4.4.4 Spay-Neuter Clinic Transports
Many spay-neuter clinics transport animals in order to increase access to veterinary services. When transporting owned animals, it is important that the organization consider legal requirements for safe transport. A release from the owner should be drafted with the assistance of an attorney and include release from liability in the event of an accident or injury during transportation. Checking with groups that offer similar programs will help streamline that process. Seeking appropriate coverage from a local insurance carrier or an insurance company that specializes in animal welfare policies will be a crucial part of protecting the

organization and shielding the individuals involved from personal liability. Awareness of the current best practices for transport will be vital to provide the safe transport of owned pets and ensure the owner is informed of the conditions their pet will experience and any pre-transport preparations that may be indicated, such as fasting. Overloading the vehicle, not having an acceptable means of fastening all kennels to the vehicle structure, or accepting inappropriate kennels or containers to transport the animals can increase risk and liability and damage the professional reputation of the organization.

20.4.4.5 Cruelty Investigations

Cruelty investigations often result in the need to transport large numbers of animals or multiple species to a safe location away from a crime scene for forensic examination and/or holding. Ensuring that those animals are documented, safely transported, and medically managed while maintaining chain of custody can be key to a successful case. When live animals are intended as evidence, each animal must be photographed (along with their living environment) in situ and documented on an evidence log. It is recommended that each animal be photographed as loaded into the transport vehicle, but at minimum, they must be logged on the evidence receipt and a transport manifest containing their identification number and description. Testimony may be required regarding the humane and professional transport of the animals, adherence to state and federal regulations, and investigators should document the conditions during the transport, the distance travelled, and any stops where animals are provided with food, water, or rest.

Some of the animals that are part of a crime scene may be a danger to each other or to investigators and transporters. Similar principles apply to both fighting dogs and fighting roosters when it comes to the importance of always keeping them physically separated, but the ability to escape is more commonly associated with fighting dogs. Whether housing animals at the scene, in a holding facility, or in a transport vehicle, care should be taken not to place animals from dog fighting scenes near each other. When determining loading order, consideration should be given to where the dogs were located on-scene; aggression is frequently worse between unfamiliar dogs than between dogs that are known to each other due to adjacent housing on-scene. Regardless, caution is necessary as strong, aggressive dogs have been known to escape from standard kennels and injure themselves or attack other dogs. Kennels must have no leverage attachments that may facilitate an escape (e.g., bowls or leashes attached to the door). Such items should be removed when preparing a vehicle for transport of these populations. Additional door security such as multiple locking latch systems, solid barriers that limit visual stimuli, and metal door liner inserts are additional considerations that may help keep both dogs and drivers safe.

Other animals that are victims of cruelty or abuse should be housed and handled in such a manner to minimize fear, anxiety, stress and frustration. The same principles apply as described above for community cats and undersocialized dogs. In some situations (e.g., hoarding, puppy mill cases), pair housing of familiar, social animals may be appropriate. Operating procedures and carefully executed plans for transport should play a key role in the planning stage of every case. More information about managing a cruelty investigation can be found at www.aspcapro.org/casetools.

20.5 Outcomes

20.5.1 Physical and Behavioral Health

A few studies have evaluated medical and behavioral outcomes in dogs and cats after relocation. One survey investigated medical and behavioral characteristics as reported by adopters of dogs imported into the United Kingdom (Norman et al. 2020). Although 20% of the dogs were imported with known health conditions, the survey was not designed to identify the development of unanticipated health concerns post-adoption. Nearly half of adopters thought their dog underwent a formal behavior "test" prior to importation. The overall prevalence of problem behaviors in the study population was thought to be similar to that of dogs from local shelters; the most common problems reported included fear of strange noises and objects, refusing to come when called, pulling on the leash, and fear of strangers. Just over two-thirds of adopters sought training or behavioral help after adoption, most commonly via the internet, and the majority of those who sought help were able to resolve those problems. Only 1% of dogs had been rehomed, primarily due to behavior problems.

Animal outcomes, the incidence of spay-neuter complications, and incidences of canine infectious respiratory disease, gastrointestinal disease, and dermatologic disease were described in a group of dogs transported by ground or air from out-of-state to a shelter in the northwestern United States (Doyle et al. 2020). Ninety-nine percent of relocated dogs were adopted after a mean length of stay of 9 days. Among adopters who were contacted 30 days post-adoption, 10% of adopted animals were returned to the shelter. Two percent of dogs developed spay-neuter complications within two weeks of relocation, though neither timing of spay-neuter (i.e., whether it was performed at the source or destination) nor method of transportation impacted the rate or likelihood of complications or disease incidence. Disease incidences were ≤5% both in the destination shelter and at 30-day follow-up, except for canine infectious respiratory disease, which was 17% at follow-up. It is worth noting that, although the timing of spay-neuter surgery did not impact disease

incidence, the authors recommend surgical sterilization be performed at the destination shelter in order to balance resources such as surgical capacity, length of stay, and community need.

A final study evaluated the prevalence and risk factors for development of upper respiratory infection (URI), feline panleukopenia, and dermatophytosis in cats transported by ground or air into a shelter in the northwestern United States (Aziz et al. 2018). The average transport time for these cats was more than 17 hours and average length of stay at the destination was 18 days. Ninety-five percent of cats were adopted and <6% were returned within 30 days. Prevalence of URI, feline panleukopenia, and dermatophytosis was 25.8%, 1.6%, and 0.9%, respectively; younger, age, longer time in transport, and longer length of stay were associated with increased URI prevalence.

Although the authors are unaware of any objective data describing post-transport acclimation practices, these undoubtedly play a key role in the ultimate impact on welfare of the individual animals relocated. Handling, housing, and husbandry practices should be designed to minimize fear, anxiety, stress, and frustration and maximize animal welfare (see Chapters 8, 10, 14, and 16).

20.5.2 Data Collection and Reporting

It is rewarding to send a vehicle of animals off on a life-saving journey to a destination partner and completing a successful transport is certainly a reason to celebrate as an organization and community. However, the success of an individual transport must be based on the experience of and outcome for each individual animal. Similarly, the success of an animal relocation program as a whole must be based on community-level animal sheltering trends. At a minimum, both source and destination partners should track the number of animals relocated, the incidence of unanticipated medical and behavioral concerns, and animal outcomes (AVMA 2020a). These data can be used to develop protocols to enhance physical and behavioral health of transported animals, inform operational protocols at the source and destination organizations, and guide strategic direction of the program. Tracking total length of stay (source + destination) provides important information about the overall duration of the animals' time in shelter, and complements other metrics, such as outcome, that are important for animal welfare and for program planning.

Data collection may be facilitated through the reporting function of various shelter management software packages. Where not feasible, logging and summarizing key data points in standard software can allow for more customized analyses. Consideration should be given to the timing of data collection relative to relocation as well as to the frequency and types of analyses needed based on the desired program outcomes. The authors have found that collecting non-urgent animal health and outcome data within 14 days of relocation and performing a quarterly analysis of aggregate data will capture the majority of concerns with individual animals, shelter partners, and programmatic trends and allow for a timely response when needed. This information should then inform programmatic decisions and operational policies regarding animal selection and preparation, thereby improving short-term success and long-term viability of the program.

Although much more difficult to quantify, the development of strong relationships between the source shelter, destination shelter, and any third-party transporters is critical to the long-term success of relocation programs. All parties must be familiar and comfortable with the operational practices of each participant, agree upon the expectations for data collection, be reliable in transportation logistics, be transparent with and adhere to characteristics of animals deemed eligible or ineligible for the program, troubleshoot issues collaboratively, and generally strive to maintain a supportive partnership.

20.6 Conclusions

Animal relocation programs serve an important function in reducing and ultimately eliminating euthanasia of safe, healthy companion animals in the United States. They are one tool in the toolbox that can help improve opportunities for and access to companion animal adoptions. Comprehensive sterilization strategies, humane education and laws, and programs to promote and enhance pet retention are also critical spokes in a comprehensive non-lethal companion animal population control plan.

Animal transport is not without risk; it can be (and often is) done poorly. Disaster and emergency scenarios, whether real or perceived by well-intentioned individuals and organizations, should strive to adhere to the same basic principles of good transportation and relocation practices. Though the means of conveyance, the application of these concepts, and operational practices may differ, the animals' needs remain the same regardless of the scenario. Disregard for such concepts promotes the spread of infectious disease, places animals and humans at risk for physical and psychological harm, and jeopardizes the feasibility and longevity of relocation programs for the animal welfare community at large.

With scientific data and knowledge of basic animal needs, relocation programs can be designed and operated with the objective of protecting and promoting physical and behavioral health. When effective, relocation programs help ensure that animals reach their ideal placement as safely and efficiently as possible until the disparity between areas of supply and demand balance out and every companion animal has found their home.

Please visit the companion website for video clips and downloadable resources associated with this chapter.

References

American Veterinary Medical Association (AVMA). (2020a). Non-emergency Relocation of Dogs and Cats for Adoption within the United States. https://www.avma.org/sites/default/files/2020-03/AWF-TransportAdoptionBestPractices.pdf (accessed 19 March 2020).

American Veterinary Medical Association (AVMA). (2020b). Air Travel and Short-Nosed Dogs FAQ. https://www.avma.org/resources-tools/pet-owners/petcare/air-travel-and-short-nosed-dogs-faq (accessed 29 April 2020).

Animals and Animal Products, 9 C.F.R. § 3.5 (2016).

The Association for Animal Welfare Advancement (AAWA). (2019). Companion Animal Transport Programs Best Practices. https://cdn.ymaws.com/theaawa.org/resource/resmgr/files/2019/BP_Updated_March2019.pdf (accessed 19 March 2020).

Association of Shelter Veterinarians (ASV). (2010). Guidelines for Standards of Care in Animal Shelters. https://www.sheltervet.org/assets/docs/shelter-standards-oct2011-wforward.pdf (accessed 19 March 2020).

Aziz, M., Janeczko, S., and Gupta, M. (2018). Infectious disease prevalence and factors associated with upper respiratory infection in cats following relocation. *Animals*. https://doi:10.3390/ani8060091.

Bergeron, R. Scott, S.L., Émond, J. et al. (2002). Physiology and behavior of dogs during air transport. *Can. J. Vet. Res.* 66: 211–216.

Blood, D.C. and Studdert, V.P. (1999). *Saunders Comprehensive Veterinary Dictionary*, 2nd ed. Edinburgh, UK: Harcourt.

Brun, A., Chappuis, G., Précausta, P. et al. (1979). Immunisation against panleukopenia:

Early development of immunity. *Comp. Immunol. Microbiol. Infect. Dis.* 1 (4): 335–339.

Carmichael, L.E., Joubert, J.C., and Pollock, R.V. (1983). A modified live canine parvovirus vaccine. *II. Immune response. Cornell Vet.* 73(1): 13–29.

Cannas S, Evangelista, M., Attilio Accorsi, P. et al. (2010). An epidemiology study on travel anxiety and motion sickness. *J. Vet. Behav.* 5 (1): 25–26.

Department of Transportation. (2010). "Short-Faced" Dogs More Prone to Death in Flight, According to DOT Data. https://www.transportation.gov/sites/dot.dev/files/docs/Canine_Deaths_Press_Release.pdf (accessed 28 April 2020).

DiGangi, B.A., Craver, C., and Dolan, E.D. (2021). Incidence and predictors of canine parvovirus diagnoses in puppies relocated for adoption. *Animals*. https://doi.org/10.3390/ani1041064.

Dillane, M. (2020). Driver Killed in SC Box Truck Crash, Dogs in Vehicle Being Assisted by Shelter. https://www.azcentral.com/story/news/local/phoenix-traffic/2020/05/15/phoenix-animal-rescuers-ann-watson-christopher-kracht-14-dogs-killed-crash-on-way-to-canada-shelter/5204207002/ (accessed 14 July 2020).

Doyle, E., Gupta, M., Spindel, M. et al. (2020). Impact of the timing of spay-neuter related to transport on disease rates in relocated dogs. *Animals*. https://doi.org/10.3390/ani10040630.

Ellis, S.L.H., Rodan, I., Carney, H.C. et al. (2013). AAFP and ISFM feline environmental needs guidelines. *J. Fel. Med. Surg.* https://doi.org/10.1177/1098612X13477537.

Frank, D., Gauthier, A., Bergeron, R. (2006). Placebo-controlled boule-blind clomipramine trial for the treatment of anxiety or fear in beagles during ground transport. *Can. Vet. J.* 47 (11): 1102–1108.

Gandia Estellés, M. and Mills, D. (2006). Signs of travel-related problems in dogs and their response to treatment with dog appeasing pheromone. *Vet. Rec.* 159: 143–148.

Gruen, M.E., Thomson, A., Clary, G. et al. (2013). Conditioning laboratory cats to handling and transport. *Lab. Anim.* 42: 385–389.

Hales, J.R.S. and Bligh, J. (1969). Respiratory responses of the conscious dog to severe heat stress. *Experientia* 25: 818–819.

Hampton, A., Ford, A., Cox, R.E. et al. (2020). Effects of music on behavior and physiological stress response of domestic cats in a veterinary clinic. *J. Fel. Med. Surg.* https://doi:10.1177/1098612X19828131

Hoffman, B. (2020). Phoenix Animal Rescuers, 14 Dogs Killed in Idaho Crash while Heading to Canada Shelter. https://abcnews4.com/news/local/driver-killed-in-sc-box-truck-crash-dogs-in-vehicle-being-assisted-by-shelter (accessed 14 July 2020)

Kronen, P.W., Ludders, J.W., and Hollis, N.E. (2006). A synthetic fraction of feline facial pheromones calms but does not reduce struggling in cats before venous catheterization. *Vet Anaesth. Analg.* 33: 258–265.

Kuhn, G., Lichtwalkd, K., Hardegg, W. et al. (1991). The effect of transportation stress on circulating corticosteroids, enzyme activities and hematological values in laboratory dogs. *J. Exp. Anim. Sci.* 34 (3): 99–104.

Larson, L.J. and Schultz, R.D. (2006). Effect of vaccination with recombinant canine distemper virus vaccine immediately before exposure under shelter-like conditions. *Vet. Ther.* 7 (2): 113–118.

Leadon, D. and Muyllins, E. (1991). Relationship between kennel size and stress in greyhounds transported short distances by air. *Vet. Rec.* 129: 70–73.

Lindig, A.M., McGreevy, P.D., and Crean, A.J. (2020). Musical dogs: A review of the influence of auditory enrichment on canine health and behavior. *Animals* 10 (1): 127.

National Research Council. (1996). Animal environment, housing, and management. In: *Guide for the Care and Use of Laboratory Animals*, 21–55. Washington DC: National Academies Press.

Norman, A., Stavisky, J., and Westgarth, C. (2020). Importing rescue dogs into the UK: Reasons, methods and welfare considerations. *Vet. Rec.* https://doi:10.1136/vetrec-2019-105380.

Ochi, T, Yamada, A., Naganuma, Y. et al. (2016.) Effect of road transportation on the serum biochemical parameters of cynomolgus monkeys and beagle dogs. *J. Vet. Med. Sci.* 78 (5): 889–893.

Overall, K. (2013). Normal canine behavior and ontogeny: Neurological and social development, signaling, and normal canine behaviors. In: *Manual of Clinical Behavioral Medicine for Dogs and Cats.* St. Louis, MO: Elsevier.

Polak, K. (2019). Dog transport and infectious disease risk: An international perspective. *Vet. Clin. N. Am. Small Anim. Pract.* 49: 599–613.

Rowan, A. and Kartal, T. (2018). Dog population & dog sheltering trends in the United States of America. *Animals.* https://doi:10.3390/ani8050068.

Shu, H. and Xianhong, G. (2021). Effect of a synthetic feline facial pheromone product on stress during transport in domestic cats: A randomized controlled pilot study. *J. Fel. Med. Surg.* https://doi:10.1177/1098612X211041305.

Stevens, B.J., Frantz, E.M., Orlando, J.M. et al. (2016). Efficacy of a single dose of trazodone hydrochloride given to cats prior to veterinary visits to reduce signs of transport- and examination-related anxiety. *J. Am. Vet. Med. Assoc.* 249 (2): 202–207.

Tefft, B. (2016). Acute sleep deprivation and risk of motor vehicle crash involvement. Washington: AAA Foundation for Traffic Safety. Report.

Tennyson, A.V. (1995). Air transport of sedated pets may be fatal. *J. Am. Vet. Med. Assoc.* 207: 684.

van Haaften, K.A., Eichstadt Forsythe, L.R., Stelow, E.A. et al. (2017). Effects of a single preappointment dose of gabapentin on signs of stress in cats during transportation and veterinary examination. *J. Am. Vet. Med. Assoc.* 251 (10): 1175–1181.

Venable E.G., Bland S.D., Holscher, H.D. et al. (2016). Effects of air travel stress on the canine microbiome: A pilot study. *Intl. J. Vet. Health. Sci. Res.* 4 (6): 132–139.

Zawistowski, S. and Morris, J. (2013). Introduction to animal sheltering. In: *Shelter Medicine for Veterinarians and Staff*, 2nd ed. (eds. L. Miller and S. Zawistowski), 3–12. Hoboken, NJ: Wiley Blackwell.

21

Behavioral Care of Animals in Disasters, Cruelty Cases, and Long-Term Holds

Victoria A. Cussen, Bridget Schoville, and Pamela J. Reid

21.1 Introduction

This chapter addresses the behavioral care of animals originating from special circumstances: rescued during natural disasters and housed in temporary field shelters; confiscated from cruel or neglectful circumstances and suffering varying degrees of behavioral challenges; and enduring long-term stays in the shelter because of legal holds. These circumstances represent substantial challenges to maintaining animal welfare and even make it challenging to alleviate suffering. Short-term challenges include: severe acute trauma (i.e., from the disaster itself); the loss of secure attachment figures (owners); and acute stressors associated with the rescue effort, including noises, equipment, handling, and transport. Long-term challenges include: chronic stress due to an inadequate social and/or physical environment prior to rescue, sometimes during sensitive developmental periods; emotional and behavioral learned responses stemming from cruelty (e.g., extreme anxiety and escape attempts); and chronic stress due to extended exposure to shelter stressors (Taylor and Mills 2007).

Time in a shelter, whether temporary or permanent, is often unavoidable and necessary to secure rescued animals' future physical and psychological well-being. The negative welfare consequences of this time can prove challenging to mitigate. The impact of stressors, including those related to the shelter environment, varies between and within individuals over time. Vulnerability to stressors is also influenced by life history and genetic predispositions. However, all sheltered animals are potentially at risk. Even when facing extraordinary circumstances and limitations, best efforts should be made to prevent, mitigate, or eliminate negative welfare consequences and to facilitate psychological well-being. This chapter focuses on how to achieve these goals when caring for animals sheltered in special circumstances.

21.2 Disasters

Sheltering animals during or following natural disasters, such as floods, wildfires, earthquakes, hurricanes, and tornadoes, can be especially challenging. While pet owners are encouraged to include their animals in evacuation plans, this is sometimes not possible, and even if they do accompany their owners, inevitably, there will be animals who need sheltering in the wake of a disaster.

Disasters vary in predictability. Seismologists can predict where an earthquake will occur but are unable to forecast when a quake is likely to happen. It is also not always possible to prepare for the possible secondary effects of

Animal Behavior for Shelter Veterinarians and Staff, Second Edition. Edited by Brian A. DiGangi, Victoria A. Cussen, Pamela J. Reid, and Kristen A. Collins.
© 2022 John Wiley & Sons, Inc. Published 2022 by John Wiley & Sons, Inc.
Companion website: www.wiley.com/go/digangi/animal

a major earthquake, such as tsunamis, floods, fires and landslides, because they follow so quickly afterwards. Wildfires typically have a rapid onset and can change path or intensity in an instant with changes in wind direction and the density of flammable materials in an area. Hurricanes, floods, and tornadoes may have a slower onset, and their paths may be more predictable, but it's often impossible to anticipate the degree of destruction they will cause.

In 2006, after Hurricane Katrina, the United States established the Pets Evacuation and Transportation Standards Act to include service animals and pets in disaster planning. The act makes it possible for the Federal Emergency Management Agency (FEMA) to provide funding to states and localities for the operation and maintenance of pet-friendly emergency shelters or animal and human colocated shelters. This act was deemed necessary after as many as 44% of pet owners refused to evacuate and remained in danger during Hurricane Katrina because they weren't willing to abandon their pets (Fritz Institute 2006). Whether animals accompany their owners out of disaster areas or are left behind to be rescued, large numbers of animals continue to need sheltering and care following a natural disaster (Green 2019).

21.2.1 Animal Population

Many animals rescued after a natural disaster and housed in a temporary shelter will be owned pets. Pet owners often intend to take their animals to safety (Day 2017) but, for any number of reasons, they may be unable to evacuate with their pets. For example, they may be caught up in the disaster and separated from their animals. Sometimes the people themselves need to be rescued, or they may even be killed. Other animals rescued in a disaster are free-roaming, such as stray and feral animals (see Box 21.1 for definitions).

If the disaster occurs in an area where rescuers anticipate that free-roaming animals are likely to be caught and brought to the shelter, it is critical to identify feral and severely undersocialized animals quickly and make alternative arrangements for them. Sometimes the local people can advise on whether the animals are known to be feral. These animals will be unaccustomed to being confined or handled and are likely to be extremely stressed when in proximity to people. If the locale requires a lengthy hold period before designating an animal as unowned, the authors advise petitioning to get the hold time reduced in the wake of a disaster primarily so that undersocialized and feral animals can be removed from the stressful shelter environment as soon as possible.

In the United States, cats are the species most likely to be feral or undersocialized, as free-roaming dogs are relatively rare. It can be a significant challenge to distinguish undersocialized and feral cats from cats who are shut down because of the trauma of the disaster, the rescue, and/or the stress of the shelter environment. The Feline Spectrum Assessment is currently the best tool available for identifying feral cats (Slater et al. 2013a, 2013b). Depending upon local regulations, adult cats may be candidates for desexing and returning to the area where they were trapped. The prognosis for taming adult feral and extremely undersocialized cats is poor, so if a return to a community cat colony is not possible and the only option is long-term confinement, euthanasia may be the most humane outcome (see Chapter 7 for additional discussion of community cat management). Box 21.2 presents a case study of feral dogs rescued in St. Croix in the aftermath of Hurricane Maria.

21.2.2 Housing and Husbandry

Regional or national organizations or coalitions of groups, such as the National Animal Rescue and Sheltering Coalition, often step in to rescue animals, particularly when local animal shelters are damaged or destroyed during a disaster. As the animals are rescued, they need safe housing and medical and behavioral care.

Transporting animals out of the disaster area to provide housing or fostering animals in individual homes may seem ideal from a welfare

---

Box 21.1   Types of Animals Encountered in Disasters

Free-roaming. An umbrella category for dogs that are not under human control. It includes feral, stray, and pet dogs. Category definitions differ across authors and are not necessarily static; depending on the definition used, dogs can move between categories during their life (Coppinger and Coppinger 2016).

Stray. Currently or recently owned dogs that are separated from their owners for any number of reasons, such as becoming lost or being abandoned. Boitani and colleagues (1995) distinguish strays from other free-roaming populations based on their social bonds with humans: in the absence of their prior attachment figure, they will seek out a new bond (Boitani et al. 1995). This is supported by recent research findings, which indicate that shelter dogs form attachments to humans more indiscriminately compared to owned dogs (a phenomenon called "disinhibited attachment"; Thielke and Udell 2020).

Feral. Feralization is a process that happens to a population of animals over several generations, involving changes in the frequency of alleles in the population due to the relaxation of artificial selection and the application of natural selection pressures (i.e., the reverse of the domestication process; Price 1984). Therefore, it is likely that feralization is characterized by an increased frequency of animals exhibiting fear and/or defensive aggression toward humans. The animal sheltering community uses the term in a looser sense, as relates to the behavior of an individual animal (Daniels and Bekoff 1989), especially where no affiliative behavior is shown toward humans (Boitani et al. 1995). This means the label could be applied both to genetically feralized animals and to strays that have lost their desire for social interaction with humans. This complicates comparisons between studies (Boitani et al. 1995) and hinders the sheltering community's ability to predict behavioral outcomes for "feral" animals and their offspring.

Undersocialized. A colloquial term used in the animal sheltering sector to refer to a cat or dog that did not receive exposure to humans and/or the human environment during their sensitive period of development. Because there is no empirically supported "optimum" level of socialization, there is no set threshold amount under which an animal becomes "undersocialized." The term is applied to animals exhibiting moderate to severe fear of people or situations commonly encountered by pet animals.

Box 21.2   The Challenge of Undersocialized Dogs in a Disaster Shelter

In 2017, the ASPCA responded to the island of St. Croix in the aftermath of Hurricane Maria. Several feral dogs, known to the locals, were trapped by rescuers and brought to the temporary shelter because they were no longer being fed by the residents and were ranging onto the roadways. These animals were unable to be handled or walked on a leash, which meant they were confined to wire crates 24/7 and constantly exposed to frightening stimuli during operational hours. The best available option for these dogs was to house them in a quieter area, next to each other. De-sexing and returning the dogs to the field was not a legal option, so once the hold time was up, special measures were taken to perform low-stress euthanasia of the adult dogs (Barton and Reid 2018). Because they were still within their sensitive period for socialization with humans, four feral pups under three months of age were transported back to the mainland United States for rehabilitation and eventual successful placement in pet homes.

perspective, but the potential impacts of these options on pet-owner reunification should be considered. The more logistically difficult it is for people to reclaim their pets, especially if they are homeless and have no ability to travel, the more likely it is that animals will remain unclaimed. Not only does this leave animals in need of new homes; pet loss following a disaster is a significant source of psychological distress for the human survivors (Hunt et al. 2008).

Thus, the best option is often to shelter the animals at a temporary central location, such as a warehouse or other large structure that wasn't designed to house animals. Due to the urgency of the situation and the lack of available resources, pets are often kept in hastily constructed enclosures, pens, or wire crates. Usually, there isn't the ability to house cats in a building or room separate from dogs, and the best that can be accomplished is to hang tarps to provide a visual and nominal sound barrier to minimize stress for the cats.

Compatible pets from the same household should be co-housed if possible. The next best option is to make sure pets from the same household are positioned next to each other. The cages or crates should be touching so that bonded animals can be in physical contact through the bars if they choose. If the pets come from a multispecies household, the best that can be done may be to assess how disruptive the dog(s) would be in the cat area or how distressed the cat(s) would be in the dog area and choose the least unsettling option.

Providing opportunities for animals to relieve themselves away from their feeding, drinking, and sleeping areas is especially important when caring for owned pets (Wagner et al. 2014). Dogs that are housed in small enclosures or crates need to be walked regularly to allow opportunities for elimination outside. Most owned dogs are housetrained and will be reluctant to eliminate in an enclosure. Some will even refuse to eliminate inside a building. Well-housetrained dogs will become distraught if unable to eliminate outside for lengthy periods of time. These individuals should be identified

as quickly as possible and prioritized for walks first and last during operational hours as well as frequently and regularly throughout the day so they can anticipate a routine schedule. Cats can have strong substrate preferences for elimination and may refuse to use a litterbox with unfamiliar litter. If possible, a variety of litter types should be on hand to offer cats who are reluctant to use the standard litter provided.

In-kennel enrichment is particularly critical for pets who are confined to small cages for much of the day. Meals should be offered in puzzle toys to keep animals occupied for periods of time. Puzzles can be commercial products or "homemade" (e.g., placing food inside a cardboard box or tube). Opportunities to engage in certain repetitive movements such as chewing and licking appropriate items are considered important for alleviating stress in dogs. Chews can be zip-tied or otherwise secured to the sides of enclosures so that, when space is limited, dogs can lie down and chew at the same time. This keeps chew items free of feces and urine. Similarly, tug toys that encourage object play can be suspended from the tops of crates to keep them clean. As with any form of in-kennel enrichment, some animals will prefer variety, while others have strong preferences for specific items. In disaster sheltering, monitoring individuals for enrichment usage typically isn't viable, so unless it's obvious that the animal is really engaged with a particular item, it's best to default to rotating items frequently (a DIY shelter-enrichment webinar is available at https://www.aspcapro.org/webinar/20180221/cheap-fun-enrichment-ideas).

By far, the most efficient and effective form of out-of-kennel enrichment for dog-social dogs, and especially puppies, is to implement playgroups as soon as dogs are medically cleared (see Chapter 13). If an outdoor enclosure is not available, a play yard can be constructed from portable steel mesh kennel panels. At one ASPCA temporary disaster shelter, a makeshift play yard was created by attaching some existing fencing to the outside of the building, as in Figure 21.1. Makeshift setups may not be secure

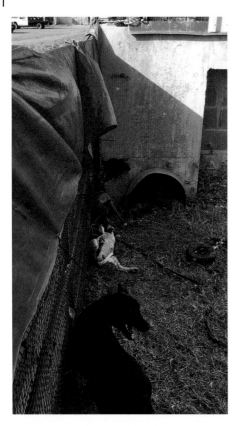

Figure 21.1 A makeshift play yard at a disaster field shelter made from existing fencing, panels, and tarps, attached to the outside of a building. *Source:* Pamela J. Reid.

so it's imperative to have dogs drag long lines (very long, lightweight leashes without loops at the end) attached to their collars to help prevent escape. Lines made of vinyl or polyurethane coated polyester webbing are preferable, as they are less likely to get caught around other dogs' limbs or on fixtures. A few structures, such as cardboard boxes, overturned chairs, crates, or folding tables, should be available inside the space to provide safe areas for dogs who need a break from the action. These should be positioned away from perimeter fencing to prevent dogs from jumping up on them to escape.

The movement of dogs through the shelter for elimination breaks, on-leash walks, and transit between their kennels and playgroup areas, can result in near-constant commotion during operational hours. Tarps hung along alleyways can help reduce the visual stimulation of dogs walking past enclosed animals and lower the stress for dogs "walking the gauntlet." Especially frightened or aggressive animals should be housed where traffic is minimal, with tarps or fiberglass reinforced panels (FRP) affixed to the fronts of their cages to serve as visual barriers. The visual barriers can be set up in a way that allows them to be opened and closed (tarps) or easily clipped on and off (FRP) to give animals access to visual stimulation when appropriate.

21.2.3 Enduring Post-Disaster Stress

Little is known about the lasting psychological impact on pets who live through a natural disaster. After the 2011 tornado in Joplin, Missouri, survivors recounted stories of having their pets swept out of their arms or sucked away through blown-out windows. Animals were trapped, some for days, under debris until rescuers were able to uncover them. As mentioned above, there are several potential sources of distress for animals affected by a disaster: the trauma of enduring the disaster itself; the experience of being displaced or abandoned; for some animals, the experience of being caught by rescuers (perhaps being lassoed or trapped); and the stay in a temporary field shelter. It is reasonable to assume that being caught and confined in a box trap is extremely stressful for some individuals, particularly undersocialized and feral animals. Wild species confined to box traps experience heightened cortisol levels, as well as increased body temperature, heart rate, and some blood metabolites associated with the physical activity of attempting to escape (Iossa et al. 2007; White et al. 1991). The administration of anxiolytics may help. Pankratz et al. (2017) demonstrated that a single dose of gabapentin reduced behavioral indications of stress in community cats trapped and brought into a clinic for sterilization. However, it remains unknown if there are long-term negative repercussions from the experience of being trapped and confined.

While animal behaviorists remain conflicted about the question of whether dogs or cats suffer something clinically analogous to human post-traumatic stress disorder (PTSD) after a traumatic event (McMillan 2020; Siegmund and Wotjak 2006), animal models of PTSD are well established in the laboratory (Flandreau and Toth 2018; Foa et al. 1992; Richter-Levin et al. 2019). Animals subjected to unpredictable and uncontrollable aversive events can exhibit generalized fear and arousal, heightened vigilance, fear of specific stimuli, and passive avoidance/resignation (Seligman et al. 1971). In a study of 14 military working dogs who failed to perform well during deployments, Burghart (2013) reported signs of hypervigilance and hyperresponsivity to normally encountered stimuli, attempts to escape or avoid previously positive or neutral environments, failure to perform previously trained responses, and changes in social interactions with their handlers. Burghart (2013) felt these behavioral changes were sufficiently like the class of behaviors suffered by human PTSD patients to dub this syndrome canine post-traumatic stress disorder (C-PTSD).

Nagasawa et al. (2012) documented physiological and behavioral effects consistent with post-traumatic stress in dogs following the 2011 earthquake in Fukushima, Japan. They compared the behavior and urine cortisol levels of 17 dogs who were abandoned after the earthquake with a control group of eight homeless dogs from Kanagawa, an area in Japan not affected by the disaster. The dogs were all housed in a rescue center and subjected to the same rehabilitation processes. Caretakers reported on the dogs' behavior through the Canine Behavioral Assessment and Research Questionnaire at one and three months into their stay. The Fukushima dogs were reported to show significantly lower levels of aggression toward unfamiliar people, poorer trainability, and less attachment to their caretakers than the control dogs. Furthermore, the Fukushima dogs' urine cortisol levels were 5- to 10-fold higher than the control dogs, and the elevation persisted even after 10 weeks in the rescue center. Nagasawa and colleagues (2012) argue that their findings suggest the dogs who endured the earthquake and the abrupt separation from their families suffered extreme and long-lasting trauma.

There is no question that companion animals suffer when separated from their primary attachment figures (Prato-Previde et al. 2003; Konok et al. 2011; Stellato et al. 2020). After Hurricane Sandy, the ASPCA established a temporary shelter where people who were displaced from their homes could bring their pets. While these animals didn't experience the trauma of being rescued by strangers, they presumably still suffered from being separated from their human families. Owners were encouraged to visit their pets at the temporary shelter and some came every day, while others were unable to come at all until they found alternative housing that would accommodate their pets. In a future disaster response, it would be enlightening to compare behavioral and physiological indicators of stress in the pets who are visited by their owners with those of animals who are only able to spend time with caretakers.

21.2.4 Reunification

Encouraging and enabling people to reclaim their pets after a disaster should be a critical component of any disaster response plan. Reuniting people and their pets not only frees up space in the temporary shelter for other animals, it also safeguards the mental health of both the pets and their owners. For example, people who permanently lost their pets after Hurricane Katrina were more likely to suffer symptoms of depression and PTSD than people who were reunited or were able to evacuate with their pets (Hunt et al. 2008). Likewise, Lowe et al. (2009) found that pet loss was a significant predictor of psychological distress in survivors of Hurricanes Katrina and Rita. At the ASPCA's temporary shelter in Joplin, Missouri after the 2011 tornado, a human psychologist was available to counsel distraught pet owners—there were people who came day after day, searching for their pets, and never found them.

Reports on the success of reunification efforts after Hurricane Katrina are mixed. According to Lowe et al. (2009), an estimated 200,000 pets were displaced in the aftermath of the hurricane, of which just 5% were reunited with their guardians. However, the Louisiana SPCA, the agency that ran a temporary shelter for more than a year after the hurricane, reported that more than 15,500 animals came through their system and that 15–20% were reunited with their families (Louisiana SPCA n.d.). After the Joplin tornado, the ASPCA housed 1,308 dogs and cats in two warehouse spaces outfitted as temporary shelters, with dogs in one building and cats in the other. A total of 526 pets (40.2%) were reunited with their owners. It's likely that the number of animals reclaimed was higher than after Hurricane Katrina because the devastation wasn't quite as widespread. At a Hurricane Sandy temporary shelter in New York City, the ASPCA cared for 164 dogs, 115 (70.1%) of which were reclaimed by their owners, and 111 cats, 65 (58.6%) of which were reclaimed. The higher rate of reunion after Sandy is undoubtedly due to the fact that most animals were brought to the shelter by their owners for temporary boarding.

From an animal behavior perspective, one of the fascinating aspects of disaster sheltering is the actual reunion between pet and owner. Most dogs seem to recognize their owners right away when they come to collect them. In the authors' experience during the Joplin tornado response, however, a few dogs appeared not to recognize their owners at first. Instead, they reacted as they would toward any unfamiliar person. But, after some time, often several seconds, each dog would suddenly seem to realize who the person was and engage in exaggerated greeting behavior, accompanied by high-pitched vocalizations. Similar anecdotes exist about dogs who have been lost in the wilderness for lengthy periods of time before being found and reunited with their families, as well as dogs greeting their owners after the owner's lengthy military deployment. Numerous examples of such dog- and cat-owner greetings can be found online. (Not surprisingly, cats are much less demonstrative!)

What could be happening here? Is the dog's recognition of her owner linked to olfaction and, for some individuals, it takes a bit of time for her to retrieve her olfactory memory? Belief in dogs' olfactory prowess is widespread (Taslitz 1990), while their visual acuity is regarded as relatively poor compared to that of humans (Byosiere et al. 2018). Perhaps because of this, it is generally assumed that dogs rely heavily on olfaction for individual recognition of conspecifics and familiar humans. However, it is unlikely dogs use olfaction as the primary means of identifying their owners. Experimental evidence suggests they also use visual and auditory cues in social recognition of con- and heterospecifics (Adachi et al. 2006; Ratcliffe et al. 2014; Taylor et al. 2011). In one study, when the cues were tested individually, visual cues were significantly better than auditory or olfactory cues for dogs engaged in a human-detection task (Fukazawa and Watanabe 2017). It seems much more likely that dogs rely on a combination of cues to create composite, multimodal "signatures" of their owners.

Perhaps the explanation for some dogs not immediately recognizing their owners lies more in the context where the reunification occurs. Research on violating expectations may be relevant here. Violation of expectation (VOE) studies assess the effect of "impossible" or incongruent scenarios—for example, a wheel rolling uphill—on cognition by measuring looking time. Longer looking times indicate increased cognitive processing of the scenario because the subject's expectations were violated. Dogs exhibit VOE in relation to incongruent physical scenarios, such as when one object is substituted for another, physically different object while out of the dog's view; in such cases, dogs look significantly longer at the incongruent object compared to congruent scenarios (Pattison et al. 2013). Could the appearance of the owner in the disaster shelter be so improbable to some dogs that they have no expectation of encountering them there? Performance of known behaviors is significantly slowed in contexts where dogs don't expect to have to perform the behavior (Fugazza et al. 2016), indicating the cognitive processing involved when expectations are violated does lead to a delay in behavior output. Therefore, it seems plausible that the appearance of a familiar human in an incongruent context could delay the processing of the owner's individual "signature," thereby slowing recognition and subsequent greeting behavior.

21.3 Cruelty Cases

21.3.1 Behavior Forensics

It is recommended that all dogs from large-scale cruelty cases undergo a formalized behavior evaluation in order to develop, over time, a behavioral profile of dogs from specific types of cruel conditions (Reid 2013). In the authors' experience, dogs from substandard commercial breeding operations (i.e., puppy mills) and hoarding circumstances, for instance, tend to show more fear of humans and environmental stimuli than shelter dogs from other backgrounds. As an example, in one population of 35 Labrador retrievers belonging to a suspected animal hoarder, the authors determined 17 (48.6%) to be so fearful that they needed behavior modification before adoption. In contrast, only 8 of 94 (9%) Labrador retrievers and Labrador mixes from other types of cruelty cases were determined to be too fearful for immediate adoption. Pit bull dogs kept for organized dogfighting, however, are more likely to be aggressive to conspecifics than pit bull dogs with no known history of organized dogfighting. Using a model dog as a stand-in for a real dog, the authors found that almost twice as many pit bull type dogs from suspected dogfighting cases exhibited aggression (45%; n = 363) than did pit bull type dogs from defunct sanctuaries (26%; n = 46) (P. Reid, ASPCA, New York, unpublished data).

By collecting and documenting these descriptive comparisons, a characteristic behavior profile of dogs from various circumstances, including puppy mills, animal hoarding situations, and organized dogfighting can be developed. These data can then lend support to the prosecution of animal cruelty in a particular case when the behavior of the animals seized in the case more or less matches the overall profile for animals from other puppy mill, hoarding, or dogfighting cases. This information is important because, while prosecutions traditionally rely exclusively on physical evidence of injury and neglect, physical insults can heal or manifest themselves in ways that are not externally apparent. In the United States and Canada, legal definitions of "cruelty" often include some reference to suffering, which opens the door to considering psychological trauma. There is a growing body of evidence that dogs living in puppy mills or intensely crowded conditions, such as animal hoarders' homes, and those exposed to chronically harsh conditions, particularly in early life, manifest epigenetic changes (Bissell 2019), physiologic changes (Lezama-García et al. 2019), and long-term behavioral deficits (McMillan et al. 2013). This suggests that dogs from these types of circumstances are likely to behave in distinctly different ways than dogs with no known history of abuse or neglect. In Canada, charges of cruelty have been based solely on the behavior of the animal when no physical injuries were present (Ledger and Mellor 2018).

21.3.2 Dogfighting

In the United States, organized dogfighting, in which dogs are pitted against each other to fight for prize money and gambling profits, almost exclusively involves the American Pit Bull Terrier and mixes of similar morphology (Miller et al. 2016). Despite it being a felony in all states, dogfighting is prevalent, and animal welfare organizations have rescued thousands of dogs destined for the fighting pit. Established dogfighters often have large numbers of dogs in their yards, even into the hundreds, which may include dogs being conditioned for fighting, proven studs and brood bitches for breeding, young dogs and puppies as future fighting prospects, and/or dogs for sale. Few dogs will be elderly unless they are especially prized for breeding.

21.3.2.1 Animal Population

Extreme conspecific aggression is common in organized dogfighting populations; these dogs characteristically direct little or no investigatory or affiliative behavior to conspecifics, instead attacking other dogs without warning behaviors. Typically, rival domestic dogs will go through a series of ritualized threat behaviors involving aggressive displays before making potentially more risky physical contact with each other. If opponents are well-matched, these displays not only provide useful information about the capabilities of the adversary but also afford the time needed for the animals to become sufficiently physiologically aroused to engage in actual fighting (Parker 1974). However, in a pit fight, there is no need to assess the opponent's abilities and determine a winner in nonviolent ways because the fight is inevitable. In fact, it is advantageous to communicate the least amount of information to one's opponent, as any behavior that signals a next move would be counterproductive. Thus, it seems that selective breeding for success in the pit has shortened the time between threat displays and physical strikes to the point that these dogs exhibit an unsignaled style of offensive aggression (Lockwood and Rindy 1987). Other species that have been bred for fighting, such as gamecocks and Siamese fighting fish (*Betta splendens*), likewise spend little time displaying, arouse quickly, and fight relentlessly (Millman and Duncan 2000; Verbeek et al. 2007).

Despite selective breeding for conspecific aggression, anywhere from an estimated 30–60% of dogs removed from suspected dogfighting cases do not exhibit it (Miller et al. 2016). Some

may have been retired from fighting and used exclusively for breeding. Most, however, tend to be puppies and juveniles who are still social and playful with other dogs. These individuals need careful pairing with playmates and shrewd guidance to increase the likelihood that they will remain affiliative as they mature.

After working with thousands of dogs from suspected dogfighting cases, it is the authors' experience that individuals from these populations are also prone to exhibiting high levels of agitation and arousal, particularly when dog movement occurs in the shelter. Even the movement of people without dogs can also create frustration. Some dogs will become highly agitated in response to the use of specific objects, brooms and mops being the most common triggers, and may be quick to bite and hold onto those same objects if they are leaned momentarily against their kennel.

Generally, dogs seized from suspected dogfighting operations are notoriously friendly with people (Lockwood and Rindy 1987). Despite this, they are prone to mouthy behavior, which can quickly escalate to hard mouthing with sustained contact. Puppies from this population can be exceptionally mouthy, both with humans and with puppy playmates (Collins et al. 2012).

21.3.2.2 Housing and Husbandry

Proper housing is critical to the successful management of dogfighting populations, due to the agitation and arousal created by sheltering numerous dog-aggressive dogs in close proximity to each other. Fighting dogs cannot be housed in regular wire crates or airline crates; they are liable to break free of these enclosures if they have visual, olfactory, or auditory contact with other dogs. Further, a highly motivated crated dog can move her crate a large distance across the floor as she thrashes about in an attempt to reach another dog or escape confinement. This is highly problematic because a crated dog can bite and cause damage through her closed crate door.

Fighting dogs must be housed in permanent or temporary kennels made of sturdy metal with secure tops, as highly motivated dogs can easily scale a wall to fight with other dogs. Most permanent and temporary kennels require additional reinforcement of the kennel door, such as a sturdy chain and carabiners, to ensure that dogs cannot break open the door or squeeze through a gap. In a temporary field shelter, care should be taken to erect kennels on a solid surface so that the dogs cannot dig and tunnel under kennel panels.

Adjacent kennels cannot be in physical contact unless they are built-in kennels with solid, permanent partitions, such as cinderblock or solid metal, because dogs can displace less sturdy kennel partitions and will take any opportunity to grab neighboring dogs' feet or tails. Dogs housed in temporary kennels may be highly agitated by the close proximity of dogs in immediately adjacent kennels. Adjacent temporary kennels should be physically separated by 1 ft. or more because dogs can slide large, heavy metal kennels across the floor as they jump with force against the side panel of their kennel toward neighboring dogs.

Visually separating adjacent kennels with a visual barrier may be necessary to further reduce agitation and the likelihood of a dog escaping or moving her enclosure in pursuit of neighboring dogs. It may be necessary to fully cover the side walls of her kennel with visual panels if she persistently leaps above the visual barriers. However, it is important to never fully eliminate her view from the kennel, leaving, at minimum, the front panel free from visual barriers. Using sturdy, rigid visual barriers, as opposed to cardboard or fabric, serves to further safeguard against dogs in adjacent kennels making physical contact with one another. For temporary shelters, a cost-effective visual barrier option is using FRP, which is relatively easy to clean and rigid (see Figure 21.2).

Subdividing housing into small sections (pods) of 10 to 12 kennels may reduce dogs' arousal and improve ease of care (see Figure 21.3). Even if dogs can see and hear activity in other pods, over time, most dogs appear to habituate to this activity and eventually stop reacting. Therefore, agitation and arousal can be reduced to only the pod in

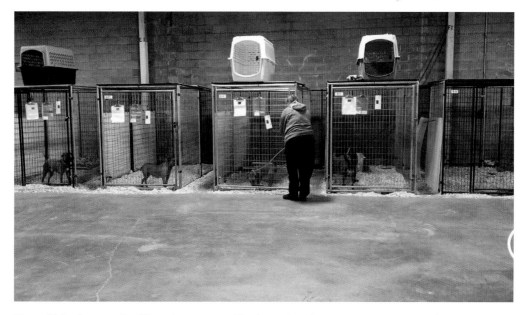

Figure 21.2 An example of kennels constructed for dogs seized from a suspected dogfighting operation. FRP panels limit the dogs' ability to become aroused at the sight of other dogs. Kennels are spaced so that dogs are unable to make physical contact with one another through the bars. *Source:* ASPCA Behavioral Sciences Team.

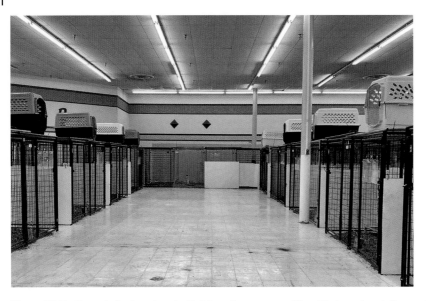

Figure 21.3 Kennels for housing dogfighting dogs arranged in a U-shaped pod. *Source:* ASPCA Behavioral Sciences Team.

which the activity (cleaning, dog movement, etc.) is happening. Because fighting dogs in a yard habituate to the sights, smells, and sounds of neighboring dogs, the authors recommend mimicking the yard layout to reduce stimulation as much as possible. Folklore has it that when a dog escapes from her chain space in a dog yard, the dog rarely fights with her neighbors; instead, she will go farther afield to a dog she cannot see from her customary vantage point. Subdividing sections of kennels into pods with a secure physical perimeter also serves to contain dogs should one escape from her kennel or escape from her handler while on leash. Due to the risk of damaging fights between dogs, it is strongly advised that only one dog is out of her kennel at a time within a secure perimeter. Secure perimeters around each pod allow for dogs in different pods to be moved simultaneously without risk of contact. To further reduce the risk of dogs contacting one another, portable two-way radios or another communication system can be used to announce dog movement.

Arranging kennels in a U-shape within each pod, as opposed to arranging kennels in rows, creates a large, open center space, ideal for kennel staff and handlers to clean and to move dogs without forced proximity to other kenneled dogs.

If kennels are arranged in rows instead of in a U-shape, care should be taken to leave wide walking aisles between the rows. Walking dogs on leash close to kenneled dogs creates intense arousal and reactivity, rendering the kennel environment highly stressful for the dog being moved as well as the dogs housed within visual or auditory range. The handler may have difficulty restraining the leashed dog to prevent her from contacting the kenneled dogs, and fights can ensue. The leashed dog may become so aroused that she redirects aggression toward the handler.

Like all dogs, fighting dogs should be provided with a bed and/or an airline crate. Crates provide a hideaway for dogs needing an escape from the stimulation of the shelter environment. In addition, crates offer an alternative vantage point and an elevated spot for resting. It is important to bear in mind, however, that fighting dogs tend to be heavy chewers and may even harm themselves chewing on kennel furnishings. Therefore, plastic airline crates, non-durable beds, and soft bedding may not be appropriate for some dogs from dogfighting populations.

Due to fighting dogs' propensity for high levels of arousal and mouthy behavior toward people, kennels should never be cleaned while dogs are inside them. If dogs cannot be shifted to the opposite side of a guillotine door during cleaning, they should be leashed and walked or moved to an alternative secure location. If they are closely supervised, it can be safe to temporarily keep fighting dogs in airline crates during the cleaning process. Care should be taken to keep the crates spatially and visually separated to reduce the dogs' motivation to escape. Some dogs cannot be safely contained in airline crates, even under close supervision, so alternative holding options should be employed to secure such dogs during cleaning.

21.3.2.3 Handling

All handlers should wear appropriate gloves when handling dogs. Gloves allow a more secure grip on the leash and afford an added layer of protection if a dog bites or mouths the handler. Handlers should be trained to hold dogs in a "control stance" when necessary (see Chapter 8, Figure 8.9). Most dogs from fighting populations are accustomed to this stance from being handled by dogfighters. The handler should first secure and control the movement of the dog's head by holding the dog's collar or a shortened leash. Then the handler straddles the dog, using the legs to apply even pressure around the dog's waist and secure the back end of the dog. If holding the collar, the handler can further control the dog's movements by gently bracing their knuckles against the base of the dog's skull. The control stance can be used proactively to prevent a dog from becoming overaroused while on leash, or it can be used to calm and manage an already aroused or aggressive dog. The restraint and even pressure applied to the dog in the control stance effectively inhibits the dog's movement and typically de-escalates the dog's arousal or aggression.

It is common for fighting dogs to bite and tug the leash as the handler attempts to leash the dog, while the handler is actively walking the dog, and/or when the handler attempts to remove the leash upon returning a dog to her kennel. One of the most effective ways to mitigate this behavior is for the handler to offer the dog a treat or toy through the neck loop of a slip leash as they slip the loop over the dog's head. Note that highly aroused dogs may grab for the objects with little regard for the handler's hand. For these dogs, a large toy or a spreadable treat (peanut butter, cheese spread, canned dog food, etc.) applied to a large piece of consumable cardboard can keep the dog's mouth occupied. For dogs who bite at the leash or the handler's hands when the leash is removed, a quick-release leash is the best solution (see Chapter 8, Section 8.6.1.2 and Figure 8.2).

If a dog does bite and hold onto a leash or another object, it might be sufficient to put her in control stance to prompt her release of an object. A dog may require the use of a startling stimulus or a break stick (see Figure 21.4) to remove an object from her mouth. A break stick is a piece of wood or very hard plastic with a handle at one end and a flattened edge at the other, which can be inserted between the dog's teeth to pry the jaw open (see Chapter 8 for an explanation of how to use a break stick). For object grabbing (including leash grabbing and tugging), it is important not to try to tug the object out of the dog's mouth, as

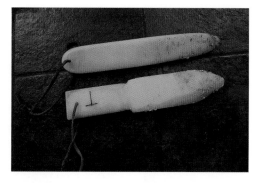

Figure 21.4 A break stick, a piece of wood or plastic with a handle at one end and a flattened edge at the other, can be used to remove an object from a dog's mouth. Training is critical to ensure that the break stick is used in an effective and humane manner. *Source:* Pamela J. Reid.

this will only encourage her to intensify tugging or to regrip the object, which may result in a bite to the handler.

For dogs that cannot be safely leashed, it may be necessary to create a temporary shift cage (see Figure 21.5). This allows for no-contact movement of the dog during the cleaning process. When possible, unsafe dogs and dogs that are exceptionally stressed by the shelter environment should be moved to a quieter, less-trafficked part of the shelter. In a calmer environment, the behavior of some of these dogs improves to the extent that they can be safely handled by experienced handlers. Care should be taken to ensure that adequate mental and physical enrichment is provided for dogs who are housed in shift cages or in isolated locations within the shelter. Psychological quality of life should be closely monitored.

21.3.2.4 Additional Safety Measures

Due to the increased risk of damaging fights between dogs from fighting populations, as well as the potential for these dogs to bite and hold on to objects or even their handlers, it is critical that safety kits are strategically placed and readily accessible throughout the shelter. Safety kits should include citronella spray, compressed air, airhorns, and break sticks.

Personnel who routinely handle fighting dogs should learn how to properly use break sticks and should carry break sticks at all times.

Untrained handlers should not attempt to intervene directly when a dog is biting an object, another dog, or a person except in extreme circumstances. They should always request the assistance of trained personnel first and then are encouraged to deploy hands-off startle tools to prompt a dog to release her bite from a safe distance. Dogs that are biting and holding may release their bite in response to a startling stimulus, such as citronella spray or compressed air. Dogs seem to find airhorns most aversive, but these can negatively impact other dogs in auditory range. Other hands-off tactics that may prove effective are shouting, banging metal bowls together, pouring a bucket of water on the dog, spraying the dog with a water hose, or placing a blanket over the dog's head. If a dog does not release her bite immediately upon deployment of any single stimulus, the handler should choose a different stimulus. Dogs that are biting and holding onto an object, dog or a person are often unfazed by startle stimuli. Experienced handlers may elect to try a startle stimulus first but should quickly change course to a hands-on approach if the dog is not immediately responsive to the startle stimulus.

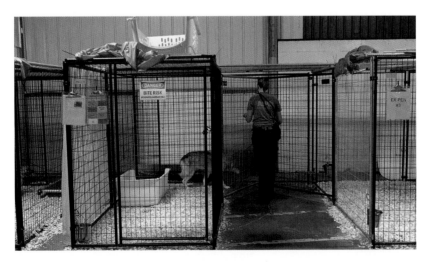

Figure 21.5 A temporary shift cage for no-contact movement of a dog during cleaning. *Source:* ASPCA Behavioral Sciences Team.

See Chapter 8 for additional suggestions on safely breaking up a dog fight.

Especially adept handlers, well-versed in fighting dog behavior, may be more successful prompting a dog to release her bite by holding the dog in a fight stance or momentarily suspending the dog in the air by the collar and the base of her tail. The former may be the most humane and appropriate way to respond to object biting. Neither might be practical if the dog is biting a human or another dog.

If a dog is biting and holding onto another dog or a human, it is prudent for trained and experienced handlers to quickly pivot to deploying a break stick. Most dogs from dogfighting populations are accustomed to being "broken" off a bite with a break stick, and it is the most surefire option. A handler who has been trained to use a break stick should always be present during operational hours in a shelter housing dogs from a dogfighting population. Training is critical to ensure that the break stick is used in an effective, humane, and safe manner.

21.3.2.5   Enrichment
21.3.2.5.1   *In-Kennel Enrichment*
Like all kenneled dogs, fighting dogs need to be routinely provided with a rotation of in-kennel enrichment items. These dogs tend to be intense chewers, so selected items should be sufficiently durable or, alternatively, safe for consumption. The authors have successfully used KONG® Extreme toys (KONG Company, Golden, CO); large, hard-plastic balls without handles or holes; bowling balls; large smoked knuckle bones; and cardboard boxes with food inside. When offering any of these or other enrichment items, initial monitoring is critical. Some dogs can chew through the KONG Extreme toys. Some dogs will bite at the large plastic or bowling balls with such vigor that they cause their gums to bleed and create jagged edges on the plastic balls that inflict cuts and scrapes. At times, fighting dogs can become so aroused and noisy playing with balls that they induce arousal and stress in dogs kenneled nearby. Additionally, they can

become overly aroused themselves. While they appear to enjoy the activity, they can become so focused and intense that they continue manipulating the object to the point of exhaustion and heat stress.

21.3.2.5.2   *Enrichment Activities*
Dogs seized from dogfighting operations tend to be athletic and highly energetic; thus, they need plenty of physical exercise and mental stimulation to keep them from becoming bored and frustrated. Weight pulling, treadmill running, flirt pole chasing, and hang time with a spring pole are particularly beneficial and enjoyable for this population and should be incorporated to the extent that shelter resources and skilled handling allow. Fighting dogs also benefit from most typical enrichment activities that should be provided to other sheltered dogs: off-leash exercise in fenced yards, games of fetch and tug, leash walks, office time, training games, and one-on-one socialization time with people. Playgroups may or may not be appropriate for fight-bred dogs (see Section 21.3.2.5.3). No matter the activity, special precautions are often needed to ensure dog and handler safety. Additionally, attention must be paid to ensure that dogs benefit from the activities; if they become agitated, hyperaroused or frustrated, the activities may backfire, causing or exacerbating stress. High-arousal activities can also ramp up other dogs in the vicinity, so it's best to hold play sessions when neighboring dogs are elsewhere.

When returning a dog to her kennel after a high-arousal activity, handlers should use caution, particularly when leashing the dog, because she may still be likely to mouth forcefully and grab indiscriminately. It is best to keep a leash attached to the dog's collar and leave it dragging throughout the activity because it provides a safe and quick means for a handler to gain control should the dog become too aroused. High-arousal activities should always be balanced by opportunities to practice impulse control exercises (e.g., "Sit," "Down," "Stay," "Wait," "Leave it," and "Drop it") and quiet, calm time socializing with people.

Modifications to enrichment activities should be made on a case-by-case basis. Some suggestions for making common enrichment activities as safe and effective as possible include:

1) One-on-one time with people: It may not be safe to socialize with a high-energy, hard-mouthing dog in her kennel, but she may calm down enough to interact safely in a quiet room or play yard, away from the chaos of kenneled dogs.

2) Fetch: Some dogs may be reluctant to release a ball or frisbee and can present a bite risk to the handler attempting to get the toy away from the dog. Throwing a second ball or frisbee often prompts the dog to drop the first. This way, the handler never has to remove a toy from the dog's mouth. To end the game of fetch, the toy can be tossed into an area that's inaccessible to the dog and, while he's searching for a way in, the handler can collect the dog. Alternatively, if a leash is left dragging on the dog during the game, the handler can pick up the handle of the leash and walk the dog back to her kennel while she is holding the toy in her mouth. Many dogs will drop the toy along the way and the handler can come back for it after securing the dog in her kennel.

3) Tug-of-war ("tug"): Playing tug can be tricky if the dog is inclined to grab at anything available, including the toy, the handler, or the handler's clothes. Adept handling and consistency are key for the game to be safe and beneficial; inexpert handling and a lack of structure to the game can worsen grabbing behavior by increasing arousal and frustration. The dog should be taught to take the tug toy only on cue, release the toy on cue, and refrain from putting her mouth on anything except for the toy. The dog can be tethered while playing tug to prevent her from lunging for the toy while it is in the handler's hands.

Despite precautions and modifications, tug and other high-arousal activities can prove counterproductive for some dogs and unsafe for handlers. For dogs like this, protected-contact tug-of-war play with experienced handlers may be necessary. The handler can interact with the dog through sturdy kennel bars so that the dog and person are not in the same physical space. Using a more complex setup, a tug toy can be suspended using a pulley system from a secure point above the dog's kennel, making the game fully contact-free. Kenneled dogs can also be enriched by target training or shaping games that the handler can conduct safely while standing outside of the dog's kennel—creative ideas can be gleaned from zookeepers who engage in protected contact interaction with exotic species.

21.3.2.5.3 Playgroups

Given the prevalence of conspecific aggression within dogfighting populations and the potential to inflict significant damage on other dogs, playgroups must be managed with extreme caution. Obviously, attempting to modify the behavior of dogs that exhibit severe aggression to other dogs in the context of playgroups is not recommended. This requires highly skilled handlers who can work with the dogs intensively and a large selection of resilient, friendly "helper dogs" who can withstand repeated exposure to aggressive dogs, which can be extremely stressful, even if the aggressive dogs are muzzled. In addition, and perhaps most importantly, in the authors' experience there is no evidence to suggest that the long-term prognosis for these supposedly "rehabilitated" dogs is anything but poor.

However, playgroups may be effective for gathering additional information about dogs who aren't clearly aggressive to other dogs but exhibit tense or awkward social behavior. Monitoring these interactions also requires highly skilled handlers. The dog being assessed should be attached to a dragline, in the event an interaction should go awry. Ideal helper dogs are social, tolerant, resilient in the face of handler corrections (in case the handler has to interrupt an interaction), and roughly the same age and size as the dog being assessed. While it is valuable to observe questionable dogs in interactions with other dogs, it is critical to consider the helper dogs' welfare. Repeated (and sometimes even a single) exposure to inappropriate or aggressive dogs, even muzzled, can have long-term or even irreparable damaging impacts on the helper dogs.

While a large percentage of dogs from dogfighting operations are typically unsafe around other dogs, a good number may be highly affiliative and playful. Some initially need guidance from handlers or other dogs to learn how to play and interact with other dogs appropriately. However, with careful playgroup management, many, especially the juveniles, will become increasingly socially adept. The play behavior of pit bull puppies from a dogfighting population (either seized as neonates or whelped in the shelter) is often indistinguishable from other terrier puppies. Collins et al. (2012) tested pit bull puppies, bred for organized dogfighting, in play dyads repeatedly, from 7 to 16 weeks of age, and observed little aggression. Some puppies, however, were persistent in biting, holding, and shaking their playmates. Often the playmates were unperturbed and continued to engage and even initiate play. Regardless, puppies who lack appropriate social behavior—do not greet but instead rush up to and relentlessly bite, hold, and shake other puppies and adult dogs and appear unfazed by corrections, either from dogs or from humans—are concerning. Unfortunately, there has been no systematic follow-up on puppies from dogfighting populations to know if their early social behavior is predictive of future aggressive behavior.

21.3.2.6 Euthanasia

As stated above, a significant percentage of dogs, particularly adults, seized from organized dogfighting operations are likely to be dangerously aggressive to other dogs and unsafe to place as companion pets in the community. Their behavior toward people is often strikingly incongruent, with many

being highly affectionate and playful. This can make it exceedingly difficult for shelter personnel to understand why dogs might be slated for humane euthanasia once the criminal case has been resolved and the shelter is awarded ownership of the dogs. Proactive and transparent communication is an especially critical strategy for mitigating compassion fatigue in those caring for fighting dog populations.

21.3.3 Puppy Mills and Animal Hoarding

Commercial breeding establishments (often referred to as "puppy mills") are facilities that keep dogs for the sole purpose of producing puppies for profit. Puppy mills that sell to pet stores, brokers, or over the internet are regulated by the United States Department of Agriculture. Federal standards of care are minimal, allowing a puppy mill to keep large numbers of dogs in small, stacked cages for their entire reproductive lives. Dogs in these facilities are typically bred at every opportunity and rarely—if ever—permitted outside of their cages to exercise. They have little to no positive interaction with people. Conditions found in substandard puppy mills include cages with excessive waste, inadequate protection from the elements, wire cage flooring that can injure dogs' paws, dogs with untreated injuries, dogs with painful matting, and contaminated food and water.

Animal hoarding, on the other hand, is a very different phenomenon. It is defined in the *Diagnostic and Statistical Manual of Mental Disorders* as "the accumulation of a large number of animals and a failure to provide minimal standards of nutrition, sanitation, and veterinary care and to act on the deteriorating condition of the animals (including disease, starvation, or death) and the environment (e.g., severe overcrowding, extremely unsanitary conditions)" (American Psychiatric Association 2013). While typically associated with older females living alone, with cats and dogs as the primary species hoarded, animal hoarding is also observed among younger individuals, males, couples, and families, and it can involve a range of companion and non-companion animal species (Lockwood 2018). In addition, sheltering organizations can sometimes be a foil for or deteriorate into a hoarding situation, although the animals won't necessarily fit the characteristic behavior profile described below because they often originate from a variety of sources. Animal hoarding poses a complex problem for both animal and human welfare due to the extent of suffering involved, challenges for stakeholder agencies in responding, and a lack of effective interventions for the people (Lockwood 2018).

21.3.3.1 Animal Population

Animals from puppy mills and hoarding situations tend to behave in similar ways and share similar needs. Dogs with these backgrounds tend to be more fearful than the general population of shelter dogs. This is because most of the animals are rarely exposed to anything beyond their enclosures. They are rarely, if ever, taken off the property even for veterinary care, so many experience severe neophobia when presented with normal, everyday stimuli. Human contact is usually limited to caretakers, although puppy mill breeding dogs may have occasional exposure to brokers or puppy buyers. Animal hoarders tend to be highly secretive, so the animals rarely encounter anyone other than their owners. Severely undersocialized, the animals can exhibit extreme fear of unfamiliar people. It's also typical for these populations to be unaccustomed to handling and restraint. They may panic when restrained and become defensively aggressive or harm themselves in their attempts to escape. Alternatively, some individuals become immobile and catatonic.

In contrast to dogs from dogfighting operations, puppy mill dogs and hoarded animals tend to be highly social or at least extremely tolerant of conspecifics. Puppy mill dogs are typically confined to pens individually, in small same-sex groups, or in groups of females housed together with a male. Dogs and cats in hoarding situations may be housed indoors or outdoors, often in large groups of reproductively intact

animals. Hoarded animals are often found in crowded conditions, sometimes with inadequate food resources, so these animals may be prone to competing with other animals over resources. Cannibalism has been documented in hoarding cases, but there is no evidence to suggest that animals that have fed on the bodies of dead conspecifics are likely to prey on or feed on their own species once adequate nutrition is available or density is reduced (Kockaya et al. 2018; Meek and Brown 2016).

21.3.3.2 Housing and Husbandry

The type of housing that is best for puppy mill dogs and dog and cats from hoarder homes is not necessarily straightforward. In the authors' experience, some animals are likely to be highly social with people and confident in novel environments while others will be extremely fearful, even within populations that appear to be closely related. Until the animals are assessed as individuals, it is probably ideal to keep them in circumstances that are relatively similar to those with which they are familiar. Puppy mills can be a lot like shelters and so puppy mill dogs may initially be most comfortable in enclosures with plenty of ongoing activity. Animals that have never been exposed to the out-of-doors are likely to be more comfortable with an indoor enclosure, whereas animals that have never been inside may find indoor housing highly stressful.

Fearful animals, particularly if they've come from a reclusive hoarder's home, may find the typical activity and commotion of a shelter environment too much to endure. While it is tempting to assume that a foster placement would be the most humane option for all fearful animals because a home is bound to be quieter and less chaotic than a shelter, for animals that have never been exposed to the sights and sounds of a home and are unaccustomed to being handled, the transition to a home may be too drastic. A shelter environment may be better equipped to provide hands-off care. Segregating fearful animals into a quieter area of the shelter, with routines that minimize activity, noise levels, and—most importantly—the number of caretakers, may be what is required to provide these animals with an acceptable quality of life until their legal case is resolved.

Because puppy mill dogs and hoarded animals tend to be fearful of humans and highly social with conspecifics, they are likely to be more comfortable when cohoused with other animals rather than when housed alone (dogs undergoing behavior modification for fearfulness are an exception). Pairs or small groups of same-sex animals are best, unless they have been sterilized, in which case male-female groups may be the most compatible (Feltes 2021). Given the potential for competition, it is advised that dogs be separated, typically by introducing barriers to split the enclosure into sections or by encouraging individual dogs to enter adjacent pens when feeding or providing edible or chewable enrichment items. Alternatively, chew items can be spaced out and affixed to the sides of the pen to encourage the dogs to spread themselves out and prevent an individual dog from amassing all the items. Social cats may be housed in pairs or groups by ensuring that they have adequate real estate, including vertical spaces and hiding spots, and by including multiple separate areas for feeding, resting, and eliminating. Some cats are prone to competing and may be more likely to guard resting areas and litter boxes, so it's important to make sure there are plenty of equally desirable options.

Fearful animals should always be housed in enclosures with secure tops and floors so that they are unable to escape confinement. They also need options for taking cover from people and normal sheltering activities going on outside their enclosures. Airline crates make good hiding spots for dogs; the tops can be zip-tied along one side and unsecured on the other to work like a clamshell if a dog needs to be removed easily. (This setup is much preferable to elevating the back end of the crate so that the dog is dumped out or pulling the dog out of the crate using a leash.) If crates are unavailable, another option is to cover part of the enclosure with FRP so the dog can retreat behind the barrier to escape the stimulation of high activity. Resist the temptation to cover the entire enclosure; complete isolation is not ideal even for extremely fearful animals because they can hear and smell but not see what's going on outside of their enclosure. They should at least have visual access to the outdoors or to other animals. Yet another possibility is a shower curtain mounted over the front of the enclosure that can be pulled across whenever there are potentially scary activities happening in the aisle. Likewise, fearful cats need airline crates, feral boxes, cardboard boxes, cave-style beds, or some other option for hiding.

21.3.3.3 Handling

Unless the animals are receiving systematic behavior modification for fearfulness, it's best to minimize the amount of direct handling by humans. In a temporary shelter environment, the authors recommend incorporating chutes (see Figure 21.6) to move animals for cleaning or for spending time in an alternative enclosure, such as a play yard. Most of these dogs will not be capable of walking on a leash at first, so a low-stress alternative for movement is to get them to go into a crate (fearful dogs will often prefer to hide in a crate anyway) that's on wheels (see Figure 21.7) so they can be slowly and gently rolled to a new location. If rolling a crate is not an option, even two people carrying the crate is preferable to handling the dog. While handling should be kept to a minimum, when it is necessary, enlist handlers skilled in low-stress handling procedures (Yin 2009; Swim et al. 2021) and, for severe cases, consider the use of sedatives and psychopharmaceuticals.

21.4 Long-Term Holds

Several animal welfare organizations have shared a similar impression with the authors: that animals entering the shelter system are frequently medically or behaviorally compromised—or both—and require medical or

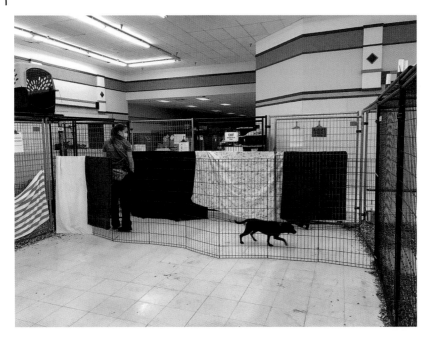

Figure 21.6 An example of a solid chute used to permit hands-free movement of a fearful dog from her kennel to the indoor exercise pen. *Source:* ASPCA Behavioral Sciences Team.

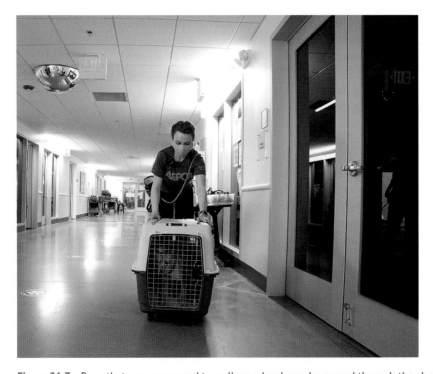

Figure 21.7 Dogs that are unprepared to walk on a leash can be moved through the shelter, with little stress, by means of a rolling crate. *Source:* Renee Dunaway.

behavioral treatment prior to placement. Perhaps because of this, there is also a perception that the average length of stay has increased for animals in shelters generally. Average length of stay aside, special circumstances can extend the amount of time an animal spends in a shelter environment. Perhaps the most common circumstance is that of animals from criminal cruelty cases. In these cases, the animals are put into the care of an animal welfare organization by law enforcement agencies and are held while the legal cases are resolved. Criminal cruelty cases can involve anywhere from an individual or a few animals to tens or hundreds of animals. Large-scale cruelty cases typically involve organized dogfighting, animal hoarding, sanctuaries or shelters that have become institutionalized hoarding situations, and puppy mills. Many factors influence how long the animals are held, including whether the case is a local or federal one, the timing of court proceedings, appeals, and so forth. It is common for animals in criminal cruelty cases to require shelter stays of months; less commonly, the case may take years to resolve. Because the animals are evidence in the criminal proceedings, some enrichment options, such as sleepovers or foster placement, may be more difficult or impossible to arrange. Outside of criminal cases, there are instances where animals become lifetime residents of sanctuaries and rescues, sometimes because they exhibit behavior that precludes their placement in a home environment.

Regardless of the reason, as length of stay increases, the question of how best to prevent or minimize shelter stress becomes even more important. Long-term stress is damaging to welfare because the deleterious effects accumulate over the duration of the stressor (Beerda et al. 2000; Winkler 2019).

Extended lengths of stay raise many questions. What happens when animals are exposed to stressors for weeks to months—or, in some cases, even years? What behavior problems are likely to develop during extended shelter stays, and how are they best mitigated? Do animals in shelters habituate to initially stressful stimuli,

rendering them benign over time? Or, rather, do animals in shelters sensitize to initially benign stimuli, rendering them aversive over time? Do behavioral interventions developed using animals that have been in the shelter for days to weeks have the same efficacy for long-term residents?

These questions, and many others, remain largely unanswered. Caution should be used before extrapolating from studies based on unknown or variable lengths of stay or based on animals with extremely different life histories (e.g., purpose-bred laboratory or working animals) than those of animals in a shelter. The remainder of this section considers what is known, but readers are encouraged to bear the above caveats in mind.

21.4.1 Behavioral Adaptation

Cortisol decreases during the first three days in the shelter (Hennessy et al. 1997). This decrease is commonly believed to indicate that the animals have regained homeostatic balance after the stresses of transport (Radisavljević et al. 2017) and the introduction to a novel environment with potentially aversive sights, smells, and sounds (Taylor and Mills 2007). During the first six days in the shelter, dogs in one study began to spend more time in the back of the kennel and less time active, which may indicate they became more comfortable in the shelter and began to relax and rest (Wells and Hepper 2000). Similarly, Van den Berg (2017) found the average rest bout duration increased significantly between day 1 and day 13 post-intake, albeit with large individual differences. These studies seem to support the common conclusion that dogs likely acclimate to the shelter environment, becoming comfortable enough to rest (and presumably sleep).

Sleep patterns are potentially useful metrics of animal welfare, because sleep is a biological need but is also sensitive to perturbation by environmental stress (Hediger 1980; Langford and Cockram 2010). For example, Powell and colleagues (1978) found sleep suppression and increased wakefulness when laboratory-housed dogs were disturbed by human activity, followed by a rebound in rapid eye movement (REM) sleep post-disturbance. More recently, the sleep architecture (the duration and sequence of various sleep stages) of pet dogs was recorded in a laboratory after brief positive and negative interactions with human researchers. Using a counterbalanced, within-subjects design, the researchers found the negative-interaction condition correlated with a decreased latency to enter REM sleep and an increased duration of the REM sleep stage (Kis et al. 2017). Similarly, when dogs went from a shelter to a short-term foster stay (a one- to two-night "sleepover"), accelerometer data indicated that they rested significantly more compared to their baseline activity in the shelter (Gunter et al. 2019). This suggests a compensatory response due to sleep disturbances in the shelter environment. These findings, along with reports of habituation and increased rest during the first week or two in the shelter in the studies cited above, suggest that when adaptation to the shelter occurs, it is variable across individuals or incomplete compared to a home environment. Because dogs in shelters are known to respond vigorously to activity in the shelter throughout the day, the rebound in "rest" in the home may be the artifact of a less stimulating environment rather than a reflection of in-shelter sleep disruption per se. However, even in their least active period, when humans were not present, dogs in a shelter were more active compared to pet dogs' least active period of the day (Hoffman et al. 2019). These findings are not necessarily contradictory, as animals may acclimate to the shelter relative to intake yet still find it more arousing or stressful relative to a home environment.

Adaptation to the shelter environment likely follows an inverted U-function. Initially, increasing time in the shelter corresponds to habituation to at least some environmental stressors, manifested by an increased willingness/ability to rest and to experience species-typical sleep patterns (or come closer to them). Beyond a certain—and currently unknown—point, increasingly lengthy

stays correspond with behavioral deterioration (e.g., Coppinger and Zuccotti 1999) and breakdown of normal activity and sleep patterns.

21.4.2 Behavioral Deterioration

Barrier aggression, high arousal, worsening reactivity to common stimuli, increasing fear, and, less frequently, the onset of abnormal behavior, are among the commonly cited examples of behavioral deterioration in the shelter environment. Behavioral deterioration seems to be an outward manifestation of progressive changes in an animal's internal motivational and emotional states as the animal fails to cope with a shelter environment that is inherently stressful (Taylor and Mills 2007).

The assumption that exposure to chronic stressors alone underpins behavioral deterioration fails to consider the potential contributory role of sensitization, which may explain some behavioral changes associated with deterioration over long-term shelter stays. Essentially the inverse of habituation, sensitization is an increasingly strong response to a given stimulus with repeated exposure. A common example from the human world is the sound of a dripping faucet, which initially evokes no response and may be filtered from higher-order processing but, over time, becomes increasingly aversive. A possible example in the shelter is a dog's progressively more vigorous response to innocuous items or actions in the environment, such as the action of sweeping with a broom or mop. Unlike chronic stress, sensitization does not require the stimulus to *begin* as a physiological or psychological stressor. Because it is driven by non-associative learning (Shettleworth 2010), neither does it require a negative event to have been paired with the stimulus as with negative conditioned emotional responses. These two aspects have important implications for maintaining the psychological well-being of long-term hold animals, as they require proactive monitoring and management of developing adverse responses to seemingly benign stimuli.

Setting aside the topic of sensitization, it is apparent that many aspects of the shelter environment do represent chronic stressors: they are stressful from the outset and remain so over time. Chronic stressors in the shelter include spatial and social restriction (Taylor and Mills 2007) and a lack of agency and predictability (Cussen and Reid 2020). Most shelter professionals believe, based on anecdotal evidence, that animals' mental well-being deteriorates over a long shelter stay because of unrelenting exposure to chronic stressors. Yet, it is surprisingly difficult to support that belief with empirical evidence.

There are many challenges associated with the existing literature on behavioral manifestations of chronic stress as pertains to long-term shelter stays. The most commonly used behavioral indicators of chronic stress come from work done with laboratory-housed dogs who had a history of participation in research studies and some of whom had relatively short exposure to chronic stressors (Beerda et al. 1999, 2000). This raises the question of whether or not the behavioral metrics are appropriate to detect welfare problems in animals experiencing long-term shelter stays. There is some limited evidence to suggest they may not be—at least not for all lengths of stay. For example, Wells and colleagues (2002) compared behaviors between groups of dogs who were in the shelter for less than one month, two months to one year, one to five years, and more than five years. Most people would consider all but the group held for less than one month to be long-term residents. Importantly, there were differences between the groups held for 2 to 12 months, 1 to 4 years, and more than 5 years in the measures of activity, kennel position, and vocalization (Wells et al. 2002). They found differences in behavior between all of the groups, which means that a long-term resident of two months doesn't necessarily behave like a long-term resident of two years, etc. These results highlight an important, seemingly obvious yet commonly overlooked point: behavioral indicators of diminished welfare likely differ across stay durations. This means that using one or a handful of "standard" stress indicators or averaging across subjects could potentially miss important welfare problems if the animals differ in the stage of their behavioral stress response trajectories.

Routinely controlling for the length of stay of all subjects involved in shelter-based research could lead to clarification of ambiguous results or generate completely novel insights on how length of stay impacts animals' behavior and welfare. Currently, however, it is unknown which behavioral indicators are best to use as metrics for any given duration. While dogs apparently acclimate to the shelter over a period of days to weeks, increasing the frequency and/or duration of resting or sleeping bouts as described earlier, some authors report an increase in activity as length of stay increases. In one study, after three to four weeks in the shelter, dogs increased the frequency of escape-related behaviors such as scratching at the kennel door, digging at the floor, and whining, and they spent less time performing rest-related behaviors such as lying and dozing (Cozzi et al. 2016). These findings are congruent with another study that found increased activity over a six-week period in the shelter (Stephen and Ledger 2005). While the frequency of certain active behaviors tended to increase, they also found age differences in the frequency of motor activities: dogs that chewed on their bedding and repeatedly play-bounced during their first two weeks in the shelter tended to be younger, while dogs that were panting and barking tended to be older (Stephen and Ledger 2005). In humans, the "temporal monotony" of an unvaryingly repetitive schedule is a cause of boredom, even in stimulating environments (Burn 2017). Dogs in shelters are known to have less variation in their activity patterns compared to pet dogs in homes (Hoffman et al. 2019); the shelter population experiences a high degree of temporal monotony because of the fixed schedule of shelter operations. This temporal monotony, together with the findings that dogs appear to acclimate to the shelter and then begin to exhibit more frequent and/or longer bouts of activity as stay duration increases, may indicate restlessness due to boredom. Repeated thwarting of goal-directed behavior can lead to frustration and, in some cases, may contribute to aggression (McPeake et al. 2019).

Behavioral deterioration can manifest actively, as just described, or passively through inactivity due to boredom and/or depression-like states (Cussen and Reid 2020). Beerda and colleagues (2000) themselves point out the contradictory findings between studies on chronic stress: some authors report increases in activity, while others report decreases. Although boredom initially increases activity, over time it can lead to wakeful inactivity and fragmented sleep (Burn 2017). Consistent with this, Owczarczak-Garstecka and Burman (2016) studied dogs who were in the shelter between ten days and two months. They found that dogs with more fragmented sleep also slept less overall, consistent with descriptions of boredom's effects on behavior (Burn 2017). During extended durations of time in the shelter, it is possible that animals may develop a depression-like affective state from chronic sleep disruption due to boredom or disruptive stimuli in the environment. The relationship is speculative for shelter animals, but it is well known that sleep deprivation can lead to depression in humans (Langford and Cockram 2010). Depression-like states can appear outwardly similar to boredom, as they are characterized by awake inactivity (Meagher et al. 2017), but they differ in that a bored animal will act on the opportunity for stimulation, whereas depression-like states are characterized by a loss in responsiveness to opportunities for reward (Fureix and Meagher 2015). Further, while boredom tends to fragment sleep, animal models of depression, which use chronic exposure to stressors to induce the depression-like state, show increased duration of sleep bouts (Cheeta et al. 1997) but without the typical changes in post-deprivation sleep patterns (Suchecki et al. 2000) described in the acclimation section above.

Thus, *changes* in activity and sleep patterns over time could indicate the onset of boredom and/or a depression-like state in individual animals. Such within-individual changes in behavior are critical in identifying stress responses and compromised welfare (Åkerberg et al. 2012). It is not sufficient to simply assess the gross amount of time spent active or spent resting or sleeping. To capture behavioral deterioration, it is necessary to track changes over time at the individual animal level, especially for those animals that respond to chronic stress passively.

21.4.3 Recommendations for Care during Long-Term Holds

Regardless of duration, following the principles outlined throughout this book will help safeguard against the broadest range of problems. Long-term holds also lend themselves to complementary management practices that help reduce the cumulative effects of chronic stress. For example, when animals are held for a longer duration, they will likely experience more medical handling because of injury/illness or simply for periodic health checks. Operant conditioning of specific behaviors can reduce handling stress during medical examinations (e.g., training a chin-rest behavior; Jones 2018). Training behaviors takes time, which may not be practical in short-stay facilities/cases, but it is possible when animals are held for longer periods of time. Proactively implementing low-stress handling and a long-term management strategy on intake can help prevent reactive interventions for behaviors associated with deterioration.

Tailoring management and intervention to animals' personalities or coping styles (Jones and Gosling 2005) is likely the best way to prevent behavioral deterioration during long-term stays (Cussen and Reid 2020). This is because recommendations for minimizing kennel stress are not necessarily generalizable across breed types or among individuals (Coppinger and Zuccotti 1999). Indeed, the authors find that very fearful dogs are less likely to acclimate to the shelter and are at high risk for behavioral deterioration over time. Identifying fearful dogs allows for tailored management, such as that provided by the "Mini-Rehabilitation Center" (MRC) in the ASPCA temporary holding facility for rescued animals. MRC operations are based on the protocols of a dedicated, specialized Behavioral Rehabilitation Center (BRC; Miller et al. 2018), where severely fearful dogs are rehabilitated to improve their quality of life and make them suitable for adoption. The MRC provides tailored management outside the context of a specialized facility; it includes modified operational protocols that minimize stress and prevent behavioral deterioration of at-risk dogs during long-term legal holds (Zverina and Cussen 2020). See Chapter 12 for a more detailed discussion of the MRC and the BRC.

For pro social animals, group housing should be seriously considered when facing a long-term hold. Studies indicate that traditional concerns regarding group housing, namely disease transmission and physical harm from aggression (Coppinger and Zuccotti 1999), are minimal in well-managed programs. Instances of abnormal behavior were extremely rare to absent, even in dogs housed for more than four years in one shelter (Dalla Villa et al. 2013), which may reflect a protective benefit of social housing. Even in dynamically changing groups, behavior stabilized within one to two days of adding a new dog (Sonderegger and Turner 1996). Short of physical or psychological harm stemming from aggression or aversion to conspecifics, the stresses of social housing are likely preferable to those of social restriction. As Coppinger and Zuccotti (1999) said, "In theory, being low on a dominance hierarchy is more healthy and rewarding than not being part of one." While group housing is not always possible due to safety risks (e.g., extremely conspecific-aggressive dogs), it is so beneficial that it ought to be considered the rule rather than the exception and should be taken into account when remodeling or building facilities. If group housing is not possible

for long-term holds, additional staff resources to manage playgroups and to walk dogs should be a standard part of capacity planning; one study found that being taken out of their kennel for walks was the single best predictor of good welfare in dogs held long term in several Italian shelters (Cafazzo et al. 2014). Playgroup opportunities are vital for any long-term hold dog that is eligible and enjoys them, because they provide opportunities for social interaction and investigation of the physical and olfactory environment of the play yard (see Chapter 13).

While much work needs to be done to validate indicators of positive welfare (Lawrence et al. 2019), it is clear that behavioral deterioration includes both the absence of reward-related behaviors and the emergence of stress-related behaviors. Therefore, some indicator(s) of positive welfare should be agreed upon and included in systematic assessments. Suggested indicators include play or other behaviors that are substantially reduced or absent in stressful conditions (i.e., they have "elastic demand"). Another proposed indicator is the animal's response to reward, specifically anticipatory behavior exhibited in response to cues associated with rewarding events (Baciadonna et al. 2020), which can indicate the valence and strength of the animal's perception of that reward (Van der Harst and Spruijt 2007).

Tracking changes in behavior from the time of intake could help distinguish whether changes in activity patterns are due to sensitization (increased activity), habituation (increased or decreased activity), or depression-like affective states (decreased activity) (Cussen and Reid 2020). Behavioral indicators associated with deterioration in the shelter can manifest for a variety of reasons, and these underlying reasons differ in their implications for future behavior. This is highly relevant to animals' likelihood of adoption and to estimations of their future quality of life. For instance, are high-arousal behaviors such as jumping, mouthing, barking, lunging, etc., which commonly develop over long-term stays, due to sustained elicitation (Mason and Latham 2004) by the shelter environment and, therefore, unlikely to continue post-placement? Or, do they instead represent an enduring change, caused by chronic stress, in the biological mechanisms organizing behavior (Garner 2006) and, therefore, are they unlikely to change when the animal is removed from the shelter environment? To date, these questions are unexplored in the shelter-behavior literature.

In the authors' experience, behavioral deterioration can be unintentionally provoked or exacerbated by poor handling choices. Examples include scaring the dog into moving from one side of her enclosure to the other, inadvertently reinforcing jumping and mouthing by leashing the aroused dog and then providing the powerful reward of exercise or social interaction, and repeatedly tugging on an item in the dog's mouth in an attempt to remove it. Although some of these handling tactics are expedient and seem like good options for that reason, over time they can add to animals' stress and endanger staff. Alternative approaches, such as requiring "four [paws] on the floor" before allowing a dog out of the kennel or using target training to facilitate a dog's movement inside the kennel, take additional time initially but pay dividends by reducing stress and maximizing safety for both humans and animals. For best results, it is important that all staff and volunteers are consistent in their interactions and expectations.

21.4.4 Quality of Life Assessment

Quality of life (QoL) is a meta-assessment of welfare in aggregate and a projection into the future on how the animal's welfare will stay constant, improve, or decline. McMillan (2007) points out the difficulties of "hitting a moving target" such as an animal's future affective state. Some of the difficulties are mitigated in special circumstances like natural disasters (e.g., when dealing with adult feral animals unsuited to life as pets) or long-term stays. A longer length of stay helps to clarify QoL assessment because it

allows for repeated monitoring to see if it is remaining consistent, improving, or declining. While decisions still include uncertainty about the animal's future affective state, predictions are generally better when based on more observations (Epstein 1979). Furthermore, in humans (and likely animals, too), some individuals are typically more or less happy than others. Their affective state can be shifted fleetingly by life events but settles back to their usual "happiness set point" (McMillan 2007). Applied to animals in shelters, individuals who consistently exhibit, for instance, behavioral indicators of extreme fear over the course of weeks or months despite environmental and behavioral interventions are unlikely to suddenly become relaxed/happy in the future.

The authors discourage the use of thresholds above or below which euthanasia is decisively triggered for several reasons. At present, there is no straightforward mathematical summation to determine the total "quantity" of QoL belonging to an animal. Further, although many QoL assessments rate the animal on a numeric Likert-like scale (e.g., 1 to 7), it is important to remember that such ratings are *ordinal* scores. That means there is an order to the ratings (e.g., a 2 is worse than a 3 is worse than a 4, etc.), but *there is no continuity of increment*—there is no expectation that a one-unit increase from, say, 2 to 3 is the same as a one-unit increase from a 5 to 6. Because we are used to operating in a world of continuous measurements (e.g., temperature, height, etc.), the default tendency is to interpret ordinal scores in the same way, even if we "know" they are not. Assigning a number gives an appearance of accuracy/consistency/precision that is at odds with the nature of the subjective score.

The authors encourage making the ordinal nature of the scores explicit by not using numbers at all. If an identifier is needed for answers, using an alphabetic identifier such as "A," "B," etc., is preferable. Each response option can be assigned to a category (e.g., "Good/Bad/Neutral" or "Acceptable/Unacceptable") based on the shelter's criteria. For a given assessment, the percentage of answers for each response category can be depicted graphically to provide a visual representation of "Acceptable" versus "Unacceptable" indicators exhibited by the animal. Change in the proportion of acceptable or unacceptable indicators would reflect improvement or decrements, respectively, in an animal's QoL over time. This approach allows shelters to document and monitor QoL in a consistent way while avoiding the pitfalls of implicit interpretation and false accuracy associated with using numeric scores.

Decision-making around QoL includes consideration of physical diagnoses and prognoses as well as the mental well-being of the animal (see Chapter 19). Temporary field shelters used in disasters and cruelty cases may require different protocols for monitoring QoL, providing additional enrichments, and making euthanasia decisions compared to long-term hold facilities. Regardless of the circumstances, though, monitoring and decision-making protocols are an important and necessary component for operations and should be in place prior to deploying to the disaster/cruelty situation.

21.5 Conclusions

Under the best of circumstances, shelter environments pose welfare challenges to animals (Taylor and Mills 2007). Disasters and cruelty cases require additional considerations related to both animal welfare and staff safety. Understanding the unique challenges posed by specific populations, such as feral animals, fighting dogs, and animals from puppy mills, is vital. Capacity planning must include the additional resources necessary for safety and good welfare in these cases. Long-term holds exacerbate any welfare challenges because chronic stress accumulates over time and has deleterious physiological and behavioral effects. Monitoring behavior from the time of intake is critical for early detection of welfare problems and for ensuring acceptable QoL for animals in shelters, particularly those held in special circumstances.

References

Adachi, I., Kuwahata, H., and Fujita, K. (2006). Dogs recall their owner's face upon hearing the owner's voice. *Anim. Cogn.* 10: 17–21.

Åkerberg, H., Wilsson, E., Sallander, M. et al. (2012). Test for personality characteristics in dogs used in research. *J. Vet. Behav.* 7: 327–338.

American Psychiatric Association. (2013). *DSM-5*. Washington, DC: American Psychiatric Association.

Baciadonna, L., Briefer, E.F., and McElligott, A.G. (2020). Investigation of reward quality-related behaviour as a tool to assess emotions. *Appl. Anim. Behav. Sci.* 225: 104968.

Barton, R.C. and Reid, P.J. (2018). Field euthanasia during Hurricane Maria disaster response efforts. *American Veterinary Medical Association's Humane Endings Symposium*, Chicago, IL.

Beerda, B., Schilder, M.B., Van Hooff, J.A. et al. (1999). Chronic stress in dogs subjected to social and spatial restriction. I. Behavioral responses. *Physiol. Behav.* 66: 233–242.

Beerda, B., Schilder, M.B., van Hooff, J.A.R.A. et al. (2000). Behavioural and hormonal indicators of enduring environmental stress in dogs. *Anim. Welf.* 9: 49–62.

Bissell, S. (2019). Cascading effects of early life stress: An integrative dog model of the hypomethylation of the glucocorticoid receptor (NR3C1). Canine Science Conference, Phoenix, AZ.

Boitani, L., Francisci, F., Ciucii, P. et al. (1995). Population biology and ecology of feral dogs in central Italy. In: *The Domestic Dog: Its Evolution, Behaviour and Interactions with*

People (ed. J. Serpell), 217–244. Cambridge, UK: Cambridge University Press.

Burghart, W.F. (2013). Preliminary evaluation of case series of military working dogs affected with canine post-traumatic stress disorder (N=14). *Proceedings of Veterinary Behavior Symposium*, American College of Veterinary Behaviorists, Chicago IL (19 July 2013).

Burn, C.C. (2017). Beastly boredom: A biological perspective on animal boredom and suggestions for its scientific investigation. *Anim. Behav.* 130: 141–151.

Byosiere, S.E., Chouinard, P.A., Howell, T.J. et al. (2018). What do dogs (*Canis familiaris*) see? A review of vision in dogs and implications for cognition research. *Psychon. Bull. Rev.* 25: 1798–1813.

Cafazzo, S., Maragliano, L., Bonanni, R. et al. (2014). Behavioural and physiological indicators of shelter dogs' welfare: Reflections on the no-kill policy on free-ranging dogs in Italy revisited on the basis of 15 years of implementation. *Physiol. Behav.* 133: 223–229.

Cheeta, S., Ruigt, G., Van Proosdij, J. et al. (1997). Changes in sleep architecture following chronic mild stress. *Biol. Psychiatry* 41: 419–427.

Collins, K., Reid, P., and Martinez, L. (2012). Bred to fight: Evaluating play in pit bull puppies from fighting lines. *ACVB/AVSAB Veterinary Behavior Symposium*, San Diego, CA (3 August 2012).

Coppinger, L. and Coppinger, R. (2016). *What Is a Dog?* Chicago, lL: University of Chicago Press.

Coppinger, R. and Zuccotti, J. (1999). Kennel enrichment: Exercise and socialization of dogs. *J. Appl. Anim. Welf. Sci.* 2: 281–296.

Cozzi, A., Mariti, C., Ogi, A., Sighieri, C., and Gazzano, A. (2016). Behavioral modification in sheltered dogs. *Dog Behavior* 2. https://doi.org/10.4454/db.v2i3.38.

Cussen, V. and Reid, P.J. (2020). The mental well-being of animals in shelters. In: *Mental Health and Well-Being in Animals*, 2nd ed. (ed. F. McMillan). Boston, MA: CABI.

Dalla Villa, P., Barnard, S., Di Fede, E. et al. (2013). Behavioural and physiological responses of shelter dogs to long-term confinement. *Vet. Ital.* 49: 231–241.

Daniels, T.J. and Bekoff, M. (1989). Feralization: The making of wild domestic animals. *Behav. Process.* 19: 79–94.

Day, A.M. (2017). Companion animals and natural disasters: A systematic review of the literature. *Int. J. Disaster Risk Reduct.* 24: 81–90.

Epstein, S. (1979). The stability of behavior: I. On predicting most of the people much of the time. *J. Pers. Soc. Psychol.* 37: 1097–1126.

Feltes, E. (2021). Characteristics of intrahousehold interdog aggression and dog and pair factors associated with a poor outcome. *Interdisciplinary Forum on Applied Animal Behavior* (1 May 2021).

Flandreau, E.I. and Toth, M. (2018). Animal models of PTSD: A critical review. *Curr. Top. Behav. Neurosci.* 38: 47–68.

Foa, E.B., Zinbarg, R., and Rothbaum, B.O. (1992). Uncontrollability and unpredictability in post-traumatic stress disorder: An animal model. *Psychol. Bull.* 112: 218–238.

Fritz Institute. (2006). Hurricane Katrina: Perceptions of the Affected. https://reliefweb.int/sites/reliefweb.int/files/resources/19D62C898E90E44B8525715C0068ED2B-fin-gen-26apr.pdf (accessed 20 June 2021).

Fugazza, C. Pogány, A., and Miklósi, A. (2016). Recall of others' actions after incidental encoding reveals episodic-like memory in dogs. *Curr. Biol.* 26: 3209–3213.

Fukuzawa, M. and Watanabe, M. (2017). Relevance of visual, auditory, and olfactory cues in pet dogs' awareness of humans. *Open J. Anim. Sci.* 7: 297–304.

Fureix, C. and Meagher, R.K. (2015). What can inactivity (in its various forms) reveal about affective states in non-human animals? A review. *Appl. Anim. Behav. Sci.* 171: 8–24.

Garner, J.P. (2006). Perseveration and stereotypy: Systems-level insights from clinical psychology. In: *Stereotypic Animal Behaviour: Fundamentals and Application to Welfare*, 2nd ed. (eds. G. Mason and J. Rushen), 141–152. Cambridge, MA: CABI.

Green, D. (2019). *Animals in Disasters*. Burlington, MA: Butterworth-Heinemann.

Gunter, L.M., Feuerbacher, E.N., Gilchrist, R.J. et al. (2019). Evaluating the effects of a temporary fostering program on shelter dog welfare. *Peer J.* 7: e6620.

Hediger, H. (1980). The biology of natural sleep in animals. *Experientia* 36: 13–16.

Hennessey, M.B., Davis, H.N., Williams, M.T. et al. (1997). Plasma cortisol levels of dogs at a county animal shelter. *Physiol. Behav.* 62: 485–490.

Hoffman, C.L., Ladha, C., and Wilcox, S. (2019). An actigraphy-based comparison of shelter dog and owned dog activity patterns. *J. Vet. Behav.* 34: 30–36.

Hunt, M., Al-Awadi, H., and Johnson, M. (2008). Psychological sequelae of pet loss following Hurricane Katrina. *Anthrozoös* 21: 109–121.

Iossa, G., Soulsbury, C.D., and Harris, S. (2007). Mammal trapping: A review of animal welfare standards of killing and restraining traps. *Anim. Welf.* 16: 335–352.

Jones, A.C. and Gosling, S.D. (2005). Temperament and personality in dogs (*Canis familiaris*): A review and evaluation of past research. *Appl. Anim. Behav. Sci.* 95: 1–53.

Jones, D. A. (2018). *Cooperative Care: Seven Steps to Stress-Free Husbandry*. Self-published.

Kis, A., Gergely, A., Galambos, A. et al. (2017). Sleep macrostructure is modulated by positive and negative social experience in adult pet dogs. *Proc. R. Soc. B.* 284: 20171883.

Kockaya, M., Ercan, N., Demirbas, Y.S. et al. (2018). Serum oxytocin and lipid levels of dogs with maternal cannibalism. *J. Vet. Behav.* 27: 23–26.

Konok, V., Dóka, A., and Miklósi, A. (2011). The behavior of the domestic dog (*Canis familiaris*) during separation from and reunion with the owner: A questionnaire and an experimental study. *Appl. Anim. Behav. Sci.* 135: 300–308.

Langford, F.M. and Cockram, M.S. (2010). Is sleep in animals affected by prior waking experience? *Anim. Welf.* 19: 215–222.

Lawrence, A.B., Vigors, B., and Sandøe, P. (2019). What is so positive about positive animal welfare? A critical review of the literature. *Animals.* https://doi:10.3390/ani9100783.

Ledger, R.A. and Mellor, D.J. (2018). Forensic use of the Five Domains model for assessing suffering in cases of animal cruelty. *Animals.* http://doi:10.3390/ani8070101.

Lezama-García, K., Mariti, C., Mota-Rojas, D. et al. (2019). Maternal behaviour in domestic dogs. *Int. J. Vet. Sci. Med.* 7: 20–30.

Lockwood, R. (2018). Animal hoarding: The challenge for mental health, law enforcement, and animal welfare professionals. *Behav. Sci. Law.* http://doi.org/10.1002/bsl.2373.

Lockwood, R. and Rindy, K. (1987). Are "pit bulls" different? An analysis of the pit bull terrier controversy. *Anthrozoös* 1: 2–8.

Louisiana SPCA. (n.d.). https://www.la-spca.org/about/katrina-dogs-animal-rescue-stories/rescuefacts (accessed 15 April 2021).

Lowe, S.R., Rhodes, J.E., Zwiebach, L. et al. (2009). The impact of pet loss on the perceived social support and psychological distress of hurricane survivors. *J. Trauma. Stress* 22: 244–247.

Mason, G. and Latham, N. (2004). Can't stop, won't stop: Is stereotypy a reliable animal welfare indicator? *Anim. Welf.* 13: S57–S69.

McMillan, F.D. (2007). Predicting quality of life outcomes as a guide for decision-making: The difficulty of hitting a moving target. *Anim Welf.* 16: 135–142.

McMillan, F.D. (2020). Psychological trauma and posttraumatic psychopathology in animals. In: *Mental Health and Well-Being in Animals*, 2nd ed. (ed. F. McMillan), 182–211. Boston, MA: CABI.

McMillan, F.D., Serpell, J.A., Duffy, D.L. et al. (2013). Differences in behavioral characteristics between dogs obtained as puppies from pet stores and those obtained from noncommercial breeders. *J. Am. Vet. Med. Assoc.* 242: 1359–1363.

McPeake, K.J., Collins, L.M., Zulch, H., and Mills, D.S., 2019. The Canine Frustration Questionnaire—Development of a new psychometric tool for measuring frustration in domestic dogs (*Canis familiaris*). *Front. Vet. Sci.* https://doi.org/10.3389/fvets.2019.00152.

Meagher, R.K., Campbell, D.L.M., and Mason, G.J. (2017). Boredom-like states in mink and their behavioural correlates: A replicate study. *Appl. Anim. Behav. Sci.* 197: 112–119.

Meek, P.D. and Brown, S.C. (2016). It's a dog eat dog world: Observations of dingo (*Canis familiaris*) cannibalism. *Aust. Mammal.* http://doi.org/10.1071/AM16018.

Miller, K., Cussen, V.A., Collins, K. et al. (2018). Optimizing treatment outcomes for extremely fearful dogs at the ASPCA Behavioral Rehabilitation Center. *Proceedings of the 55th Annual Conference of the Animal Behavior Society,* Milwaukee, WI.

Miller, K.A., Touroo, R., Spain, C.V. et al. (2016). Relationship between scarring and dog aggression in pit bull-type dogs involved in organized dogfighting. *Animals.* http://doi:10.3390/ani6110072.

Millman, S.T. and Duncan, I.J.H. (2000). Strain differences in aggressiveness of male domestic fowl in response to a male model. *Appl. Anim. Behav. Sci.* 66: 217–233.

Nagasawa, M., Magi, K., and Kikusui, T. (2012). Continued distress among abandoned dogs in Fukushima. *Sci. Rep.* http://doi:10.1038/srep00724.

Owczarczak-Garstecka, S.C. and Burman, O.H.P. (2016). Can sleep and resting behaviours be used as indicators of welfare in shelter dogs (*Canis lupus familiaris*)? *PLOS ONE.* http://doi: e0163620.

Pankratz, K.E., Ferris, K.K., Griffith, E.H. et al. (2017). Use of single-dose oral gabapentin to attenuate fear responses in cage-trap confined community cats: A double-blind, placebo-controlled field trial. *J. Fel. Med. Surg.* http://doi:10.1177/1098612X17719399.

Parker, G.A. (1974). Assessment strategy and the evolution of fighting behaviour. *J. Theor. Biol.* 47: 223–243.

Pattison, K.F., Laude, J.R., and Zentall, T.R. (2013). The case of the magic bones: Dogs' memory of the physical properties of objects. *Learn. Motiv.* 44: 252–257.

Powell, E.W., Lucas, E.A., and Murphee, O.D. (1978). Influence of human presence on sleep-wake patterns in nervous pointer dogs. *Physiol. Behav.* 20: 39–42.

Prato-Previde, E., Custance, D.M., Spiezio, C. et al. (2003). Is the dog-human relationship an attachment bond? An observational study using Ainsworth's strange situation. *Behaviour* 140: 225–254.

Price, E.O. (1984). Behavioral aspects of animal domestication. *Q. Rev. Biol.* 59: 1–32.

Radisavljević, K., Vučinić, M., Becskei, Z. et al. (2017). Comparison of stress level indicators in blood of free-roaming dogs after transportation and housing in the new environment. *J. Appl. Anim. Res.* 45: 52–55.

Ratcliffe, V.F., McComb, K., and Reby, D. (2014). Cross-modal discrimination of human gender by domestic dogs. *Anim. Behav.* 91:127–135.

Reid, P.J. (2013). Animal behavior forensics: Evaluation of dangerous dogs and cruelty victims. In: *Shelter Medicine for Veterinarians and Staff*, 2nd ed. (eds. L. Miller and S. Zawistowski), 559–568. Hoboken, NJ: Wiley Blackwell.

Richter-Levin, G., Stork, O., and Schmidt, M.V. (2019). Animal models of PTSD: A challenge to be met. *Mol. Psychiatry* 24: 1135–1156.

Seligman, M.E.P., Maier, S.F., and Solomon, R.L. (1971). Unpredictable and uncontrollable events. In: *Aversive Conditioning and Learning* (ed. F.R. Brush), 347–400. Cambridge, UK: Academic Press.

Shettleworth, S. (2010). *Cognition, Evolution, and Behavior*, 2nd ed. New York: Oxford University Press.

Siegmund, A. and Wotjak, C.T. (2006). Toward an animal model of posttraumatic stress disorder. *Ann. N.Y. Acad. Sci.* 1071: 324–334.

Slater, M., Garrison, L., Miller, K. et al. (2013a). Practical physical and behavioral measures to assess the socialization spectrum of cats in a shelter-like setting during a three day period. *Animals.* http://doi:10.3390/ani3041162.

Slater, M., Garrison, L., Miller, K. et al. (2013b). Physical and behavioral measures that predict cats' socialization in an animal shelter environment during a three day period. *Animals.* http://doi:10.3390/ani3041215.

Sonderegger, S.M. and Turner, D.C. (1996). Introducing dogs into kennels: Prediction of social tendencies to facilitate integration. *Anim. Welf.* 5: 391–404.

Stellato, A.C., Dewey, C.E., Widowski, T.M. et al. (2020). Evaluation of associations between owner presence and indicators of fear in dogs during routine veterinary examinations. *J. Am. Vet. Med. Assoc.* 257: 1031–1040.

Stephen, J.M. and Ledger, R.A. (2005). An audit of behavioral indicators of poor welfare in kenneled dogs in the United Kingdom. *J. Appl. Anim. Welf. Sci.* 8: 79–95.

Suchecki, D., Duarte Palm, B., and Tufik, S. (2000). Sleep rebound in animals deprived of paradoxical sleep by the modified multiple platform method. *Brain Res.* 857: 14–22.

Swim, A., Smart, C., and Staton, A. (2021). Low stress handling techniques in shelter animals and the overall effects on physiological parameters. Speech presented at the 2021 Celebration of Student Scholarship in Morehead, KY (April). https://scholarworks. moreheadstate.edu/celebration_ videos_2021/10 (accessed 23 June 2021).

Taslitz, A.E. (1990). Does the cold nose know— The unscientific myth of the dog scent lineup. *Hastings Law J.* 42: 15–134.

Taylor, A.M., Reby, D., and McComb, K. (2011). Cross modal perception of body size in domestic dogs (*Canis familiaris*). *PLOS ONE* 6: e17069. http://doi:10.1371/journal. pone.0017069.

Taylor, K.D. and Mills, D.S. (2007). The effect of the kennel environment on canine welfare: A critical review of experimental studies. *Anim. Welf.* 16: 435–447.

Thielke, L.E. and Udell, M.A.R. (2020). Characterizing human–dog attachment relationships in foster and shelter environments as a potential mechanism for achieving mutual wellbeing and success. *Animals.* https://doi.org/10.3390/ani10010067.

Van den Berg, A.C.M. (2017). Good welfare or a nightmare? Resting behaviour at night of dogs over an acclimatization period after intake at the shelter. Report on a Research Project, Faculty of Veterinary Medicine, Utrecht University, The Netherlands.

Van der Harst, J.E. and Spruijt, B.M. (2007). Tools to measure and improve animal welfare: Reward-related behaviour. *Anim. Welf.* 16: 67–73.

Verbeek, P., Iwatmoto, I., and Murakami, N. (2007). Differences in aggression between wild-type and domesticated fighting fish are context dependent. *Anim. Behav.* 73: 75–83.

Wagner, D., Newbury, S., Kass, P. et al. (2014). Elimination behavior of shelter dogs housed in double compartment kennels. *PLOS ONE* 9: e96254. https://doi.org/10.1371/journal. pone.0096254.

Wells, D.L., Graham, L., and Hepper, P.G. (2002). The influence of length of time in a rescue shelter on the behaviour of kennelled dogs. *Anim. Welf.* 11: 385–393.

Wells, D.L. and Hepper, P.G. (2000). The influence of environmental change on the behaviour of sheltered dogs. *Appl. Anim. Behav. Sci.* 68: 151–162.

White, P.J., Kreeger, T.J., Seal, U.S. et al. (1991). Pathological responses of red foxes to capture in box traps. *J. Wildl. Manag.* 55: 75–80.

Winkler, C. (2019). Assessing animal welfare at the farm level: Do we care sufficiently about the individual? *Anim. Welf.* 28: 77–82.

Yin, S. (2009). *Low Stress Handling, Restraint and Behavior Modification of Dogs and Cats.* Davis, CA: Cattle Dog Publishing.

Zverina, L. and Cussen, V.A. (2020). Report on a program to improve outcomes for fearful dogs: The ASPCA in-shelter Mini-Rehabilitation Center (MRC). *Proceedings of the 57th Annual Conference of the Animal Behavior Society.* Milwaukee, WI.

22

Behavioral Pharmacology

Sara L. Bennett

22.1 Appropriate Use of Behavioral Pharmacology in the Shelter Setting

Medications for sheltered pets can be used to address immediate welfare concerns, often stemming from the shelter environment itself. Addressing these early can help to improve adoptability, facilitate a smoother transition to the new home, and often lead to a shorter-term treatment overall. They can also be used to address behavior disorders present in a pet within a shelter, whether the pet entered the shelter with the problem or the stress of the shelter became a trigger for an already at-risk animal. Addressing these disorders as soon as they are recognized can improve welfare short and long term, help to make a less adoptable pet more adoptable, and help to facilitate that pet being successfully maintained in a home long term. In this chapter, the indications and goals for behavior medication use, factors to consider prior to prescribing, requirements to prescribe, monitoring, and medication choices will be discussed. A medication formulary will also be included. To understand the medications and how to select them, a brief discussion about neurotransmitters is presented. Additionally, some tips on how to set up behavior medication protocols, along with some examples, will be reviewed. And lastly, a brief

discussion on non-pharmaceutical or adjunct treatment options will wrap up this chapter.

22.1.1 Indications for Behavioral Pharmacology

General goals of behavioral medication use include addressing specific underlying neurotransmitter alterations; to decrease underlying anxiety, fear, and emotional arousal; and to make behavioral and environmental modification easier to implement. It is important to remember that these medications do not change the animal's behavior itself, as the behavior patterns have been learned and practiced as coping strategies. The negative emotional states underlying the motivations for the behavior are what is being affected.

This chapter is not intended to provide a comprehensive list of behavioral diagnoses, clinical signs, differentials, or comprehensive treatment plans. The reader is referred to other resources for such details (see Landsberg et al.'s *Behavior Problems of the Dog and Cat*, 3rd ed. [2013], Overall's *Manual of Clinical Behavioral Medicine for Dogs and Cats* [2013a], or Horwitz and Mills's *BSAVA Manual of Canine and Feline Behavioural Medicine*, 2nd ed. [2009]). On a general level, at minimum, a working diagnosis should be made prior to prescribing pharmaceuticals. This can include

Animal Behavior for Shelter Veterinarians and Staff, Second Edition. Edited by Brian A. DiGangi, Victoria A. Cussen, Pamela J. Reid, and Kristen A. Collins.
© 2022 John Wiley & Sons, Inc. Published 2022 by John Wiley & Sons, Inc.
Companion website: www.wiley.com/go/digangi/animal

a succinct description of the problem—for example, a dog that cowers, tries to hide, and struggles to get away when approached by men can be given a working diagnosis of "fear of men." This working diagnosis can then be the basis of setting up a treatment plan, including environmental management (e.g., a hiding spot from passing men), behavior modification (all men toss treats to the dog no matter what—classical conditioning), and a fast-acting behavior medication that does not impede learning (e.g., trazodone or gabapentin).

The keys to making a working diagnosis are to identify the behavior, trigger, target (if different), and motivation for the behavior (e.g., fear or frustration being the most common in shelters). By recognizing the motivation, a more informed decision on medication choice—fast-acting short-term, long-term baseline, or both—can be made, along with an understanding of which specific neurotransmitters to target. For example, the dog reacting with high physiologic arousal—hackles up, pupils dilated, panting hard, salivating heavily—with poor recovery might benefit more from clonidine than the dog previously described who might do well on trazodone.

Suzanne Clothier, an experienced, qualified, force-free trainer has an excellent article that helps to describe when to consider medications for a behavior problem (Clothier 2019). She discusses the Three Ps—provocation, proportion, and persistence, which complement the identifiers listed above when making a working diagnosis. The provocation can be considered along the same lines as the trigger—the event or environment that incited the behavior of interest. The proportion considers the intensity of the dog's reaction to a trigger: is the behavior response extreme to a minor trigger? That is an important observation to note. Persistence can be thought of as ability to recover. A normal dog should be able to recover from a mild to moderately stressful situation within a couple of minutes at most. Longer than that, and we should consider whether that behavior pattern is abnormal or impairing

welfare. By taking a few minutes to make a list of the pet's unwanted behavior, triggers and targets for it, and the suspected motivation, and layering the Three Ps over each behavior pattern of concern, one can then create a working diagnosis and also determine if the behavior(s) in question are severe enough to warrant adding behavior medication to the treatment plan. This process is often best accomplished using a team approach in the shelter. Animal care staff play an important role in identifying behaviors of concern, and also helping to clarify targets and triggers. The shelter behavior staff (if available) can also be instrumental in helping to determine motivation and applying the Three Ps. In an ideal world, the animal care staff recognize a problem, notify the shelter behavior team, and then if they identify behaviors that are more than just a training or management problem, they can notify the shelter veterinarian that this particular case might also need their input for a diagnosis and behavioral medication intervention.

22.1.2 Things to Consider before Prescribing

A risk assessment should be performed for every pet with behavioral complaints before an outcome decision and treatment plan are created. Things that should be considered include:

- Safety. What is the risk to the patient, the other animals and staff at the shelter, and the people and animals in the community? Does this pet pose a safety risk to himself, perhaps by self-injury from self-inflicted behaviors, or as a consequence of his behavior directed toward another target? Does he pose a safety risk to other animals in the shelter or to the staff and volunteers that care for him? Does he pose a safety risk that is unacceptably high to the community if he were to be placed in a foster or adoptive home? Remember, aggression is not the only problem that can cause a safety risk. Chasing, escaping, and some frustration-related behaviors such as extreme jumping and mouthing might be considered too risky for some communities. Each organization must develop their own level of risk sensitivity that balances their responsibility to the pets in their care and to their community.

- Emotional risk. What is the emotional risk to the potential adopter being asked to take on this problem long term? Are you asking them to change their lifestyle to an unrealistic and unreasonable level? Are you placing them in a situation where a healthy human-animal bond will be difficult to form? Are you setting them up for a negative experience and therefore losing a supporter of your sheltering organization?
- Quality of life assessment. Does the pet have a reasonably good quality of life? Can it be improved to a life worth living and even enjoyed? Are you sacrificing the potential owner's quality of life for the pet's? This should be re-evaluated at regular intervals.
- Risk of continued behavioral deterioration. If you do not intervene, what is the likelihood the pet will continue to deteriorate? Have you already tried to intervene with environmental adjustments, or can they be made? Has behavior modification been attempted? Is the pet continuing to worsen despite these? This potential complication should be considered when deciding whether to add medication to a behavior treatment plan. What is the risk of waiting? Can the problem worsen to a point where it becomes dangerous or the welfare of the pet is so severely compromised that they may not be able to recover? Can you make enough adjustments that progress is likely to be made? It is unacceptable to keep a pet in a situation where improvement cannot be made and deterioration is inevitable.
- Shelter resources. Does your organization have the resources to address this behavior problem?
- Shelter's community. Does your community have individuals who are truly equipped and willing to manage this problem? What is

their perception of behavior medications in general?

22.1.3 Requirements for Prescribing Medication

The same requirements for prescribing any medications can be applied to those intended to modify behavior. A valid veterinarian-client-patient relationship (VCPR) should be established. To make an accurate diagnosis or working diagnosis, a medical evaluation, which includes a behavioral examination in addition to a physical examination, needs to be completed. This will help to ensure the practitioner is addressing the motivation for the behavior and the accompanying diagnosis rather than just trying to treat the clinical signs. For example, if one tries to treat feline housesoiling (previously called inappropriate elimination) (Carney et al. 2014) by shutting a cat in the bathroom with his own litterbox and amitriptyline, the social conflict that might be the main contributor to the problem has been neglected. Though the problem might "resolve" while the cat is sequestered in the bathroom, it will recur as soon as the cat is reintroduced to the household and the social interactions that led to the housesoiling occur again. Always consider other treatments that can be implemented prior or in addition to pharmaceutical therapy. There should always be some type of environmental management and behavior modification included in any behavior treatment plan. These do not have to be complex, as both can be implemented in simple, inexpensive, and efficient ways (see Chapters 12 and 18).

What about labwork? Although ideal, and typically recommended for an owned pet prior to prescribing pharmaceuticals, is labwork a reasonable use of shelter resources? What is the risk of prescribing without it? Do the benefits potentially outweigh the risks? Does it change what medication one might choose for a particular pet? The answers to these questions often depend on the pet and the medications considered. Realistically, the risk of an underlying problem is low in an otherwise healthy young adult pet, especially if they have already undergone surgical sterilization under anesthesia without complication. However, if a problem were to occur, there would not be a baseline available for comparison. If labwork is not available, the shelter may consider medications that have a lower risk of complications and side effects (e.g., using gabapentin instead of a benzodiazepine in cats; Hughes et al. 1996). If medications are available but labwork is not, it would not be fair to the sheltered pet to refuse medication that could help save them suffering from a behavioral problem just because pre-medication labwork could not be performed.

Prescribing medication and formulating a plan is only the beginning, never the end: a follow-up plan must be created. There should always be a plan for monitoring the pet's response to treatment and welfare status at regular intervals. Additionally, outcome options available to that pet might change as their behavior, shelter resources, environment, or community change. One big benefit from continuing to monitor a pet on a behavior treatment plan is that as more information about that pet's problem is identified, including what is and is not helping the problem, additional creative transfer solutions can be considered. Perhaps a breed rescue can now take a specialized breed with separation anxiety treatment already underway, or a herding dog can be more manageable on leash in a suburban environment whereas he is still too risky to try to manage in a dense urban environment. Additionally, starting treatment of a behavior problem immediately upon identification can help the next party, regardless of role, continue to set that pet up for success. The shelter is able to clearly inform "this is what we know," advise "this is what we've done so far," and counsel "this is what you can continue to do" so the next person/organization responsible for that pet has a better understanding of what that pet needs

and from what information the plan was created. Creating a follow-up plan for behavior treatment, regardless of whether behavior medication is used, is no different than setting up a follow-up plan for a pet diagnosed with a urinary tract infection or other medical problem.

Requirements to prescribe medication can vary widely state by state. In some states, there are no requirements except for controlled substances. Additionally, the list of medications subject to controlled substance scheduling also varies state by state. For example, gabapentin is currently a schedule V drug in Kentucky, Virginia, West Virginia, Michigan, and Tennessee. It is important to check laws and regulations in your local jurisdiction and state of practice and to work within them. Additional regulatory considerations pertinent to animal shelters are presented elsewhere (Newbury et al. 2010).

22.1.4 Medication Choices

When deciding which medication to use for a particular pet, the goal(s) of treatment, administration requirements, cost and availability, abuse potential, and legal requirements should all be considered.

What is your goal? What do you plan to accomplish by adding behavior medication to the treatment plan? If trying to manage kennel stress or an immediate welfare concern, often a short onset (fast-acting) medication would be a rational choice. If you suspect you are dealing with an underlying behavior disorder, expect this pet to have a longer length of stay (LOS), or anticipate management of a significant behavior disorder or problem in the future, such as in a home, perhaps a longer-term baseline medication might be more appropriate (see Table 22.1). Along with considering the goal of medication administration, one must consider what neurotransmitter system is most appropriate to address when determining which specific behavioral medication to use (see Section 22.3).

Table 22.1 Behavioral medicines for shelter use.

Medication category	Dosing frequency	Indications	Drug classes and examples
Baseline medications	Daily; Longer-term use; several weeks to effect	Chronic, daily, or unpredictable events

Example conditions: Anxiety, fear, impulsivity, compulsive disorder, aggression (majority based in fear/anxiety), cognitive dysfunction syndrome | *Selective serotonin reuptake inhibitors (SSRIs)* Fluoxetine, sertraline

Tricyclic antidepressants (TCAs) Clomipramine, amitriptyline

Monoamine oxidase inhibitors (MAOIs) Selegiline |
| Situational, adjunct, or secondary medications | PRN; daily short term; combination with baseline | Short duration; predictable events; bridging medication while waiting for baseline to take effect; additional support with baseline long term

Example conditions: Transitional or travel stress, kennel stress (short term), noise aversion, fear on walks, etc. | *Benzodiazepines*

Alpha-2 agonists Clonidine, dexmedetomidine

Trazodone

Gabapentin |

Administration requirements should take into account both the frequency and route of delivery as well as the stress that may be associated with administration. Does the organization have the manpower to medicate multiple times per day? Generally, a lower frequency of administration leads to better compliance. Most behavioral pharmaceuticals are given by an oral route, with varying levels of palatability and distaste. Some options to make administration easier for staff and increase acceptance and reduce stress for the pet include mixing oral medications in canned food, pill pockets, peanut butter, cheese, etc.

Staff should consider if the stress caused by administering medication to aggressive or fearful animals is worth the benefit potentially gained by the pet, such as is often the case with fearful cats. Creative strategies or smart choice of formulation can be helpful to minimize stress and maximize success. For example, one creative strategy is to give liquid oral medications to fearful cats via a tom cat catheter attached to a syringe. This can be gently guided into the cat's mouth without restraint and the liquid administered quickly. An excellent description of this can be found in Pankratz et al. (2018) where the researchers administered gabapentin pre-operatively to community cats housed in humane traps when presented for sterilization (see Figure 14.15). Another option is to consider offering medication in a highly palatable food just before leaving for the evening, giving the fearful pet the opportunity to eat it overnight.

Money and time are common limiting factors for sheltering organizations. What is the cost and ease of availability of the medication to be prescribed? Unfortunately, the cost of generic medications can still vary widely depending on production and sometimes surprisingly may be higher than FDA-approved formulations (e.g., at the time of writing, the cost of generic clomipramine is frequently higher than the cost of the veterinary formulation, Clomicalm®, Elanco Animal Health, Inc., Greenfield, IN), for many canine patients. This is particularly important if a pet is likely to go to their final outcome on medication that needs to be continued long-term. One option to set the pet and adopter up for success is giving options for price shopping of the medication after adoption. There are several websites that are set up for consumers to price shop prescriptions between retail pharmacies, such as GoodRX.com.

Does the medication you wish to prescribe have staff or volunteer diversion risk? What protocols are in place to monitor and manage this risk? Are there other medications available that could meet the same need with lower risk? Always be sure to check local and state jurisdictions for an up-to-date list of what medications are subject to controlled drug scheduling.

Similarly, depending on the state and municipality, there might be some constraints on which cases medication may be used as part of a treatment plan, even if you determine the pet's behavior indicates a need. For example, if the medication being considered has behavioral side effects that could mimic neurologic changes seen with the rabies virus, it may not be permissible to use in pets under bite quarantine. Neurological changes, such as sedation, ataxia, altered mentation, and hypersalivation are uncommon side effects of many behavioral pharmaceuticals. However, side effects such as these will often resolve within a few days of discontinuation of the medication, whereas a primary neurologic complaint, such as rabies, would not.

In the case of court-ordered holding of animals, organizations may be required to hold the "evidence" in a manner to prevent deterioration. This should include not only physical health but also mental health. Many of these cases end up with extended LOS and managing

them in a way to prevent behavioral deterioration can be challenging. It can be helpful to have discussions with the investigators, legal team, and other professionals involved in the case about welfare concerns identified and what role management options, including medications, might play in maintaining the pet's behavioral health for the duration of the hold (see Chapter 21).

22.1.5 Monitoring

There should always be a designated person or persons responsible for the regular monitoring of pets under pharmacologic therapy. In private practice, this team usually is made up of the owner, the veterinarian, and possibly an additional staff member such as a veterinary technician or assistant. In the shelter, this often consists of the team doing daily behavior and wellness rounds and might include a veterinary technician, behavior team member, or experienced handler or caregiver. This might or might not include the veterinarian. This team should know what to watch for with the particular medication prescribed and know to whom they report any concerns or observations. These observations should include monitoring appetite, water intake, urination, defecation, activity level, and level of undesired and anxiety/stress-related behaviors, specifically noting frequency, duration, and intensity of those behaviors of interest. Post-outcome planning is also an integral part of monitoring. Each pet prescribed medication should have a plan to go with them through their anticipated outcome, including after they leave the shelter and enter the home environment. This plan should be reviewed regularly. If progress is not being made, the diagnosis and plan should be re-evaluated and adjusted. If resources are available, the shelter can also reach out to other qualified behavior professionals, including force-free trainers, Certified Applied Animal Behaviorists, or veterinary behavior specialists, dependent on the individual case and where the challenges are being identified.

22.1.6 Outcome Considerations

Finally, the post-outcome plan for animals undergoing behavioral pharmaceutical treatment should be considered prior to instituting therapy. Who performs the adoption counseling or advises the next group of the pet's current status? These requirements vary, with some states requiring such advice to be given by the prescribing veterinarian. A written management/education plan should always accompany verbal instructions. Full disclosure of the pet's problem and current treatment needs should be provided in a thoughtful and compassionate manner in order to fully educate the caregiver without creating undue alarm about the problem. Such plans could even include offering a recommendation for follow-up care with a veterinarian; animal behaviorist; a member of your organization familiar with the pet; or a qualified, humane, force-free trainer.

If the pet is made available for adoption or placed in a foster home, the new owner/caregiver counseling should include education about medication, including the goals of treatment, how to give it, what side effects to watch for, and who to follow up with. A plan for continuation or weaning of the medication should be discussed and should include any risks of stopping the medication abruptly. If the new owners/caregivers have concerns about the medication or treatment at any time, they should be encouraged to speak with a veterinarian before making decisions about the medication on their own. Some organizations might consider weaning the pet's medication before adoption; this decision should be made on an individual animal basis with consideration of the risks of prolonged stay in shelter care versus those associated with abrupt discontinuation of therapy.

When animals undergoing treatment are transferred to another organization, such as another shelter or rescue group, the new organization's philosophy and policies on behavioral medications should be considered and discussed prior to transfer. A plan for continuation or weaning should be made prior to transfer. The discussion of the risk of stopping medication abruptly should be included in this plan, as it would be for an adopter or foster home.

22.2 Developing a Medication Protocol

Some organizations might consider adding behavior medications to their standard operating procedure or developing protocols for their use in specific cases that the shelter is equipped to manage. In some organizations, animals can be treated by trained staff via protocols provided by a veterinarian (Association of Shelter Veterinarians 2018). Protocols should include information about the specific problem to be addressed, including accompanying behavioral observations. How the medication can be used as part of the treatment should be briefly discussed, but other aspects of the treatment plan such as environmental management, enrichment, and behavior modification should also be included. It should be emphasized that medication alone is not the sole treatment for the problem. Doses based on body weight, time to effect, side effects, and adjustments based on side effects can also be mentioned. If dosed chronically (i.e., longer than daily for four weeks) a weaning plan should be made. This will be imperative if medication is anticipated to be reduced or discontinued after the pet has moved to their final outcome. For most medications, a weaning plan of reducing the dose (not dosing frequency) by 25–33% every one to two weeks is judicious. If at any time the pet's behavior deteriorates, the caregiver should be instructed to go back to the last previously effective dose and contact a veterinarian for further instructions. It is prudent for the welfare organization to have a few recommendations of veterinarians within their organization or community who are well versed in common behavior medications and can be referred to in these situations.

Appendices 22.A–22.E contain a formulary and example behavior medication protocols for select scenarios common in shelter practice. It will be important to keep in mind that these are merely examples, and the environmental management and behavior modification skills, tools, and resources will vary widely between organizations. The intent of these resources is to guide practitioners on how to incorporate behavioral medication into a behavior treatment protocol.

22.3 Neurotransmitters

Glutamate, an amino acid, is the primary excitatory neurotransmitter in the central nervous system (CNS). This is where NMDA receptor blockers, such as ketamine and memantine, act creating analgesia and addressing anxiety associated with pain. At high doses, a dissociative and/or cataleptic state can be induced (Overall 2013b; Plumb 2018).

Gamma (γ)-aminobutyric acid (GABA) is synthesized from glutamate and is the major inhibitory neurotransmitter in the CNS (Murray 2019a). It plays a role in vigilance, anxiety, muscle tension, seizure activity, and memory. Benzodiazepines have their effect via this neurotransmitter by binding to the GABA A receptor site to enhance the effect of GABA (Plumb 2018.)

The monoamines make up another class of neurotransmitters, containing several well-known compounds commonly used in behavioral pharmacology: dopamine, norepinephrine, and serotonin. Along with epinephrine, melatonin, and histamine, which will not be discussed further, these compounds make up the biogenic amines.

Dopamine (DA) plays a major role in reward systems. It is released in anticipation of and response to natural rewards such as food, water, and sex, or synthetic rewards (dopamine agonists) such as amphetamines, cocaine, opioids, and nicotine. Excess dopamine transmission is associated with stereotypic/compulsive behavior and schizophrenia in humans. Decreased dopamine transmission is associated with decreased alertness, anxiety, and depression as well as cognitive deficits and Parkinsonian-like tremors in people. Dopamine and acetylcholine have an inverse relationship (Murray 2019b).

Norepinephrine (NE) is synthesized from dopamine and plays a role in the control of emotions (such as the intensity of the emotional response), arousal, and reward systems. The α-adrenergic receptors, especially the α2 adrenergic class, are particularly useful in behavioral pharmacology. Alpha-2 agonists such as xylazine, dexmedetomidine, and clonidine inhibit NE release via action at presynaptic autoreceptors, resulting in sedation, analgesia, muscle relaxation, and at lower doses, anxiety control. Alpha-2 antagonists such as yohimbine, atipamezole and amphetamines, stimulate NE release, hence their role as reversal agents (Murray 2019b).

Serotonin (5-HT) is synthesized from tryptophan obtained by dietary intake. Dietary levels of tryptophan can alter brain serotonin levels, though it is not a simple linear relationship and simply supplementing tryptophan to the diet will not necessarily increase serotonin levels in the brain (Dodman et al. 1996). There are many serotonin receptors, not just in the brain but throughout the body, including the heart, gastrointestinal (GI) tract, smooth muscle lining, and platelets (see Table 22.2). Consequently, serotonin plays a role in the control of mood, impulsivity, anxiety and panic, satiety, nausea, cognition, aggression, sex drive, sleep, pain, coagulation, and even thermoregulation (Murray 2019c).

Acetylcholine (Ach) is the only neurotransmitter not directly synthesized from an amino acid. It is synthesized by linking choline with acetyl coenzyme A (acetyl CoA). It is involved in signal transmission at postganglionic parasympathetic synapses (muscarinic), autonomic ganglia (Nicotinic n), and neuromuscular junctions (Nicotinic m). Anticholinergic effects such as dry mouth, dry eyes, urine retention,

Table 22.2 Location and function of serotonin (5-HT) receptors.

Receptor	Location/function
5-HT 1A	Prereceptor, autoreceptor—inhibits firing of neuron; synthesis and release of 5-HT; postreceptor
5-HT 1B	Autoreceptor—inhibits additional 5-HT release
5-HT 2A	Platelet aggregation and smooth muscle contraction
5-HT 2B	Found on human heart valves
5-HT 2C	Regulates appetite
5-HT 3	GI tract, chemoreceptor trigger zone (vomiting, nausea)
5-HT 4	GI tract (secretion and peristalsis)
5-HT 6	Limbic system
5-HT 7	Limbic system

constipation, pupil dilation (mydriasis), and an increase heart rate can occur with medications that affect this neurotransmitter, such as tricyclic antidepressants (TCAs). This neurotransmitter's effect at the muscarinic receptors can play a role in memory. Its effect at the nicotinic-n receptors in the brain, adrenal medulla, and autonomic ganglia also affect learning and memory. Nicotine also binds nicotinic-n receptors, activating the reward and dependence systems, but also improving mental alertness and memory (Crowell-Davis 2019). This makes sense when one considers the effect of cigarettes on emotion and focus as well as addiction. Degeneration of cholinergic pathways is implicated in learning and memory decline, as occurs in Alzheimer's disease.

22.4 Impact of Psychopharmaceuticals on Behavior

There is a great breadth of literature on psychopharmaceuticals' impact on behavior though the majority of studies involving animals were performed during safety studies for humans. While some medications have been more extensively reviewed, particularly with regard to use in dogs and cats, some of those with the most data may be challenging to apply to shelter behavior cases due to cost, duration of action, frequency of dosing, or route of administration. These data will be reviewed where pertinent while going through the different classes of behavior medications available. If the reader should want more extensive information about any of the below, the author recommends *Veterinary Psychopharmacology*, 2nd ed., by Crowell-Davis et al. (2019), for the most extensive review in veterinary behavioral medicine.

22.4.1 Selective Serotonin Reuptake Inhibitors and Tricyclic Antidepressants

22.4.1.1 Selective Serotonin Reuptake Inhibitors (SSRIs)
The general mechanism of action for SSRIs is inhibit reuptake of serotonin molecules from the synaptic space back into the presynaptic neuron. This prevents "recycling" of the neurotransmitter and a net increase in serotonin available in the synaptic space. However, clinical effects of this increased availability often take as long as four to eight weeks to detect. This delay is attributed to an SSRI-induced desensitization of the serotonin 1A autoreceptors blocking negative feedback, which leads to a more normalized release of serotonin (Blier and de Montigny 1998). Common medications in this class used to help treat veterinary behavior problems include fluoxetine, paroxetine, sertraline, citalopram and escitalopram. Fluoxetine will be discussed below as it has the most extensive research background, lowest dosing frequency, and is consistently inexpensive and easily available, therefore making it suitable for shelter use. Additional information about the other SSRIs can be found in other references (Ogata 2019; Plumb 2018; Overall 2013b; Landsberg et al. 2013).

Fluoxetine, an SSRI, is one of the most extensively researched behavioral medications for dogs and cats. Studies have described its use and evaluated its efficacy in generic and branded form (Reconcile®, PRN® Pharmacal, Pensacola, FL) for the treatment of separation anxiety in dogs (Simpson et al. 2007; Landsberg et al. 2008; Ogata 2016), territorial and other forms of aggression in dogs (Haug 2008, 2014; Sherman et al. 1996; Reisner 2003; Houpt and Virga 2003), urine marking in cats (Pryor et al. 2001), and compulsive disorder in dogs (Wynchank and Berk 1998; Luescher 2009; Mills and Luescher 2006; Irimajiri et al. 2009; Houpt and Virga 2003). Fluoxetine has been used clinically for many other behavior problems, with the justification of treating the underlying fear and anxiety contributing to the behavior problem. This use is due in part to genetic studies on serotonin receptors that indicate receptor polymorphism may play a role in susceptibility to affective (mental illness) diseases in people. This important change, that effectively leads to a functional difference with the serotonin autoreceptor, correlates with the degree of response to fear in the amygdala (the part of the brain that manages and immediately processes primitive emotions). Those with a particular allele for this gene may be more vulnerable to stress and at higher risk of developing clinical depression (Caspi et al. 2003; Hariri et al. 2002). In other words, a large proportion of behavior disorders with underlying fear and anxiety as motivators (including several types of aggression) are suspected to be due to low serotonin levels in the brain.

Due to the extensive literature available in people, dogs, cats, and other species, the mechanism of action, effects, and side effects of fluoxetine are well known. Just as with its use in humans, though the reuptake effect is immediate, it may take several weeks (at least four to six) to see the full behavioral effect due, in part, to later presynaptic auto-receptor downregulation (Blier and de Montigny 1998). The half-life of fluoxetine is very long in dogs, at least five days (Ogata et al. 2019; Plumb 2018), so changes in behavioral effect, and time for it to be completely cleared from the body is much

longer than other antidepressants. For example, when switching from fluoxetine to a monoamine oxidase inhibitor (MAOI), a five-week washout period is recommended to help reduce the risk of serious side effects, including serotonin syndrome (de Souza Dantas and Crowell-Davis 2019a; Murray 2019b, Ogata et al. 2019) (see Section 22.4.1.4).

Fluoxetine is typically dosed at 1–2 mg/kg by mouth once daily for dogs and 0.5–1 mg/kg by mouth once daily for cats (Landsberg et al. 2013; Plumb 2018; Ogata et al. 2019). The most common side effects include a decrease in appetite or lethargy, though these typically are mild and should not last longer than one to two weeks. If they are severe, or if other more serious side effects such as vomiting, diarrhea, tremors, increased fear or anxiety (often identified as new fears of objects or noises), or increased irritability are noted, the veterinarian managing the case should reduce the dose or stop the medication. If given daily for more than four weeks, this medication should be weaned gradually, if possible, rather than discontinued abruptly. Because fluoxetine can alter blood glucose levels, it should be avoided, or blood glucose and insulin doses monitored carefully, in diabetic patients (Ogata et al. 2019; Plumb 2018).

22.4.1.2 Tricyclic Antidepressants (TCAs)
Tricyclic antidepressants work by inhibiting the reuptake of norepinephrine and serotonin by the presynaptic plasma membrane transporters. Additionally, they will alter the conformation and enhance the sensitivity of postsynaptic serotonin 1A receptors, which makes them more efficient. As with SSRIs, it may take several weeks to see the full effect. Because TCAs impact norepinephrine receptors in addition to serotonin receptors, this class of medication is less specific than the SSRIs. Not only is norepinephrine altered, but other neurotransmitter systems are impacted, with anticholinergic, antihistaminic and $\alpha2$ antagonistic effects (Crowell-Davis 2019). This can lead to a greater breadth of side effects,

including anticholinergic effects and antihistaminic effects such as dry mouth, changes in urination pattern (increased or decreased), constipation, decreased tear production, increased ocular pressure, mydriasis, and cardiovascular changes such as arrhythmias, syncope, or hypostatic congestion. This class of medication might also reduce a patient's seizure threshold (Crowell-Davis 2019; Plumb 2018). However, these alternate receptor side effects can be beneficial sometimes, depending on the case. For example, a pet that urinates frequently or suffers from atopy might benefit from mild urine retention or antihistaminic effects of a TCA.

The most common TCAs used in veterinary behavior include clomipramine, amitriptyline, and doxepin. It is important to note that these medications have variable effects relative to each neurotransmitter that must be considered prior to selection (Crowell-Davis 2019). Clomipramine has the greatest serotoninergic effect and hence is one of the better choices for anxieties or behaviors whose suspected underlying pathology includes low serotonin. Though amitriptyline has historically been recommended for cats urinating outside the litterbox, this recommendation was likely initially due to cost and familiarity. There are other medications that are now easily available at a reasonable cost if the underlying motivation is anxiety (such as fluoxetine or clomipramine) (Crowell-Davis 2019). Amitriptyline may also have some beneficial effect on feline interstitial cystitis due to pain reduction via the effect on norepinephrine, rather than anxiety reduction via the effect on serotonin (Hanno et al. 1989). Doxepin has a high antihistaminic effect relative to the others, so is more frequently used for pruritis relief, though it has a relatively low effect on serotonin (Crowell-Davis 2019).

Clomipramine is an extensively researched behavioral medication for dogs and cats. Studies have described its use and evaluated its efficacy in generic and branded form (Clomicalm) for the treatment of separation

anxiety in dogs in conjunction with a behavior modification plan (King et al. 2000; Sherman and Mills 2008; Cannas et al. 2014), some forms of aggression in dogs, urine marking and other behavior problems in cats (Hanno et al. 1989; Litster 2000; Landsberg and Wilson 2005; Ellis and Wells 2010), and compulsive disorder in dogs (Luescher 2009; Mills and Luescher 2006; Seksel and Lindeman 2001). Of all of the TCAs, clomipramine has the strongest serotonin reuptake effect, which is why it is a popular and effective choice for the former and for several other behavior problems, with the justification of treating the underlying fear and anxiety contributing to the behavior problem. As mentioned above, it may take up to four to eight weeks to see the full effect of this medication, although some pets will show response earlier. Clomipramine is better tolerated with a lower rate of side effects in dogs than in people, likely due to the difference in proportion of clomipramine and its metabolite desmethylclomipramine (clomipramine is higher in dogs, vs. lower in people) (Crowell-Davis 2019). The half-life of clomipramine is shorter than fluoxetine, and is highly variable, reported at 16 hours (Crowell-Davis 2019) up to 32 hours (Plumb 2018). It should be noted that a two-week washout is recommended when switching from clomipramine to an MAOI (Landsberg et al. 2013; Plumb 2018; Crowell-Davis 2019).

Clomicalm label dose is 2–4 mg/kg PO q 24 hours; however, most clinicians have found a q 12-hour dosing strategy more clinically effective in dogs. The current standard dose range is 1–2 mg/kg PO q 12 hours, up to 3 mg/kg PO q 12 hours (Landsberg 2013; Plumb 2018; Crowell-Davis 2019). Similar side effects as expected with fluoxetine might be noted such as a decrease in appetite or lethargy for the first one to two weeks. Side effects such as vomiting, diarrhea, constipation, changes in urination, tremors, increased anxiety, or increased irritability are indications that the veterinarian managing the case should reduce the dose or stop the medication. If given daily for more than four weeks, this medication should be weaned gradually if possible, rather than discontinued abruptly. Clomicalm should not be given to pets with a history of dry eye, glaucoma, urinary retention, constipation, abnormal blood pressure or arrythmias due to the potential for anticholinergic and antihistaminic side effects (Crowell-Davis 2019; Plumb 2018). Unfortunately, generic clomipramine has drastically increased in cost and the branded Clomicalm is sometimes less expensive than the generic formulation. This puts Clomicalm/clomipramine out of range for rational use in most sheltered pets due to financial constraints.

22.4.1.3 Thyroid Hormone Measurements

It should be noted that any SSRIs or TCAs can affect thyroid hormone measurements, causing cats with hyperthyroid disease to appear euthyroid and euthyroid dogs to appear hypothyroid. This does not preclude the use of these medications in patients with thyroid disease, but it can superficially complicate diagnosis and management. It is always prudent to check thyroid hormones prior to administration, when possible, and to reassess the patient for clinical signs associated with thyroid disease prior to instituting or adjusting treatment, especially if they are already on an SSRI or TCA (Martin 2010; Shelton et al. 1993; Gulikers and Panciera 2003).

22.4.1.4 Serotonin Syndrome

Sometimes referred to as serotonin toxicity, serotonin syndrome is a serious side effect that consists of a collection of physiologic, behavioral and neuromuscular side effects that can range from mild to fatal. The clinical signs most easily observed in the dog or cat include agitation, confusion, anxiety, restlessness, tremors, increased heart rate, vomiting or diarrhea. These signs can worsen in severity to include seizures, hyperthermia, blood pressure changes, coma and death (Almgren and Lee 2013; Sinn 2018; de Souza Dantas and Crowell-Davis 2019b). Typically,

serotonin syndrome occurs when a pet accidentally ingests a large amount of their owner's medication, or when an individual is given a combination of two or more medications/supplements that both have some impact on the level of serotonin. The most notable combination is an antidepressant (SSRI or TCA) combined with an MAOI; however, this can occur with any combination of serotoninergic medications and/or supplements. Rarely, in some sensitive individuals, serotonin syndrome can occur at standard dose ranges. Additionally, medications such as tramadol, trazodone, and mirtazapine all have some effect with serotonin, even if it is not included in their primary intended effect.

It is important to note that some supplements sold over the counter, such as St. John's Wort and Griffonia seed extract (5-HTP), have serotoninergic effects and can be quite potent, especially in smaller animals (Gwaltney-Brant et al. 2000). This is one of many reasons it is always important to pay attention to what other medications, supplements, herbal remedies, or other over-the-counter treatments a pet is being given when creating a behavior treatment plan. Especially when a pet is likely to move on to a different caregiver (foster, adoption, transfer), it should be noted that serotonin syndrome is a side effect that must always be considered and discussed proactively any time any medication or supplement that works to increase serotonin is used (Almgren and Lee, 2013; Sinn 2018; de Souza Dantas and Crowell-Davis 2019b; Overall 2013b). For more information regarding the neurotransmitter and behavioral effects of herbal and natural remedies, *Psychoactive Herbs in Veterinary Behavior Medicine* by Stefanie Schwartz (2005) is an excellent resource.

Diagnosis of serotonin syndrome is generally based on the pet's history of a high dose of serotoninergic medication, or a combination of medications and supplements. Most frequently, this will occur relatively soon (e.g., within days) after starting a medication, supplement, or dose change. It must be noted that some of the signs of serotonin syndrome overlap with those of expected side effects of serotonin-modifying medications. However, if these changes, such as severe GI upset, agitation, irritability, etc., are occurring secondary to a therapeutic dose for the pet, this is indicative that the dose or medication plan itself should be changed. If clinical signs are suspected to be due to serotonin syndrome, the medication that is implicated should be discontinued. If clinical signs are mild or are due to anticipated initial side effects of the medication, they will often resolve within 48 hours if the dose is reduced by ~one-half or discontinued. Larger overdoses or toxicity from multiple serotoninergic medications, and more severe clinical signs may require immediate medical attention. Symptomatic treatment, in addition to some reversal and support agents, can be implemented. Aggressive treatment in-hospital is described elsewhere (Almgren and Lee 2013; Sinn 2018).

22.4.2 Benzodiazepines

Benzodiazepines (BZDs) are a class of medication that can be used to help treat intense anxiety or panic associated with events such as storms, separation anxiety, car ride anxiety, and others. They work by potentiating the inhibitory effect of GABA by binding to the GABA-A receptor. Typically, the anxiolytic effect can occur within 1–2 hours of dosing, and dependent on the specific medication used, the effect can last from a few hours up to 8–10 hours. The most common side effects include increased appetite, changes in urination, sedation, muscle relaxation, loss of inhibition of behavior, increased friendliness, paradoxical excitation, and, rarely, acute liver failure in cats (de Souza Dantas and Crowell-Davis 2019c; Overall 2013b).

This class of medication is also known to help with seizure control and is often used in emergency situations to help manage status epilepticus or seizures of extended duration. This effect on seizure control may be reduced with chronic dosing, so it may be prudent to use BZDs only on an as-needed basis in patients with a seizure history or increased risk of seizure. Other side effects include increased appetite and consequent polydipsia, elimination, and food seeking. This can actually be a very helpful side effect when managing a patient that is so fearful they have difficulty eating or taking treats, or who is experiencing anorexia from an antidepressant (de Souza Dantas and Crowell-Davis 2019c).

It has been reported that administration of BZDs can cause memory deficits, leading to difficulty in learning new material. This can be challenging if behavior modification is a goal during reduced anxiety, though it can also be helpful to prevent additional negative learning during frightening events, such as veterinary procedures or events occurring while the pet is alone. At higher doses where sedation is achieved (such as during sedation or pre-medication for anesthesia), there can also be a short amnesic effect, where the pet does not really remember the few minutes prior to onset of effect (de Souza Dantas and Crowell-Davis 2019c).

Sedation as a result of BZD administration is typically dose dependent. Generally, the anxiolytic effect will occur prior to sedation with increasing doses. A good monitoring exercise for this medication class, as well as other fast-acting behavior medications, is to start a pet on a low dose and increase it incrementally. Continue to increase the dose within the dosing range, until either appropriate anxiety control is observed, or sedation occurs. If sedation occurs and anxiolysis has not, it is not likely that this particular medication will be suitable for anxiety control for that patient. Caution should be used when combining BZDs with other sedating medications.

Behavioral disinhibition is an important construct to consider when using BZDs. Essentially, this side effect occurs when the forebrain's conscious inhibition of specific behaviors is reduced. The pet might normally consider a behavioral response, then decide that a different option is a safer or more reasonable choice. However, with the addition of the medication, that forebrain inhibition is reduced. This same effect occurs in people with BZDs and with alcohol consumption. For example, you might consider dancing on the bar when out with friends, but decide it is not the best idea in the company of someone you don't know well. However, after a couple of martinis, now dancing on the bar seems like a great idea, regardless of who you are with! This can result in behaviors not typically observed in the pet, such as extended food seeking, reduced fear and retreat response, and most importantly, increased likelihood of reacting with aggression. Therefore, the prescribing veterinarian must consider their level of risk sensitivity regarding the prospect of disinhibition when prescribing. In general, caution should be used when treating a pet with a history of aggressive responses. Safety tools, such as basket muzzles and crate confinement, can be set up if this is a concern but a BZD is deemed the best choice for that pet and problem.

Paradoxical reactions to BZDs need to be differentiated from behavioral disinhibition. The former refers to an idiosyncratic reaction demonstrated by extreme excitation, agitation, and restlessness and has been reported in dogs and cats. In general, the dose that leads to this is lower than the dose that causes anxiolysis and sedation. If a pet experiences paradoxical excitation, theoretically the dose should be increased and, if sedate, the dose decreased. However, talking owners or caregivers into giving a BZD again to a pet in which they witnessed paradoxical excitation is a challenging conversation indeed (de Souza Dantas and Crowell-Davis 2019c).

Acute hepatic necrosis is a rare but often fatal idiosyncratic side effect in cats, reported after oral administration of diazepam (Hughes et al. 1996). Though reports have only been published with oral diazepam, this is a potential risk with other BZDs. Some consider those BZDs that do not have secondary hepatic metabolites (e.g., oxazepam and lorazepam) (de Souza Dantas and Crowell-Davis 2019c) to be relatively safer, as cats are well-known to have poor efficiency of

medication metabolism via glucuronidation. However, BZDs can be extremely helpful in reducing and managing fear, anxiety, and panic in cats, such as is experienced when a cat is taken into a sheltering situation. There have been clinical reports of very effective in-shelter use for management of transitional fear for cats, with few reported side effects without labwork performed pre administration (L. Jacobson, personal communication). Therefore, the clinician managing the case must consider their own level of risk sensitivity regarding use. It is the author's standard recommendation to evaluate the cat's liver values prior to and within five days of starting a BZD if it is to be used on a daily basis for more than three days.

BZDs are controlled substances throughout the United States. Risk of abuse and diversion must be considered prior to prescribing. In the shelter, just as in a veterinary clinic, stock supplies must be kept in a locked box and quantities closely reported consistent with DEA regulations. When considering whether to use this medication, the clinician should consider who will have access to it, who will be responsible for administering the medication, and whether it might be sent home with a foster or a new adopter.

Dependence on BZDs can occur even in nonhuman species. Therefore, to prevent withdrawal, it should be weaned down gradually when dosing chronically. Signs of withdrawal can vary between the specific BZDs given, but include increased anxiety, anorexia, tremors, and seizures. Additionally, if given chronically, tolerance can occur (de Souza Dantas and Crowell-Davis 2019c).

22.4.3 Alpha-2 Agonists

This class of medication works to bind to presynaptic (negative feedback) α2 receptors, which then reduces the release of NE. This neurotransmitter is important behaviorally and physiologically in the immediate panic response that occurs during fight or flight, at the primitive level of the brain. Though frequently used for sedation, analgesia can also be produced, and anxiolysis can occur at doses lower than required for sedation. Alpha-2 agonists of clinical importance in veterinary behavioral pharmacology include clonidine and dexmedetomidine/detomidine.

Clonidine is an α2 agonist historically used to control blood pressure in people that has antianxiety effects in both people and animals. This effect typically lasts four to six hours in most dogs. It can be dosed one to two hours prior to a stressful event and then again after about six hours as needed or given chronically up to three times daily. It can be given alone as a fast-acting situational medication, or in conjunction with a longer-term baseline anxiety reducing medication, such as fluoxetine (Ogata and Dodman 2011). Side effects are uncommon, but excess sedation might be noted at higher doses. Theoretically, hypotension can occur, but this has not been recognized clinically as a frequent side effect of concern. However, it is prudent to caution caregivers that if an uncoordinated gait or collapse occurs, the pet might be experiencing low blood pressure. If concerned, heart rate can be monitored at home or during care. Typically, heart rate will increase to compensate for hypotension, and this is an easier physiologic parameter to measure than blood pressure in dogs and cats. This finding should be taken with the perspective of the pet's overall behavior including their anxiety level and other behaviors, as anxiety can also lead to tachycardia. Additionally, occasional vomiting, diarrhea, changes in urination, tremors, increased anxiety, or increased irritability are noted. If these are identified, the dose should be reduced, or the medication discontinued. If hypotension or other severe side effects are noted, or overdose occurs, this medication can be reversed using atipamezole.

Dexmedetomidine has been a popular and useful medication for sedation for a long time in veterinary medicine. Detomidine, a close relative, has been used for equine sedation via transmucosal absorption for some time as well.

Detomidine has been used in the same manner to help control fractious behavior (i.e., fear and panic-based aggression) in dogs during veterinary examination. However, dosing must be done very carefully as there is a very real risk of overdosage due to the concentration of the equine formulation (Hopfensperger et al. 2013). More recently, dexmedetomidine oromucosal gel (Sileo®, Zoetis, Parsippany, NJ) has been labeled for noise aversion in dogs. It is administered in the buccal pouch so that it can be absorbed transmucosally, either one hour prior to a noise event, as soon as the noise trigger is heard, or as soon as the pet begins to show a fear response (Korpivaara et al. 2017). It can be re-dosed after two to three hours, up to five times in a row if needed. In the author's experience, few patients need to be re-dosed during an acute event, and if they do, often they can be given a lower dose that still provides appropriate anxiolytic effect. Though it may be cost-prohibitive for some organizations, this product has, in the author's opinion, the most beneficial niche in that it can be given even after a dog has begun to show signs of fear, or the noise event has already started, and still have a beneficial effect with reducing fear. With any of the other fast-acting oral formulations listed in this chapter, the time to effect is at a minimum 30 minutes and, more reasonably, 1–2 hours; if the pet has not been medicated appropriately ahead of time, they will not gain much benefit from the medication given after the fact and will continue to suffer high anxiety throughout the event. Dexmedetomidine oromucosal gel can catch those surprise events, which can be particularly important when housing and managing pets that one does not know well because triggers may often be a surprise, at least the first time. The author has discussed using this medication for sheltered dogs who are not coping well upon intake, especially with the ambient noises of the shelter, or for those dogs who are showing distress during transport. Fear responses during vehicle transport often have a large noise component with the engine, barking dogs, rattling crates and doors, traffic, etc., in addition to the fear and instability associated with acceleration forces (see Chapter 20).

This medication may not be suitable to administer to dogs with severe fear (leading to aggression) with handling, as it must be given oromucosally. It is important to warn caregivers that the mucous membranes at the site of administration will become pale due to the vasoconstrictive action of the medication, but this does not indicate a systemic concern. If swallowed, the effect of the medication will be lowered to non-existent, depending on the amount swallowed, due to the high level of first pass metabolism. Therefore, the risk of overdosing is low, provided the administrator understands how to properly use the dosing syringe. Just as with oral clonidine, the oromucosal gel formulations of the α2 agonists can also be reversed using atipamezole if overdosage is suspected (Sinn 2018).

22.4.4 Other Medications

22.4.4.1 Trazodone

Trazodone, an atypical antidepressant, is a serotonin antagonist/reuptake inhibitor (SARI) that can be used to help decrease anxiety. It is also considered a hypnotic at higher doses and has been reported to have some antiepileptic effect. It can be used alone as a fast-acting situational medication, as a bridging agent while waiting for the baseline medication to take effect or combined longer term with a baseline medication for synergistic anxiety management.

Trazodone has been the topic of several research studies in the last 10–12 years and has rapidly gained popularity for behavioral management in veterinary and shelter behavioral medicine. Retrospective and open label studies for use as an adjunct to baseline antidepressants or for short-term confinement demonstrated behavioral improvement (Gruen and Sherman 2008; Gruen et al. 2014). However, a more recent placebo controlled, blinded study on dogs during post-operative confinement did not show a difference between trazodone and a placebo (Gruen et al. 2017).

Because of the rapidly increasing popularity and additional research that continues to be published regarding trazodone use, it is important for the practitioner to keep in mind appropriate ways to use this medication. First, it is imperative to keep in mind that the dosing matters. When reviewing the literature, there is a vast range of doses used. This medication, as is the case with many, has anxiety reducing effects at the lower end of the dosing range. At higher doses, the effect of the medication at the serotonin receptors becomes less specific, so more side effects can be observed, and the hypnotic effect is enhanced. This is important when dosing and advising caregivers on what to expect from the medication. The clinician must have a goal in mind for this medication and for the dose. In general, it should be to help reduce anxiety quickly, without excess sedation, on a short-term basis. If an appropriate baseline anxiety reducing medication is not enough and additional anxiety control is needed, trazodone can be used as an adjunct by being mindful of the dose range used. It is not fair to the pet or to the public to give high doses to take advantage of the hypnotic effect. It is also not the best use to give only trazodone long term. If it helps, but the pet still will likely have a longer LOS or has an underlying behavior disorder, that pet will be better served starting a longer-term baseline sooner rather than later, using trazodone as the bridging agent to the antidepressant's time to effect. Also, it is not good practice to just continue to increase the dose, or to simply add medications, if the trazodone is not having a beneficial effect. For trazodone, as with all medications used to help manage behavior, the effect should be monitored. If it helps, it can be continued, along with a longer-term plan. If it doesn't help and is dosed at an appropriate level, then it should be discontinued and replaced with another medication instead.

When dosing trazodone, to avoid GI upset, the dose may be gradually increased over the first few days to week. Mild sedation when first giving this medication may be noted. Pets should be monitored for side effects of excess sedation, vomiting or diarrhea, changes in urination, tremors, increased anxiety, or increased irritability. As discussed with other medications, these signs are indications to reduce the dose or discontinue the medication. Dosing recommendations for trazodone can be found in Appendix 22.A or medication protocol examples (see Appendices 22.B–22.E).

A recent study investigated giving trazodone to dogs upon shelter intake in order to reduce transitional stress, smooth acclimation to the shelter, and help reduce physical illness. This interesting study hypothesized that if the dogs' stress upon intake could be reduced, there would be less pressure on the pet's immune system and these dogs would experience lower levels of infectious disease. The results were promising, with statistical improvements in rates of illness, LOS, and adoption rates for those dogs who received trazodone during the first 48 hours of intake versus those who did not (Abrams et al. 2020). This would be considered a reasonable use of trazodone—at an appropriate dose, short-term, with a goal in mind (to reduce transitional stress during the first two days of intake). Similar protocols have been discussed for sheltered cats, using gabapentin on intake (van Haaften 2018).

Trazodone has also been studied in cats. One study investigated dosing effect and safety. Notable findings include that the time to effect for cats is longer than dogs—one to two hours for dogs versus at least three hours for cats (Orlando et al. 2015). Dosing up to 100 mg per CAT was determined safe but, in the author's experience, lower doses generally are just as effective with fewer side effects. When used for transport to the veterinary clinic and examination, a 50 mg per CAT dose was determined to help reduce anxiety and improve handling (Stevens et al. 2016). In the author's experience, the effect of trazodone in cats is highly variable, so dosing trials should be performed prior to the stressful event if this medication is to be used situationally in cats.

22.4.4.2 Gabapentin

Gabapentin is a medication that has been used for neuropathic pain and seizure control, but also has antianxiety properties. It is known as an alpha-2 delta-1 ligand because it binds to that receptor, which prevents the release of excitatory neurotransmitters such as glutamate and norepinephrine (see Section 22.3), and also Substance P (Sinn 2018). Though it has a similar structure to GABA, it does not act at that neurotransmitter, or GABA receptors, whereas the BZDs do. It can be used alone or in combination with other medications for anxiety and it can be helpful if there is concern for a pain or seizure component to the abnormal behavior. In general, for behavioral use, it is dosed within the same range as used for pain control, 10–30 mg/kg PO. It can be dosed as needed, up to three times daily, and can be used chronically. The most common side effect is sedation, which often resolves after several days. Rarely, GI upset might be noted. If any of these side effects are severe or prolonged, the dose should be reduced, or the medication discontinued. It is important to note that the human liquid formulation of gabapentin contains xylitol, so if liquid is needed for dogs, it should be compounded, or the capsules opened and the contents mixed in a small amount of water.

Gabapentin has recently been most popular as a pre-veterinary-pharmaceutical, especially for cats. However, it can be very useful for dogs and has been reported to have some impact on impulsivity (Overall 2013b). Two recent studies evaluated its effect for managing fear and anxiety-related behavior in cats. In one study, cats were dosed orally prior to being placed in a carrier for transport to the veterinary hospital and examination. In the treatment group, behavioral signs of stress were reduced and the cats were able to tolerate the exam better than those receiving the placebo (van Haaften et al. 2017). In the other study, community cats were dosed on intake for sterilization while still in their cat traps. Cats given 50 or 100 mg of gabapentin versus placebo showed lower stress scores (Pankratz et al. 2018). The route of administration was creative: the researchers administered liquid gabapentin via a tom cat catheter in a 3-cc syringe while the cat remained in their cage (see Figure 14.15). The process, reviewed by video, was quite smooth; this strategy can be used to administer any liquid medication to cats in a lower stress manner with less restraint than is usually required (K. Ferris, personal communication).

Just as trazodone was used on intake to try to manage transitional stress in dogs, some shelters report using gabapentin in this same manner for cats though, at this time, no data has been published in the peer-reviewed literature. Gabapentin used situationally for cats can also facilitate handling, such as during ringworm treatments or other more invasive procedures. In addition to the situational uses described above, gabapentin can be used as a bridging medication dosed twice to three times daily, or as an adjunct to longer-term baseline medications, just as described with trazodone and clonidine.

22.5 Non-Pharmaceutical Interventions

Beyond traditional medication, some shelter organizations might consider complementary or non-pharmaceutical interventions instead of, or in addition to, behavioral medication. Complementary products include natural products such as herbal products, hyperdiluted flower remedies, vitamins or minerals, nutraceuticals and probiotics. Additionally, some would include treatments such as therapeutic touch, acupuncture, massage therapy, and magnets in this category. Additional nutraceutical and alternative therapy products and supplements are commercially available and indicated to help reduce fear and anxiety in dogs and cats, though their practical use in sheltered pets is limited due to questionable efficacy and cost. A full discussion of herbal remedies to impact behavior concerns is beyond the scope of this chapter, see *Psychoactive Herbs*

in Veterinary Behavior Medicine by Stefanie Schwartz (2005) for more information on this topic.

It is important to note that studies evaluating efficacy of these therapies may only apply to the brand and product tested, as quality, ingredients, standardization, and concentrations may vary greatly between brands. Though there are many natural and complementary products marketed or sold for the treatment of fear and anxiety, very few have any evidence of effectiveness. Therefore, it is important to critically review the information available and consider the level of evidence and the expected effect on the negative emotional states the welfare organization intends to treat, just as one would using a behavioral medication. The National Center for Complementary and Integrative Health can be a helpful resource when considering quality and effect of non-pharmaceuticals (nccih.nih.gov).

Given the overwhelmingly frightening and stressful environments of even well-run shelters, and the mild to moderate effect expected from most complementary and alternative products, it will often be the case that the cost of these products is not worth the benefit to the pets needing the behavioral support. Investigating the use of generic or low-cost versions of supplements can be useless at best and dangerous at worst due to the lack of regulation of what is actually in the product purchased if not from a reputable source. Additionally, diverting resources into products or treatment that are not likely to have a clinical impact on the animal's welfare can have additional consequences when one considers that the funds for these could be used instead for longer term interventions with far reaching impacts, such as providing hiding spots, sound absorbing panels, or portals, for example.

22.5.1 Pheromone Therapy

Pheromones are chemical signals that aid in communication between individuals of the same species. Pheromones are generally not detected by the olfactory epithelium—they act mainly through an accessory pathway involving the vomeronasal organ. There, they bind to receptors on nerve cells, which causes emotional, behavioral, or physiological changes in the individual sensing the pheromones.

Pheromone therapy uses analogues of natural pheromones to help reduce negative emotional states. There is weak to moderate evidence that dog appeasing pheromones and some synthetic cat pheromones (cheek gland-F3 and appeasing-F4) help to reduce anxiety in some settings (Frank et al. 2010; DePorter et al. 2018). In general, pheromones are very safe for pets of all ages and health issues because they are not systemically absorbed and do not interact with other medications.

Most pheromones are available commercially as sprays, wipes, or as plug-in diffusers. The sprays and wipes can be used for topical application to treatment area tables, in housing enclosures and in carriers; these applications usually only have a short-term effect—up to about 6 hours. Diffusers spread over ~650 ft^2 or 50–70 m^2 for 30 days. In shelter, these might be a good option for some smaller housing rooms, but it is important to consider the room's air flow system. If there is an effective negative outflow air system, it is possible that much of the pheromones could be pulled out of the room after release from the diffuser, never having the chance to land on surfaces near the animal, therefore having little to no effect on the pet. The dog appeasing pheromone also comes in a collar formulation. The collar diffuses for 30 days once removed from the package and placed on the dog. It may take up to 24 hours for the pheromones from the collar to take effect. Dog and cat products, and multiple cat products can be used concurrently in the same environment, though this is not a remedy for mixing species in the same space.

22.5.2 Milk Protein Derivatives

Alpha-casozepine is a milk protein derivative that has been studied in several formulations

(Royal Canin® Veterinary Diet Calm, Royal Canin, St. Charles, MO; Zylkene®, Vetoquinol, Ft. Worth, TX) to help reduce anxiety in dogs and cats (Beata, Beaumont-Graff, Coll et al. 2007; Kato et al. 2012; Beata, Beaumont-Graff, Diaz et al. 2007 Palestrini et al. 2010). When the product in Zylkene was compared to standard antidepressant therapy (positive control) in Europe, no difference between anxiety reduction was seen between the two products, indicating the same level of efficacy between the two treatments (Beata, Beaumont-Graff, Diaz et al. 2007). When the diet was compared using a case-control methodology, reductions in owner perceived anxiety signs and physiologic signs were correlated with the α-casozepine group (Kato et al. 2012). The dose is ~15–30 mg/kg daily and should be started one to two days in advance of anticipated stressors. It does not have any reported adverse effects or contraindications, though in the author's experience, some patients might experience mild GI upset or somnolence. It has a structure similar to GABA, which is the neurotransmitter that is affected by BZDs such as diazepam. There are several different products that include this derivative, though the research published is for specific brands of products and cannot be extrapolated to all formulations. For the specific dietary formulations, it is important to consider it is challenging to get a dog larger than ~9 kg (20 lbs) to eat enough of the food to get a therapeutic dose. In the author's experience, the dietary formulation has been helpful in some feline patients only.

22.5.3 L-Theanine

L-theanine is a green tea derivative that may help to reduce fear and anxiety in dogs and cats in stressful settings, such as during loud noises, travel, and frightening social interactions. It is suspected to reduce the effect of glutamate (the main excitatory neurotransmitter) and increase GABA (the main inhibitory neurotransmitter) and dopamine. L-theanine does not have any reported adverse effects or contraindications, though in the author's experience, some patients might experience mild GI upset or somnolence. This neutroceutical typically is used for chronic anxiety relief with some benefit, but some products have been labeled for acute relief if dosed 12 hours before and again 2 hours before the fearful event. The author has found less effectiveness used acutely. This derivative can be found alone (Anxitane®, Virbac, Carros, France); Araujo et al. (2010) found that a small sample of fearful dogs treated with Anxitane spent more time near unfamiliar people and interacted with them more frequently than placebo. Berteselli and Michelazzi (2007) found similar findings with a reduction in fear-related behaviors in a small sample of phobic dogs with Anxitane in conjunction with a behavior modificiation plan or in combination with other alternative supplements (Solliquin®, Nutramax, Lancaster, SC).

22.5.4 Probiotics

Recently, there has been much discussion surrounding the communication between the GI tract and the nervous system, including the specific bacterial population within the gut and its impact on anxiety, depression, and behavior in people and dogs. This is described as the microbiota-gut-brain axis (Foster and McVey Neufeld 2013). A new study investigated the use of a novel probiotic strain intended to help reduce anxiety in dogs (Purina® Pro Plan® Veterinary Supplements Calming Care, Nestlé Purina PetCare Company, St. Louis, MO). Using a randomized, blinded, crossover design, the addition of the supplement showed statistically significant improvements in anxiety-related behaviors, heart rate variability, and cortisol levels in one study (McGowan 2018), though the findings have not been published in a peer-reviewed journal. Though the cost is significantly more than other probiotic products at the time of writing, the author's clinical experience is in line with the findings of this study. This could be a route that can be considered for individual dogs at risk for side effects

with medication, or with owners, fosters, or communities that are medication-averse but need anxiety support. Additionally, a formulation of this same product has just been released for cats (Purina Pro Plan Veterinary Supplements Calming Care, Nestlé Purina PetCare Company, St. Louis, MO), although there is no peer-reviewed literature available on the efficacy of this product in cats either.

22.5.5 Olfactory and Auditory Enrichment

Other complementary products that might help to reduce some fear, anxiety, and unwanted behaviors in sheltered pets include aromatherapy scents. Graham et al. (2005) investigated the effect of scents including chamomile, lavender, peppermint, and rosemary on dogs. They found that dogs exposed to chamomile and lavender spent more time resting and vocalized less, whereas peppermint and rosemary led to more standing and moving. More recently, Binks et al. (2018) found similar results with the scents of ginger, coconut, vanilla, and valerian: these scents were associated with reduced levels of vocalization and movement versus controls. It must be noted that these findings cannot be extrapolated across species. Ellis and Wells (2010) performed similar studies with cats, finding no behavioral effect with lavender but more relaxation behaviors with catnip and prey scents and more play-like behavior with catnip. When exposing sheltered pets to aromatherapy, the same restrictions on surface area treated with the diffusers and impact of an efficient air flow system that might affect the use of pheromone diffusers should be considered here also. Alternate methods to expose the pets to these scents for enrichment and stress reduction should be implemented where surface area and air flow concerns are present.

Classical music and species-specific modified music may also be considered to help reduce fear and anxiety in dogs (Kogan et al. 2012; Bowman et al. 2017) and cats (Snowdon et al. 2015; Mira et al. 2016) in a home, hospital, or shelter environment. There is also evidence of a calming effect with an audiobook on dogs in a shelter environment (Brayley and Montrose 2016). An important concept to keep in mind when using this therapy to reduce negative emotional states is that it is not just the type of music or book used: a nocturne by Chopin is not the same as the *1812 Overture* by Tchaikovsky. In the audiobook study, *The Lion, the Witch and the Wardrobe* by C. S. Lewis was read—it is unknown if reading any book will have the same effect. Additionally, when any type of auditory enrichment devices are used, these should be played at a volume no louder than at conversational level (50–60 dB) and should not be played 24 hours a day. Habituation can occur if the audio enrichment is played consistently over time. Do not forget the importance of a little quiet time for distress and anxiety relief in any setting!

While olfactory and auditory enrichment can be widely implemented in a cost-effective, efficient, and humane manner, and other nutraceutical or natural products might help to reduce negative emotional states during the shelter stay for some mildly affected pets, they must still be critically evaluated before widespread implementation. When setting up behavior treatment and management plans at a herd health level, which is often required for efficient treatment of all pets affected in a shelter setting, these products might not produce enough beneficial effect for the majority of the population to justify the cost associated with commercial products generally intended for the private consumer.

22.6 Conclusions

Behavioral medications can be a life-saving addition to behavioral treatment plans for dogs and cats in shelter settings. They can be useful for those pets experiencing acclimation and kennel stress (distress solely resultant from the shelter environment) or for those pets that pass through the shelter system with underlying behavior disorders. Behavioral medications should not be used alone, without a working diagnosis and other aspects of a treatment plan (environmental management, behavior modification). Not only do these steps help to outline a clear treatment plan, they also help to create a clear idea of the behavioral and physiologic signs to monitor for the effectiveness of the treatment plan. Just medicating a behavioral complaint, such as barking dogs, is inappropriate. There are many motivations for barking, and medication may not be appropriate for all of them. Also keep in mind that behavior medications and behavior treatment should not be reserved for only the excessively well-resourced shelter or the most severe of cases. Even a limited-resource shelter can do something simple to meet the requirements of a comprehensive behavior treatment plan, including medication use—often via a population-level protocol. And all pets, once a problem has been identified, deserve the benefit of a comprehensive treatment plan. Follow-up is important in all cases, because if improvement is not noted, or if not enough improvement is noted, the pet or population should be reassessed and the plan should be updated.

Not only are fast-acting short-term medications helpful in a shelter, but also baseline antidepressants. Remember, some of these animals come in with preexisting behavior disorders, and we need to treat them when recognized. If shelter personnel suspect a problem is related to kennel stress and are working diligently to get that pet out of the shelter (which is the best goal and outcome for this problem and should be for all that are safe, really), then consider adding another adjunct to the short-term medication or switching to a different one. If the first medication helped some but not enough, consider adding a second to it. If it didn't help or had negligible impact, consider switching to a different one. And when it comes to the baseline, once it's had time to take effect, consider trying to taper the short-term medications to see if the pet can remain stable on the fewest medications possible. However, if a pet needs both while in the shelter, that is okay, provided the pet has a plan to follow it as they leave.

References

Abrams, J., Brennan, R., and Byosiere, S-E. (2020). Trazodone as a mediator of transitional stress in a shelter: Effects on illness, length of stay, and outcome. *J. Vet. Beh.* 36: 13–18.

Almgren, C.M. and Lee, J.A. (2013). Serotonin syndrome. *Clinician's Brief.* https://files.brief.vet/migration/article/16151/serotonin-syndrome-16151-article.pdf (accessed 15 June 2020).

Araujo, J.A., de Rivera, C., Etheir, J.L. et al. (2010). ANXITANE® tablets reduce fear of human beings in a laboratory model of anxiety-related behavior. *J. Vet. Behav.* https://doi.org/10.1016/j.jveb.2010.02.003.

Association of Shelter Veterinarians. (2018). Veterinary Supervision in Animal Shelters. https://www.sheltervet.org/assets/docs/position-statements/Veterinary%20Supervision%20in%20Animal%20Shelters%202018.pdf (accessed 6 July 2020).

Beata, C., Beaumont-Graff, E., Coll, V. et al. (2007). Effect of alpha-casozepine (Zylkene) on anxiety in cats. *J. Vet. Behav.* https://doi.org/10.1016/j.jveb.2007.02.002.

Beata, C., Beaumont-Graff, E., Diaz, C. et al. (2007). Effects of alpha-casozepine (Zylkene) versus selegiline hydrochloride (Selgian, Anipryl) on anxiety disorders in dogs. *J. Vet. Behav.* https://doi.org/10.1016/j.jveb.2007.08.001.

Berteselli, G.V. and Michelazzi, M. (2007). Use of L-theanine tablets and behavior modification for treatment of phobias in dogs: A preliminary study. *6th International Veterinary Behavior Meeting*, Riccione, Italy.

Binks, J., Taylor, S., Wills, A. et al. (2018). The behavioural effects of olfactory stimulation on dogs at a rescue shelter. *Appl. Anim. Behav. Sci.* https://doi.org/10.1016/j.applanim.2018.01.009.

Blier, P. and de Montigny, C. (1998). Possible serotonergic mechanisms underlying the antidepressant and anti-obsessive-compulsive disorder responses. *Biol. Psychiatry* 53: 193–203.

Bowman, A., Scottish SPCA, Dowell, F.J. et al. (2017). The effect of different genres of music on the stress levels of kennelled dogs. *Physiol. Behav.* https://doi.org/10.1016/j.physbeh.2017.01.024.

Brayley, C. and Montrose, V.T. (2016). The effects of audiobooks on the behaviour of dogs at a rehoming kennels. *Appl. Anim. Behav. Sci.* https://doi.org/10.1016/J.APPLANIM.2015.11.008.

Cannas, S., Frank, D., Minero, M. et al. (2014). Video analysis of dogs suffering from anxiety when left home alone and treated with clomipramine. *J. Vet. Behav.* https://doi.org/10.1016/j.jveb.2013.12.002.

Carney, H.C., Sadek, T.P, Curtis, T.M. et al. (2014). AAFP and ISFM guidelines for diagnosing and solving house-soiling behavior in cats. *J. Fel. Med. Surg.* https://doi.org/10.1177/1098612X 14539092.

Caspi A., Sugden, K., Moffitt, T.E. et al. (2003). Influence of life stress on depression: Moderation by a polymorphism in the 5-HTT gene. *Science* 301 (5631): 386–389.

Clothier, S. (2019). the Three P's: Does Your Dog Need Medication? https://suzanneclothier.com/article/3-ps-dog-need-medication/ (accessed 15 June 2020).

Crowell-Davis, S. (2019). Tricyclic antidepressants. In: *Veterinary Psychopharmacology*, 2nd ed. (eds. S. Crowell-Davis, T.F. Murray, and L.M. de Souza), 231–256. Hoboken, NJ: Wiley.

Crowell-Davis, S., de Souza Dantas, L.M., and Ogata, N. (2019). Combinations. In: *Veterinary Psychopharmacology*, 2nd ed. (eds. S. Crowell-Davis, T.F. Murray, and L.M. de Souza), 281–290. Hoboken, NJ: Wiley.

DePorter, T.L., Bledsoe, D.L., Beck, A. et al. (2018). Evaluation of the efficacy of an appeasing pheromone diffuser product vs placebo for management of feline aggression in multi-cat households: A pilot study. *J. Fel. Med. Surg.* https://doi.org/10.1177%2F1098612X18774437.

de Souza Dantas, L.M. and Crowell-Davis, S.L. (2019a). Monoamine oxidase inhibitors. In: *Veterinary Psychopharmacology*, 2nd ed.

(eds. S. Crowell-Davis, T.F. Murray, and L.M. de Souza), 185–199. Hoboken, NJ: Wiley.

de Souza Dantas, L.M. and Crowell-Davis, S. (2019b). Combinations. In: *Veterinary Psychopharmacology*, 2nd ed. (eds. S. Crowell-Davis, T.F. Murray, and L.M. de Souza), 281–288. Hoboken, NJ: Wiley.

de Souza Dantas, L.M. and Crowell-Davis, S. (2019c). Benzodiazepines. In: *Veterinary Psychopharmacology*, 2nd ed. (eds. S. Crowell-Davis, T.F. Murray, and L.M. de Souza), 67–102. Hoboken, NJ: Wiley.

Dodman, N.H., Reisner, I., Shuster, L. et al. (1996). Effect of dietary protein content in dogs. *J. Am. Vet. Med. Assoc.* 208: 376–379.

Ellis, S.L.H. and Wells, D.L. (2010). The influence of olfactory stimulation on the behaviour of cats housed in a rescue shelter. *Appl. Anim. Behav. Sci.* https://doi.org/10.1016/j.applanim.2009.12.011.

Foster, J.A. and McVey Neufeld, K.A. (2013). Gut-brain axis: How the microbiome influences anxiety and depression. *Trends Neurosci.* https://doi.org/10.1016/j.tins.2013.01.005.

Frank, D., Beauchamp, G., and Palestrini, C. (2010). Systematic review of the use of pheromones for treatment of undesirable behavior in cats and dogs. *J. Am. Vet. Med. Assoc.* 236: 1308–1316.

Graham, L., Wells, D.L., and Hepper, P.G. (2005). The influence of olfactory stimulation on the behavior of dogs housed in a rescue shelter. *Appl. Anim. Beh. Sci.* 91 (1–2): 143–153.

Gruen, M., Roe, S.C., Griffith, E. et al. (2014). Use of trazodone to facilitate postsurgical confinement in dogs. *J. Am. Vet. Med. Assoc.* 245: 296–301.

Gruen, M.E., Roe, S.C., Griffith, E.H. et al. (2017). The use of trazodone to facilitate calm behavior after elective orthopedic surgery in dogs: Results and lessons learned from a clinical trial. *J. Vet. Beh.* 22: 41–45.

Gruen, M. and Sherman, B. (2008). Use of trazodone as an adjunctive agent in the treatment of canine anxiety disorders: 56 cases (1995–2007). *J. Am. Vet. Med. Assoc.* 233: 1902–1907.

Gulikers, K.P. and Panciera, D.L. (2003). Evaluation of the effects of clomipramine on canine thyroid function tests. *J. Vet.*

https://doi.org/10.1892/0891-6640(2003)017<0044:eoteoc>2.3.co;2.

Gwaltney-Brant, S.M., Albretsen, J.C., and Khan, S.A. (2000). 5-Hydroxytryptophan toxicosis in dogs: 21 cases (1989–1999). *J. Am. Vet. Med. Assoc.* 216: 1937–1940.

Hariri A.R., Mattay, V.S., Tessitore, A. et al. (2002). Serotonin transporter genetic variation and the response of the human amygdala. *Science* 297: 400–403.

Hanno, P.M., Buehler, J., and Wein, A.J. (1989). Use of amitriptyline in the treatment of interstitial cystitis. *J. Urol.* https://doi.org/10.1016/s0022-5347(17)41029-9.

Haug, L.I. (2008). Canine aggression toward unfamiliar people and dogs. Vet. *Clin. N. Am. Small Anim. Pract.* https://doi.org/10.1016/j.cvsm.2008.04.005.

Haug, L.I. (2014). Territorial aggression in dogs. *Clinician's Brief* April, 23–25.

Hopfensperger, M.J., Messenger, K.M., Papich, M.G. et al. (2013). The use of oral transmucosal detomidine hydrochloride gel to facilitate handling in dogs. *J. Vet. Beh.* 8 (3): 114–123.

Horwitz, D.F. and Mills, D.S. (2009). *BSAVA Manual of Canine and Feline Behavioural Medicine*, 2nd ed. Gloucester, UK: British Small Animal Veterinary Association.

Houpt, K.A. and Virga, V. (2003). Update on clinical veterinary behavior. *Vet. Clin. N. Am. Small Anim. Pract.* https://doi.org/10.1016/S0195-5616(02)00134-1.

Hughes D., Moreau, R.E., Overall, K.L. et al. (1996). Acute hepatic necrosis and liver failure associated with benzodiazepine therapy in six cats, 1986–1995. *J. Vet. Emerg. Crit. Care.* https://doi.org/10.1111/j.1476-4431.1996.tb00030.x.

Irimajiri, M., Luescher, A.U., Douglass, G. et al. (2009). Randomized, controlled clinical trial of the efficacy of fluoxetine for treatment of compulsive disorders in dogs. *J. Am. Vet. Med. Assoc.* https://doi.org/10.2460/javma.235.6.705.

Kato, M., Miyaji, K., Ohtani, N. et al. (2012). Effects of prescription diet on dealing with stressful situations and performance of anxiety-related behaviors in privately owned anxious dogs. *J. Vet. Behav.* https://doi.org/10.1016/j.jveb.2011.05.025.

King, J.N., Simpson, B.S., Overall, K.L. et al. (2000). Treatment of separation anxiety in dogs with clomipramine: Results from a prospective, randomized, double-blind, placebo-controlled, parallel-group, multicenter clinical trial. *Appl. Anim. Behav. Sci.* https://doi.org/10.1016/S0168-1591(99)00127-6.

Kogan, L.R., Schoenfeld-Tacher, R., and Simon, A.A. (2012). Behavioral effects of auditory stimulation on kenneled dogs. *J. Vet. Behav.* https://doi.org/10.1016/j.jveb.2011.11.002.

Korpivaara, M., Laapas, K., Huhtinen, M. et al. (2017). Dexmedetomidine oromucosal gel for noise-associated acute anxiety and fear in dogs—a randomised, double-blind, placebo-controlled clinical study. *Vet. Rec.* 180 (14): 356.

Landsberg, G., Hunthausen, W., and Ackerman, L. (2013). *Behavior Problems of the Dog and Cat*, 3rd ed. Edinburgh, UK: Saunders.

Landsberg, G.M., Melese, P., Sherman, B.L. et al. (2008). Effectiveness of fluoxetine chewable tablets in the treatment of canine separation anxiety. *J. Vet. Behav.* https://doi.org/10.1016/j.jveb.2007.09.001.

Landsberg, G.M. and Wilson, A.L. (2005). Effects of clomipramine on cats presented for urine marking. *J. Am. Anim. Hosp. Assoc.* https://doi.org/10.5326/0410003.

Litster, A.L. (2000). Use of clomipramine for treatment of behavioural disorders in 14 cats—Efficacy and side-effects. *Aust. Vet. Pract.* 30 (2): 50–54.

Luescher, A.U. (2009). Repetitive and compulsive behaviour in dogs and cats. In: *BSAVA Manual of Canine and Feline Behavioural Medicine* (eds. D.F. Horwitz and D.S. Mills.), 236–244. Gloucester, UK: British Small Animal Veterinary Association.

Martin, K.M. (2010). Effect of clomipramine on the electrocardiogram and serum thyroid concentrations of healthy cats. *J. Vet. Behav.* https://doi.org/10.1016/j.jveb.2009.12.019.

McGowan, R.T.S. (2018). Tapping into those "Gut Feelings": Impact of BL999 (*Bifidobacterium longum*) on Anxiety in Dogs. https://www.purinaproplanvets.com/media/521317/086602_vet1900-0918_cc_abstract.pdf (accessed 17 July 2021).

Mills, D. and Luescher, A. (2006). Veterinary and pharmocological approaches to abnormal repetitive behaviour. In: *Stereotypic Animal Behaviour: Fundamentals and Applications to Welfare* (eds. J. Rushen and G. Mason), 286–324. https://doi.org/10.1079/9780851990040.0286.

Mira, F., Costa, A., Mendes, E. et al. (2016). Influence of music and its genres on respiratory rate and pupil diameter variations in cats under general anaesthesia: Contribution to promoting patient safety. *J. Fel. Med. Surg.* https://doi.org/10.1177/1098612X15575778.

Murray, T.F. (2019a). Amino acid neurotransmitters: Glutamate, GABA, and pharmacology of benzodiazepines. In: *Veterinary Psychopharmacology*, 2nd ed. (eds. S. Crowell-Davis, T.F. Murray, and L.M. de Souza Dantas), 11–19. Hoboken, NJ: Wiley.

Murray, T.F. (2019b). Biogenic amine neurotransmitters: Acetylcholine, norepinephrine, and dopamine. In: *Veterinary Psychopharmacology*, 2nd ed. (eds. S. Crowell-Davis, T.F. Murray, and L.M. de Souza Dantas), 29–42. Hoboken, NJ: Wiley.

Murray, T.F. (2019c). Biogenic amine neurotransmitters: Serotonin. In: *Veterinary Psychopharmacology*, 2nd ed. (eds. S. Crowell-Davis, T.F. Murray, and L.M. de Souza Dantas), 21–28. Hoboken, NJ: Wiley.

Newberry, S., Blinn, M.K., Bushby, P.A. et al. (2010). *Guidelines for Standards of Care in Animal Shelters*. Apex, NC: Association of Shelter Veterinarians.

Ogata, N. (2016). Separation anxiety in dogs: What progress has been made in our understanding of the most common behavioral problems in dogs? *J. Vet. Behav.* https://doi.org/10.1016/j.jveb.2016.02.005.

Ogata, N., de Souza Dantas, L.M., and Crowell-Davis, S. (2019). Selective serotonin reuptake inhibitors. In: *Veterinary Psychopharmacology*, 2nd ed. (eds. S. Crowell-Davis, T.F. Murray, and L.M. de Souza Dantas), 103–128. Hoboken, NJ: Wiley.

Ogata, N. and Dodman, N.H. (2011). The use of clonidine in the treatment of fear-based behavior problems in dogs: An open trial. *J. Vet. Behav.* https://doi.org/10.1016/J. JVEB.2010.10.004.

Orlando, J.M., Case, B.C., Thomson, A.E. et al. (2015). Use of oral trazodone for sedation in cats: A pilot study. *J. Fel. Med. Surg.* https://doi.org/10.1177/1098612X15587956.

Overall, K.L. (2013a). *Manual of Clinical Behavioral Medicine for Dogs and Cats*. St. Louis, MO: Elsevier.

Overall, K.L. (2013b). Pharmacologic approaches to changing behavior and neurochemistry. In: *Manual of Clinical Behavioral Medicine for Dogs and Cats* (ed. K.L. Overall), 474. St. Louis, MO: Elsevier.

Palestrini, C., Minero, M., Cannas, S. et al. (2010). Efficacy of a diet containing caseinate hydrolysate on signs of stress in dogs. *J. Vet. Behav.* 5 (6): 309–317. doi: 10.1016/j.jveb.2010.04.004.

Pankratz, K.E., Ferris, K.K., Griffith, E.H. et al. (2018). Use of single-dose oral gabapentin to attenuate fear responses in cage-trap confined community cats: A double-blind, placebo-controlled field trial. *J. Fel. Med. Surg.* https://doi.org/10.1177/1098612X 17719399.

Plumb, D.C. (2018). *Plumb's Veterinary Drug Handbook*, 9th ed. Hoboken, NJ: Wiley.

Pryor, P.A., Hart, B.L., Cliff, K.D. et al. (2001). Effects of a selective serotonin reuptake inhibitor on urine spraying behavior in cats. *J. Am. Vet. Med. Assoc.* https://doi.org/10.2460/javma.2001.219.1557.

Reisner, I. (2003). Differential diagnosis and management of human directed aggression in dogs. *Vet. Clin. N. Am. Small Anim. Pract.* 33: 303–320.

Schwartz, S. (2005). *Psychoactive Herbs in Veterinary Behavior Medicine*. Ames, IA: Blackwell.

Seksel, K. and Lindeman, M.J. (2001). Use of clomipramine in treatment of obsessive-compulsive disorder, separation anxiety and noise phobia in dogs: A preliminary, clinical study. *Aust. Vet. J.* https://doi.org10.1111/j.1751-0813.2001.tb11976.x.

Shelton, R.C., Winn, S., Ekhatore, N. et al. (1993). The effects of antidepressants on the thyroid axis in depression. *Biol. Psychiatry.* https://doi.org/10.1016/0006-3223(93)90311-Z.

Sherman, B.L. and Mills, D.S. (2008). Canine anxieties and phobias: An update on separation anxiety and noise aversions. *Vet. Clin. North Am. Small Anim. Pract.* 38 (5): 1081–1106.

Sherman, C.K., Reisner, I.R., Taliaferro, L.A. et al. (1996). Characteristics, treatment, and outcome of 99 cases of aggression between dogs. *Appl. Anim. Behav. Sci.* https://doi.org/10.1016/0168-1591(95)01013-0.

Simpson, B.S., Landsberg, G.M., Reisner, I.R. et al. (2007). Effects of Reconcile (fluoxetine) chewable tablets plus behavior management for canine separation anxiety. *Vet. Ther.* 8 (1): 18–31.

Sinn, L. (2018). Advances in behavioral psychopharmacology. *Vet. Clin. N. Am. Small Anim. Pract.* 48: 457–471.

Snowdon, C. T., Teie, D., and Savage, M. (2015). Cats prefer species-appropriate music. *Appl. Anim. Behav. Sci.* https://doi.org/10.1016/j.applanim.2015.02.012.

Stevens, B.J., Frantz, E.M., Orlando, J.M. et al. (2016). Efficacy of a single dose of trazodone hydrochloride given to cats prior to veterinary visits to reduce signs of transport- and examination- related anxiety. *J. Am. Vet. Med. Assoc.* 249: 202–207.

van Haaften, K. (2018). Case report: Under-socialized cats from an animal hoarding case. *BCSPCA Speaking for Animals.* https://spca.bc.ca/wp-content/uploads/Spring-2018-Veterinary-Update.pdf (accessed 28 July 2021).

Van Haaften, K.A., Eichstadt Forsythe, L.R., Stelow, E.A. et al. (2017). Effects of a single preappointment dose of gabapentin on signs of stress in cats during transportation and veterinary examination. *J. Am. Vet. Med. Assoc.* https://doi.org/10.2460/javma.251.10.1175.

Wynchank, D. and Berk, M. (1998). Fluoxetine treatment of acral lick dermatitis in dogs: A placebo-controlled randomized double blind trial. *Depress. Anxiety* https://doi.org/10.1002/(SICI)1520-6394(1998)8:1<21::AID-DA4>3.0.CO;2-8.

Appendix 22.A   Behavioral Medicine Formulary

Drug class	Drug name and strength	Dog dose	Cat dose
Baseline (Long-term)			
Selective serotonin reuptake inhibitor (SSRI)	**Fluoxetine (Reconcile®)** 8, 16, 32, 64 mg tablets **Fluoxetine (generic)** 10 mg tablets, capsules 20, 40 mg capsules	**Reconcile** is FDA approved for canine separation anxiety 1–2 mg/kg PO q 24 hours	0.5–1.0 mg/kg PO q 24 hours
Tricyclic antidepressant (TCA)	**Clomipramine (Clomicalm®)** 20, 40, 80 mg tablets **Clomipramine (generic)** 25, 50, 75 mg capsules	**Clomicalm** is FDA approved for canine separation anxiety. Label 2–4 mg/kg PO q 24 hrs 1–2 mg/kg PO q 12 hours, up to 3 mg/kg PO q 12 hours	2.5–5 mg/CAT PO q 24 hours
Situational, adjunct, secondary			
Benzodiazepine (BZD)	**Alprazolam** 0.25, 0.5, 1.0, 2.0 mg tablets	0.02–0.1 mg/kg PO PRN or q 8–12 hours Author doses at 0.25 mg/small DOG, 0.5 mg/medium DOG, 1–2 mg/large DOG	0.125–0.25 mg/CAT PO PRN or q 12 hours
BZD	**Lorazepam** 0.5, 1.0, 2.0 mg tablets	0.02–0.1 mg/kg PO PRN or q 8–24 hours	0.25 mg/CAT PO PRN
Alpha-2 agonist	**Dexmedetomidine OTM gel (Sileo®)**	**Sileo** is FDA approved for canine noise aversion. See packet insert	
Alpha-2 agonist	**Clonidine** 0.1, 0.2, 0.3 mg tablets	0.01–0.05 mg/kg PO q 8-12 hours or PRN	
Gabapentin	**Gabapentin** 100, 300, 600 mg capsules or 100 or 50 mg/ml suspension (must be xylitol-free suspension for dogs)	10–30 mg/kg PO PRN or q 8–12 hours	50–100 mg/CAT PO PRN or q 8–12 hours
Atypical antidepressant (SARI)	**Trazodone** 50, 100, 150, 300 mg tablets	2–5 mg/kg PO PRN or q 12 hours; author uses 3–4 mg/kg PO q 12 hours for kennel stress; generally try to keep dose below 10 mg/kg per day If situational, can go up to 7–10 mg/kg PO 1–2 hours prior to event (e.g., physical exam, medical treatment, noise event, etc.)	12.5–50 mg/CAT PO PRN

Appendix 22.B Shelter Behavior Medication Information Sheet

Behavioral presentation

Dogs will present with fearful, anxious, and/or frustrated body language and behavior in a variety of situations. (See appropriate behavior protocols for additional description of clinical signs and body language.) No one signal should be relied upon solely for determining the emotional state of fear, stress, anxiety, and/or frustration, but the pet's entire body observed and available history reviewed to create a comprehensive picture of the pet's behavioral and emotional state.

Assessment

Many dogs will show some degree of stress or anxiety upon experiencing the new environment of a shelter setting, regardless of how well set up or enriched. Some dogs will acclimate within a few days, other might take longer, and yet another subset might continually deteriorate and stay in a chronically negative emotional state, leading to reduced quality of life and poor welfare. Some dogs might enter the shelter with the history of a behavior problem in the previous home. In addition to compassionate, patient, and empathetic caregivers, behavior management, and modification, some animals require additional medical support to acclimate and recover in this environmental setting and improve their behavior concerns in order to be successful in a new home.

Working differential diagnostic list

Kennel stress, generalized anxiety, global fear, phobias, other fears, separation anxiety, barrier frustration

Recommendations

Trazodone can be used immediately twice daily to try to reduce the dog's current anxiety and stress. After a week of the trazodone and a long length of stay (>1 month) is anticipated,

fluoxetine can be added to try to further reduce anxiety and fear and is often needed for longer-term baseline anxiety control. If it is determined that the dog's level is still severe and compromising his welfare after one week of trazodone, clonidine can also be added to help give more immediate control of anxiety and stress. This medication might be particularly helpful for dogs experiencing sympathetic nervous arousal when anxious (pacing, panting, whining, jumping, mouthing, lack of focus during training/play), in addition to body language signs consistent with stress or anxiety. Clonidine can also be used instead of trazodone if side effects occur or the dog's body weight prevents him from being safely dosed with trazodone. If the pet is already on two medications with serotoninergic effects, or if there is a pain component suspected to be involved in the undesired behavior or the pet has another reason to be painful, gabapentin is a reasonable option to add to the above medications or used by itself for immediate anxiety, stress, and pain relief. This would also be a very safe option for any pet with suspected neurologic disease or seizure concerns. The mechanism of action for gabapentin's anxiolytic effects is unknown, but it has been found to be effective for this use in both dogs and cats. This is also an excellent medication choice for cats experiencing situational or chronic stress and anxiety since it can be given orally without having to directly administer a pill. If there is concern regarding liver function, this may also be a safer option, as it is excreted essentially unchanged in the urine. It is also a safe option for diabetics. The human liquid formulation should not be used in dogs because it contains xylitol.

Trazodone: 3–4 mg/kg PO q 12 hrs

This is a serotonin 2A antagonist/reuptake inhibitor (SARI) that can be used to help decrease anxiety, often in combination with another medication. To avoid GI upset, your pet's dose may be gradually increased over the first week. Mild sedation when first giving this medication may be noted. Please stop the medication and contact your primary care veterinarian immediately if you note excess sedation, vomiting or diarrhea, changes in urination, tremors, increased anxiety, or increased irritability. *This medication should not be discontinued abruptly after being administered longer than one month, as serious side effects can occur.*

Fluoxetine: 1–2 mg/kg PO q 24 hrs

This medication can be added in one week

This medication is a selective serotonin reuptake inhibitor (SSRI) to help decrease your pet's anxiety. It may take up to 4–6 weeks to see the full effect of this medication, although some pets will show response earlier. This medication should not be combined with other SSRIs, tricyclic antidepressants (TCAs), or monoamine oxidase inhibitors (MAOIs) (including amitraz, an ingredient in some topical tick control products or collars), as a serious side effect, serotonin syndrome, could occur. You may note a decrease in appetite or lethargy (quiet) for the first one to two weeks; these are usually mild and resolve on their own. If they are severe, or if you notice vomiting, diarrhea, tremors, increased anxiety, or increased irritability, please stop the medication and contact your primary care veterinarian immediately. *This medication should not be discontinued abruptly after being administered longer than one month, as serious side effects can occur.*

Fluoxetine should not be used in diabetes mellitus as it can interfere with blood glucose and insulin management.

Clonidine 0.02–0.04 mg/kg PO q 8–12 hrs PRN

Generally, this medication is most effectively and efficiently used in the shelter either as a situational medication (e.g., 1–2 hours prior to a walk) or given 2–3 times daily, at a minimum of 6–8 hour intervals, at minimum first thing in the morning and mid-afternoon.

This is an alpha-2 agonist medication historically used to control blood pressure in people that has an antianxiety effect in both people and animals. This antianxiety effect typically lasts 4–6 hours in most dogs. Side effects are uncommon, but if you note excess sedation, uncoordinated gait or collapse, vomiting, diarrhea, changes in urination, tremors, increased anxiety, or increased irritability, please stop the medication and contact your primary care veterinarian immediately.

Gabapentin 10–30 mg/kg PO q 8–12 hrs PRN

If needed, the capsule can be opened and the contents mixed with a small amount of canned food. A liquid formulation can be used in cats for administration directly into the mouth using a 3-cc syringe and a tom cat catheter.

Gabapentin is a medication that has been used for neuropathic pain or seizure control but also has antianxiety properties. It can be dosed as needed, up to three times daily. Most common side effects are GI upset and sedation. If any of these side effects are severe, please stop the medication and contact your primary care veterinarian immediately. *This medication should not be discontinued abruptly after being administered longer than one month, as serious side effects can occur.*

Appendix 22.C   Fearful/Phobic Behavior Protocol

Behavioral presentation

Dogs will present with fearful body language in a variety of situations. This includes ears back, eyes wide, vigilant darting gaze, whale eye, furrowed brow, tightened lips, lowered body, trembling, cowering, tail tucked, panting, lip licking, frequent yawning, pacing, avoidance, hiding, whining, barking, howling, and sometimes growling and lunging. Defensive aggression might be displayed if the dog feels threatened enough that he feels he must defend himself from a substantial threat. No one signal should be relied upon solely for determining the emotional state of fear, but the pet's entire body observed, and the many signals put together and taken for interpretation within the context of the situation.

Triggers for this fearful behavior could include going outside for a walk, entering a new/novel area or situation (e.g., stairs), exposure to new people, unfamiliar dogs or sounds (loud barking, trains, buses, etc.)

Assessment

Many dogs' level of fear and avoidance are profound and present a significant concern for quality of life upon entering the shelter, a new environment, or an urban setting. Many of these dogs come from rural backgrounds, and particularly those that experienced impoverished or barren environments during behavioral development will likely always be very fearful and will need careful lifelong management to help them remain safe and have a reasonable quality of life. Improvement in fear will likely be a very slow process, and any interested adopters need be made aware of the commitment to patience and management that will be needed for this dog.

Working differential diagnostic list

Kennel stress, generalized anxiety, global fear, neophobia, environmental/situational fear, or phobias

Recommendations

Trazodone can be used immediately to try to reduce the dog's current anxiety and stress. If needed, after a week of the trazodone, fluoxetine can be added to try to further reduce anxiety and fear and is often needed for longer-term baseline anxiety control. If possible and behaviorally appropriate, the fearful dog should remain in the company of another dog, as this makes the fearful dog more comfortable and can facilitate observational learning. Counterconditioning (pairing events and interactions with treats) should be used in every interaction; even if the fearful dog doesn't eat the treat right away when tossed, it should still be implemented.

These fearful dogs should be made a high priority for a foster home, preferably one with another dog. This home (and any adoptive home) would have a fenced-in yard so that exposure to other environments can be done slowly and leash walks off property for elimination are not required. Typically, dogs with this level of fear can be challenging to call in and out of thresholds and doorways, so a leash should be used to walk though doorways (such as in and out of the home to the yard). The fearful dog can drag a long light leash in the yard so he can be brought inside without having to grab his collar or corner him.

Interactions should be minimal and occur on his terms as he is comfortable enough to approach. Continuing to approach him and interact because he doesn't try to defend himself will only heighten his fear of people.

Discontinue punishment

Please discontinue any punishment, verbal reprimands, or negative interactions with _____, including the word "No." These interactions are ineffective in decreasing the undesired behavior and, additionally, increase fear and anxiety. This often will actually increase the motivation for the undesired behavior and therefore the likelihood of its performance. These techniques are contra-indicated with aggression. Please also advocate for _____ and do not allow other people to use these methods with him/her either.

Neutral interactions

Because _____ has had such a traumatic past, and previous interactions with people approaching him/her are perceived by him/her as not safe, even though he/she does not protest, remember that he/she is in a high state of anxiety, called learned helplessness. For now, please avoid approaching him/her when he/she has retreated away (unless he/she needs to eliminate or it is meal time) and do not pet, hug, kiss, carry, or otherwise force interactions with him/her. Right now that is very frightening to him/her. Please advocate for him/her as well and do not allow guests, friends, or passersby on walks to do this either.

If _____ begins to venture out to see where family members are, do not look at him/her, talk to him/her, or approach him/her. Instead, drop a treat on the ground nearby. You may have to walk out of the room initially for him/her to feel safe to take it. But, if he/she does pick it up, this is a way to reward him/her for his/her bravery of venturing out of his/her safe spot without further frightening him/her.

Daily routine

Please maintain a consistent and predictable daily routine for your pet. This includes meals, walks, play, and training sessions that occur in the same order each day. Knowing what to expect next during the day is beneficial to decrease anxiety in your pet.

Safe spot

Please make additional safe spots throughout the home where your dog can go to retreat but still be part of the family as he/she feels brave enough to venture out. This should be a place that is out of the high-traffic area and a place that he/she is unlikely to be inadvertently bothered or bumped. You can take him/her by the area when he/she is on leash and show it to him/her, but do not force him/her there. Additionally, children and guests should be taught to never approach the dog while he/she is in his/her safe spot. Children should be monitored closely by a responsible adult to ensure they follow this rule any time they are near the dog.

1 hand 1 second rule for interactions

If _____ begins to approach to solicit interaction, you can begin to set up a 1 hand 1 second rule for interactions. If he/she is showing body language that is relaxed and social, you can pet him/her under his/her chest for a length of 1 second, then pause and wait to see what _____ does next. If he/she shows that he/she wants to continue the inter-action, the person can do so for another 1 second. If he/she does not solicit more attention or walks, moves, or looks away, then end the interaction. You can find examples of this at this link: http://www.youtube.com/watch?v=-cGDYI-s-cQ. Dog body language says yes or no to petting.

Target training, often called "touch," where _____ touches your hand with his/her nose is also a good place to start with interactions.

Additional resources

Fearful Dog website by Debbie Jacobs: http://fearfuldogs.com/

Decoding Your Dog, edited by Debra Horwitz, John Ciribassi, and Steve Dale

The Culture Clash, by Jean Donaldson

The Other End of the Leash, by Patricia B. McConnell

Don't Shoot the Dog! by Karen Pryor

Trazodone: 3–4 mg/kg PO q 12 hrs

Trazodone ___ mg tablets: Please give your pet ___ tablet by mouth ___. This is a serotonin 2A antagonist/reuptake inhibitor (SARI) that can be used to help decrease anxiety, often in combination with another medication. To avoid GI upset, your pet's dose may be gradually increased over the first week. Mild sedation when first giving this medication may be noted. Please stop the medication and contact your shelter organization's veterinarian immediately if you note excess sedation, vomiting or diarrhea, changes in urination, tremors, increased anxiety, or increased irritability. *This medication should not be discontinued abruptly after being administered longer than one month, as serious side effects can occur.*

Fluoxetine: 1–2 mg/kg PO q 24 hrs

If needed, this medication can be added in one week

Fluoxetine ___ mg tablets/capsules: Please give your pet ___ tablet/capsule by mouth once daily. This medication is a selective serotonin reuptake inhibitor (SSRI) to help decrease your pet's anxiety. It may take up to 4–6 weeks to see the full effect of this medication, although some pets will show response earlier. This medication should not be combined with other SSRIs, tricyclic antidepressants (TCAs), or monoamine oxidase inhibitors (MAOIs) (including amitraz, an ingredient in some topical tick control products or collars), as a serious side effect, serotonin syndrome, could occur. You may note a decrease in appetite or lethargy (quiet) for the first 1–2 weeks; these are usually mild and resolve on their own. If they are severe, or if you notice vomiting, diarrhea, tremors, increased anxiety, or increased irritability, please stop the medication and contact your shelter organization's veterinarian immediately. *This medication should not be discontinued abruptly after being administered longer than one month, as serious side effects can occur.*

Appendix 22.D   Kennel Stress Protocol

Behavioral presentation

Dogs will present with fearful, anxious, and/or frustrated body language and behavior in a variety of situations. However, kennel stress can be considered when these negative emotional states and associated behaviors and body language signs are present in a pet in the care of a shelter, whereas they were not present in the previous environment prior to entering the shelter.

Body language consistent with fear and distress includes ears back, eyes wide, vigilant darting gaze, whale eye, furrowed brow, tightened lips, lowered body, trembling, cowering, tail tucked, panting, lip licking, excessive drooling, frequent yawning, pacing, whining, barking, or howling. Frustrated and active anxious dogs might jump and mouth frequently and have difficulty focusing during play and training. Abnormal repetitive behaviors might be observed with both emotional states, such as circling, tail chasing, shadow/reflection chasing, weaving, or other patterned movements (pacing). No one signal should be relied upon solely for determining the emotional state of fear, stress, anxiety, and/or frustration, but the pet's entire body observed, and the many signals put together and taken for interpretation within the context of the situation.

Assessment

Many dogs will show some degree of stress or anxiety upon experiencing the new environment of a shelter setting, regardless of how well set up or enriched. The dramatically new environment in addition to the loud novel sounds, intense smells, exposure to unfamiliar people and animals, and lack of control of schedule and interactions is incredibly stressful. Some dogs will acclimate within a few days, others might take longer, and yet another subset might continually deteriorate and stay in a chronically negative emotional state, leading to reduced quality of life and poor welfare. In addition to compassionate, patient, and empathetic caregivers, a daily routine, and variety of enrichment, some animals require additional medical support to acclimate and recover in this environmental setting.

Working diagnosis

Kennel stress, generalized anxiety, fears, barrier frustration

Dogs that should be considered to be experiencing high levels of kennel stress include those showing increased barking, jumping, and lunging at passersby; those hiding, trembling, cowering, or excessively drooling in their current housing system; and those showing abnormal repetitive behaviors such as patterned pacing, circling, tail chasing, shadow chasing, stereotyped pouncing, or other repeated behaviors. A key diagnostic criteria for kennel stress is that the pet was not showing these specific abnormal behaviors prior to entering the shelter environment.

Recommendations

It has been documented that stress due to environmental and social factors can increase susceptibility to infectious disease, allow more severe disease to occur, and prolong recovery time.

Trazodone can be used immediately to try to reduce the dog's current anxiety and stress. If needed after a week of the trazodone and a long length of stay (>1 month) is anticipated, fluoxetine can be added to try to further reduce anxiety and fear and is often needed for longer-term baseline anxiety control. If needed or due to size, clonidine or another adjunct can be used in addition to or instead of trazodone. (See behavior medication information sheet and associated handouts.)

Some options for additional behavioral management to consider are as follows:

- For those dogs still exhibiting a normal appetite: meals can be prepared in KONGS rather than bowls. Meals can be prepared ahead of time (e.g., evening meals can be prepped when normal morning meals for those dogs are served) and then frozen. This allows the preparation time for meals to remain relatively unchanged and on the same staff schedule. The only change is the vessel the meals are served in and the time of preparation. Tomorrow's breakfast is prepped this evening.

- Daily walks, runs, or indoor play sessions with a caregiver can be very helpful for mental and physical stimulation and enrichment. Treadmill training and sessions can be added to the enrichment schedule as needed.

- Daily quiet time can be added for those dogs that could benefit from a quieter low-key environment and interactions. This can be provided by a reading program (volunteers sit quietly with the dog and read aloud to him) or by offering time in office foster as time, staffing, and space permits.

- Positive reinforcement-based training can also be another form of excellent physical and mental enrichment as well as having the benefit of increasing knowledge of basic obedience and manners that makes the pet more adoptable. One-on-one sessions with a trained volunteer using clicker training, group training classes, agility classes, or other activity classes such as Fit Paws or Nosework can be included as staff time and resources permit.

- If possible and behaviorally appropriate, the stressed dog can remain in the company of another dog by being paired with a roommate. Additionally or alternatively, group play sessions with other dogs can be added to the dog's routine.

- The above behavior management can be implemented for all dogs as time, space, and manpower allow to help prevent the development of kennel stress and reduce behavioral deterioration while the dog awaits his forever home.

Appendix 22.E Gabapentin Protocol

Behavioral presentation

Dogs and cats diagnosed with ringworm are likely to face a prolonged length of stay while under quarantine and treatment. At this time, the current treatment recommendations include a minimum of two lime sulfur dips before being made available for adoption and quarantine until two negative fungal cultures have been completed. Unfortunately, foster homes for pets with this condition can be challenging to find, so it is expected that much of this time will be in isolation in the shelter. Additionally, most of the pets affected are young adolescent pets in some of the most critical periods of their behavioral development. It is expected that kennel stress, frustration, and fear due to lack of exposure will be sequelae from a prolonged period of isolation. Details of how this presents can be found in the kennel stress protocol. The treatment protocol of lime sulfur dips can also be unpleasant for person and pet alike, creating an environment of negative learning that handling and bathing are something to be frightened of. Details of this can be found in the fearful dog protocol. Cats will generally demonstrate fear by trying to hide, retreat or escape, or use defensive aggression, which can become extremely intense.

Assessment

Because oral antifungals are often used for the canine ringworm patients and cats can be notoriously challenging to medicate orally on a daily basis, most chronic antianxiety medications used for long-term chronic stressors are not appropriate for these patients. There is risk of drug interaction between most selective serotonin reuptake inhibitors (SSRIs), serotonin 2A antagonist/reuptake inhibitors (SARIs), tricyclic antidepressants (TCAs), and the oral antifungal medications.

However, other behavior medications might be useful either for chronic or situational use during ringworm treatment and quarantine.

The lack of positive exposure to other people, animals, and environments, in addition to the lack of control of schedule and interactions, is incredibly stressful for dogs and cats in quarantine. Some of these pets might enter quarantine in a positive emotional state but over time continually deteriorate and stay in a chronically negative emotional state, leading to reduced quality of life and poor welfare. In addition to compassionate, patient, and empathetic caregivers, a daily routine, and variety of enrichment, some animals require additional medical support to acclimate and recover in this environmental setting.

Working diagnosis

Kennel stress, generalized anxiety, fears, barrier frustration

Recommendations

It has been documented that stress due to environmental and social factors can increase susceptibility to infectious disease, allow more severe disease to occur, and prolong recovery time.

Gabapentin can be used orally every 8–12 hours as needed for chronic or persistent levels of kennel stress or fear in dogs or cats housed in isolation. Alternatively, gabapentin can be administered 2 hours prior to a stressful event such as a lime sulfur dip to try to reduce the stressful impact of this event for the dog or cat.

Dogs

Gabapentin can be administered orally at 10–30 mg/kg 1–2 hours prior to a stressful event or given chronically every 8–12 hours as needed. *This medication should not be discontinued abruptly after being administered longer than one month, as serious side effects can occur.*

Cats

Gabapentin can be administered orally generally at 100 mg PER CAT 2 hours prior to a stressful event, or 10–30 mg/kg chronically every 8–12 hours as needed. Given that cats are notoriously challenging to medicate, some professionals have had luck mixing the powder from the capsules into a small amount of wet food, tuna juice, or anchovy paste. Alternatively, recently a study has demonstrated an effective way to administer gabapentin in a liquid suspension orally when given through a 3-cc syringe with a tom cat catheter attached to the tip. The tom cat catheter can be gently placed in the oral cavity with little to no restraint and the medication administered in a low-stress manner. This study used community cats as the subjects successfully, so it is anticipated this could be used on fearful socialized cats as well. *This medication should not be discontinued abruptly after being administered longer than one month, as serious side effects can occur.*

The gabapentin was suspended using a 50/50 mix of ORA-Plus and ORA-Sweet from Perrigo.

Additional behavioral management to consider are those recommendations included in the kennel stress protocol. It is expected that these recommendations can and should be modified to meet the quarantine requirements for this particular disease process. If possible, cats should be group-housed in an all in–all out system. Each and every cat should be given a place to hide as well.

23

Caring for Small Mammals

Elise Gingrich

23.1 Introduction

Small mammals are becoming more frequently encountered in shelters than ever before. However, shelters may not be accustomed to dealing with some of these animals and their unique behaviors, which can differ significantly from those of the cats and dogs shelters historically serve. An in-depth discussion of every small mammal species that could be encountered in the shelter setting is beyond the scope of this chapter; therefore, this chapter will focus on the most frequently encountered small mammals: rabbits, ferrets, guinea pigs, and a collective overview of common small rodents.

Small mammals enter the shelter through a variety of pathways similar to most other species. As with these other animals, if they are surrendered or transferred from another sheltering organization, medical and/or behavioral information may be available; however, if the animal is stray there is no information other than the immediate history observed by the finder. Unfortunately, another common entry pathway for some small mammals is through confiscation (or, less often, surrender) of large numbers of a single species when hoarding or uncontrolled breeding cases are investigated.

Just as with other animals that enter shelters, there should be standard protocols in place for small mammal handling and care. These protocols should encompass aspects of intake such as examination, parasite treatment, and vaccination as well as aspects of basic husbandry including enclosures, bedding options, nutrition, location within the shelter, and enrichment. Since there are a large variety of small mammals that could potentially enter the shelter, creation of protocols should be prioritized for the most frequently encountered species. Shelter intake data can be used to help determine which species are most common at a specific location. One other factor to consider with these species is whether there are local rules and regulations that limit or prohibit care of specific species; for example, ferrets and gerbils cannot be kept as pets in California (*California Fish and Game Code* 2019).

The intake period—and associated processes—is perhaps the most critical period in the animal's shelter stay. It provides an opportunity to initiate a physical and behavior care plan based on the animal's condition. Every small mammal should be evaluated on intake just as any cat or dog would be; this includes an exam to assess for physical and behavioral

Animal Behavior for Shelter Veterinarians and Staff, Second Edition. Edited by Brian A. DiGangi, Victoria A. Cussen, Pamela J. Reid, and Kristen A. Collins.
© 2022 John Wiley & Sons, Inc. Published 2022 by John Wiley & Sons, Inc.
Companion website: www.wiley.com/go/digangi/animal

abnormalities that require further evaluation by appropriate staff.

It is important to understand the basic needs and behavior of the various species encountered so the shelter can ensure adequate welfare. Understanding normal behavior is of particular importance; without this understanding, staff may confuse normal species-specific behavior with problematic behavior or, worse, may overlook abnormal behavior because they do not understand what they are observing.

23.2   Small Mammal Housing and Husbandry

While specific housing requirements will vary by species, there are some generalizations to keep in mind when housing small mammals in a shelter setting. First and foremost, it is important to remember all housing decisions should be made to provide for an animal's physiologic and psychosocial well-being. The initial considerations should include the larger environment that is external to the animal's individual enclosure. One important consideration at this level is where to place these animals within the shelter. While it is likely not possible to have different rooms for each species that may be encountered, care should be taken when deciding which species to house in the same room. Many small mammals are prey species and should never be housed in the same room as predator species such as cats. As predators, ferrets are a notable exception to this rule and they should not be housed in the same room as many of the other small mammals. The ambient temperature of the housing location also needs to be considered. While the specific temperature range will vary slightly for each species a general guideline to follow is that most small mammals are much more cold tolerant than heat tolerant. High temperatures can lead to heat stress and even death. It also important to make sure the housing areas are protected from excessive moisture and drafts. Laboratory

animal temperature recommendations can provide guidance for creating appropriate housing protocols for the shelter. The *Guide for Care and Use of Laboratory Animals* recommends ambient temperature of 61–72° F for rabbits and 68–79° F for guinea pigs and other rodents commonly encountered in the shelter (Garber et al. 2011).

The next housing consideration is the primary enclosure. A primary enclosure must be appropriate for the species, allow for normal movement and posturing, prevent escapes, allow for good ventilation (especially when ammonia levels are likely to be high), and be easy to clean. The enclosures should be as large and as enriched as possible for the shelter. In addition to protecting the animal's mental well-being while at the shelter, this will help to set an example for adopters and encourage appropriate housing after adoption. Some shelters may even choose to send the primary enclosures with the adopter to set them up for success.

Even though several species of small mammals are social animals that do well when housed with other members of the same species, this does not mean animals from different sources should be housed together automatically. These animals must have the same criteria used for cats and dogs applied before co-housing is attempted. The animals should be evaluated and determined to be at low risk for transmitting or contracting infectious diseases before housing them with other animals (of the same species). In addition to disease status concerns, the animals' sterilization status should also be considered. Just as with cats and dogs, small mammals should not be co-housed with the opposite sex once the animals reach breeding age. This is a very important consideration for small mammals, many of which are capable of breeding as young as eight weeks of age. The behavior of each animal should be considered also, to help make the housing choices as suitable as possible for every animal involved.

Several general husbandry recommendations are applicable to all small mammals. When considering nutrition, it is imperative to feed a diet specific to the species of interest. Some species have very specific nutrient requirements, for example, guinea pigs cannot produce vitamin C so it must be added in their diet. It is best to avoid diets with brightly colored supplements, which are typically fruit and seed. Animals often preferentially eat these supplements, which typically have lower nutritional value. Since many of these small mammal species will enter the shelter infrequently it may not be feasible to keep food stocked for every species. Instead, the shelter should have basic feeding protocols available, so if one of these less frequent species does arrive at the shelter staff will know what type of food to obtain.

23.3 Rabbits

23.3.1 Behavior

Domestic rabbit behavior is very similar to that of its wild rabbit ancestor, the European rabbit (*Oryctolagus cuniculus*), with few exceptions. The primary difference is response to confinement; domestic rabbits have adapted well to confinement whereas wild rabbits are stressed by confinement and often fail to breed (Bays 2006). In the wild they live in large groups known as warrens and tend to be nocturnal. The population of the warrens can range from dozens of rabbits to more than 100; there tends to be an equal number of females and males (Parer 1977). The other significant difference is that domestic rabbits have become crepuscular and are most active in the morning and evening (Jilge 1991). Rabbits are prey species, which is an important factor to consider in their care because the highly developed flight response dictates a large portion of their behavior; for example, rabbits spend a significant amount of time sniffing as a way of surveying their environment even when frightened (Jenkins 2001).

Due to their crepuscular activity, rabbits spend large portions of the afternoons resting.

When rabbits are relaxed and resting, they stretch out on their sides or abdomens with hind legs stretched out behind them. Extremely relaxed rabbits may lay on their backs with their feet extended in the air. While they are resting, it is not unusual to witness thrashing and twitching movements; these movements are often mistaken as seizures by individuals unfamiliar with rabbit behavior.

Rabbits will scratch and bite if nervous or not accustomed to being held; this is especially true when the rear limbs are not properly supported. When not properly restrained they will kick, which can easily lead to spinal fractures due to the high ratio of muscle to bone. The "football hold" describes a technique where the rabbit is kept close to the handler's body with their whole body supported and their head directed toward the handler's elbow (see Figure 23.1). This hold is ideal for nervous rabbits; it keeps the eyes covered, thus reducing struggling secondary to fear.

The whiskers beneath the mouth are extremely sensitive, which is beneficial for grazing, but means rabbits do not like to have their noses touched. They also do not like to have hands placed below their noses or chins; when this happens rabbits often startle and can snort and scratch in response. This aggressive behavior is first seen at the onset of puberty, around four to eight months of age, depending on the breed of rabbit. At this age, intact male rabbits also begin urine spraying similar to intact male cats; they may mount other rabbits, objects, and even other pets. Intact, litter trained rabbits often start urinating and defecating outside the litterbox to mark territory. In order to prevent or decrease these behaviors, all rabbits should be surgically sterilized prior to adoption. This also tends to make the rabbits better pets and thus more likely to remain in the home. Sterilization also provides a health benefit for females as it eliminates the risk of the most common neoplasia in female rabbits, uterine adenocarcinoma; incidence varies by age but can be as high as

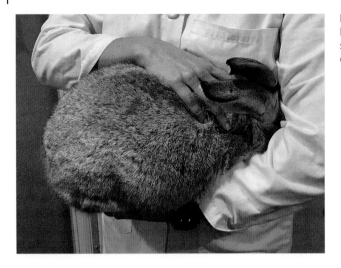

Figure 23.1 Example of a "football hold" for rabbits. The rabbit's body is supported by the handler and its head directed toward the handler's elbow.

50–80% in certain breeds (Klaphake and Paul-Murphy 2012).

Rabbits are very territorial and use scent to mark territory. Rabbits will mark their territory with urine and feces; they also have three sets of scent glands on the body that secrete substances used in scent marking. One common form of scent marking is chin rubbing, which disperses secretions from the glands under the chin. Rabbits will rub their chins on inanimate objects to mark territory. Another scent marking behavior, which is frequently misinterpreted, is the deposition of fecal pellets. Fecal pellet deposits serve as a carrier for anal gland sections and can occur in an apparently random pattern throughout the rabbit's territory or, in the case of intact males, along the periphery of their territory; fecal deposition can also occur in a common "latrine" site (Bell 1980) shared by multiple rabbits. The chin and inguinal scent glands are also used by female rabbits ("does") to mark their young ("kits"). Does are aggressive to, and may even kill, kits that are not their own. For this reason, attempting to cross-foster young rabbits can be very difficult.

Rabbits are relatively quiet animals but will use specific noises to communicate a range of emotions, including fear, aggression, and contentment. It is important to be aware of the various sounds rabbits can make because several are similar but indicate very different affective states. For example, rabbits may make a low-pitched purr by lightly chattering teeth when they are content. This noise is often accompanied by quivering whiskers. Teeth grinding, in contrast, produces a louder, crunching noise that is indicative of pain or discomfort, especially gastrointestinal pain. Sounds related to fear are typically high-pitched screams, whereas those associated with aggression are often low grunting noises. Fear responses may also be denoted by a specific body language: the rabbit's pupils are dilated, eyes are bulging, ears are flattened against the head, and the body is pressed flat against the ground with feet underneath it as the rabbit remains motionless. Rabbits also frequently thump their back feet in response to aversive stimuli to alert other rabbits.

Rabbits are social animals and often do better in groups of two to three rather than individually housed. They exhibit behaviors such as grooming one another, lying together, and nuzzling (see Figure 23.2). While rabbits generally benefit from social groups, certain pairings can lead to significant aggression between the rabbits. Therefore, attempts to co-house them must undergo careful consideration (see Section 23.3.2).

Rabbits, especially juveniles, are extremely curious and can be chewers and diggers.

Figure 23.2 Co-housed rabbits lying next to each other, a behavior frequently displayed in bonded pairs.

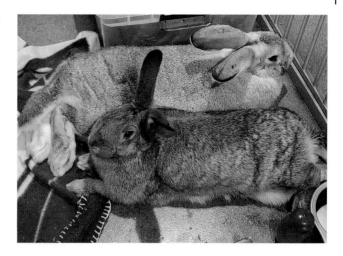

These behaviors are common reasons for owner relinquishment. While the behavior is normal and cannot be stopped, it can be redirected to appropriate outlets. These include appropriate rabbit-safe toys for chewing such as woven or wicker baskets, cardboard, or heavy plastic toys designed for large birds or dogs. These toys can be combined with food to encourage normal foraging behavior. For example, empty cardboard tubes can be stuffed with hay and a few pellets mixed in, or a small quantity of pellets can be put in a cardboard or tissue box that the rabbit can rip apart. These activities also serve as wonderful enrichment opportunities in the shelter environment. As with other species, it is important to rotate enrichment objects as interaction with objects decreases over time. Enrichment can help decrease boredom and destructive behaviors as well as encourage exercise; providing enrichment to maintain mental health is just as important as veterinary care is in maintaining physical health.

23.3.2 Housing

Rabbits have traditionally been kept in small cages or enclosures; however, giving rabbits access to more space, such as a small room or escape proof dog enclosure, promotes normal movement. Regardless of the type of enclosure, it is very important the housing allows for adequate ventilation. Rabbits produce large amounts of urine daily, so ventilation is necessary to prevent the build-up of ammonia. When used, individual cages should consist of coated wire or steel bars instead of solid walls such as those found in glass aquariums or some cat cages. Ideally the entire floor of the enclosure should be solid; if a wire floored enclosure is used, then a significant portion needs to be covered with solid material, such as carboard or wood to allow time off the wire. This will help prevent the development of pododermatitis, a painful ulceration of the bottom of the feet that often results in infection and can be difficult to treat (see Figure 23.3). The enclosure should be large enough for the rabbit to hop three times and to stand up on its hind feet (Love 1994).

Ideally rabbits should have space to demonstrate normal behavior. Exercise is important for both medical and behavioral well-being of rabbits; those not given the opportunity to exercise are prone to obesity and pododermatitis. When rabbits have the ability to roam freely, such as in a large room, they will demonstrate typical rabbit "antics" such as running and kicking their hind feet up or jumping off the ground with twisting and sideways kicks in the air. When giving rabbits this opportunity, it is important to ensure the flooring is a

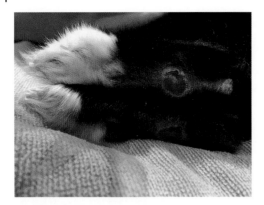

Figure 23.3 Example of pododermatitis in a rabbit. *Source:* Dr. Miranda Sadar.

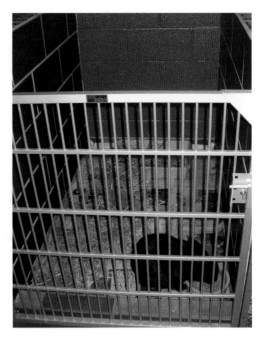

Figure 23.4 Example of a small run originally designed for puppies that was converted to rabbit housing with adequate space and ventilation.

non-slip surface. Placing towels or thin foam mats can provide traction and prevent injuries in playful rabbits. Rabbits will also often stand on their hind legs with ears erect to check out the surroundings. It is important for rabbits to have space to perform these normal behaviors along with platforms to climb on. Accommodating these needs can be difficult in a traditional shelter environment, especially in older facilities that were typically designed to house cats and dogs. Many shelters have modified existing enclosures, such as those designed for puppies, to house rabbits (see Figure 23.4). If this is not possible and rabbits must be housed in small enclosures, shelters should aim to allow rabbits time out of their primary enclosures each day and explore other housing options such as foster homes if rabbits are not quickly adopted.

Outdoor access is a great way to provide environmental enrichment opportunities to engage in the more complex behaviors described above. If provided with outdoor access, it is imperative there is a cover over the outdoor enclosure to provide shade and to protect rabbits from predators, such as hawks. The outdoor temperature must also be considered. Overall, rabbits tolerate cold better than heat; they do not tolerate temperatures above 80° F. Exposure to high temperatures can lead to heat stress and even death.

Rabbits can and should be housed together if possible; however, there are very important considerations that must be addressed, especially in the shelter setting. Co-housing works best when rabbits can be housed together from an early age. In this case it is extremely important to spay and neuter before puberty not only for the obvious benefit of population control but also to prevent aggressive behavior. Intact males will become very aggressive toward other intact males at puberty and, if not separated, serious injury can result. This aggressive behavior is not typically noted in females housed together from a young age. Older rabbits who have been individually housed may not adapt well to co-housing, so attempts at this set up should only occur slowly and under direct supervision. More specific information about pairing rabbits can be found on the National House Rabbit Society website (www. rabbit.org). If a shelter does not have the resources to ensure rabbit introductions are completed with proper supervision it may be more beneficial for the shelter to house rabbits individually and focus efforts on promoting rabbit adoptions. The animals will spend less time in the shelter and quickly move into a home setting where adopters can devote the necessary time to rabbit introductions.

23.3.3 Husbandry

Rabbits require high fiber diets due to the anatomy of their gastrointestinal system, which closely resembles that of a horse. Therefore, their diets should consist primarily of grass hay, with the exception of juvenile rabbits and pregnant or lactating does who benefit from the higher protein and calcium content of alfalfa hay. Hay should be available at all times. Rabbits are crepuscular, meaning they are most active and eat mostly at dawn and dusk. A small amount of leafy greens, such as romaine, red, or green lettuce (not iceberg, which has little nutritional value), mustard greens, collard greens, or cilantro, should be offered twice daily when rabbits are most active. Greens should be prepared as for human consumption. Commercially formulated rabbit pellets should be limited, if offered at all because they are low in fiber and can lead to obesity, decreased gastrointestinal motility, and cheek teeth overgrowth. When pellets are offered, adults should be fed timothy-based pellets and no more than ¼ cup per 5 lbs of body weight per day. Pellet mixes that contain added treats, such as seeds and dried fruits, should be avoided. These added treats are high in carbohydrates and sugars, which can lead to serious gastrointestinal problems as well as obesity. Obesity is a common problem in pet rabbits.

Providing objects suitable for chewing is also important for the rabbit's dental health. Rabbits have open-rooted teeth, which means they continually grow throughout life. If rabbits do not have an appropriate diet along with items to chew on, they can develop serious dental problems.

Rabbits have a much higher water intake compared to other animals: an average of 120 ml of water per kilogram of body weight per day (Harkness and Wagner 1995). Water should be provided in a sipper bottle or bowl depending on the rabbit's preference, and intake should be monitored just as with any other species. If the rabbit's preference is unknown, as in the case of a stray rabbit, make sure to monitor the rabbit's drinking behavior if bowls are offered, as a rabbit unfamiliar with bowls may not immediately drink from them. When bowls are used, ensure they are heavy enough to prevent rabbits from tipping them over, as rabbits may attempt to play with the bowls, which can lead to the water becoming dirty very easily and needing to be changed frequently.

Due to their unique digestive system, rabbits produce small fecal pellets throughout the day. They also produce large amounts of urine, due to their high water intake. Rabbits tend to deposit urine and feces in one location within their enclosure and can, therefore, be litter trained fairly easily. In the shelter setting, litterbox use can be encouraged by placing the litterbox in the location the rabbit has selected to use as a latrine, which is typically in a corner. These litter habits can be interrupted with the onset of puberty when rabbits begin marking their territory; surgical sterilization can significantly reduce this problem. Traditional clay, clumping, or corn-based cat litters should not be used with rabbits. If ingested, this material can lead to gastrointestinal stasis (decreased movement of material through the gastrointestinal tract) or obstruction. Pine, cedar, and other soft wood shavings should be avoided as the aromatic compounds in these products can cause skin and respiratory problems as well as increases in liver enzymes. Safe options include recycled paper products, which are available in a pellet form, towels, newspapers, and straw; however, straw does not absorb urine well.

23.4 Ferrets

Ferrets have historically been used for rodent control and hunting; however, in the United States they are primarily kept as companion animals and also used as laboratory animals. As their historical use indicates, they are predators; for this reason, it is important they are not housed near any prey species in the shelter, such as rabbits, rodents, or birds.

23.4.1 Behavior

Like other carnivores, ferrets tend to sleep frequently between bursts of activity. When they sleep, they like to burrow under a blanket or other cozy spot. Their eyes have difficulty adjusting to bright light, so they need time to adjust to bright light before being removed from their sleeping spot; otherwise, the handler risks startling the ferret, which may result in a bite.

When they are active, ferrets like to burrow and need material to dig in, such as shredded paper or litter, along with tunnel-like structures to crawl through, like cat play tunnels, suspended hammocks, or cardboard tubes. The strong instinct to dig provides numerous opportunities for enrichment, such as hiding toys in a box filled with pelleted litter or rice. When not burrowing, ferrets can become very playful and will hop or bounce around excitedly. They enjoy chasing moving objects, such as balls or small toys pulled around in front of them. The predatory sequence of stalking and pouncing on the "prey" is often elicited when such toys are offered, similar to cats. This predatory behavior explains why ferrets should not be allowed around smaller mammals, which they may perceive as prey. Ferrets are playful, but play can become aggressive toward humans or other ferrets when threatened. Signs of aggression include lunging, sideways attacks, dancing, and clucking sounds. As mentioned, they may bite if scared or startled. When scared, defensive threats can include hissing, screaming, and snapping of the jaws.

Ferrets are extremely curious and appear almost fearless when exploring! When provided with space to play and exercise, they require close supervision or a ferret-proofed area to explore. They will chew on almost any material and can easily develop gastrointestinal obstructions if foreign material is ingested.

When providing enrichment it is important to make sure the items cannot be chewed into small pieces that could be swallowed; for example, foam and soft rubber toys should be avoided. The benefit of this curiosity is that ferrets do not appear to be significantly stressed when introduced to novel situations and environments. Their curiosity can help ferrets adapt quickly to a shelter environment and subsequently to an adopter's home. Ferrets also have a very keen sense of smell. They will spend a lot of time investigating the environment with their noses. This sense can be capitalized upon when considering types of enrichment to include in the enclosure. Food or animal scents, like those found at hunting supply stores, rubbed on toys or favorite areas of the enclosure can serve as excellent enrichment for ferrets (Harris 2015; Meredith 2017).

Ferrets use urine, feces, and anal gland secretions to mark territory, even when sharing an enclosure with other ferrets. They typically choose a corner to defecate in, just as rabbits do. Once it is clear where the ferret has chosen to defecate, a litterbox can be placed in that spot to encourage litterbox training. They train very easily, as rabbits do. Ferrets enjoy digging, so litterboxes can quickly become a place to play and can easily be tipped over. Securing the litterbox to the side of the enclosure can help prevent tipping of the litterbox. There are no toxicity concerns with litter choice as there are with rabbits; however, dusty litter should be avoided as it can lead to respiratory irritation.

Ferrets can be housed as pairs or in small groups, which is beneficial as they like to play and interact with one another. They can often be found curled up and sharing the same sleeping spot. Unfamiliar ferrets can be housed together as long as they are sterilized, but introductions must be monitored as aggression is more likely to occur between unfamiliar ferrets (Staton and Crowell-Davis 2003). It is uncommon to encounter an unaltered ferret in the United States due to routine surgical sterilization at six weeks by commercial breeders (Pollock 2012). Determining the sex of a ferret is relatively straightforward; the males have a prepuce on the ventral abdomen just caudal to the umbilical area. A more in-depth description can be found in *Ferrets, Rabbits, and Rodents: Clinical Medicine and Surgery,* 4th ed. (see "Additional Resources").

Like rabbits, ferrets tend to be fairly quiet, but they do have a range of vocalizations. The high-pitched scream can denote fear or a startle response. Ferrets will also hiss, typically as a sign of anger or, when used in a prolonged fashion, to indicate frustration. It can also be used as a warning signal directed at a perceived threat.

23.4.2 Housing

In the United States, ferrets are primarily housed indoors; this is different from Europe and Australia where it is more common to house the species outside. A solid bottom is preferred for the primary enclosure to prevent trauma to the feet, which can easily get caught in a wire bottom. Glass enclosures are not appropriate as they do not allow for adequate ventilation. The need for a secure enclosure cannot be overstated. Ferrets are extremely flexible and can escape through extremely small openings, even openings that may appear too small for escape to be possible.

Ferrets also need to have a dark place to sleep. Providing blankets or beds they can crawl into is preferred, because they like to burrow. Many ferrets will curl up in a hanging hammock that has a blanket over it. They will often sleep on top of each other if multiple ferrets are housed together. A dark area also provides a safe place for the ferret to retreat to if they are stressed. Although ferrets appear to be less affected by change and novel situations than other small mammals, it is still important to provide them hiding space in a shelter environment, where change and potentially aversive stimuli may be frequent.

As discussed earlier, ferrets can be litter trained, so they should be provided with an appropriate litterbox. The litterbox should have a low entry but high back and sides to prevent accidental defecating and urinating outside the litterbox; ferrets like to back into the corner where they choose to eliminate. Ferrets will not cover feces after defecating as a cat does, so the litter does not have to be very deep. It is important to avoid clay and clumping litters that can be dusty and lead to respiratory problems. Pelleted litters are preferred.

23.4.3 Husbandry

Ferrets are very fastidious; therefore, waste must be removed daily. The enclosure should be cleaned and disinfected regularly, at a minimum, whenever there is visible soiling. They should have fresh water available at all times provided from a sipper bottle or in a bowl; if water is provided in a bowl, the bowl must be heavy enough to prevent tipping as ferrets tend to play in their water. This behavior can lead to the water quickly becoming dirty, so it must be monitored regularly.

Ferrets are obligate carnivores that require diets high in protein and fat and low in fiber. Dry ferret food should be available at all times, as they eat small, frequent meals throughout the day. Ferrets rarely become obese unless fed very high fat foods. High sugar treats should be avoided, because ferrets cannot easily digest these foods. Ferrets can be finicky eaters, so it is important to change diets slowly to avoid anorexia. This can be a challenge with stray animals where diet history is unavailable, or in surrendered ferrets if the previously fed diet is unavailable or was inappropriate. In these situations, more than one diet could be offered to determine which diet the ferret prefers.

23.5 Guinea Pigs

23.5.1 Behavior

Like rabbits, guinea pigs are crepuscular and most active at dusk and dawn. When resting, their behavior is also similar to rabbits; they may lay on their sides with feet extended or remain sternal with feet tucked under them. Unlike rabbits, they frequently seek out a hide box or other hiding spot to lay in when they are resting. If they are disturbed during a rest period they may startle easily.

If guinea pigs are startled or excited, they will stampede or circle. This can be dangerous when young are present in the enclosure, as they can be trampled. It can also be dangerous if the animals are not in an enclosure; if they stampede, they can easily fall from any height because they do not have a good sense of the edge when placed on an exam table or other raised surface.

Ideally, guinea pigs should have space to exercise out of their primary enclosure. As with other species, exercise is important for both medical and behavioral well-being. Just as with rabbits, guinea pigs not given the opportunity to exercise are prone to obesity and pododermatitis. Providing space to exercise can be relatively easy due to guinea pigs' small size and lack of propensity to climb. Something as basic as setting up an exercise pen with enrichment items can meet their exercise needs.

Guinea pigs rarely bite and scratch. These behaviors are only seen if they are threatened and do not have a place to hide. They tend to tolerate frequent handling very well. However, if they are not well supported in the hind end when carried, they will struggle and squeal and could injure themselves. Anecdotally, it appears to be comforting and calming for the guinea pig to be held near the handler's body.

Guinea pigs are very social and benefit from being around other guinea pigs; therefore, they should be housed in pairs or small groups whenever possible. They will often stay close to one another when resting and eating. When housing guinea pigs together, sufficient space must be provided to allow for hiding spaces for each animal and sufficient quantity and density of food provided to allow all animals access to food at the same time to prevent potential food guarding. When attempting to house two unfamiliar animals, it is important to closely monitor the introduction as is the case with any species.

As opposed to rabbits and ferrets, guinea pigs are extremely vocal. Anyone familiar with guinea pigs will attest they have numerous vocalizations, which vary considerably depending on situation. Vocalizations range from purrs and chirps to whistles and squealing. They can be quite entertaining to listen to!

Guinea pigs often develop rigid preferences as they age, which need to be accommodated or there will be negative consequences such as anorexia and gastrointestinal upset. This is important in the shelter environment when the guinea pig's preferences may be unknown. When attempting to make changes, such as introducing new food, it may take up to a week for the guinea pig to accept the new item. They may also refuse to drink water if it is dirty or tastes different, therefore adding supplements to water is not recommended.

23.5.2 Housing

Guinea pigs do not frequently climb like other rodents, so there is less risk of escape via that route; however, care should be taken to ensure the enclosure is secure. Guinea pigs require enclosures with solid floors to prevent their small feet from becoming trapped between wire slats and to help prevent pododermatitis, a painful condition resulting from the ulceration of the bottom of the feet. Some substrate, such as shredded paper, recycled newspaper pellets, or hardwood shavings, should be used for bedding because guinea pigs urinate and defecate indiscriminately. Pine and cedar shavings should be avoided due to aromatic compounds in soft woods, which can cause respiratory problems. The bedding helps provide additional padding to protect the feet and aids in absorbing urine. Guinea pigs produce large volumes of urine, so the enclosure also needs to be well ventilated to prevent ammonia levels from building up. Glass aquariums are not appropriate enclosures. The enclosure must also contain a hiding place should they feel threatened; this can be as simple as a small cardboard box.

Due to their high metabolism, guinea pigs defecate and urinate frequently, so bedding becomes soiled very quickly. Soiled bedding should be removed daily, and the cage completely cleaned frequently (i.e., at least once weekly). They can be very messy and often scatter feed and bedding; a high-sided base to the enclosure helps to contain most of the debris. Their scattering behavior also leads to contamination of food bowls, so these must be cleaned frequently.

23.5.3 Husbandry

Guinea pigs should be fed grass hay free-choice, along with a limited amount of fresh veggies and greens twice daily. Due to their high metabolic rate, guinea pigs eat throughout the day; therefore, it is imperative that they have hay available at all times. Feeding recommendations are similar to those of rabbits; adults should be offered grass hay, but juveniles can be fed alfalfa hay. Pellets can also be offered daily (and may be used to supplement vitamin C as discussed below), but the quantity should be limited.

Vitamin C supplementation is a unique nutritional requirement of guinea pigs. They cannot produce vitamin C, so it must be supplemented in the diet. The easiest method of providing vitamin C is to supplement the diet with fruits or vegetables high in vitamin C (see Table 23.1). However, as previously mentioned, guinea pigs may not readily adapt to changes in diet, so they may snub these foods if they have not been previously offered. In a shelter setting, a guinea pig's preferences may not be known; offering novel or potentially novel foods in the morning, before giving any other fruit or vegetables, may increase the likelihood of consumption.

For shelters that do not frequently take in guinea pigs, they may not regularly stock these foods, and therefore it may be tempting to rely

Table 23.1 Supplemental sources of vitamin C for guinea pig diets.

Ideal sources of vitamin C	Poor sources of vitamin C
Oranges	Vitamin C drops added to water
Red bell peppers	Vitamin C tablets
Kiwi	Guinea pig pellets—when not following strict storage requirements
Beet greens	
Parsley	
Broccoli	
Tomatoes	
Kale*	
Cabbage*	
Spinach*	

* These vegetables are high in oxalates, which could contribute to urinary calculi formation and should be fed sparingly.

on guinea pig specific pellets that are supplemented with vitamin C. The pelleted food may be a viable option for these shelters; however, if food is not stored properly or stored for more than 90 days past milling date the vitamin C levels in the food can drop significantly. Another option for supplementation is to offer a chewable vitamin C tablet designed for guinea pigs, but only if staff can ensure each guinea pig is consuming one. Vitamin C should not be added to the water because, as mentioned earlier, guinea pigs may refuse to drink water that looks or tastes abnormal. It can also be difficult to ensure each guinea pig is consuming enough supplemented water to meet vitamin C needs.

Guinea pigs have a high water intake requirement: approximately 100 ml per kilogram of body weight per day. Water should be provided via a sipper bottle to prevent spilling and contamination of the water bowl. They will stand on the edge of bowls when drinking and eating and can easily tip or soil the water. Guinea pigs are notorious for playing with and chewing on sipper tubes, which may cause the water to leak. They also tend to block the sipper tube because they mix food and water in their mouths and pass the slurry back into the tube.

It is important staff check water bottles frequently, to ensure water is available and accessible. The bottles must also be cleaned frequently to prevent build-up of scale from the slurry and to prevent bacterial contamination.

Guinea pigs have open-rooted teeth, which means the teeth continually grow, so they must have appropriate items for chewing to prevent the development of dental abnormalities. Free-choice feeding of hay fulfills this requirement; but providing other items to chew not only provides an outlet for a motivated behavior but can also fulfill enrichment needs. The chewing items recommended for rabbits are also suitable for guinea pigs: cardboard, hay mats, wicker baskets. Hiding pellets and greens inside an empty cardboard tube or box can also serve the additional purpose of encouraging normal foraging behavior.

23.6 Other Small Rodents

Numerous other species of small mammals may be encountered by shelters. These can include small rodents like hamsters, rats, mice, and gerbils and less common animals like chinchillas, degus, and sugar gliders. Specific detail on each of these species is beyond the scope of this chapter; this section will highlight some general housing and husbandry considerations that can affect, and be impacted by, the behavior of the most common small rodents (rats, mice, hamsters, and gerbils). Unless otherwise noted, the discussions below apply to these four species.

If shelters anticipate encountering these animals, they need to be prepared to provide the appropriate care. As previously mentioned, it is important to have references and basic protocols readily available in the event these species enter the shelter (see "Additional Resources").

23.6.1 Behavior

In general, these small rodents are incessant chewers, due to the fact that their incisor teeth are continually growing. If they do not have objects to gnaw on, then severe dental complications will result. They tend to be nocturnal, except for gerbils, which are fairly active during the day.

For small rodents, their sense of smell is the most acute of the senses. It is the primary sense they use to investigate their environment. When they are restrained they will immediately smell the handler. Therefore, shelter staff must wash their hands or change gloves before handling rodents, especially after handling predator species. If the rodent is stressed by an unfamiliar scent during handling, they will struggle to get away and may bite. Assigning staff to care for rodents prior to other species may help to decrease stress.

Small rodents mark their territories through use of scent glands. Gerbils and hamsters have obvious scent glands on the ventral abdomen and flanks, respectively (see figures in Evans 2006). They rub the scent glands on objects they are attempting to mark. These scent glands are often mistaken for skin lesions or even tumors by individuals not familiar with these species.

Gerbils are the least vocal of these species but still make sounds, especially when frightened or in pain. The other three species have a range of vocalizations to express everything from pleasure to fear to pain.

Rats and gerbils are the least likely of this group to bite when startled. Hamsters have a lower startle threshold, likely a result of their heavy reliance on structure as compared to the other species. For example, they typically have separate areas for different activities such as sleeping and eating within the same enclosure (Evans 2006). It is important to avoid sudden movements when approaching and handling hamsters, giving them time to adjust to the situation, thus preventing aggressive behaviors. When they sleep, they tuck their head under their abdomen so they cannot hear or see anything in their environment. For this reason, they are easily startled when suddenly awakened. When this happens, they typically roll onto their back, bare their teeth, and make a "gritching" noise that is assumed to be an attempt to intimidate the threat. Gently waking the hamster, by lightly tapping on the enclosure or making noise, prior to attempting to handle them is the best way to avoid being bitten.

23.6.2 Housing

Small rodents are adept at escaping and, given their small size, can fit through extremely small openings. Therefore, their primary enclosures must be escape proof. They are prolific chewers and have been known to chew through plastic enclosures. It is important to routinely check enclosures for areas of damage that could allow for escape.

These species are very social and can often live together in groups; however, the size of the enclosure can limit the number that can be housed together. Each animal needs space to burrow and hide, as well as enough objects to chew on. As is true with most species, housing intact males together after puberty can lead to aggression and in general should be avoided, unless the animals were housed together prior to puberty. Gerbils are the most social of these species and are more tolerant of large social groups. Given the prolific breeding in these species, it is advisable to house only same gender groups.

These animals are very active and are good climbers. It is important to provide them a variety of surfaces to crawl through and on. This can be accomplished by providing objects as simple as empty cardboard boxes and tubes they can crawl through. The added benefit of these items is they also provide the rodents items to chew on. There are also durable plastic items such as ramps and small cave-like structures that can provide climbing and perching opportunities in the enclosure.

23.6.3 Husbandry

Small rodents are primarily nocturnal, mostly eating and drinking at night. They should be fed a pelleted rodent diet instead of mixes that contain seeds and fruit, as they will preferentially eat the seeds and fruit. This results in nutrient imbalances with obesity being the most common sequela. Mice and rats will often cover food bowls with bedding. If fresh fruits or vegetables are offered the enclosure needs to be checked daily to remove any leftovers, as the animals may eat spoiled food resulting in gastrointestinal upset.

Gerbils are a desert animal, and so their water intake is very low, especially compared to other rodents. If they are given high-moisture fruits or vegetables, they may not even need to drink from their water bottles. If staff do notice gerbils drinking large volumes of water, they should notify shelter veterinary staff, because this could indicate an underlying medical condition.

Hamsters have large cheek pouches, which are pockets of the oral cavity alongside the head and neck extending to the shoulder blades. The pouches are used to transport food and filled cheek pouches can easily be mistaken for tumors by individuals not familiar with hamsters. Hamsters will move food from the bowl to a different location of the enclosure where they will hide and hoard it. It is important to check enclosures daily and remove this hoarded food as it can quickly spoil and cause gastrointestinal upset if consumed.

Enclosures need to be cleaned regularly for each of the species (at least weekly), but this can probably occur less frequently for gerbils since they produce so little urine. The low urine production means there is less odor than with the other species. Hamsters are the one species in this group that tend to urinate in one location, typically in a corner. Hamster urine is very concentrated and more odorous than the other rodent species; therefore, their soiled bedding may need to be removed more frequently.

23.7 Conclusions

With the increased intake of small mammals, shelters must be ready to appropriately care for these animals. It is important that shelters understand how the needs of small mammals differ significantly from those of traditional shelter animals and, in some cases, from one another. By being prepared and understanding the behavior of each species, shelters will be able to provide the care necessary to elevate the welfare of small mammals, both in the shelter and the adoptive home.

Additional Resources

Exotic Pet Behavior: Birds, Reptiles, and Small Mammals
Edited by Teresa Bradley Bays, Teresa Lightfoot, and Jörg Mayer
Saunders Elsevier, 2006

Manual of Exotic Pet Practice
Edited by Mark M. Mitchell and Thomas N. Tully Jr.
Saunders Elsevier, 2009

Ferret Medicine and Surgery
Edited by Cathy A. Johnson-Delaney
Taylor & Francis, 2017

Ferrets, Rabbits, and Rodents: Clinical Medicine and Surgery, 4th ed.
Edited by Katherine Quesenberry, Connie J. Orcutt, Christoph Mans, and James W. Carpenter
Saunders Elsevier, 2020

References

Bays, T. (2006). Rabbit behavior. In: *Exotic Pet Behavior: Birds, Reptiles, and Small Mammals* (eds. T.B. Bays, T. Lightfoot, and J. Mayer), 1–49. St. Louis, MO: Saunders Elsevier.

Bell, D.J. (1980). Social olfaction in lagomorphs. *Symp. Zool. Soc. London* 45: 141–164.

California Fish and Game Code, § 2118 (b) (2019).

Evans, E. (2006). Small rodent behavior: Mics, rats, gerbils, and hamsters. In: *Exotic Pet Behavior: Birds, Reptiles, and Small Mammals* (eds. T.B. Bays, T. Lightfoot, and J. Mayer), 239–261. St. Louis, MO: Saunders Elsevier.

Garber, J.C., Barbee, R.W., Bielitzki, J.T. et al. (2011). *Guide for the Care and Use of Laboratory Animals*, 8th ed. Washington, DC: National Academies Press.

Harkness, J.E. and Wagner, J.E. (1995). *The Biology and Medicine of Rabbits and Rodents*, 4th ed. Philadelphia, PA: Williams and Wilkins.

Harris, L.M. (2015). Ferret wellness management and environmental enrichment. *Vet. Clin. North Am. Exot. Anim. Pract.* 18 (2): 233–244.

Jenkins, J.R. (2001). Rabbit behavior. *Vet. Clin. North Am. Exot. Anim. Pract.* 4 (3): 669–679.

Jilge, B. (1991). The rabbit: A diurnal or nocturnal animal? *J. Exp. Anim. Sci.* 34 (5–6): 170–183.

Klaphake, E. and Paul-Murphy, J. (2012). Disorders of the reproductive and urinary systems. In: *Ferrets, Rabbits, and Rodents: Clinical Medicine and* Surgery (eds. K. Quesenberry and J. Carpenter), 217–231. St. Louis, MO: Saunders Elsevier.

Love, J.A. (1994). Group housing: Meeting physical and social needs of the laboratory rabbit. *Lab. Anim. Sci.* 44: 5–11.

Meredith, A. (2017). Ferret behaviour, housing and husbandry. In: *Ferret Medicine and Surgery* (ed. C. Johnson-Delaney), 31–46. New York: Taylor & Francis.

Parer, I. (1977). The population ecology of the wild rabbit, *Oryctolagus cuniculus* (L.), in a Mediterranean-type climate in New South Wales. *Aust. Wildl. Res.* 4: 171–205.

Pollock, C. (2012). Disorders of the urinary and reproductive systems. In: *Ferrets, Rabbits and Rodents: Clinical Medicine and* Surgery (eds. K. Quesenberry and J. Carpenter), 46–61. St. Louis, MO: Saunders Elsevier.

Staton, V.W. and Crowell-Davis, S.L. (2003). Factors associated with aggression between pairs of domestic ferrets. *J. Am. Vet. Med. Assoc.* 222 (12): 1709–1712.

24

Equine Care
Sue McDonnell

24.1   Introduction

A considerable number of horses find their way into shelter care in farm animal facilities commonly referred to as farm animal rescues or sanctuary farms as well equine-specific rescue and rehabilitation or retirement farms. Although current numbers are not readily available, the trend in recent decades has appeared to be a growing number of unwanted horses as well as farm animal rescue and sanctuary farms providing for their care and/or rehoming. Many factors account for this trend in unwanted horses, including increasing cost of maintenance, health care, euthanasia, and carcass disposal, along with changing societal attitudes toward humane euthanasia and humane slaughter of horses for human consumption or as a source of protein for zoo or pet animal feed (American Association of Equine Practitioners 2008).

Farm animal rescue facilities vary in the number and types of species accepted. Some specialize in horses, while others accept a variety of farm animal species. Some rescue organizations now not only accept neglected or abused horses confiscated by humane authorities but also actively seek horses for rescue and/or rehabilitation and re-sale. One common rescue scenario involves purchase of horses from equine auction barns known to serve the export meat market. Rescues typically advertise specific horses for emergency rescue, soliciting monetary donations specifically to save a particular horse from purchase for transport to slaughter.

Whether an equine specialist rescue/rehabilitation for adoption or re-sale, or a general farm animal rescue or sanctuary facility, it is not uncommon for well-meaning staff caring for these special needs horses to have limited skill and knowledge in care of horses in general or the particular needs common to unwanted horses. This chapter addresses the basic needs particularly relevant to behavior concerns of horses in rescue, rehabilitation, and farm animal sanctuary care. Comprehensive health care guidelines particular for horse rescue and rehabilitation facilities have been outlined by the American Association of Equine Practitioners and are available online (American Association of Equine Practitioners 2012).

24.2   Basic Husbandry Needs of Horses Relevant to Behavior

Horses evolved in open plains as a grazing, herd-living prey species. Their behavior and physiology have remained, for the most part, unchanged despite centuries of domestic management.

Animal Behavior for Shelter Veterinarians and Staff, Second Edition. Edited by Brian A. DiGangi, Victoria A. Cussen, Pamela J. Reid, and Kristen A. Collins.

Accordingly, their basic health and behavioral welfare needs are similar to their wild ancestors. Although relatively simple, horses' behavior and health needs are not always understood or intuitive to well-meaning care staff, whether at shelters or in the equine industry at large. To the extent that these basic needs can be accommodated, welfare will be maximized (Lesimple 2020; Parker and Yeates 2012). The following are key husbandry recommendations.

24.2.1 Free Access to High-Fiber, Calorie-Sparse Forage

Horses are trickle feeders, in that their digestive system is adapted to continuous through-put of relatively high-fiber, calorie-sparse forages and browse. The natural behavior pattern of horses alternates periods of eating and resting around the clock, with rarely more than 30 to 60 minutes of rest before they resume foraging. For domestically managed horses, these basic behavioral and physiological needs are not always appreciated or easily accommodated. This is likely the principal factor in the high incidence of gastrointestinal disorders in domestically managed horses (Cohen et al. 1999; Buchanan and Andrews 2003). Recent estimates of the prevalence of squamous gastric ulcer disease, for example, vary among breeds and disciplines from 17 to 39% before or when not being trained or worked to 66 to 100% when being trained or competed; estimates of prevalence of glandular ulcer disease are less well known but likely almost as high (Sykes et al. 2015). Colic is another common gastrointestinal condition, with estimates of incidence of more than 4% annually among the general horse population (Traub-Gardatz et al. 2001).

Under free-roaming/foraging and natural social organization conditions, eating and resting activities are conspicuously synchronized, with all herd members eating or resting at the same time. These activities are obviously socially facilitated, with transitions from one to another initiated by a leader animal within a lead band (McDonnell 2003). Similar social facilitation of eating has been observed in domestically stabled horses with ad lib forage, even when individually stalled (Sweeting et al. 1985). Stabled horses often appear stressed when not fed at the same time as stablemates are fed. Stress behaviors commonly seen in this context include agitated pawing, head or other aggressive threats, frustration head shaking, weaving or stomping, teeth grinding, and stress vocalization. Some grab anxiously at their empty feed tubs, or may grab bites of bedding or gnaw at wood. Some may show other more dangerous food-urgent/food-aggressive behaviors such as guarding food tubs, charging and biting caretakers or kicking feed containers they carry to deliver a meal. This is particularly the case for horses fed infrequent, calorie-dense highly palatable grain meals. Horses with gastric ulcers often seem particularly uncomfortable in this regard. Horses with gastric ulcers typically show specific behaviors indicating gastric discomfort, particularly before and during grain feeding. These can include nuzzling or swatting or nipping the abdomen just behind the shoulder, gazing caudally, ears focused caudally, pawing, stamping, tail swishing, and head shaking (Torcivia and McDonnell 2021). When anticipating feeding, or when neighboring horses are fed and they are not fed or are awaiting their feed, these horses typically display an animated outburst of their particular cluster of gastric discomfort behaviors. For these various reasons, it is recommended that whenever other horses are fed, all in the stable should be fed with as little delay as possible. Those not receiving certain meals should be provided something; for example, a small amount of fresh hay.

In addition, as a grazing animal, digestive physiology of equids has evolved for continuous locomotion while ingesting (Houpt 2006). Horses naturally graze in a characteristic foraging style of locomotion, moving along taking bites, chewing and swallowing with their head down at ground level most of the time. For horses with limited grazing opportunities, it is helpful to provide forage at ground level in multiple locations around their enclosure rather than using raised stationary hay racks or feeders. Chewing and swallowing are most efficient with the head in that normal low grazing posture (Clauss 2013). When horses have a good 360-degree view of the environment with the head low to the ground, they will likely continue chewing and swallowing with the head in that grazing position. If their view is occluded many will take a bite and then raise the head to monitor threats while chewing and swallowing, reducing efficiency of chewing and swallowing (Houpt 2006).

24.2.2 Free Access to Fresh, Clean Water

Horses eating natural forage, typically high in water content, may not drink water at regular intervals, but it is standard of care for domestically managed horses to be provided free access to water. Horses generally adapt to various watering methods (buckets, tubs, automatic water bowls) and to variation in water quality (chemical characteristics affecting taste or odor). Although rare, some horses are reluctant to drink water with particular characteristics, especially chemically treated municipal water or inadvertently chemically adulterated water. Care should be taken to avoid disinfectant or soap residues in water buckets or automatic watering bowls. When first caring for a particular horse, carefully monitor drinking behavior and total water intake. When water level cannot be used to measure water intake, as with automatic watering systems and group housed horses sharing water tubs or buckets, manure consistency should be monitored as an indication of adequate hydration. Freshly voided fecal balls should appear slightly moist rather than dry and crumbly. Reduced water intake is a common cause of gastrointestinal discomfort and can lead to dehydration colic. In cold weather, particularly with a sudden change in ambient temperature from above to below freezing, horses tend to drink less (Kristula and McDonnell 1994). To maintain good hydration during subfreezing weather, it is advisable to provide only warm water (several degrees above freezing). That is because when both ambient icy cold and warmer water are simultaneously available, horses preferentially drink the colder water but drink a smaller volume than if only warm water were available. In subfreezing ambient conditions, plastic water buckets filled with water as warm as 100° F will often remain above freezing for several hours and longer if insulated.

24.2.3 Social Companionship

Herd vigilance is the natural predator avoidance strategy of horses with escape as a group the first response to threat. Therefore, horses appear to be most comfortable psychologically when with other compatible horses and with as little confinement as possible. Horses are typically more comfortable when kept in outdoor enclosures with or within sight of other horses. Whether in stall confinement or in outdoor paddocks, horses seem most relaxed with a 360-degree open view.

24.2.4 Protection from Harsh Environmental Conditions

Healthy horses are remarkably adaptable to various climates and extremes in environmental conditions. Their natural hair coat (undisturbed by clipping, blanketing, or frequent bathing) is sufficient to enable adequate thermoregulation under a broad range of weather conditions. Natural (e.g., trees, hedges, boulders, gullies) or artificial (e.g., sheds, lean-tos) means for horses to protect themselves from changes in the environmental condition should be available in open pastures or paddocks.

24.2.5 Sufficient Space

Horses should be provided with sufficient space to exercise freely at the walk or greater gait, comfortably lie down for uninterrupted rest, and to roll. The standard indoor box stall measures at least 100 sq. ft., in a roughly square configuration. Ideally, stabled horses are given at least one to several hours daily turn-out into a pasture or paddock, not confined 24/7 to an indoor stall (Lemarchand et al. 2019). Outdoor paddocks typically range in size from less than one acre to many acres. Larger paddocks have the advantage of safely allowing exercise at more than a walk or slow trot.

24.3 Quarantine

It is customary and recommended to quarantine newly arriving horses from resident equids, typically for at least two to three weeks. Equine herpes myeloencephalopathy and salmonella are two examples of diseases with a large percentage of latently infected individuals that tend to shed microorganisms in association with the usual stress of change in physical and social environment, transport, and management. Strangles, an often lethal bacterial (*Streptococcus equi*) infection, is common in auction and other holding facilities through which rescue horses may pass. More comprehensive summaries of health care concerns and quarantine recommendations for rescued horses are available (American Association of Equine Practitioners 2012; Boswell 2020).

For many reasons, quarantine itself can be a particularly stressful time for relocated horses. Biosecurity concerns typically require physical isolation of newly arriving horses from direct contact with other equids during the quarantine period, as well as dedicated equipment and staff so as not to transmit infectious diseases. For some horses, isolation from other horses can be quite stressful. Visual contact with one or more other equids usually appears to provide some comfort. When not within visual contact of other horses, a mirror, poster, or virtual companion video featuring a calm horse can, in many cases, be a helpful substitute (see Figure 24.1). For some individuals, other species can appear to provide positive companionship during the quarantine period.

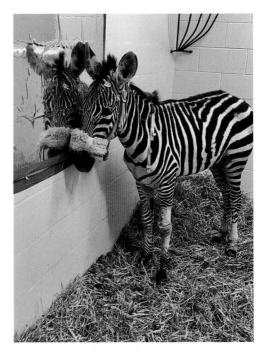

Figure 24.1 Hospitalized zebra foal with a mirror as a substitute companion.

For example, if a horse is familiar with goats, which are often kept at horse stables, a goat can serve as a stall or paddock companion.

Horses generally seem to acclimate to new environments more efficiently when human handling is limited. During a quarantine period, minimum handling is advisable for biosecurity reasons, of course, but it will also minimize stress from human-animal interaction while the horse is acclimating to other aspects of the new environment. While admission protocols may require early veterinary examinations and behavior evaluations, these interactions with new people, often with different human-animal interaction styles and equine skills, can be stressful to a recently relocated horse. Any human-animal interactions, either of a newly arriving horse or any other animal within sight or sound, should involve quiet, calm, respectful low-stress handling and care. Particularly for health care procedures, all personnel should be skilled with and/or supportive of primarily non-confrontational, positive reinforcement-based techniques as detailed below for the most common health care procedures (Foster 2017; McDonnell 2017; Watson and McDonnell 2018).

24.4 Environmental Enrichment

Environmental enrichment for horses can take many forms, including, for example, hay balls and pillows that slow the intake and/or require "foraging behaviors," hanging licks, rolling balls, and grab and toss toys (see Figure 24.2). Experience indicates that initial interest in and duration of use of any particular form of environmental enrichment varies among individual horses. Enrichment in the form of daily, simple training sessions, for example, target training with obstacle courses, reverse round pen training, or simple trick training, can provide positive human-animal interaction. For horses with experience-related handling difficulties, or for previously unhandled horses, these activities can build trust in human handling and build basic skills that will make the horse more appealing to potential future owners.

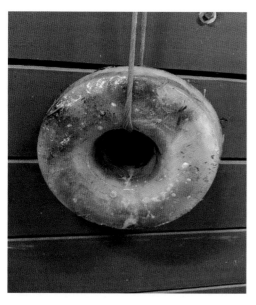

Figure 24.2 Simple water ice lick with pieces of hay and carrot frozen in a ring cake pan mold.

24.5 Common Behavior Problems Relevant to Shelter Environments

24.5.1 Unfamiliarity/Fear of Other Species

Domestic horses are reared, trained, and kept under a variety of environmental conditions in which they may or may not have been exposed to other common farm species and pets. Horses, particularly adult horses that have not been previously exposed to other species, normally react with fear when first exposed. When unable to flee, as would be the natural reaction of horses as a prey species, exposure to unfamiliar species may result in a cowering retreat to the extent possible, or defensive aggression, and often includes an initial "blow" alarm vocalization and stance (McDonnell 2003). These normal fear/alarm behaviors can occur at a distance, often before visual contact, or even when approaching an area where the novel species had been; presumably such responses are mediated via current or residual olfactory stimuli.

If leading a horse, fear may result in displaced (also known as redirected) aggression toward the handler rather than the inciting source. A common scenario is for a fearful horse to hesitate, stop, or pull away. When handlers misinterpret the horse's fear behavior as disobedience or stubbornness, they may respond with coercive methods to move the horse toward or past the feared species. In this situation the fearful horse may bite or lunge at the handler rather than the feared species. Forced exposure to a feared species, for example, housing near or in the same barn, without gradual introduction, can result in behaviors associated with distress (e.g., locomotor stereotypies, frantic self-injurious attempts to escape, inappetence, restlessness, cowering depression).

For these reasons, care should be taken when exposing a horse with unknown species experience history. Any novel species may elicit an adverse response, but it is most common with first exposure to pigs, llamas, alpacas, cattle, exotic equids (e.g., zebra or equid crosses), sheep, or goats.

24.5.2   Aggression

One of the most common root causes of aggression of horses toward their caretakers or herd mates is underlying physical discomfort or illness (Fureix et al. 2010; Hausberger et al. 2016). In many cases, the aggression is easily interpreted as misbehavior. Therefore, whenever aggression is observed, particularly if uncharacteristic for that individual horse, physical discomfort or illness should be ruled out. Horses also readily learn to be aggressive to humans when subjected to punitive handling and/or inadvertent negative reinforcement of ordinary avoidance behaviors or fear-related defensive responses. Intact adult male horses (stallions) are particularly vulnerable to learned aggressive responses, as they typically have a lower threshold for aggression. In addition, their aggressive responses are typically more animated, and therefore inherently more dangerous, so more likely to be negatively reinforced. For these reasons, stallions require specialized housing and especially skilled, non-confrontational handling. Shelter staff inexperienced with stallions should not handle or directly interact with them. Stallions not intended for breeding, which is likely the case for most in shelters, should be castrated. Following castration, it may take several weeks or more for stallion-like aggression and sexual behavior to dissipate to gelding levels. Many geldings continue to retain some level of residual stallion-like sexual behavior when exposed to mares, independent of age or previous breeding experience (Line et al 1985; McDonnell, 1992). For geldings of unknown history with problematic levels of stallion-like sexual and/or aggressive behavior, cryptorchidism or testicular remnant should be ruled out (McCue 2021).

24.5.3   Food Urgency/Aggression

Some horses, particularly those that have experienced poorly managed nutrition or periods of starvation, become food urgent (anxiously active at feeding time) and/or food aggressive. Anticipation of feeding can incite aggressive guarding of the feeding area and these horses may direct aggression at herd mates and may kick barriers when in separate enclosures. They may also show aggressive guarding of feed from approaching care staff. These problems tend to be more severe when the horse is fed infrequent, highly palatable, grain meals, whether or not forage is available between meals. Horses exhibiting food aggression do best with continuous access to an all-forage diet and salt/trace mineral licks. Occasionally, a group housed horse will similarly guard a point water source. In some instances, horses will mark their feed or water with feces, as is the case for wild and feral horses; in domestic horses, this can result in fecal soiling of the water containers. In such cases water must be checked for soiling frequently. Sometimes fecal soiling of water can be prevented by repositioning the bucket or installing an apron around the bucket or waterer that prevents soiling.

24.5.4   Wood Chewing/Object Licking

Although repetitive behaviors, wood chewing and object licking in horses are considered the result of nutritional (salt/mineral) deficiencies. These typically subside when salt/trace mineral licks are provided. These behaviors are distinct from stereotypies.

24.5.5   Stereotypies

Stressed horses can easily develop locomotor stereotypies (Houpt and McDonnell 1993; Roberts et al. 2017; Mills 2005). In horses, the most common locomotor stereotypies include pacing, circling, weaving, and pawing. These are not misbehaviors but rather the natural result of physical and/or psychological discomfort. The behaviors should not be punished or otherwise discouraged. Rather, efforts should be made at improving environmental conditions to minimize stress as described in Sections 24.2 and 24.4.

Cribbing is an unusual behavior that is one of the more common problems in horses. It is considered an oral stereotypy, although it is distinct from other stereotypies in several aspects.

It involves grasping onto a surface with the upper incisors, arching the neck, contracting the neck muscles to facilitate taking in a gulp of air, then expelling that air with a characteristic audible grunt-like sound. It occurs in cluster of a few to many events at intervals of a few seconds. In many cases it occurs with greater frequency at the time of highly palatable grain meals, immediately before, during and/or immediately after eating. Estimates of the prevalence of cribbing range from 2% to as high as 10% among various populations studied (Escalona et al. 2014). The population with the highest prevalence of cribbing is race horses, particularly those trained and housed at racetrack facilities.

24.5.6 Intraspecies Social Incompatibilities

While the common expectation is that horses should be compatible with one another, even when undergoing frequent group housing changes, many horses have difficulties adjusting to new social companions and groups. As mentioned, not all geldings are free of sexual drive, and may herd and harass mares or fight off other geldings. Some mares express certain aspects of harem stallion social behavior, herding and guarding mare herd mates. In some cases this results from exposure to androgens, either due to steroid secreting tumors or purposeful administration of steroid hormones (McDonnell 2004). In mare only groups, sometimes a mare takes on a role of resource guarding or other dominance behavior that can resemble certain aspects of harem stallion behavior.

24.5.7 Sleep Deprivation

Although horses can remain standing during light sleep, they require some recumbent rest in order to experience rapid eye movement

(REM) sleep, which is important for physical and psychological well-being. Horses may be reluctant to lie down for various reasons, most commonly due to physical discomfort and/or disability associated with getting down and/or rising (Bertone 2005; Fuchs 2017). Another category of causes is termed "environmental insecurity." For any number of reasons, a horse may not feel comfortable or secure in a particular environment. For example, it is quite normal for horses in a new environment not to lie down when resting for two to three days or longer. After long periods (usually two to three weeks) without recumbent rest, most horses have a tendency to go into deeper sleep while standing and partially or fully collapse. Some horses experiencing this typical sleep deprivation response also show other associated behavior changes. These can include a general somnolence and or dull attitude, hyperreactivity to ordinary stimuli, general ill-at-ease, frequent abandoned attempts to lie down, and other various changes in attitude and interaction with other animals and caretakers. These behavior changes typically resolve once the horse resumes normal recumbent rest patterns. For detailed discussion of sleep deprivation in horses, see Aleman et al. (2008).

24.5.8 Overhandled Foal Syndrome

Occasionally shelters become caretakers for foals that are either born at a shelter or are presented as orphans. Foals, particularly orphan foals in shelter environments or those rescued from poor conditions, tend to attract considerable attention from caretakers. Foals that are closely handled by humans (daily or more frequent direct contact/interaction beyond momentary interaction necessary for husbandry, playing, grooming) often become what is described as overly bonded to humans (McDonnell 2012; Grogan and McDonnell 2006). This is particularly the case for hand-fed orphan foals. It can be tempting for staff to frequently spend long hours with foals, cuddling and playing with the foal, without realizing that this can lead to abnormal behavior that often limits their subsequent trainability, and often leads to unsafe behavior toward humans. In extreme cases, this behavior becomes so dangerous as the foal matures that euthanasia is recommended.

Signs of a foal becoming overly human-bonded include following people as a dog would, attempting to suckle clothing, vocalizing to humans as a foal would when separated and rejoining its dam, and initiating play (rearing, bucking, circling the human, mounting) with the human as if it were a horse. As the foal matures, they may have mild to severe handling problems associated with what appears to be interacting with people as if they were a horse, including playful and serious aggression and sexual interaction. Mild forms are described as "dull to discipline," "bargey," and "ill-socialized with horses."

To avoid over-bonding of a hand-reared foal to people, it is recommended to limit human interaction as much as possible, and particularly to disassociate human presence with mealtime (McDonnell 2012). For this reason, bucket feeding is preferred to bottle feeding. Remote filling of the bucket can be arranged to further disassociate humans from milk delivery. For orphans to develop normal intraspecies social behavior, equine companions are essential. While other young equids are likely ideal companions for an orphan, adult or juvenile horses, ponies, or donkeys can also provide opportunity for normal equine interaction and behavior as well as stimulate exercise. Mares with or without foals, geldings, and even stallions, are good caretakers of orphan foals. Equine companions of foals typically take on the parenting tasks of lingering near the foal (particularly when recumbent), intervening between the foal and perceived threats, and, geldings and stallions in particular, may play with the foal. Before openly exposing a foal to a potential companion group, their response can be assessed along a safe fence line, or with the foal confined initially to a safe enclosure within the pasture group. A goat can be used if no equine companions are available.

Orphan foals have a tendency for nonnutritive sucking, either sucking on their own or other's body or on inanimate objects, and tongue sucking. This can be directed to safe objects such as rubber equine toys or equine licks sold for environmental enrichment.

24.5.9 Self-Mutilation

Repetitive self-injurious behavior in horses includes self-biting, incessant kicking or slamming body parts against objects, pawing, and in some cases extreme frenetic locomotor behavior (weaving, pacing). These behaviors reflect extreme psychological and/or physical discomfort. It can be challenging for veterinarians and staff to distinguish the source of discomfort, and humane euthanasia should be considered in cases where a diagnosis and relief is not provided in a timely manner (McDonnell 2008).

24.6 Behavior and Skills Assessment

Many horses are unwanted because of handling difficulties or other unsolved behavior concerns. In addition, the route to a shelter may have included experiences that tend to induce and/or exacerbate behavior problems. Accordingly, the incidence of behavior problems is likely higher than in the general horse population. Example problems include aggression to humans or herd mates, locomotor stereotypies or cribbing, handling difficulties (e.g., difficulty catching, rearing, biting, learned aversions to routine health care, transportation difficulties, bolting, bucking, repeatedly unseating riders). Many of these behavior problems are due to underlying physical discomfort that is often undiagnosed, and these problems are not always accurately relayed or otherwise known to organizations receiving unwanted horses.

Once the horse has settled into an environment, it is recommended that a behavior evaluation be undertaken to identify any management, handling, and health care–related behavior problems as well as to assess the level of basic training the horse has had for ordinary care and management. Examples of assessments have been presented by Berger, Madigan et al. (2013) and Foster (2018).

24.7 Calming Medications/ Supplements

While there are many commercially available products marketed as calming agents for horses, few have been scientifically tested for efficacy. One product that has shown efficacy in blind studies is alpha-casozepine. For previously unhandled semi-feral ponies being introduced to domestic care and veterinary procedures, animals treated with alpha-casozepine progressed more efficiently and comfortably than placebo controls (McDonnell et al. 2013). For horses with established aversions undergoing rehabilitation, treated horses progressed more rapidly than placebo treated controls (McDonnell et al. 2014). A synthetic pheromone product with purported calming properties that is used widely for small animals is also available in an equine formulation, although systematic placebo-controlled blind studies have not demonstrated beneficial effects (Berger, Spier et al. 2013; de Paula et al. 2019).

24.8 Auction Rescue Considerations

In recent years, rescue and rehabilitation organizations increasingly purchase horses from auctions where they are at high risk of entering the slaughter market. These horses often present health or behavior challenges, as many are sent to slaughter auctions due to intractable medical or behavior problems. In addition, the auction environment and process can be especially traumatic psychologically and physically and, in some instances, horses are moved from auction to auction over a period of days or weeks. This makes it difficult to assess core temperament and training or trainability until long after the horse is returned to a reasonable environment and care.

Data shared from one organization that specializes in the purchase of slaughter auction horses for rehabilitation for adoption indicate that about half of their purchased prospects are found to have serious medical or behavior problems that preclude adoption. Of 187 prospects purchased by this rescue organization in two recent years, 66 were euthanized for medical problems and 26 for behavior problems. A few of those with potentially treatable medical problems also had behavior problems that were judged too dangerous and stressful both for the horse and caretakers to undertake full diagnostics and treatment. For the 26 horses euthanized primarily for behavior reasons, the specific problems included bucking and/or rearing under saddle that were not responsive to available training, severe anxiety or aggression that did not improve with time, and, less commonly, severe food-related aggression (N. M. Sherrer, Omega Horse Rescue and Rehabilitation, personal communication).

24.9 Low-Stress Positive Reinforcement-Based Handling of Horses for Health Care

Horses in shelters should be handled using positive reinforcement training methods based on scientifically sound learning and behavior modification principles (see Chapter 3). Although not commonly employed with horses, or other farm animals in general, low-stress cooperative care and protected contact techniques as applied with other large animals work very well with horses (Torcivia and McDonnell 2018). Appendices 24.A–24.E describe behavior modification principles and approaches toward common preventive care and husbandry needs of horses.

24.9.1 Restraint and Assistance

A substantial part of the "art" of positive reinforcement-based behavior modification for gaining compliance with a mildly aversive procedure involves judging and implementing the most helpful restraint for the particular horse, procedure, environment, and skill of personnel. For many horses, it is worthwhile arranging for some "wiggle" room and planning to safely ride out some movement. The horse's ability to move, even a little bit, as opposed to being trapped, typically reduces the risk of explosive escape or defensively aggressive responses. Care should be taken to survey the environment in anticipation of obstacles, for example, water buckets or other implements, that if contacted could cause a commotion that essentially represents a fear increasing negative consequences that will potentiate fear and avoidance. Particularly when rehabilitating a horse that has developed dangerous avoidance responses, personal safety gear, such as safety shoes, vest, and helmet can be helpful.

The benefit of one or more assistants will similarly vary with the procedure, the environment, and the skills of available assistants. When positive distraction and or/reward (food or scratching) (Watson and McDonnell 2018) is needed during the procedure, as opposed to only before and after, an assistant can be very helpful to hold the horse and deliver the distraction.

24.9.2 Shaping Compliance with Mildly Aversive Procedures

When *shaping* compliance with a mildly aversive procedure, attention should focus on maintaining the animal's relaxation and tolerance of the procedure rather than on any undesirable avoidance behavior. This enables recognition and well-timed reinforcement of relaxation with each increment of tolerance. While it helps to be prepared for any anticipated undesirable behaviors, simply ignoring undesirable responses whenever possible will speed progress. The most efficient results can be expected when assistants (as well as any observers) remain calm, relaxed, and non-reactive to any undesirable responses. Those working with the horse should maintain focus on prompting, anticipating, and immediately positively reinforcing relaxation and progress. Any response that can be perceived as punishment, such as verbal or physical reprimand or punitive restraint, should be avoided.

24.9.3 Avoiding the "Avoidance Cycle"

It goes without saying that reactivity to aversive stimuli is a natural adaptive response. When the reaction interrupts the procedure, a common inadvertent mistake is to keep repeating the same approach. This is essentially a negative reinforcement (pressure and release) paradigm, which is particularly effective at teaching avoidance. A good rule of thumb is that if the horse successfully avoids more than once, it is best to discontinue or significantly modify the approach. Successful rehabilitation often requires a toolbox of multiple approaches to various procedures, along with a variety of positive distractors and generous rewards to off-set the aversive aspect.

24.9.4 Primary and Secondary Positive Reinforcer/Distractor Options

For most horses, a small food tidbit can be offered both routinely to prevent development of an aversion or for positive reinforcement for relaxation and compliance during rehabilitation of an established aversion. For extended rehabilitation sessions, a variety of treat items can be alternated to maintain interest and higher motivation than a single type of treat. Example treats that most horses appear to enjoy include apple pieces, carrot pieces, peanuts in shells, pretzel pieces, sugar cubes, grain pellets, alfalfa cubes, hard candy pieces, cookie pieces, and commercial horse treats. If for any reason food is not an option, vigorous rhythmic scratching at the withers for most horses may be an effective substitute (Watson and McDonnell 2018).

When treats are used routinely for mildly aversive procedures, many horses quickly learn to associate the health care provider with food treats. To prevent a food urgent horse from becoming nudgy or nippy, food reinforcement can be delivered from a small feed pan, always reaching under the head to deliver the treat on the off side (i.e., the side of the horse opposite the handler delivering the treat). Most horses will readily learn to anticipate food only when the pan is presented, and will also turn the head to the off side, rather than toward the person, when expecting the treat. While food treats are typically quite effective, some horses may become too excited or animated in anticipation of the treat. In that case, changing from food to scratching at the withers as the primary reinforcement may be almost as effective without inducing problematic excitement. An auditory secondary reinforcer (e.g., a clicker sound or a word or short phrase spoken in consistent volume and tone), if paired with the primary reinforcer, will quickly take on positive value (conditioned positive reinforcer), such that it can be effective when used alone intermittently, as needed.

24.9.5   Caretaker "Homework"

Caretakers with reasonable horse handling comfort can often work effectively on their own to introduce horses to a battery of potential health care procedures, or even to perform systematic desensitization procedures for horses with established or developing aversions. Working at times other than when the veterinarian is present or when the procedure must otherwise be completed without delay can allow more gradual shaping of desired behavior.

24.10   Conclusions

There are a number of reasons that horses may find themselves in a shelter or rescue setting. Just as with the care of other animals in these environments, steps must be taken to ensure both psychological and physical well-being. Measures to both prevent problem development and mitigate the impact of those that are preexisting should take into account the unique physiology of equine species as well as their history as a grazing, herd-living, prey-species. Understanding the basic husbandry needs of horses and developing familiarity with common behavior concerns and their management strategies can help optimize a horse's experience while in the shelter environment.

Please visit the companion website for video clips and downloadable resources associated with this chapter.

References

Aleman, M., Williams, C., and Holliday, T. (2008). Sleep and sleep disorders. *Proceedings of the AAEP 54th Annual Convention*, San Diego, CA (6–10 December 2008). Lexington, KY: American Association of Equine Practitioners.

American Association of Equine Practitioners. (2008). The Unwanted Horse. https://aaep.org/issue/unwanted-horse-us (accessed 29 July 2021).

American Association of Equine Practitioners. (2012). *Care Guidelines for Equine Rescue and Retirement Facilities*, 3rd ed.). Lexington, KY: American Association of Equine Practitioners.

Berger, J., Madigan, J., and Holcomb, K. (2013). Equine care in the animal shelter. In: *Shelter Medicine for Veterinarians and Staff*, 2nd ed. (eds. L. Miller and S. Zawistowski), 262–277. Hoboken, NJ: Wiley Blackwell.

Berger, J., Spier, S.J., Davies, R. et al. (2013). Behavioral and physiological responses of weaned foals treated with equine appeasing pheromone: A double-blinded, placebo-controlled, randomized trial. *J. Vet. Behav.* 8: 265–277.

Bertone, J.J. (2005). Excessive drowsiness secondary to recumbent sleep deprivation in two horses. *Vet. Clin. North Am. Equine Pract.* 22 (1): 157–162.

Boswell, S.G. (2020). *Ultimate Guide for Horses in Need*. North Pomfret, VT: Trafalgar Square.

Buchanan, B.R. and Andrews F.A. (2003). Treatment and prevention of equine gastric ulcer syndrome. *Vet. Clin. North Am. Equine Pract.* 19: 575–597.

Clauss, Marcus (2013). Digestive physiology and feeding behaviour of equids—A comparative approach. *Proceedings of the European Equine Health and Nutrition Congress*, Gent, Belgium (1–2 March 2013). Hombeek, Belgium: European Equine Health and Nutrition Congress.

Cohen, N.D., Gibbs, P.G., and Woods, A.M. (1999). Dietary and other management factors associated with colic in horses. *J. Am. Vet. Med. Assoc.* 215 (1): 53–60.

De Paula R.A., Aleixo, A.S., DaSilva, L.P. et al. (2019). A test of the effects of the equine maternal pheromone on the clinical and ethological parameters of equines undergoing hoof trimming. *J. Vet. Behav.* 31: 28–35.

Escalona, E.E., Okell, C.N., and Archer, D.C. (2014). Prevalence of and risk factors for colic in horses that display crib-biting behaviour. *BMC Vet. Res.* https://doi.org/10.1186/1746-6148-10-S1-S3.

Foster, R. (2017). Understanding and implementing principles of learning in the equine veterinary practice. *Proceedings of the AAEP 63rd Annual Convention*, San Antonio, TX (17–21 November 2017). Lexington, KY: American Association of Equine Practitioners.

Foster, R. (2018). The Basic Behaviors Profile. https://therighthorse.org/basic-behaviors-profile-dr-foster/ (accessed 15 November 2020).

Fuchs, C. (2017). Narkolepsie oder REM-Schlafmangel?: 24-Stunden-Überwachung und polysomnographische Messungen bei adulten „narkoleptischen" Pferden. PhD dissertation. LMU München, Faculty of Veterinary Medicine.

Fureix, C., Menguy, H., and Hausberger, M. (2010). Partners with bad temper: Reject or cure? A study of chronic pain and aggression in horses. *PLOS ONE* 5: e12434.

Grogan, E. and McDonnell, S.M. (2006). Mare and foal bonding and problems. *Clin. Tech. Equine Pract.* 4: 228–237.

Hausberger, M., Fureix, C., and Lesimple, C. (2016). Detecting horses' sickness: In search of visible signs. *Appl. Anim. Behav. Sci.* 175: 41–49.

Houpt, K.A. (2006). Mastication and feeding in horses. In: *Feeding in Domestic Vertebrates from Structure to Behavior* (ed. V. Bels), 195–209. Wallingford, UK: CABI.

Houpt, K.A. and McDonnell, S.M. (1993). Equine stereotypies. *Compendium* 15 (9): 1265–1271.

Kristula, M.A. and McDonnell, S.M. (1994). Drinking water temperature affects consumption of water during cold winter weather in ponies. *Appl. Anim. Behav. Sci.* 41: 155–160.

Lemarchand, J., Parias, C., Mach, N. et al. (2019). Housing horses in individual boxes is a challenge with regard to welfare. *Animals* 9: 621–639.

Lesimple, C. (2020). Indicators of horse welfare. *Animals* 10 (2): 294–313.

Line, S.W., Hart, B.L., and Sanders, L. (1985). Effect of prepubertal versus postpubertal castration on sexual and aggressive behavior in male horses. *J. Am. Vet. Med. Assoc.* 186 (3): 249–251.

McCue, P.M. (2021). Diagnostic tests for cryptorchidism. In: *Equine Reproductive Procedures*, 2nd ed. (eds. J. Dasciano and P. McCue), 655–657. Hoboken, NJ: Wiley.

McDonnell, S.M. (1992). Normal and abnormal sexual behavior. *Vet. Clin. North Am. Equine Pract.* http://doi.org/10.1016/s0749-0739(17)30467-4.

McDonnell, S.M. (2003). *The Equid Ethogram: A Practical Field Guide to Horse Behavior.* Lexington, KY: Eclipse Press.

McDonnell, S.M. (2004). Mare behavior problems. In: *Current Therapy in Equine Medicine*, 5th ed. (ed. N.E. Robinson), 264–265. Philadelphia, PA: Saunders.

McDonnell, S.M. (2008). Practical review of self-mutilation in horses. *Anim. Reprod. Sci.* 107: 219–228.

McDonnell, S.M. (2012). Mare and foal bonding behavior and problems and raising an orphan foal. *Proceedings of the AAEP 58th Annual Convention*, Anaheim, CA (2–5 December 2017). Lexington, KY: American Association of Equine Practitioners.

McDonnell, S.M. (2017). Preventing and rehabilitating common healthcare procedure aversions. *Proceedings of the AAEP 63rd Annual Convention*, San Antonio, TX (17–21 November 2017). Lexington, KY: American Association of Equine Practitioners.

McDonnell, S.M., Miller, J.L. et al. (2014). Modestly improved compliance and apparent comfort of horses with aversions to mildly-aversive routine healthcare procedures following short-term alpha-casozepine supplementation. *J. Equine Vet. Sci.* 34: 1016–1020.

McDonnell, S.M, Miller, J.L., and Vaala, W. (2013). Calming benefit of short-term alpha-casozepine supplementation during acclimation to domestic environment and basic ground training of adult semi-feral ponies. *J. Equine Vet. Sci.* 33 (2): 101–106.

Mills, D. (2005). Repetitive movement problems in horses. In: *The Domestic Horse: The Origins, Development and Management of Its Behaviour* (eds. D.S. Mills and S.M. McDonnell), 212–227. New York: Cambridge University Press.

Parker, R.A. and Yeates, J.W. (2012). Assessment of quality of life in equine patients. *Equine Vet. J.* 44: 244–249.

Roberts, K., Hemmings, A., McBride, S. et al. (2017). Causal factors or oral versus locomotor stereotypies in the horse. *J. Vet. Behav.* https://doi.org/10.1016/j.jveb.2017.05.003.

Stull, C. (2003). Nutrition for rehabilitating the starved horse. *J. Equine Vet. Sci.* 23: 456–457.

Sweeting, M.P., Houpt, C.E., and Houpt, K.A. (1985). Social facilitation of feeding and time budgets in stabled ponies. *J. Anim. Sci.* https://doi.org/10.2527/jas1985.602369x.

Sykes, B.W., Hewetson M., Hepburn, R.J., Luthersson, N., *and* Tamzali, Y. (2015). European College of Equine Internal Medicine Consensus Statement—Equine gastric ulcer syndrome in adult horses. *J. Vet. Intern. Med.* 29: 1288–1299.

Torcivia, C.A. and McDonnell S.M. (2018). Case series report: Systematic rehabilitation of specific health care procedure aversions in five ponies. *J. Vet. Behav.* https://doi.org/10.1016/j.jveb.2018.02.003.

Torcivia, C.A. and McDonnell S.M. (2021). Equine discomfort ethogram. *Animals.* https://doi.org/10.3390/ani11020580.

Traub-Dargatz, J.L., Kopral, C.A., Hillberg Seitzinger A. *et al. (*2001*).* Estimate of the national incidence of and operation-level risk factors for colic among horses in the United States, spring 1998 to spring 1999. *J. Am. Vet. Med. Assoc.* 219: 67–71.

Watson, J.K. and McDonnell, S.M. (2018). Effects of three non-confrontational handling techniques on the behavior of horses during a simulated mildly aversive veterinary procedure. *Appl. Anim. Behav. Sci.* https://doi.org/10.1016/j.applanim.2018.02.007.

Young, T., Creighton, E., Smith, T. et al. (2012). A novel scale of behavioural indicators of stress for use in domestic horses. *Appl. Anim. Behav. Sci.* 140 (1–2): 33–43.

Appendix 24.A Needle Sticks

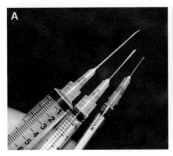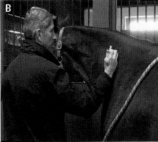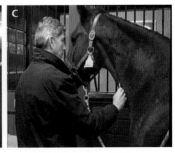

Routine Preventive

Equipment and Supplies

1) Finest needle practical (21 gauge or 22 gauge for blood withdraw; 22 gauge to 25 gauge for low viscosity aqueous solutions) (Panel A).
2) Small feed pan with highly palatable treat(s) (carrot, candy, apple, alfalfa).

Behavior Modification Principles

1) Select least stressful environment available, both for animal and technician.
2) Consider minimal restraint necessary, allowing some safe movement.
3) Ensure all personnel present are relaxed and calm.
4) Make the needle stick as comfortable as possible (Panels B and C).
   a) Stabilize hand against horse, maintaining contact with any movements of the horse during the stick.
   b) Proceed with smooth steady piercing (without hesitation or stabbing motion) through skin.
5) Ignore any undesirable behavior. With relaxed restraint, dangerous response is less likely, but should a dangerous response occur, try not to react in any way that would represent punishment or otherwise heighten fear.
6) Offer highly palatable food treat immediately before and immediately after, always preceded by verbal secondary reinforcement (e.g., the word "good" spoken in a consistent tone).
7) Scratch vigorously and rhythmically at the withers, simulating mutual grooming, for at least 30 seconds before and if possible continuing during skin stick (psychologically distracts, maintains positive motivational state, releases endorphins, and may compete with afferent transmission).

Established Aversion

Rehabilitation

Specific Behavior Modification Approaches to Consider, Alone or in Combination

1) Systematic desensitization and counter-conditioning: pair reward with each step in the process, first simulating injection with a skin pinch and then actual sticks of varying increasing levels of discomfort (30 g 5/8" to 20 g 1" needle). Ten sticks per increment is usually adequate.
2) Positive reinforcement-based operant counter-conditioning as needed to eliminate effective avoidance behaviors (e.g., stationary target training, teaching the horse to hold muzzle to target for several seconds or until actively released to receive food positive reinforcement).

Emergency Care "Get it done immediately with least further harm"

1) Overshadowing. It may be effective to perform the needle stick while leading the horse forward.
2) Respectfully applied skin twitch, gum chain, or lip twitch.

Appendix 24.B Oral Dosing

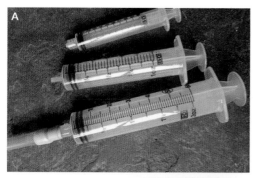
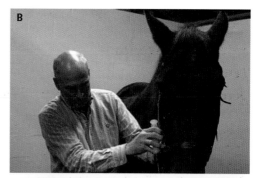
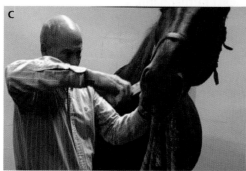
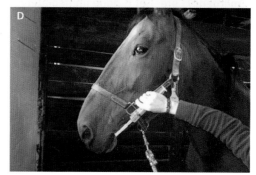

Routine Preventive

Equipment and Supplies

1) Smallest diameter dose syringe practical, with mouth-friendly tip (if tip is sharp, an extension of soft tubing can be secured over the tip) (Panel A).
2) Sweet liquid (molasses, corn syrup, maple syrup, applesauce, simple syrup).
3) Small feed pan with highly palatable treat(s) (carrot, candy, apple, alfalfa).

Behavior Modification Principles

1) Select least stressful environment available, both for animal and technician.
2) Consider minimal restraint necessary, allowing some safe wiggle room.
3) Select personnel who can remain relaxed and calm, safely ignoring any undesirable behavior.
4) Interact for a minute or so with goal of relaxing the horse (e.g., soothing rhythmic scratching at withers, rubbing of face).
5) Make the dosing itself as comfortable and palatable as possible.
   a) Use smallest dose syringe practical, with most mouth-friendly tip.
   b) Add sweet liquid to treatment, and coat the tip of syringe with sweet liquid.
   c) Respectful, unrushed insertion, avoiding contact of syringe tip with palate, gums, or teeth.
6) Suggested technique: Stabilize hand and dose syringe against cheek piece of halter, with tip near crease of the lips, maintaining stability of the syringe and contact with the horse should it move (Panel B); maintain a relaxed arm and ride-out any raising or shaking of the head until horse relaxes; then advance tip to gently contact crease of lips, which typically stimulates voluntary opening of the mouth and licking of the sweetened tip; then gently rotate syringe, aiming the tip ventrally onto tongue; calmly express liquid onto tongue, avoiding an explosive bolus (Panel C).
7) Offer highly palatable food treat immediately before and immediately after, always preceded by verbal secondary reinforcement (e.g., the word "good" spoken in a consistent tone).

Caretaker "Homework" (Discretionary)

Frequent doses of 10 cc of sweet liquid, alternating flavors following suggested routine procedure (initially daily for 10 days, then weekly or monthly) to maintain positive interest in oral dosing.

Established Aversion

Rehabilitation

Specific Behavior Modification Approaches to Consider, Alone or in Combination

1) Systematic desensitization, first gaining tolerance of placement of the syringe along cheek piece of halter by distracting and drawing head low with food (Panel D).
2) Positive reinforcement-based operant counter-conditioning as needed to displace head lifting or shaking (e.g., stationary target training, teaching horse to hold muzzle to target positioned at low convenient height).

Emergency Care "Get it done immediately with least further harm"

1) Respectfully applied skin twitch or gum chain.

Appendix 24.C Eye Medications

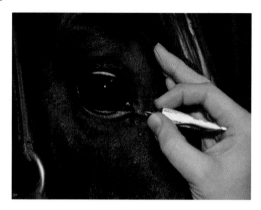

Routine Preventive

Equipment and Supplies

1) Eye-friendly applicator options: ophthalmic tube, soft rounded tip tuberculin syringe, or clean disposable glove.
2) Small feed pan with highly palatable treat(s) (carrot, candy, apple, alfalfa).

Behavior Modification Principles

1) Select least stressful environment available, both for animal and technician.
2) Consider minimal restraint necessary, allowing some safe wiggle room.
3) Select personnel who can remain relaxed and calm, safely ignoring any undesirable behavior.
4) Direct application: make the application itself as comfortable as possible.
   a) Rub face in soothing manner, rhythmically stroking approaching the medial canthus.
   b) Stabilize hand on face with relaxed arm so that hand maintains contact should the head move.
   c) When horse is relaxed, gently advance applicator to medial canthus to apply treatment.
   d) Repeat soothing rubbing of face around eyes.

   Subpalpebral catheter:

   a) Avoid pushing air through catheter.
   b) Express treatment slowly.
5) Offer highly palatable food treat immediately before and immediately after, always preceded by verbal secondary reinforcement (e.g., the word "good" spoken in a consistent tone).

Caretaker "Homework" (Discretionary)

Daily routine of rubbing face near each eye in soothing manner, maintaining hand contact while approaching and touching medial canthus in respectful, soothing manner (initially with fingertip, then with more rigid item such as tuberculin syringe or needle cap), offering a highly palatable food treat immediately before and after, as well as during as needed, paired with the verbal secondary reinforcement (e.g., "good") spoken in consistent tone just before food delivery.

Established Aversion

Rehabilitation

Specific Behavior Modification Approaches to Consider, Alone or in Combination

1) Systematic desensitization to touching of face approaching the medial canthus; food can be used to simultaneously draw the head to a comfortable position, distract, and then reward relaxation and increments of tolerance.
2) Positive reinforcement-based operant counter-conditioning as needed to displace disruptive avoidance behaviors (e.g., stationary target training, teaching horse to hold muzzle to target positioned at low convenient height).

Emergency Care "Get it done immediately with least further harm"

1) Respectfully applied skin twitch, gum chain, or lip twitch.
2) Examination stocks to limit body movement.

Appendix 24.D Intranasal Vaccination

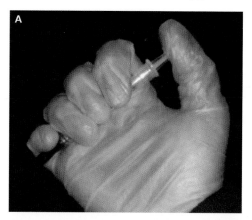

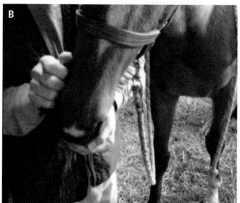
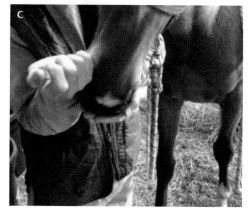

Routine Preventive

Equipment and Supplies

1) Intranasal-friendly mist applicator.
2) Small shallow feed pan with highly palatable treat(s) (carrot, candy, apple, alfalfa).

Behavior Modification Principles

1) Select the least stressful environment available, both for animal and technician.
2) Consider minimal restraint necessary, allowing some safe wiggle room.
3) Select personnel who can remain relaxed and calm, safely ignoring any undesirable behavior.
4) Make the treatment itself as comfortable as possible.
   a) Hold syringe in palm with thumb on plunger and applicator tip extending no more than ¼ inch beyond little finger (Panel A).
   b) Rest hand on face just above nostril with applicator tip pointing toward nostril; relax that arm to move with the horse, so that hand maintains stable contact (Panel B).
   c) When horse relaxed, while maintaining steady contact, rotate the hand to direct tip into nostril, simultaneously expressing the mist (Panel C).
5) Give highly palatable food treat immediately before and immediately after, always preceded by verbal secondary reinforcement (e.g., the word "good" spoken in a consistent tone).

Caretaker "Homework" (Discretionary)

Daily routine of rubbing face near each nostril in soothing manner, with simultaneous food treat.

Established Aversion

Rehabilitation

Specific Behavior Modification Approach to Consider

1) Positive reinforcement-based systematic desensitization and classical counter-conditioning to manipulation of the muzzle and nostril.

Appendix 24.E Rectal Temperature

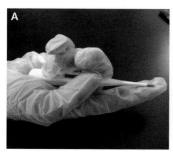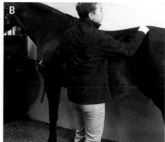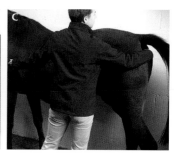

Routine Preventive

Equipment and Supplies

1) Rectal thermometer.
2) Long cotton lead (10–12 ft.) looped around a bar or ring as a sliding tether.

Behavior Modification Principles

1) Select the least stressful environment available, both for animal and technician.
2) Consider simple sliding tether to maintain and direct control of the head while standing at the hip.
3) Remain relaxed and calm, safely ignoring any undesirable behavior.
4) Make the procedure itself as comfortable as possible.
   a) Hold thermometer in palm with tip along index finger, about ½ inch proximal to fingertip held in place by thumb (Panel A).
   b) Slowly and rhythmically massage in soothing manner just lateral to base of tail, gradually approaching perineum and anus while continuing massage; this typically induces simultaneous relaxation of the anus and lifting of the tail; as that happens, give verbal secondary reinforcement (Panel B).
   c) With the index finger on the relaxed anus, advance the thermometer tip along the finger into the anus (no need to hold tail or visualize anus) (Panel C).
5) Give highly palatable food treat immediately before and immediately after, always paired with verbal secondary reinforcement (e.g., the word "good" spoken in a consistent tone).

Caretaker "Homework" (Discretionary)

Daily soothing massage of tail head, perineum, and anus as above, with food treat before and after. To teach the horse to relax the anus and lift tail upon verbal request, add spoken word or phrase to prompt the horse (e.g., "lift tail" or "tail up") while massaging the tail head and perineum. After only a few pairings of the prompt with physical stimulation of tail lifting and anus relaxation, most horses respond to just the spoken prompt and even your typical approach.

Established Aversion

Rehabilitation

Specific Behavior Modification Approaches to Consider, Alone or in Combination

1) Positive reinforcement-based systematic desensitization and classical counter-conditioning including massaging gradually from mid-back toward tail head; as horse relaxes at each increment, deliver primary and secondary reinforcement.
2) As needed for distraction and/or primary reinforcement for tolerance, have assistant offer a small food pan during the soothing massage and approach to perineum.

25

Animal Placement and Follow-Up
Alexandra Protopopova and Kelley Bollen

25.1 History and Philosophy of the Adoption Process

In this chapter, we will discuss both the experiences of the adopter as they navigate the selection and adoption process, as well as outline empirically based strategies that animal shelters can pursue to both improve adoption likelihood of their animals (Section 25.2) as well as ensure a successful adoption (Section 25.3). The concept of adopting out ownerless animals is fairly recent. Prior to the 1950s, the role of animal shelters was largely to remove loose animals from city streets in order to provide a quick death, with methods now understood as inhumane. Only later did animal shelters and humane societies begin exploring the concept of adoption rather than death as the outcome, and by the 1970s many facilities had adoption criteria in place (Troughton 2015).

In the last two decades, there has been a shift in the adoption process within animal sheltering to focus on removing barriers to adoption—the philosophy of *conversational adoptions*. Previously, many municipal animal shelters required adopters to fill out lengthy applications and have the whole family present at the time of the application, conducted home visits and income checks, and set out many barriers to adoption. However, such an approach had

serious consequences: the possibility of prejudice, limiting adoption, increasing unnecessary euthanasia, and ultimately not serving the community well. In fact, research has shown that adopter screening policies rarely match up with scientific rationale (Griffin et al. 2020). The alternative new philosophy entails seeing each adopter as an individual with personal strengths and weaknesses, as well as recognizing that adopters inherently mean well and are capable of gathering knowledge for appropriate animal care (Moulton 2003). In other words, the role of the adoption counselor, as discussed in Section 25.3, is to counsel and create a partnership rather than screen out adopters. Instead of finding reasons to deny an adoption, counselors now focus on aligning expectations of new adopters with the animals' characteristics. This shift in thinking was prompted by a demonstration of two respected leaders in animal sheltering who showed that if they were truthful about their living circumstances, they would be denied an adoption application in many shelters. This demonstration of the impossible adoption criteria led professionals to reconsider the adoption process at an Adoption Forum, hosted first by the American Humane Association in 1999 and again by PetSmart Charities in 2003, and ultimately led to the shift in philosophy that we

Animal Behavior for Shelter Veterinarians and Staff, Second Edition. Edited by Brian A. DiGangi, Victoria A. Cussen, Pamela J. Reid, and Kristen A. Collins.
© 2022 John Wiley & Sons, Inc. Published 2022 by John Wiley & Sons, Inc.
Companion website: www.wiley.com/go/digangi/animal

see today in many sheltering organizations (Troughton 2015).

In fact, research shows that adopters from animal shelters that had an open adoption policy did not differ in the quality of care or retention of the adopted animal, compared to animal shelters with the older policy-based adoption programs (Weiss et al. 2014). However, these philosophies seem to systematically vary depending on the total intake numbers in the region. Many communities with few animals coming into the shelters often have the privilege to conduct more matching to or screening of adopters simply due to having more resources available per animal. Additionally, due to increased resources, these communities are often able to admit and care for behaviorally challenging animals, thus a more thorough matching and screening program can reduce the chance of adverse outcomes such as injury to the family and the possibility of subsequent litigation. In contrast, for communities that are inundated with very large populations of companion animals serviced at the shelter, barrier-free adoption is essential to avoid the substantial welfare risks of overcrowding and in-shelter neglect.

An additional emerging theme in adoption programs is to not view the return of the adopted animal as a fundamental harm. Instead, returns may be viewed as learning opportunities about that specific animal, which can make the next placement match easier. Additionally, new research shows that time outside of the animal shelter is beneficial to dogs and that returning back to the shelter does not seem to be more traumatic than coming to the shelter in the first place (Gunter et al. 2019). Similar research has not yet been conducted with other species, such as cats and small mammals. However, a recent study found that fecal cortisol concentration, a physiological marker of stress, was largely the same in a pet home three months after adoption, compared to the concentration while at the shelter, suggesting that cats may take longer to habituate to new environments (Fukimoto et al. 2020). Because we know that transport (e.g., to a veterinary clinic) is a highly stressful experience for cats (Quimby et al. 2011), returns or short-term fostering may be more challenging for cats than for dogs. That being said, cats can learn to become accustomed to cat carriers and transport by car (Pratsch et al. 2018).

Returns may also be beneficial for an additional reason—creating a partnership with the adopter. Rather than putting blame on the adopter for a failed placement, a return can be an opportunity to adopt out a different animal to the same adopter or at least create a new foster family or an animal shelter advocate. The field of marketing shows that establishing a new customer is much more costly than retaining an existing customer (Gallo 2014). Thus, it is logical to put effort into retaining the returning adopter as an adopter for that specific animal shelter rather than driving that adopter away. Allowing adopters to try out their new animal in their home through a "trial adoption" or "foster-to-adopt" program may also be beneficial in removing the stigma associated with returning the animal, as well as creating lifelong community partners who will recommend adoption to friends and family. Throughout the chapter, we will be echoing the theme of working together with the adopter in a partnership to help them find their animal and assist them in building a relationship with their chosen animal.

25.2 Improving Adoption Likelihood

It is generally beneficial to consider the adoption process from a customer's perspective and use the science of marketing. By focusing on consumer behavior, we can describe and predict how adopters make decisions when choosing to adopt an animal. Additionally, we can learn how to determine what adopters want and need and by doing so, improve our ability to "sell" our "product"—or, in other words, increase adoptions. Kristen Auerbach, in a 2016 blog post, said it perfectly by highlighting the fact that most shelters do not use marketing approaches to their full potential. Instead, many tend to default to counseling (Auerbach 2016). For example, statements such as, "Lucky needs an active home with no children," only function to scare adopters rather than increase interest in the dog. Whereas counselling has a necessary role to play in an adoption program, marketing needs to come first to bring the adopter into the shelter and open the door for the possibility of an adoption.

In Section 25.2, we will describe the adoption process from the perspective of marketing science. We will cover how adopters make decisions when adopting animals and which animal factors predict adoption likelihood, as well as outline certain effective marketing strategies.

25.2.1 Adopter Characteristics and Behavior

To ensure high adoption rates, we must have a good understanding of our customer base—the adopter. Whereas research on the decision-making processes of adopters is still in its infancy, scientists already have generated some data, which animal shelters can use to improve their adoption programs.

25.2.1.1 Visiting the Animal Shelter

The percentage of people who would consider adopting from an animal shelter seems to be on the rise as evidenced by continuous increases in dog adoptions over the years (Rowan and Kartal 2018). The main reported reasons for not considering the shelter as a source of the next companion dog are (i) believing that the shelter will not have the specific animal wanted and (ii) wanting a purebred dog, whereas the main motivations for adoption were reported as helping the animal (Maddalena et al. 2012 cited in Garrison and Weiss 2015) and it being the right thing to do (Zito et al. 2015).

Survey research shows that whereas some adopters might be willing to drive more than 90 miles to get to an animal shelter, most will restrict their search within a 30-mile radius (Garrison and Weiss 2015). This means that the majority of the adopters are coming from the local community of a shelter. It is important for the animal shelter to have an understanding of the demographics of their local community to both tailor adoption programs as well as ensure that no sectors of the community are neglected. Ensuring the animal shelter provides equitable services to all members of the community is essential. Previous policy-based adoption programs were particularly poor at ensuring all community members were served by their animal shelter, as many adoption programs required moderately high family income in order to adopt. Income requirements as well as high adoption prices were justified by the flawed thinking that high family income was necessary to ensure good quality of life for the adopted animal. However, research shows that these concerns are unfounded; there were no differences in the attachment of adopters to their adult cats nor changes to return rates when adoption fees were reduced (Zito et al. 2015). In fact, a low advertised price of adoption was an important predictor of coming to a specific shelter as reported in a visitor survey (Crawford et al. 2017; Zito et al. 2015). One easy way to monitor whether the animal shelter provides services to all may be to request zip codes from visitors and subsequently ensure that the distribution across zip codes matches the overall population within those zip codes. If not, adoption programs may need to adjust accordingly.

Many visitors to animal shelters will not adopt. In fact, as many as two-thirds of visitors have no intention of taking an animal home that day (Southland et al. 2019). Most of these visitors do want to adopt in the future, but some have no intention to adopt at all. While many animal shelter staff are frustrated by these visitors as they may be viewed as taking staff's valuable time for seemingly no reason, they present important opportunities for the shelter. If visitors have a good experience while they are visiting, they will come back to the shelter once they are ready to adopt. Additionally, even if they do not have any intention to adopt, the shelter may still recruit these visitors as volunteers. Ultimately, these visitors may be excellent future animal welfare advocates for their community. Thus, it is important to accommodate these visitors within the shelter. Finally, some visitors end up adopting an animal even when they had no original intention to adopt. These spontaneous adoptions should be encouraged as there is no difference between retention in spontaneous compared to thought-out adoptions (American Humane Association 2013). Perhaps one way to mitigate the frustrations of overworked staff is for animal shelters to create volunteer positions that directly engage with the "just" visitors in order to capitalize on these available opportunities.

25.2.1.2 Decision-Making at the Shelter

In brick-and-mortar animal shelters, adopters seem to be making decisions in systematic ways. Of course, adopters already come with preconceived notions of their ideal animal (Garrison and Weiss 2015). However, once in the shelter, the majority of adopters seem to first browse all of the available animals and evaluate these animals initially based on morphology and, subsequently, on behavior.

On average, visitors tend to stop and look at approximately one-third of the available dogs and, once stopped, spend approximately 15–70 seconds looking at that dog (Protopopova and Wynne 2016; Wells and Hepper 2001). The interactions between the visitors and kenneled dogs can be grouped into distinct categories of behaviors: general affiliative interaction with the dog (e.g., speaking to, bending down, and reaching toward the dog) and actual interest in the dog (e.g., asking for more information about the dog and taking the dog out of the kennel). Ultimately, a given visitor, on average, takes about 1% of the dogs outside of the kennel for further interaction (Protopopova and Wynne 2016).

Less research exists on understanding adopter behavior when browsing cats. Frequency of viewing the same cat predicted ultimate adoption but the duration of viewing did not (Fantuzzi et al. 2010). Adopters showed more interest in cats when they were housed in top-tier cages and the cages contained a toy (Fantuzzi et al. 2010). Additionally, cats that displayed higher activity in their cages and lower stress (Gouveia et al. 2011) as well as human-directed social behavior had a shorter length of stay at the shelter (Brown and Stephan 2020). Singly housed cats in traditional horizontal cages had the fewest adoption outcomes as well as the most stress behavior; even a simple re-orientation of the cage to a vertical position and the addition of a shelf and towel to create a hiding area resulted in lower stress and higher adoptions (Gourkow and Fraser 2006).

Whereas some behaviors of dogs inside their kennels were predictive of overall length of stay in the shelter (Protopopova et al. 2014), closer experimental evaluations demonstrated that in-kennel training has no effect on adopter behavior. In fact, in an experimental study, only morphology of the dogs while in their kennel predicted visitor behavior (Protopopova and Wynne 2016). This suggests that the initial level of selection during the browsing phase is largely guided by evaluations of morphology. Whereas people have individual preferences for morphology, and thus, a variety of animals must be displayed, there are also overall population preferences for certain morphologies. Adopters seem to consistently prefer small-sized dogs, puppies, certain breed types, long coat length, and perhaps a light coat color (Protopopova and Gunter 2017).

Kittens, exotic breed status, unique coat patterns, and lighter colors are routinely preferred by cat adopters (Brown and Morgan 2015). Cat adopters seem to succumb to several notable biases when initially selecting cats for adoption. Black cats had a longer time to adoption (Kogan et al. 2013; Brown and Morgan 2015; Miller et al. 2019) and are judged to be less friendly and playful and more aggressive than light-colored cats. These judgments were found to be driven by superstition as well as a perceived inability to read the cat's emotion (Jones and Hart 2019). Cats that were labeled as owner-surrendered were adopted faster than those labelled as stray, even if the two groups did not differ in their latency to approach a person and even when the only difference was the label rather than the cat (Dybdall and Strasser 2014).

While seemingly superficial in their initial selection, we cannot be too annoyed with adopters—after all, even in romantic relationships, initial selection is based on appearance. People readily make judgements of character based on appearance; beautiful people are rated as being morally good, friendlier, kinder, more honest, and more trustworthy. In fact, we even choose political candidates based on appearance and give reduced prison sentences to beautiful people (Tsukiura and Cabeza 2011).

Not enough research has been conducted on decision avoidance of adopters when they encounter numerous animals in the shelter. In a famous experiment, Iyengar and Lepper (2000) found that people were more likely to purchase a jam or a chocolate when offered a choice of 6 flavors rather than 30. Because of the fear of inducing this decision avoidance, some may be inclined to recommend limiting the number of animals that the public may see. This practice, for several reasons, may not be the best approach. Previous research has shown that adopters prefer variety and even choose to avoid shelters if they perceive that selection is limited (Maddalena et al. 2012 cited in Garrison and Weiss 2015). Additionally, allowing the public to view all animals, even those that are not ready for adoption, is likely to increase the public's trust in the shelter and may establish the public as a partner. Ultimately, the research on the topic of decision avoidance in animal shelters is currently lacking thereby not supporting a recommendation to reduce the number of animals that the public can see. That being said, reduction of crowding and maintaining a shelter population within capacity for humane care is crucial to a successful adoption program in a given animal shelter. Crowding leads to unacceptable welfare concerns, including poor physical and mental health thereby reducing adoption rates (Janke et al. 2017; Hobson 2020). In summary, research supports limiting intake to ensure that the shelter is operating within its capacity for humane care; however, there is no published research to date that limiting the display of animals will reduce the supposed decision avoidance phenomenon.

After the initial browsing phase, adopters pick about one to two dogs, on average, for a meet and greet. During this phase, morphology no longer plays a role, which makes sense considering that the initial selection already screened the animal for desirable morphology. During the meet and greet phase, adopters spend about eight minutes, on average, interacting with the dog, and about one-third of the dogs are adopted following the meet and greet. For dogs, reciprocal play and lying down in proximity are the biggest behavioral predictors of subsequent adoption. Additionally, interacting in a small enclosed area led to the highest proportion of adoptions (Protopopova and Wynne 2014). Ultimately, adopters want to feel a connection to the animal—that the animal chooses to be with them, which is accomplished more easily if the dog is not distracted by other environmental variables. In an experimental study, when dogs were encouraged to stay in proximity and lie down next to adopters and only the dog's favorite toy was allowed in the meet and greet room (in order to encourage reciprocal play), adoptions nearly doubled (Protopopova et al. 2016).

While we do not have the same level of understanding of adopter behavior when it comes to cats, several researchers have asked adopters to reflect on their adoption decisions. Adopters reported that being able to interact with the cat by entering the enclosure as well as seeing their cat of interest interacting with other cats was important in their decision to adopt. Additionally, adopters reported selecting cats based on friendliness and playfulness (Gourkow and Fraser 2006). Latency to approach an unfamiliar person additionally predicted a shorter length of stay (Dybdall and Strasser 2014).

25.2.2 Marketing Approaches

Getting people into the animal shelter is crucial. While simplistic, we can estimate based on previous visitor behavior data that an animal shelter needs about 300 in-person visitors per dog adoption. As 30% of visitors will visit online sites such as Petfinder® (www.petfinder.com) prior to coming to the animal shelter and 50% of adopters reported seeing their adopted cat's online page (Workman and Hoffman 2015), any marketing approaches to increase adoption must start with the shelter's online presence. In fact, having up-to-date information on available animals online is crucial—the number of clicks on an online profile of the animal had an inverse relationship with that animal's length of stay at the shelter (Workman and Hoffman 2015)!

A good online profile for an animal is up to date and has a good-quality photo, perhaps a short video highlighting the animal's best quali- ties, and an appropriate description. The ani- mals preferably should be depicted outdoors, standing, making eye contact, and cats should have toys; having a person in the photo or hav- ing bandanas did not seem to make a difference to adopters (Lampe and Witte 2015; Schoenfeld- Tacher et al. 2019; Workman and Hoffman 2015). Participants who viewed videos rather than photos of cats rated the cats as more adoptable (Schoenfeld-Tacher et al. 2019), perhaps because they could better understand the cat's personality. Additionally, removing breed labels did not seem to create any adverse conse- quences. Instead, after the removal of breed labels, one shelter in New York saw the length of stay reduced for all dogs and no changes in the return rates (Cohen et al. 2020).

Researchers in Australia found that the fol- lowing descriptive words predicted a shorter length of stay: "make you proud," "independ- ent," "lively," "eager," and "clever." However, words like "only dog," "dominant," "sensitive," and "happy-go-lucky" actually increased length of stay (Nakamura et al. 2019). In addition, experimental research has demonstrated that adoption ads that use concrete and analytic lan- guage, rather than narrative language, resulted in higher interest from potential adopters (Markowitz 2019). Although more research is needed to clarify how language affects adopters, shelter staff must make conscious decisions when drafting the profile and focus on market- ing the animal's best qualities. The online

profile should not contain warnings about potential matching issues (e.g., that the dog needs more training, needs to be an only dog, best in a home with no children, etc.). These issues, although critical, should be brought up with individual adopters during the counseling phase and not included in the initial marketing of the animal. When creating descriptions of the animal, take care to not be too negative about the previous circumstances of that ani- mal. While sympathy is certainly a motivator for adoption, public-facing animal profiles must be considerate of larger societal issues and avoid language that puts blame on the previous owner. Research has now rather conclusively shown that surrendering an animal is a deeply emotional decision and is tied to larger societal issues such as housing or financial insecurity (Ly et al. 2021). Likewise, animal profile crea- tors must be mindful of not contributing to fur- ther discrimination by blaming entire groups of people. For example, phrases like "rescued from a lifetime on a reservation" are clearly inappro- priate. Taking from human literature of what generates the most interest in profiles in roman- tic match-making websites, descriptions should also be short, humorous, memorable, and, most importantly, focused on what the dog brings to the adopter.

Additionally, the animal's profile must be repeatedly posted on social media and frequently updated. People are susceptible to the "mere exposure effect," by which simply seeing the same face repeatedly makes us perceive that face as more attractive. Additionally, updating the animal's profile might also showcase that the animal shelter provides individualized care to each animal as well as improving the relation- ship with the community—community mem- bers may share the profile on their own social media platforms and perhaps even take a per- sonal interest in the animal. However, take care not to accidently make the animal less desirable by including phrases like, "overlooked by adop- ters," "still at the shelter," or "waiting for over six months." These phrases may indicate to adop- ters that since others do not want them, there may be something wrong with that animal.

Instead, updates may include short cute stories. For example, if a volunteer took the dog for a ride in the car to get ice cream, a photo with the dog eating ice cream with a few words about his favorite flavor and overall experience may be included. Example "bad" and "good" profiles for dogs and cats are found in Boxes 25.1–25.4.

Dog training with a mind to increasing adoption likelihood should focus on the meet and greet rather than in-kennel presentation as that is where decisions based on behavior take place. Dog training should focus on teaching a dog to lie down next to a bench or a chair, where an adopter will subsequently sit. Additionally, volunteers may take the time to determine which toy and treats each dog likes best so as to provide this information to the potential adopter and thus increase reciprocal play (Protopopova et al. 2016). Dogs may also be taught to lie down and relax through

---

Box 25.1 Example of a "Bad" Online Dog Profile

Note: Information is updated by volunteers so may not be up to date. Please call the shelter directly to request information.

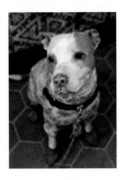

Photo source: Courtesy of Dr. Kelsea Brown.

Name: Trouble
Breed: Pit bull mix
Age: 18 months
Sex: Female
Size: 30 lbs

Special Requirements:
- NO other pets in the home
- NO apartments/condos
- HIGH energy level
- Bully breed experience

Are you looking for a fantastic jogging or hiking partner? If so, Trouble might just be the dog for you! She is a higher-energy gal who would be best suited with a family who lives an active lifestyle and has no other dogs.

Trouble is a very smart girl but does require a firm handler as she is a bit dominant. Even though she is pint sized, she is quite strong and will definitely pull on leash to chase squirrels. She just needs time and training and you will see why she is a volunteer favorite.

Problems:

- Information not up to date.
- Low-quality picture.
- No video.
- Dog is indoors, avoiding eye contact.
- Name may evoke unpleasant emotions. If staff named the animal, consider changing.
- Breed label may reduce chance of adoption.
- Starting with negatives and restrictions may reduce chance of adoption.
- Restrictions on housing are discriminatory.
- Descriptive words, such as "fantastic jogging partner," "active lifestyle" allow the adopter to assume that the dog is easily aroused and too hyperactive, which are not preferred qualities. Such language will reduce the chance of adoption.
- Negative descriptions of the dog's behavior, such as "requires a firm handler," "dominant," "will definitely pull on leash," "will chase squirrels," "needs time" will certainly be off-putting for adopters.
- Narrative language with a focus on the volunteer-dog connection will likely reduce interest from adopters.

Box 25.2   Example of a "Good" Online Dog Profile

Updated: today

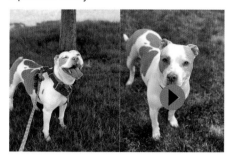

Photo source: Courtesy of Dr. Kelsea Brown.

Name: Rosie
Age: 18 months
Sex: Female
Size: 30 lbs

Meet Rosie, a playful sweetie pie who dreams of being a full-time family dog! This happy girl will trot by your side wherever you go. When she's not giving out all the kisses, she's making friends with any human she meets! Click here to learn more about how to visit us and meet Rosie: *Link here.*

Qualities of a good profile:

- Up-to-date information.
- High-quality picture.
- Video is present.
- Dog is outdoors, standing, making eye contact.
- No breed label.
- No restrictions or barriers listed.
- Descriptive words that are entirely positive.
- No descriptive words that allow adopter to "read between the lines."
- Limited use of narrative language, not unnecessarily verbose.
- Focuses on what the dog will bring to the adopter.
- Ends with a call to action.

Box 25.3   Example of a "Bad" Online Cat Profile

Note: Information is updated by volunteers so may not be up to date. Please call the shelter directly to request information.

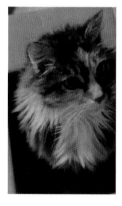

Photo source: Courtesy of Dr. Kelsea Brown.

Prissy is a pretty cat with big green eyes. She is about seven years old. She came to us from another shelter where she had been returned three times for inappropriate peeing. We have had her checked out and it is not a medical issue. Cats can be very sensitive and their stress often manifests itself in inappropriate peeing.

Clearly something in her previous homes stressed her out. Even though she is human-friendly, to be on the safe side we are looking for a quiet, adult-only home for Prissy where she can live a relaxed and stress-free life. Prissy seems to be okay with the other cats in her room so it seems that a feline roommate would be okay. Prissy is such a sweet and loving cat and we hope that someone will give her a chance to prove what a great companion she is.

Problems:

- Information not up to date.
- Low-quality picture.
- No video.
- Cat is avoiding eye contact.
- Name may evoke unpleasant emotions. If staff named the animal, consider changing.
- Starting with negatives (i.e., she was returned three times) will reduce the adopter's interest.
- Negative descriptions of the cat's behavior, such as "inappropriate peeing," "sensitive" will certainly be off-putting for adopters.

- Narrative language that describes the requirements of the adoptive family (e.g., "stress-free" home, "adult-only") severely reduces adopter interest. Who can honestly say that their home is "stress-free?" Such language will reduce the chance of adoption.
- Ending with a sentence to indicate that the shelter hopes that someone will give her a chance indicates that she is a particularly difficult and undesirable pet.

Box 25.4   Example of a "Good" Online Cat Profile

The following information is up to date.

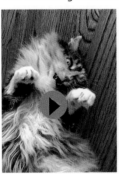 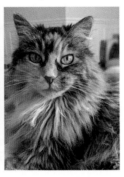

Photo source: Courtesy of Dr. Kelsea Brown.

Name: Suzie
Age: Adult
Sex: Female

Suzie is a gorgeous, affectionate cat and is very much a kitten at heart—always playing with her friends! When you enter her room, she instantly runs over for some cuddles. She's sweet and chatty and would love to meet you. Learn more about Suzie and how to adopt here: *Link here.*

Qualities of a good profile:

- Up-to-date information.
- High-quality picture.
- Video is present (eye-catching).
- Cat is making eye contact.
- No restrictions or barriers listed.
- Descriptive words that are entirely positive.
- Omission of any negative words.
- Limited use of narrative language, not unnecessarily verbose.
- Focuses on what the cat will bring to the adopter.
- Ends with a call to action.

relatively unstructured activities such as reading a book to the dog in the meet and greet area. The key is to not provide too much play and attention to the dog. Teaching a dog to relax in the presence of a person may not only improve their behavior in the meet and greet room, but may also be useful for the dog's mental health. When showing the dog to the potential adopter, care must be taken to encourage the adopter to feel that the dog chooses them. Research has shown that when a person believes that they are liked by a stranger, that stranger becomes more attractive to them (Hove and Risen 2009). Additionally, joint attention and synchrony have been implicated in successful human relationships—shared activities lead to higher feelings of affiliation. Thus, encouraging shared activities such as reciprocal play is beneficial.

Clicker training of cats using food treats to approach the front of the kennel was successful at increasing the time in the front of the cage, increasing exploratory behavior, and decreasing inactivity (Grant and Warrior 2019). Future research must experimentally demonstrate that this training affects visitor behavior; for the time being, animal shelter staff and volunteers should consider this approach as the best-practice as it improves cat well-being. See Chapter 18 for information on clicker training cats.

Cats who approached an unfamiliar experimenter had a shorter time to adoption, although this effect was only seen for cats labeled as stray (Dybdall and Strasser 2014). Additionally, people reported that they preferred cats who were friendly toward them (Dybdall and Strasser 2014). Thus, out of the cage cat training should focus on reinforcing approach behavior toward visitors, perhaps using food and play.

Staff and volunteers must be careful to not accidently disrupt the building of a connection between the animal and adopter through demonstrations of what the animal can do. For example, for fearful dogs, volunteers should not attempt to demonstrate that the dog is capable of trust by showing the adopter how much the dog trusts that volunteer. The obvious and not productive response of the adopter following such a demonstration may be to feel personally rejected and to ask why that volunteer does not take that dog home themselves. Adopters need to feel preferred by their chosen animal, and that is not possible with staff and volunteers showing off a special connection with that animal.

25.3 Increasing the Likelihood of Successful Adoptions

While we never know if an adoption will work out successfully for the adopter, a shelter's goal should be to provide adopters with as much information about the animal as possible so that they can make an informed decision about whether the dog or cat will fit into their life and family. As discussed in Section 25.2, people typically first choose a potential adoptee based on how the animal looks, and, later, the animal's behavior during the meet and greet session. During that meet and greet session, it is also important for the shelter to give the potential adopter information about the personality traits and behavioral characteristics of the animal. Knowing these things requires adoption agencies to make an effort to learn as much about the animals in their care as possible through thorough behavioral history gathering and monitoring during the animals' stay at the facility.

While it is not the shelter's place to determine if an animal is right for a family, there are two situations that, for dog adoptions, sometimes need to be considered prior to placement—the presence of young children and the presence of other animals in the home. In a survey study of 370 animal shelters and rescues across the United States, respondents indicated that the most common information used to match dogs to adopters included child safety and the safety of other pets in the home (Reese 2021).

There are dogs in every shelter that present with behaviors that may not be ideal for homes with young children. Having the behavioral propensity to guard resources, having handling sensitivities/intolerances, or becoming hyper-aroused during play may be problematic or even dangerous around young children. Studies have found that having children in the home negatively influences adoption success due to improper expectations placed on both the animal and the children (Diesel et al. 2008; Shore 2005; Kidd et al. 1992). Shelters need to be mindful of the vulnerability of young children around dogs with certain behavioral propensities and guide parents to appropriate individuals for adoption consideration.

There are also dogs in every shelter that present with behaviors that may not be ideal for homes with other animals. Behavioral propensities such as a high prey drive, resource guarding, or offensive/defensive aggression to other dogs can be problematic or even dangerous around cats and other dogs in a home. Research has shown that incompatibility between new and current animals results in increased risk of adoption failure (Shore 2005; Salman et al. 2000; Kidd et al. 1992). That being said, while shelters have a duty to provide as much information as possible about the dog to the potential adopter, the ultimately responsibility of determining whether a dog is a good match for the family will lie with the adopter.

At times other things such as the experience of the adopter as an animal caregiver and their expectations for their new companion should be discussed during the counseling session. Previous research has shown that many caregivers and people who relinquish animals, lack knowledge regarding animal behavior (New et al. 2010; Salman et al. 1998). As adopters' animal care knowledge increased, so did their expectations for the effort required in animal guardianship. Caregiver expectations can affect bonding and satisfaction with an animal, so exploring an individual's expectations of their adopted animal will be beneficial in identifying and allocating educational resources that are specific to their needs during the adoption process (O'Connor et al. 2016).

The respondents in the Reese (2021) study on adoption matching programs in shelters and rescues indicated a number of positive outcomes from their use of a matching program, the most commonly reported being a lower return rate. Some respondents also reported a positive reaction from the public and an increased overall adoption rate. Several elements of matching programs appeared to have stronger associations with positive outcomes: conducting matching conversations before potential adopters see any dogs, showing only dogs that are a good match, and limiting choice to those dogs that are deemed the best fit. They did find, however, that matching programs can be associated with longer average length of stay.

Once the adopter has chosen an animal that they feel is appropriate for them to take home, the next step is for shelter staff to provide the adopter with information to ensure the best possible transition for both the animal and the family. As discussed by Troughton (2015), understanding how adults learn is important regarding adoption counseling in a shelter. Respecting the adopters experience, knowledge, and skill is critical if we hope to add to their body of knowledge pertaining to having a new pet in their home. Adults will put the time into learning and will be motivated to acquire a deeper understanding when the benefits are clear and they can use what they have learned right away. Practical, immediately applicable, and useful information is an adult's preference. The adult learner also needs to be engaged in the process, feel motivated to learn, and receive both intrinsic (the thrill of developing greater understanding) and extrinsic (positive reinforcement) rewards for having learned something new.

Adoption counselors should try to develop a relationship with the adopter that supports their learning regarding their current needs and those of the specific cat or dog they have selected (Troughton 2015). The most important subject matter to add to an adopter's knowledge base concerns the behavior of the animal. Research tells us that behavioral concerns are on the minds of many people considering adopting from an animal shelter. In interviews of prospective adopters, it was found that the animal's behavior was the predominant consideration and pre-adoption concern for all participants (O'Connor et al. 2017). Allowing the adopters to ask questions first can set the stage for improved learning. When counselors provide the adopter with the answers to the questions they feel are important, they open the adopter to receiving additional information they may not have known to ask about.

There is a large body of research to indicate that behavioral challenges are a commonly described reason stated for relinquishment of an animal to a shelter (Patronek et al. 1996; Miller et al. 1996; Houpt et al. 1996; Salman et al. 1998; New et al. 2010; Wells and Hepper 2000). Likewise, problematic behavior has been found to be the leading cause of non-retention of adopted animals. Neidhart and Boyd (2002) reported that 64% of animals were no longer in the same home one year post-adoption due to behavior problems. Mondelli et al. (2004) found that 54% of returned dogs were returned for behavioral issues and Casey et al. (2009) found that 38% of returned cats were returned due to their behavior. Shore

(2005) interviewed 78 adopters returning their newly adopted animal, and in 59% of the cases the return was due to behavior problems. Diesel et al. (2008) stated that behavioral issues are the primary driver of adoption failure after finding that 74.1% of returned animals were returned due to behavior problems. They further noted that post-adoption returns of dogs to the shelter might have been prevented by providing the caregiver with more education in advance, including realistic expectations of the effort required in caring for an animal.

Most of the post-adoption survey studies conducted in the last 20 years have reported that behavioral issues are the biggest challenge adopters face with their newly adopted animal; see Table 25.1 (Gates et al. 2020; Scott et al. 2018; Vitulová et al. 2018; Gates et al. 2018; American Humane Association 2013; Casey et al. 2009; Lord et al. 2008; Diesel et al. 2008; Mondelli et al. 2004; Neidhart and Boyd 2002; Wells and Hepper 2000). Behavioral concerns can affect the bond that the adopter forms with their new companion and, when unresolved, can result in the return or rehoming of the animal. Adoption counseling should therefore include information on preventing, managing, or resolving the most commonly reported

Table 25.1 Commonly reported post-adoption behavioral concerns in dogs and cats.

Dogs	Cats
House damage (destructiveness/chewing)	Inappropriate elimination (housesoiling)
Inappropriate elimination (housetraining issues)	Scratching furniture
Aggression	Fearful behavior/hiding
Excessive barking	Aggression to people
Hyperactivity (high energy)	Aggression to other cats
Escapes (running away)	Problems associated with dogs
Poor manners (disobedient/pulling/jumping)	
Fearfulness	
Intolerance to other animals	
Separation anxiety	

From Mondelli et al. 2004; Scott et al. 2018; Vitulová et al. 2018; Wells and Hepper 2000; Gates et al. 2018, 2020; American Humane Association 2013; Lord at al. 2008; Diesel et al. 2010; Neidhart and Boyd 2002; Casey et al. 2009.

behaviors of concern for each species. Providing the adopter with more behavioral education at the time of adoption could increase adoption success and prevent returns to the shelter.

Previous research has looked at the usefulness of providing adoption counseling on certain behavioral issues. Herron et al. (2007) found that significantly more adopters who were provided with a five-minute counseling session on housetraining at the time of adoption reported success one month post-adoption than did adopters who did not receive such information. Herron et al. (2014) evaluated the effectiveness of providing dog adopters with a written handout on reducing the risk of separation anxiety post-adoption. They reported that 30% of the 178 adopted dogs exhibited some form of separation anxiety related behaviors in the new home; however, the prevalence of these behaviors was lower in the treatment group (adopters who received the handout) than the control group. The researchers concluded that the provision of the written advice appeared to be effective in reducing separation-related anxious behaviors. Compliance was low for most of the recommended strategies with the exception of advice to not interact with the dog before leaving and to provide the dog with a food-filled enrichment toy when alone. They suggested that these two simple strategies may help prevent the development of separation anxiety-related behaviors in shelter dogs. The researchers state that it is possible that the efficacy of the program may be enhanced if the advice was presented to the adopters verbally at the time of adoption rather than in a written handout. However, an earlier study that involved providing some adopters with a 5-min counseling session on separation anxiety prevention concluded that there was no difference between the treatment group that received the counseling and the control group that did not in the occurrence of separation anxiety related behaviors post-adoption (Herron et al. 2014). Interestingly, they found that both groups of adopters were just as likely to perform most of the recommendations

received by the treatment group anyway. The strategy that was most likely to be followed by both groups was the presentation of a food-filled toy upon departure.

Based on these findings, it seems prudent to provide behavioral information during the adoption counseling session. However, it is important to not overwhelm the adopter with too much information. Focusing on only a few issues and keeping it short and simple will help the adopter retain the information (Troughton 2015). The authors have identified five important species-specific behavioral points (three if the adopter has no other pets in the home) to discuss with adopters during their counseling session (Appendices 25.A and 25.B). For dogs, these points include information on:

- Housetraining
- Safeguarding against separation anxiety
- How to properly introduce the dog to the resident cat(s)
- How to properly introduce the dog to the resident dog(s)
- Importance of physical and mental stimulation and training.

For cats, these points include information on:

- Litterbox use
- Providing appropriate scratching posts
- Settle-in time when first home (i.e., expect some hiding the first few days)
- How to properly introduce the cat to the resident cat(s)
- How to properly introduce the cat to the resident dog(s).

The combination of in-person adoption counseling accompanied by written take-home tip sheets can improve the learning experience for the adopter. For this reason, verbally communicating these three to five most important behavior topics during the adoption counseling session and then giving the adopter a handout that details the same information should improve retention of the material.

A survey study asked adopters about the usefulness of the different types of information that was provided to them at the time of adoption as take-home tip sheets and/or provided on the website. Information about normal animal behavior, methods to train the animal, and how to introduce the animal to the household were all rated as very useful (Gates et al. 2020). In addition to providing some general behavioral information to adopters, imparting information about the personality and behavioral characteristics of the individual animal being adopted is also important. Often the shelter knows about certain behavioral propensities in the animal that could affect the bond and adoption success if the adopters are not informed and given strategies to effectively manage potentially problematic behaviors.

O'Connor et al. (2017) found that aggressive behavior was the most commonly identified undesirable behavior mentioned by cat and dog adopters. Dog adopters felt that having a dog that exhibited aggressive behavior to people or other dogs would limit their ability to enjoy and include the companion animal in leisure activities and might put a strain on their social life. Adopters discussed the importance of feeling comfortable inviting visitors to their house and having their dog behave well during interactions with people or other animals outside of the home. While both dog and cat adopters felt that aggressive behavior displayed by the animal could negatively impact their relationship, getting along with other people and animals was a greater priority for dog adopters than cat adopters because of plans to include the dog in activities outside of the home, which rarely occurs for cats.

Past studies have also shown that animal aggression is a common behavioral concern for caregivers and a commonly reported reason for relinquishment (Salman et al. 2000; Diesel et al. 2010). One of these studies showed that caregivers who received no behavioral advice regarding their dogs' aggressive behavior toward people were 11 times more likely to return the dog. These odds fell to 5.5 when caregivers received management advice regarding their dog's aggressive behavior. It is therefore extremely important to provide specific counseling when an adoptive animal is known to have aggressive propensities.

Adults learn best by playing an active role in the learning process, so allowing the adopter to interact with the animal while discussing the behaviors of concern can be a priceless learning experience (Troughton 2015). For example, if a dog exhibits behavior such as jumping up or pulling the leash, teaching the adopter how to best modify those behaviors and allowing them to practice the skills will enhance learning. Likewise, for potentially more serious problematic behaviors such as aggressively guarding resources such as food, bones, and toys or on-leash reactivity toward other dogs, showing the adopter exactly what to do to address the issues and having them practice will help to ensure they are able to successfully perform these skills at home. Simply telling them to avoid giving the dog a valuable possession or not to walk their dog near other dogs would not be as helpful.

25.3.1 New Home Experience

Millions of dogs and cats are adopted from animal shelters each year. With each adoption comes the hope that the placement will lead to a loving and long-lasting relationship between the pet and the adoptive family. The reality, however, is that many shelters have no idea how "successful" their adoptions actually are because they lack the resources to do any kind of meaningful follow-up.

For many shelters, the only gauge they have for adoption success is their return rate. Although it is inevitable that some animals will be returned to the shelter for a variety of reasons, the hope is always that unsuccessful adoptions are the exception. However, several studies have reported return rates ranging from 7% to as high as 24% (Marston et al. 2004; Diesel et al. 2008; Mondelli et al. 2004).

The return rate reflects only a portion of failed adoptions. Neidhart and Boyd's (2002) survey found that 20% of all adopters no longer had their pet within one year of adoption but that only 49% of these animals were returned to the shelter. Likewise, a large survey of six shelters in three US cities revealed that out of re-relinquished animals, only half were returned to the shelter of acquisition, while the other half had alternative outcomes (American Humane Association 2013). The reality is that adopters who choose not to keep their newly adopted pets have many other options for rehoming, and some may purposely choose not to return to the shelter for fear of being judged as a failure by the organization. To build a partnership with adopters, it is important that they view the animal shelter as a resource. Adopters should feel safe to seek help from the shelter rather than relying on other sources that may ultimately lead to less ideal outcomes for the animal.

The fact that some adoptions do not result in long-lasting relationships should not reflect failure on the part of the shelter or the adopter. The most difficult aspect of adopting an animal is that adopters cannot know for certain if that animal will fit into their life. In addition to behavioral or health concerns that may arise with the new pet, mismatched personalities (between the humans and/or the other pets in the home), unrealistic expectations on the part of the adopter, and a general lack of knowledge about animal behavior can prevent the formation of a long-lasting bond. This is why adoption matching and counseling as described above are so important.

Shelters should encourage adopters to return the animal if things are not working out, and these returns should not be considered as failures. When an animal is returned, shelters have the opportunity to learn more about that animal's behavior in a home environment, and this information can help improve the next adoption. Additionally, as stated earlier, recent research indicates that, at least for dogs, time out of the shelter is beneficial (Gunter et al. 2019).

The first few weeks and months in a new home are critical for bonding to occur between the human family and the adopted animal. When adopters experience unexpected health and/or behavioral concerns shortly after they bring their new pet home, this crucial bonding is jeopardized, and many decide to return the animal to the shelter rather than seek assistance or give the animal time to heal or adjust. Mondelli et al. (2004) reported that 41% of returned dogs came back within one week of adoption, and others have reported that 54% and 39% of the returned animals were brought back to the shelter within two weeks of adoption (Shore 2005 and Diesel et al. 2008, respectively). The American Humane Association (2013) study found that of the dogs and cats not retained in homes following adoption, 27% left the home within two weeks of adoption and another 37% between two weeks and two months. This is why it is critical to provide behavior-related adoption counseling that will help both the animal and the family with the transition.

Even for those adopters who still have their new pet, survey studies revealed that behavioral issues were the biggest challenge they faced. This finding appears to be universal across many countries. A US survey of 2,500 adopters found that nearly 51% reported that the pet had a behavioral issue of concern one week following acquisition (Lord et al. 2008). In a Northern Ireland survey, 68% of respondents who adopted a dog from a shelter reported behavioral concerns (Wells and Hepper 2000), and in an Australian study that looked at adopter satisfaction, undesirable behaviors were present in 53% of the dogs and 14% of the cats (Scott et al. 2018). Surveys of adopters in New Zealand found that 48% of the kittens and cats had at least one behavioral problem (Gates et al. 2020), and 70% of dog adopters reported the same (Gates et al. 2018). Almost 200 adopters from 84 different shelters in the Czech Republic were surveyed, and the researchers found that 72% of the dogs exhibited behavioral problems in the first week after adoption (Vitulová et al. 2018). A companion animal's personality and good behavior are keys to retention and adopter satisfaction. Half of those adopters that cited problems with their adopted animal's behavior said that bad habits were their biggest challenge (Neidhart and Boyd 2002). These studies support the necessity of good behavioral adoption counseling as well as being a resource for adopters needing behavioral help post-adoption, especially during the first few weeks and months.

The follow-up survey conducted by Vitulová et al. (2018) did reveal significant positive changes in the behavior of dogs six months after leaving the shelter. This suggests that mere patience and time spent in a family can be a solution to at least some of the behavioral problems encountered soon after adoption. The researchers suggest that if professional post-adoption behavioral counseling were provided, it could decrease the amount of time required for the solution. The only problematic behavior that did not simply improve with time was aggressive behavior. It would seem from this finding that professional post-adoption behavioral counseling is especially critical when animals are exhibiting aggressive behavior that persists over time.

25.3.2 Post-adoption Support Programs

Providing post-adoption support ensures that adoption agencies are doing everything they can to help their adopters successfully develop a loving, long-term relationship with the animals they place. The primary goal is to be available to provide assistance to adopters who may be experiencing problems with their new companion. While most shelters tell their adopters to call if they have any questions or problems, that may not be the most effective support strategy. Shelters often do not have the staff available to take incoming calls or even to return calls should the adopter leave a message. Furthermore, many staff members do not have the knowledge needed to offer sound advice to an adopter seeking resolution to a health or behavior problem they are experiencing with their new pet.

Shelters need to make more of an effort to support their adopters than simply telling them to call if they need help. The first step is for shelters to understand the kind of post-adoption health and behavioral issues that adopters commonly experience with their new companion. From there, creating or obtaining informational tip sheets that address these common medical and behavioral issues and making them available on the shelter's website is the minimum that a shelter can do. The information tip sheets need to be easily and quickly found on the website; there should be tabs on the home page directing the adopter to "Behavioral Help" and "Medical Help." Adopters should be shown the website links during the adoption counseling session so that they know that resources are available should they experience a problem.

Beyond website tip sheets, shelters can set up a designated phone line and email address as the next level of support. Providing the helpline phone number and email address at the time of adoption, in addition to having it on the shelter's home webpage, is critical. If these avenues for contact are set up, however, it is imperative that someone monitor and respond to incoming phone or email messages in a timely fashion or the adopter will become frustrated with the agency. Simple behavior questions that come into the system could be directed to staff or volunteers with some degree of behavioral/training knowledge. For more serious behavioral concerns, the caller should be referred to a certified behaviorist. All medical concerns need to be referred to a veterinarian.

The next level of post-adoption support involves proactively reaching out to adopters periodically to inquire about how things are going with their new companion. Reaching out to adopters allows shelters to answer any questions the adopter may have and provide assistance with problems they may be experiencing with their new companion. This effort serves to not only reduce returns or other forms of rehoming but will increase the goodwill adopters have toward the adoption agency.

This type of proactive post-adoption support program is unfortunately not very common-place. A survey of 56 animal shelters in the United States and Canada revealed that half of the shelters reported that they did not have the time or resources to conduct post-adoption fol-low-up of any kind. When follow-up did occur, there was a significant amount of variability regarding how often and when checks were conducted. The most significant challenge to good post-adoption support seems to be a lack of resources (Burch et al. 2006). However, perhaps the challenge is not necessarily a *lack* of resources but rather a poor allocation of available resources. Committing resources to provide post-adoption support will likely reduce other needed resources should the adopter decide to return the animal to the shelter.

There are several ways that adoption agen-cies can proactively reach out to their adopters. Conducting post-adoption follow-up phone calls is the most resource-dependent option, as it often takes several calls to contact the adop-ter, and when an adopter is actually contacted, the phone call could require a significant time commitment. During their follow-up study, Gates et al. (2018) found that, on average, each telephone interview took approximately 35 minutes to complete (range: 13–58 min-utes). Due to the significant time constraints encountered with conducting the survey by telephone, this option was discontinued four weeks into the study period. Most shelters do not have the time or personnel to conduct fol-low-up phone calls to their adopters.

Using email as a form of proactive contact is a less resource-intensive alternative. This approach may be better received by adopters, as they generally indicated a preference to be contacted by email (Gates et al. 2020). The ability to conduct post-adoption support via email requires that agencies attain the adopter's cur-rent email address at the time of the adoption. The post-adoption support email survey should not contain too many questions so that it can be completed in only a few minutes to maxi-mize the response rate. The categories of questions asked in the survey should include animal adjustment, animal health, animal behavior, need for assistance with post-adoption problems, and adopter satisfaction with animal match (Reider 2015a).

The returned email surveys will need to be reviewed daily to ensure timely responses to requests for help. Some of the requests can be responded to with a return email that includes advice and instructional material. Other adop-ter requests for help will need to be followed up with a phone call. Calling the adopters whose questions or problems require more extensive assistance will require additional time and effort by the shelter. Being able to offer adopters behavior counseling and training; guidance for health problems; referrals to pet-related ser-vices in the community; and programs to assist financially struggling adopters with items such as veterinary care, food, and supplies will be necessary (Reider 2015a). If the shelter does not have the needed services in-house, they need to have a list of outside organizations that can provide such assistance (e.g., local behavior professional or training facility, low-cost veteri-nary practice, food bank address) and offer these resources to the adopter.

Some shelters are fortunate enough to have the resources for a more robust adoption support program. The four main components of a com-prehensive program include not only proactively contacting and assisting adopters with issues but also gathering and analyzing adopter feedback and using the information gained to improve the organization's programs and services. In the first edition of this text, Reider (2015a) discusses the comprehensive adoption support program developed at the Michigan Humane Society (MHS). The MHS program, which contacts adopters at one week, one month, and one year post-adoption, is managed and conducted by a team of trained volunteers. A formula to deter-mine how many volunteers are needed to run such a program is presented (Reider 2015a).

A good adoption support program should strive to contact all adopters and to identify adop-tions that are in danger of being unsuccessful for the adopter or the animal (see "What is 'Adoption Success?'" in Reider 2015a). The survey that is sent to adopters should therefore contain questions that will inform the shelter if there are any issues relating to the health, behavior, or quality of life of the animal. A comprehensive post-adoption support program such as the one developed by MHS will be most effective if an online survey tool (SurveyMonkey®, Constant Contact®, SoGoSurvey, etc.) is used to collect the responses from adopters. These tools allow comprehensive analysis of the collected data that can be used to improve existing programs, develop new programs, or attain additional resources to help their adopters (Reider 2015a). It is important to understand that even the most comprehensive proactive post-adoption support programs will be unable to reach every adopter. Response rates for all types of survey research are typically very low. MHS reported that only one-quarter of the total number of adopters over a four-year period responded to the emailed surveys.

Each shelter has to determine what they are capable of providing in terms of post-adoption support. Comprehensive post-adoption support programs are very resource dependent. As Reider stated while describing the MHS program, "Adopter support must be sustainable. If you can't keep up or manage adopter support it can become a burden. If you find out about problems adopters are having you need to help people fix them. If the data is collected but never used, then what is the point?" (Reider 2015b).

Gates et al. (2018) suggested that it would be worth assessing greater use of technologies to help provide post-adoption support in a less resource-intensive manner. They suggested using text, emails, social media platforms, and other emerging technologies. The newest use of technology to help support adopters is the Maddie's Pet Assistant (MPA). Developed by Maddie's Fund and launched at the HSUS Expo in May of 2017, MPA is a free application for mobile phones and tablets to help animal shelters provide support to and communication with adopters. This program has the potential to assist a great many adopters without straining the resources of the shelter. Since 81% of people living in the United States now

own a smartphone (Pew Research Center 2019) and most smartphone users understand how to download and use applications, MPA is an extremely valuable tool for shelters.

Adopters who download the MPA app are sent regular check-in surveys throughout the first month post-adoption. If the adopter reports a concern in a survey, they receive an immediate response on the app and in an email that provides them with helpful tips, advice, and resources created by shelter medicine veterinarians and behaviorists to help them understand and resolve the issue they are experiencing with their pet. While more serious problems are flagged in the system to alert the shelter that additional assistance is needed, the fact that the adopter is provided with an immediate response containing helpful suggestions is extraordinary.

The shelter still has work to do on their end when using MPA. They will need to check the submitted survey responses from adopters every day. The MPA system color-codes responses so that the shelter can easily see which adopters are in need of further assistance (red = serious issue, yellow = mild to moderate issue, blue = question or comment). This allows the shelter to prioritize which adopters need immediate assistance and which may be able to wait a bit longer.

According to the Director of Client Experience at Pethealth, Inc., the company that now manages the MPA program, as of March 31, 2021, 876 organizations have registered for the MPA application with 212 organizations actively using the system. A total of 147,353 adopters or foster caregivers have downloaded the app, and 124,622 have submitted at least one health or behavioral survey (J. Gorton, personal communication).

25.4 Conclusions

Considering the perspective of the adopter and using empirically based marketing strategies can improve adoption programs by increasing the number of visitors coming into animal shelters as well as the overall adoption numbers. These strategies include ensuring that the animal shelter is serving all members of the community by not imposing unnecessary barriers to adoptions, using appropriate animal profile ads on social media, and understanding the needs and behaviors of adopters within the animal shelters as they search for their new family members. Training programs to increase the likelihood of adoption must follow the needs and desires of the adopters: to feel chosen and needed by their prospective animals. Therefore, behavioral training should focus on creating physical proximity and social interactions between adopters and their chosen animals.

Ultimately, the best adoption support that can be offered to adopters is a combination of all of the efforts discussed in this chapter. The pre-adoption measures consist of matchmaking, adoption counseling, and providing written take-home information tip sheets. Post-adoption support includes having medical and behavioral information tip sheets available on the organization's website and having some way for adopters to contact the shelter for assistance. Additionally, shelters should make efforts to proactively reach out to adopters to check in and offer assistance if they are experiencing any issues of concern with their new companions. Taking these steps will result in the best outcomes for adopters and the companion animals they take into their homes.

Please visit the companion website for video clips and downloadable resources associated with this chapter.

References

American Humane Association. (2013). Keeping pets (dogs and cats) in homes: Phase II: Descriptive study of post-adoption retention in six shelters in three U.S. cities. Denver, CO: American Humane Association. Report

Auerbach, K. (2016). Marketing Is Not Adoption Counseling: Keep 'Em Separate, Save More Lives. https://animalfarmfoundation. blog/2016/02/18/marketing-not-adoption-counseling/ (accessed 20 December 2019).

Brown, W.P. and Morgan, K.T. (2015). Age, breed designation, coat color, and coat pattern influenced the length of stay of cats at a no-kill shelter. *J. Appl. Anim. Welf. Sci.* https://doi.org/10.1080/10888705.2014.971156.

Brown, W.P. and Stephan, V.L. (2020). The influence of degree of socialization and age on length of stay of shelter cats. *J. Appl. Anim. Welf. Sci.* https://doi:10.1080/10888705.2020.1733574

Burch, M., Ganley, D., and Nugent, J. (2006). Follow up procedures in animal shelters: A survey of current practices. http://deesdogs. com/documents/ShelterFollowUpProcedures. pdf (6 accessed January 2020).

Casey, R.A., Vandenbussche, S., Bradshaw, J.W.S. et al. (2009). Reasons for relinquishment and return of domestic cats (*Felis silvestris catus*) to rescue shelters in the UK. *Anthrozoös* 22 (4): 347–358.

Cohen, N.P., Chodorow, M., and Byosiere, S.E. (2020). A label's a label, no matter the dog: Evaluating the generalizability of the removal of breed labels from adoption cards. *PLOS ONE* 15 (9): e0238176.

Crawford, H.M., Fontaine, J.B., and Calver, M.C. (2017). Using free adoptions to reduce crowding and euthanasia at cat shelters: An Australian case study. *Animals* 7 (12): 92.

Diesel, G., Brodbelt, D., and Pfeiffer, D.U. (2010). Characteristics of relinquished dogs and their owners at 14 rehoming centers in the United Kingdom. *J. Appl. Anim. Welf. Sci.* 13: 15–30.

Diesel, G., Pfeiffer, D., and Brodbelt, D. (2008). Factors affecting the success of rehoming dogs in the UK during 2005. *Prev. Vet. Med.* 84 (3): 228–241.

Dybdall, K. and Strasser, R. (2014). Is there a bias against stray cats in shelters? People's perception of shelter cats and how it influences adoption time. *Anthrozoös*. https://doi.org/10.2752/089279314X14072268688087.

Fantuzzi, J.M., Miller, K.A., and Weiss, E. (2010). Factors relevant to adoption of cats in an animal shelter. *J. Appl. Anim. Welf. Sci.* https://doi.org/10.1080/10888700903583467.

Fukimoto, N., Melo, D., Palme, R. et al. (2020). Are cats less stressed in homes than in shelters? A study of personality and faecal cortisol metabolites. *Appl. Anim. Behav. Sci.* 224: 104919.

Gallo, A. (2014). The Value of Keeping the Right Customers. https://hbr.org/2014/10/the-value-of-keeping-the-right-customers (accessed 20 December 2019).

Garrison, L. and Weiss, E. (2015). What do people want? Factors people consider when acquiring dogs, the complexity of the choices they make, and implications for nonhuman animal relocation programs. *J. Appl. Anim. Welf. Sci.* https://doi.org/10.1080/10888705.2014.943836.

Gates, M.C., Mancera, K., Dale, A. et al. (2020). Preliminary analysis of post-adoption outcomes for kittens and adult cats rehomed through a New Zealand animal shelter. *N.Z. Vet. J.* 68 (1): 38–45.

Gates, M.C., Zito, S., Thomas, J. et al. (2018). Post-adoption problem behaviours in adolescent and adult dogs rehomed through a New Zealand animal shelter. *Animals* 8: 93.

Gourkow, N. and Fraser, D. (2006). The effect of housing and handling practices on the welfare, behaviour and selection of domestic cats (*Felis sylvestris catus*) by adopters in an animal shelter. *Anim. Welf.* 15: 371–377.

Gouveia, K., Magalhães, A., and De Sousa, L. (2011). The behaviour of domestic cats in a shelter: Residence time, density and sex ratio. *Appl. Anim. Behav. Sci.* 130 (1–2): 53–59.

Grant, R.A. and Warrior, J.R. (2019). Clicker training increases exploratory behaviour and time spent at the front of the enclosure in shelter cats: Implications for welfare and adoption rates. *Appl. Anim. Behav. Sci.* https://doi.org/10.1016/j.applanim.2018.12.002

Griffin, K.E., John, E., Pike, T. et al. (2020). Can this dog be rehomed to you? A qualitative analysis and assessment of the scientific quality of the potential adopter screening policies and procedures of rehoming organisations. *Front. Vet. Sci.* 7: 617525.

Gunter, L.M., Feuerbacher, E.N., Gilchrist, R.J. et al. (2019). Evaluating the effects of a temporary fostering program on shelter dog welfare. *Peer J.* https://doi.org/10.7717/peerj.6620.

Herron, M.E., Lord, L.K., Hill, L. et al. (2007). Effects of preadoption counseling for owners on house-training success among dogs acquired from shelters. *J. Am. Vet. Med. Assoc.* 231: 558–562.

Herron, M.E., Lord, L.K., and Husseini, S.E. (2014). Effects of preadoption counseling on the prevention of separation anxiety in newly adopted shelter dogs. *J. Vet. Behav.* 9: 13–21.

Hobson, S. (2020). Examining potential impacts of Capacity for Care (C4C) as a strategy to manage shelter cat populations. Master's thesis. University of Guelph.

Houpt, K.A., Honig, S.U., and Reisner, I.R. (1996). Breaking the human–companion animal bond. *J. Am. Vet. Med. Assoc.* 208 (10): 1652–1659.

Hove, M.J. and Risen, J.L. (2009). It's all in the timing: Interpersonal synchrony increases affiliation. *Soc. Cogn.* https://doi.org/10.1521/soco.2009.27.6.949.

Iyengar, S.S. and Lepper, M.R. (2000). When choice is demotivating: Can one desire too much of a good thing? *J. Pers. Soc. Psychol.* https://doi.org/10.1037/0022-3514.79.6.995.

Janke, N., Berke, O., Flockhart, T. et al. (2017). Risk factors affecting length of stay of cats in an animal shelter: A case study at the Guelph Humane Society, 2011–2016. *Prev. Vet. Med.* https://doi.org/10.1016/j.prevetmed.2017.10.007.

Jones, H.D. and Hart, C.L. (2019). Black cat bias: Prevalence and predictors. *Psychol. Rep.* https://doi.org/10.1177/0033294119844982

Kidd, A.H., Kidd, R.M., and George, C.C. (1992). Successful and unsuccessful pet adoptions. *Psychol. Rep.* 70: 547–561.

Kogan, L.R., Schoenfeld-Tacher, R., and Hellyer, P.W. (2013). Cats in animal shelters: Exploring the common perception that black cats take

longer to adopt. *Open Vet. J.* https://doi.org/1
0.2174/1874318820130718001.

Lampe, R. and Witte, T.H. (2015). Speed of dog
adoption: Impact of online photo traits.
J. Appl. Anim. Welf. Sci. https://doi.org/10.108
0/10888705.2014.982796.

Lord, L.K., Reider, L., Herron M.E. et al. (2008).
Health and behavioral problems in dogs and
cats one week and one month after adoption
from animal shelters. *J. Am. Vet. Med. Assoc.*
233 (11): 1715–1722.

Ly, L.H., Gordon, E., and Protopopova, A. (2021).
Exploring the relationship between human
social deprivation and animal surrender to
shelters in British Columbia, *Canada. Front.
Vet. Sci.* 8: 213.

Maddalena, S.D., Zeidman, S., and Campbell,
K. (2012). An empirical look at public
perceptions and attitudes about pet adoption
and spay/neuter. Society of Animal Welfare
Administrators, St. Petersburg. Report.

Markowitz, D.M. (2019). Putting your best pet
forward: Language patterns of persuasion in
online pet advertisements. *J. Appl. Soc.
Psychol.* https://doi.org/10.1111/jasp.12647.

Marston, L.C., Bennett, P.C., and Coleman,
G.J. (2004). What happens to shelter dogs? An
analysis of data for 1 year from three
Australian shelters. *J. Appl. Anim. Welf. Sci.* 7
(1): 27–47.

Miller, D.D., Staats, S.R., Partlo, C. et al. (1996).
Factors associated with the decisions to
surrender a pet to an animal shelter. *J. Am.
Vet. Med. Assoc.* 209 (4): 738–742.

Miller, H., Ward, M., and Beatty, J.A. (2019).
Population characteristics of cats adopted
from an urban cat shelter and the influence of
physical traits and reason for surrender on
length of stay. *Animals.* https://doi.
org/10.3390/ani9110940.

Mondelli, F., Prato Previde, E., Verga, M. et al.
(2004). The bond that never developed: Adoption
and relinquishment of dogs in a rescue shelter.
J. Appl. Anim. Welf. Sci. 7 (4): 253–266.

Moulton, C. (2003). Report on Adoption Forum
II. https://aspcapro.org/sites/default/files/
adoption-forum_0.pdf (accessed 20
February 2020).

Nakamura, M., Dhand, N.K., Starling, M.J. et al.
(2019). Descriptive texts in dog profiles
associated with length of stay via an online
rescue network. *Animals.* https://doi.
org/10.3390/ani9070464.

Neidhart, L. and Boyd, R. (2002). Companion
animal adoption study. *J. Appl. Anim. Welf.
Sci.* 5 (3): 175–192.

New, J.C., Salman, M.D., King, M. et al. (2010).
Characteristics of shelter-relinquished animals
and their owners compared with animals and
their owners in U.S. pet-owning households.
J. Appl. Anim. Welf. Sci. 3 (3): 179–201.

O'Connor, R., Coe, J.B., Niel, L. et al. (2016).
Effect of adopters' lifestyles and animal-care
knowledge on their expectations prior to
companion-animal guardianship. *J. Appl.
Anim. Welf. Sci.* 19 (2): 157–170.

O'Connor, R., Coe, J.B., Niel, L. et al. (2017).
Exploratory study of adopters' concerns prior
to acquiring dogs or cats from animal shelters.
Soc. Anim. 25: 363–383.

Patronek, G.J., Glickman, L.T., Beck, A.M. et al.
(1996). Risk factors for relinquishment of dogs
to an animal shelter. *J. Am. Vet. Med. Assoc.*
209 (3): 572–581.

Pew Research Center. (2019). Mobile Fact Sheet.
https://www.pewresearch.org/internet/
fact-sheet/mobile/ (accessed 6 January 2020).

Pratsch, L., Mohr, N., Palme, R. et al. (2018).
Carrier training cats reduces stress on
transport to a veterinary practice. *Appl. Anim.
Behav. Sci.* 206: 64–74.

Protopopova, A., Brandifino, M., and Wynne,
C.D.L. (2016). Preference assessments and
structured potential adopter-dog interactions
increase adoptions. *Appl. Anim. Behav. Sci.*
https://doi.org/10.1016/j.
applanim.2015.12.003.

Protopopova, A. and Gunter, L.M. (2017).
Adoption and relinquishment interventions at
the animal shelter: A review. *Anim. Welf.*
https://doi.org/10.7120/09627286.26.1.035.

Protopopova, A., Mehrkam, L.R., Boggess,
M.M. et al. (2014). In-kennel behavior predicts
length of stay in shelter dogs. *PLOS ONE.*
https://doi.org/10.1371/journal.pone.
0114319.

Protopopova, A. and Wynne, C.D.L. (2014). Adopter-dog interactions at the shelter: Behavioral and contextual predictors of adoption. *Appl. Anim. Behav. Sci.* 157: 109–116.

Protopopova, A. and Wynne, C.D.L. (2016). Judging a dog by its cover: Morphology but not training influences visitor behavior toward kenneled dogs at animal shelters. *Anthrozoös.* https://doi.org/10.1080/08927936.2016.1181381.

Quimby, J.M., Smith, M.L., and Lunn, K.F. (2011). Evaluation of the effects of hospital visit stress on physiologic parameters in the cat. *J. Fel. Med. Surg.* 13 (10): 733–737.

Reese, Laura A. (2021). Make me a match: Prevalence and outcomes associated with matching programs in dog adoptions. *J. Appl. Anim. Welf. Sci.* 24 (1): 16–28.

Reider, L.M. (2015a). Adopter support: Using postadoption programs to maximize adoption success. In: *Animal Behavior for Shelter Veterinarians and Staff* (eds. E. Weiss, H. Mohan-Gibbons, and S. Zawistowski), 292–357. Hoboken, NJ: Wiley Blackwell.

Reider, L.M. (2015b). Adopter Support: Helping Adopters Succeed. https://www.aspcapro.org/webinar/20151209/adopter-support (accessed 6 April 2021).

Rowan, A. and Kartal, T. (2018). Dog population & dog sheltering trends in the United States of America. *Animals.* https://doi.org/10.3390/ani8050068.

Salman, M.D., Hutchison, J., Ruch-Gallie, R. et al. (2000). Behavioral reasons for relinquishment of dogs and cats to 12 shelters. *J. Appl. Anim. Welf. Sci.* 3 (2): 93–106.

Salman, M.D., New, J.C., Scarlett, J.M. et al. (1998). Human and animal factors related to relinquishment of dogs and cats in 12 selected animal shelters in the United States. *J. Appl. Anim. Welf. Sci.* 1 (3): 207–226.

Schoenfeld-Tacher, R., Kogan, L.R., and Carney, P.C. (2019). Perception of cats: Assessing the differences between videos and still pictures on adoptability and associated characteristics. *Front. Vet. Sci.* https://doi.org/10.3389/fvets.2019.00087.

Scott, S., Jong, E., McArthur, M. et al. (2018). Follow-up survey of people who have adopted dogs and cats from an Australian shelter. *Appl. Anim. Behav. Sci.* 201: 40–45.

Shore, E.R. (2005). Returning a recently adopted companion animal: Adopters' reasons for and reactions to the failed adoption experience. *J. Appl. Anim. Welf. Sci.* 8 (3): 187–198.

Southland, A., Dowling-Guyer, S., and McCobb, E. (2019). Effect of visitor perspective on adoption decisions at one animal shelter. *J. Appl. Anim. Welf. Sci.* https://doi.org/10.1080/10888705.2018.1448275.

Troughton, B. (2015). The adoption process: The interface with the human animal. In: *Animal Behavior for Shelter Veterinarians and Staff* (eds. E. Weiss, H. Mohan-Gibbons, and S. Zawistowski), 286–291. Hoboken, NJ: Wiley Blackwell.

Tsukiura, T. and Cabeza, R. (2011). Shared brain activity for aesthetic and moral judgments: Implications for the beauty-is-good stereotype. *Soc. Cogn. Affect. Neurosci.* https://doi.org/10.1093/scan/nsq025.

Vitulová, S., Voslářová, E., Večerek, V. et al. (2018). Behaviour of dogs adopted from an animal shelter. *Acta Vet. Brno* 87: 155–163.

Weiss, E., Gramann, S., Dolan, E.D. et al. (2014). Do policy based adoptions increase the care a pet receives? An exploration of a shift to conversation based adoptions at one shelter. *Open J. Anim. Sci.* https://doi.org/10.4236/ojas.2014.45040.

Wells, D.L. and Hepper, P.G. (2000). Prevalence of behaviour problems reported by owners of dogs purchased from an animal rescue shelter. *Appl. Anim. Behav. Sci.* 69 (1): 55–65.

Wells, D.L. and Hepper, P.G. (2001). The behavior of visitors towards dogs housed in an animal rescue shelter. *Anthrozoös.* https://doi.org/10.2752/089279301786999661.

Workman, M.K. and Hoffman, C.L. (2015). An evaluation of the role the internet site Petfinder plays in cat adoptions. *J. Appl. Anim. Welf. Sci.* https://doi.org/10.1080/10888705.2015.1043366.

Zito, S., Paterson, M., Vankan, D. et al. (2015). Determinants of cat choice and outcomes for adult cats and kittens adopted from an Australian animal shelter. *Animals.* https://doi.org/10.3390/ani5020276.

Appendix 25.A Behavioral Adoption Counseling—Cats

1) **Settle-In Time**

   Cats don't really like change, so going to a new house might be stressful for your new cat. The best thing to do to help him settle in is to set up a special room, complete with everything he needs (food, water, litterbox, toys), making sure there is also a place to hide. Bring the carrier into the room and open the door. Do not force the cat to come out; let him take his time.

   Your new cat needs time to adjust to his new surroundings. He will most likely hide for the first few days. Don't worry! Hiding is the coping strategy that cats use in a new environment. Do NOT try to pull him from the hiding place. Just be patient, and as soon as he feels comfortable, he will start coming out.

   Visit your new cat often but don't force any interaction. Simply sit in the room with him. Bringing in a dish of tuna fish or other yummy treat can also help lure the cat out and help to form a positive association with you. Once the cat stops hiding and comes out to you when you visit, you can let him out into the whole house.

2) **Litterbox**

   You don't need to teach a cat to use a litterbox—just let her know where it is. Cats prefer unscented litter, and the clumping varieties are preferred by most. Some cats do fine with covered boxes, but they trap odor and some cats won't use them. Make sure the litterbox is not too small for the cat to "do her business." And the most important thing is to keep the litterbox clean—scoop daily and change completely once a week.

3) **Scratching**

   Cats need to scratch on things for claw maintenance and to mark their territory—this is very normal cat behavior. To safeguard against damage to your furniture, provide your cat with a few scratching posts. Make sure the posts are placed in a prominent area in the house. The post should be tall and stable (though some cats prefer horizontal marking posts instead of the vertical type). The posts covered in sisal rope are preferred, but cats also like corrugated cardboard or even natural wood like a log (loop carpeting is not preferred by cats).

4) **Introduction to Resident Cat(s)**

   Your new cat and the resident cat(s) will be able to smell each other from under the door where the new cat is living. Putting treats near the door will help form a positive association between the cats. To help them get to know each other, do some "scent exchange" by rubbing each cat with a washcloth or a sock on your hand several times a day (without washing the cloth in between).

   After a few days, start putting your resident cat in the new cat's room and let the new cat explore the house for an hour or so each day. This will allow the resident cat to get to know the new cat's scent and will allow the new cat to get the lay of the land in the rest of the house.

   Next, set up a baby gate at the door so the cats can see each other for a couple of days before you let them in the same room together (one baby gate on top of another will prevent them from jumping over). Putting treats on either side of the gate will add some positive association. Several short sessions each day of allowing them to see each other is best.

   The next step is to set up some short, controlled introductions. Bring the cats into the same room and provide them each with a dish of tuna fish. At first the dishes should be at opposite sides of the room. Do this daily, moving the dishes closer each day.

   This process can take a few days, several weeks, or even a few months. Go at the cats' pace. A slow introduction will go a long way to improve the future relationship of the cats.

5) **Introduction to Resident Dog(s)**

Make sure to have that special room for your new cat. After she is coming out from hiding in that room, you can start to introduce her to the house *while the dog is outside*. When you are ready for the dog and cat to meet, make sure the dog is behind a baby gate and can't get to the cat. Any time you are going to introduce them without the gate, the dog should be on leash so that he doesn't learn that chasing the cat is fun. Even after you think the dog and cat are okay together, make sure the cat has an escape route should the dog ever trigger to chasing the cat. You can do this using a baby gate in a doorway that the cat can jump over or run under for safe escape.

Appendix 25.B Behavioral Adoption Counseling—Dogs

1) **Housetraining**

   Before you bring your new dog into your home, take her for a walk so that she is "empty." Keep your new dog on a leash when you go into the house for the first time. Walk her around on leash so she gets to know the house. Take your new dog outside regularly and reward all incidents of outdoor elimination. When inside, supervise your dog for the first week or so until you know her elimination schedule. If you catch the dog starting to eliminate in the house, say "et et" sharply and then take her outside to finish. If you do not catch her in the act of eliminating in the house you cannot punish because the dog will not connect the punishment with the crime. Clean the soiled area and remove the odor with a neutralizing cleaning product.

2) **Safeguard against Separation Anxiety**

   Dogs bond quickly to their new owners, a quality we love but that may lead to separation issues if you spend 24/7 with your dog the first few days and then suddenly go back to work. To help your dog adjust to your schedule, make sure that you leave him alone for bits of time starting on the very first day you bring him home. When you leave, turn the radio on and give the dog a food-filled KONG or other hollow item or hide treats around the house to keep him busy. This will also help to form a positive association with your departure. Don't make a big deal about leaving, and greet your dog calmly when you get home.

3) **Introduction to Resident Cat(s)**

   Make sure that your new dog never has the opportunity to chase your cat. Have her on a leash when in the house for the first few days and keep her behind a baby gate when you are not able to supervise. Once your new dog and cat seem fine together, you should still make sure that your cat always has an escape route to get away from your dog. A baby gate in a doorway that your cat can jump over or run under to escape from the dog is best.

4) **Introduction to Resident Dog(s)**

   You should introduce your new dog to your resident dog(s) away from your house. Take them for a walk in the neighborhood to get started. After the walk, take them into your yard and let them wander around together (still on leash). If all goes well, you can remove the leashes and let them play. Then put the leashes back on and take them into the house. Walk them around the house together. If all looks okay, you can let them off leash. Supervise the dogs well for the first few weeks as they learn to share the house and other resources.

5) **Physical Exercise, Mental Stimulation, and Training**

   All dogs need aerobic exercise (a leash walk is NOT aerobic to a dog). Make sure your new dog gets at least 20 minutes of aerobic exercise each day. Suggested activities include fetch with a ball, going for a jog with you, and playing the recall game where the dog runs back and forth between two people for treats. A tired dog is a good dog!!

   A bored dog can get into trouble as he tries to entertain himself, so you want to provide your dog with some mental exercise too. The best mental stimulation for a dog is using his nose. Take your dog for a walk and let him sniff things. Hide treats around the house for him to search for. Additionally, putting your dog's meal inside puzzle feeders, feeder balls (an empty soda bottle will do), or a KONG toy can make it a challenge to get the food, thus providing mental stimulation each day at feeding time.

   Dogs do not come knowing what you want them to do. You need to teach them to be polite members of the family and the community. Reward the behaviors you like (with praise and/or a food treat) and ignore the behaviors you don't like. Dogs learn through the consequence of their behavior—if the behavior is rewarded it will happen again, if it's not it will go away. Resist the urge to simply punish the behaviors you don't like or your dog will learn that's the only way to get your attention. Find a good positive reinforcement training class to help you understand how to communicate with and train your dog.

Appendix A

Canine Body Language

A Neutral Relaxed

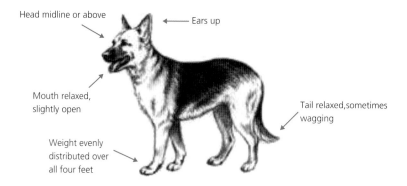

Head midline or above

Ears up

Mouth relaxed, slightly open

Tail relaxed, sometimes wagging

Weight evenly distributed over all four feet

B Greeting Behavior

A dog may show deference or "no fight" behavior while greeting another dog by approaching them with lowered body, ears back, tail down (may be wagging), and soft squinty eyes. Some overly shy or fearful dogs will start with this behavior and then move into Roll Over, as part of their greeting to people or dogs.

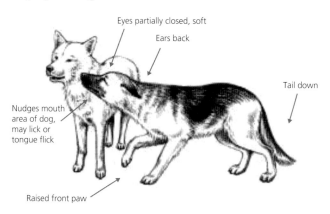

Eyes partially closed, soft

Ears back

Tail down

Nudges mouth area of dog, may lick or tongue flick

Raised front paw

Animal Behavior for Shelter Veterinarians and Staff, Second Edition. Edited by Brian A. DiGangi, Victoria A. Cussen, Pamela J. Reid, and Kristen A. Collins.
© 2022 John Wiley & Sons, Inc. Published 2022 by John Wiley & Sons, Inc.
Companion website: www.wiley.com/go/digangi/animal

C Initial Greeting

Normal canid greeting behavior includes sniffing each other's genital and anal region to gather valuable information about each other. Observing how their body language changes, both during and after this greeting, can determine if the dogs want to spend more or less time together.

Dog stands still
while being
approached, ears
back

Dog approaches with ears
forward, sniffing

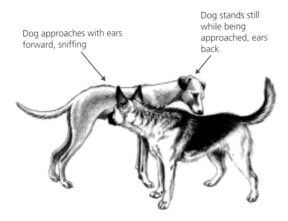

D Play Solicitation

The play bow is a combination of many behaviors. It is used to invite another dog or person to play and can also be seen during courtship behavior. The body is soft and wiggly, the front part of the dog may flatten down to the ground, and the dog may use fast, soft, popping body movements. The face has little to no tension, the mouth is typically open, and one can often hear a panting "laughing" sound. When dogs are playing with each other, it is expected to see this before play starts from one or both dogs, and they may be seen during play after some short pauses in motion.

Tail up, loose body

Ears up

Eyes soft

Mouth open and
relaxed, tongue
exposed

Front end lowered,
ready to leap forward

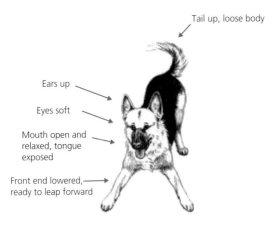

E Arousal

The dog has been stimulated by something in the environment. The hackles may raise, the tail is above spine level, body weight may shift to the front legs in a "forward" position, facial tension often increases, and the dog will typically look toward the object of interest.

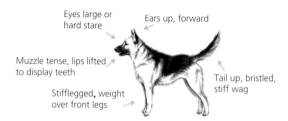

Eyes large or hard stare

Ears up, forward

Muzzle tense, lips lifted to display teeth

Tail up, bristled, stiff wag

Stifflegged, weight over front legs

F Offensive Aggression

This threatening posture is used to drive away a threat to self, a resource, or another animal.

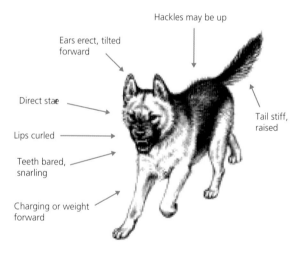

Hackles may be up

Ears erect, tilted forward

Direct stare

Tail stiff, raised

Lips curled

Teeth bared, snarling

Charging or weight forward

G Defensive Aggression

When fearful or faced with conflict, dogs will give warning signals to indicate they do not wish to be approached. If not heeded, many dogs will bite to protect themselves.

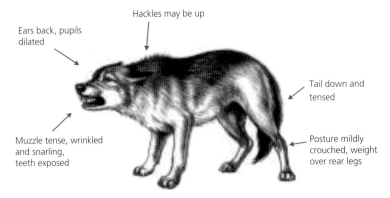

Hackles may be up

Ears back, pupils dilated

Tail down and tensed

Muzzle tense, wrinkled and snarling, teeth exposed

Posture mildly crouched, weight over rear legs

H Maternal Aggression

A mother may attempt to change behavior in her pup by using a firm muzzle hold. This is normal communication between canids. Some people try to mimic this behavior when training; however, since humans are not dogs, it is not appropriate.

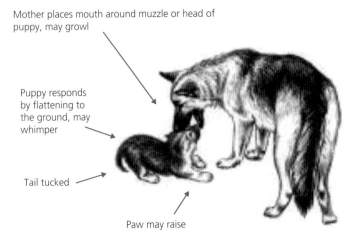

Mother places mouth around muzzle or head of puppy, may growl

Puppy responds by flattening to the ground, may whimper

Tail tucked

Paw may raise

I Crouch

This pacifying posture is a way for a dog to diffuse conflict. They make their body smaller, back is often hunched, ears are back, head often drops, tail is usually low or tucked and may be wagging slowly, and some dogs will raise their paw. If the threat continues, some dogs will progress to Roll Over.

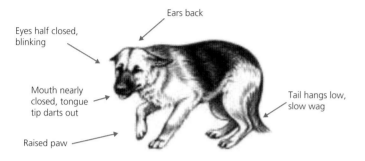

Eyes half closed, blinking

Ears back

Mouth nearly closed, tongue tip darts out

Tail hangs low, slow wag

Raised paw

J Roll Over

This is a more pacifying behavior than Crouch, and also used to diffuse conflict. Dogs will voluntarily roll over, exposing their belly. Ears are back, lips are often long, they will avoid eye contact with the person or dog who is directing their displeasure in their direction and some dogs will dribble urine. Overly shy, fearful, and some young dogs may display this as a greeting behavior to people and other dogs until they become more confident.

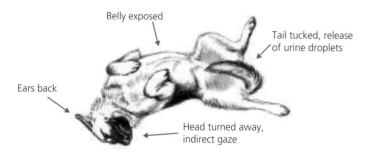

Belly exposed

Tail tucked, release of urine droplets

Ears back

Head turned away, indirect gaze

Appendix B

Feline Body Language

A The Confident Cat

The confident cat purposefully moves through space, standing straight and tall with tail erect. He is ready to explore his environment and engage those he meets along the way. His upright tail signifies his friendly intentions, while his ears are forward and erect, adding to the cat's alert expression.

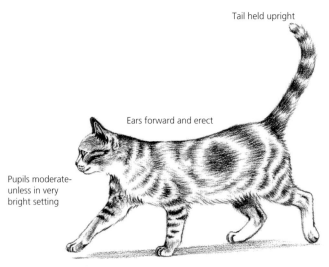

Tail held upright

Ears forward and erect

Pupils moderate-
unless in very
bright setting

Purposeful upright walk

Animal Behavior for Shelter Veterinarians and Staff, Second Edition. Edited by Brian A. DiGangi, Victoria A. Cussen, Pamela J. Reid, and Kristen A. Collins.

B The Confident Cat: At Ease

When relaxed, a confident cat stretches out on his side or lies on his back, exposing his belly. He is in a calm but alert state and accepts being approached. His entire posture is open and at ease; but beware, not every cat that exposes his abdomen will respond well to a belly rub. Some will grasp your hand with their front paws, rake your forearm with their hind feet, and bite your hand.

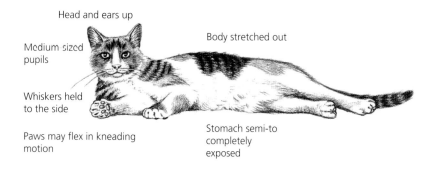

Head and ears up

Body stretched out

Medium-sized pupils

Whiskers held to the side

Paws may flex in kneading motion

Stomach semi-to completely exposed

C Distance-Reducing Behaviors

Distance-reducing behaviors encourage approach and social interaction and are meant to telegraph to others that the cat means no harm. The act of rubbing against a person's hand or another cat (scent marking) to distribute glandular facial pheromones from the forehead, chin, or whisker bed is calming and seems to guarantee friendly interaction immediately afterward. The tail is usually held erect while the cat is scent-rubbing.

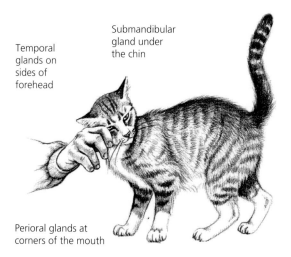

Temporal glands on sides of forehead

Submandibular gland under the chin

Perioral glands at corners of the mouth

Interdigital glands on the bottoms of all four paws

D Distance-Increasing Behaviors

The goal of distance-increasing behaviors is to keep others from coming closer. Aggressive interactions are avoided when the warnings are heeded. Conflicted cats lack the confidence to stare down and charge others. Instead, they assume a defensive threat posture, warning others away by appearing as formidable as possible by arching their backs, swishing their tails, and standing sideways and as tall as possible. Fear and arousal cause their fur to stand on end (piloerection) and pupils to dilate.

Arched back   Pilo-erect fur

Ears held flat

Pupils
dilated

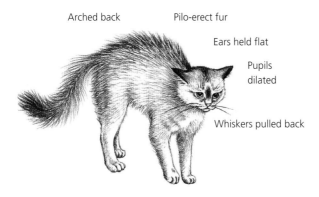

Whiskers pulled back

E The Anxious Cat

When a cat becomes anxious, he crouches into a ball, making himself appear smaller than usual. Muscles are tensed and the cat is poised to flee if necessary. The tail is held close to the body, sometimes wrapped around the feet. The head is held down and pulled into the shoulders.

Body hunched, muscles
tensed

Rolling over on one
side to better expose
claws

Ears
Swiveled
sideways

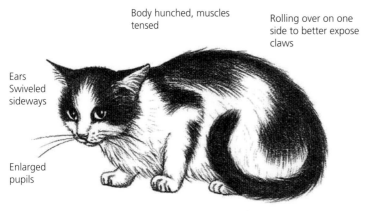

Enlarged
pupils

Tail held close to body, may flick
out

F Defensive Aggression

The pariah threat is another distance-increasing posture. When a cat determines that he cannot escape an unwanted interaction with a more dominant animal, he prepares to defend himself. The ears are pulled back and nearly flat against the head for protection, and the head and neck are pulled in tight against the body. Facial muscles tense, displaying one weapon—the teeth. The cat rolls slightly over to one side to expose the rest of his arsenal—his claws. He is now ready to protect himself.

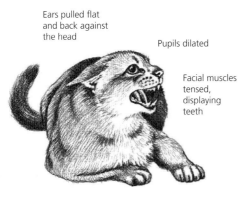

Ears pulled flat and back against the head

Pupils dilated

Facial muscles tensed, displaying teeth

Paw ready to swat with claws exposed

G The Predator

Even when fed two meals a day, cats are still predators. The predatory sequence is stalk, pounce, kill, remove, and eat. When stalking prey, a cat may stealthily move forward or lie in wait, shifting his weight between his hind feet. When movement is detected, the cat pounces on his prey and delivers a killing bite. He may then take the fresh-killed prey to a quiet place to eat—or a female may take it to her kittens. Even cats that don't hunt for their meals still enjoy chasing moving objects, including toys and, in some cases, human body parts.

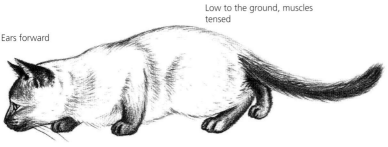

Low to the ground, muscles tensed

Ears forward

May shift weight between back feet, readying to pounce

H The Groomer

Cats spend 30–50% of their waking time grooming. Backward-facing barbs on the tongue act as a comb to loosen tangles and remove some parasites. Beyond maintaining the cat's coat, grooming also relieves tension and promotes comfort. Licking also facilitates cooling off in warm weather.

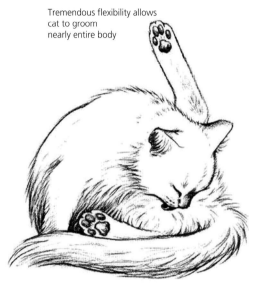

Tremendous flexibility allows cat to groom nearly entire body

Backward-facing barbs on tongue

Appendix C

Animal Behavior Professionals

Academy of Veterinary Behavior Technicians— www.avbt.net

The Academy of Veterinary Behavior Technicians (AVBT) is recognized by the National Association of Veterinary Technicians in America (NAVTA) to award certification to licensed/certified veterinary technicians as Veterinary Technician Specialists in Behavior (VTS-Behavior) who demonstrate superior knowledge of behavioral health, problem prevention, training, management, and behavior modification. Certification requires NAVTA and Society of Veterinary Behavior Technicians membership, two letters of recommendation from a veterinarian or VTS-Behavior certified technician, completion of a clinical or research skills assessment form, 3 years (minimum 4,000 hours) work experience and a minimum of 40 hours of continuing education in animal behavior within 5 years of application, maintenance of a case log demonstrating at least 50 clinical cases or 1 year of behavioral research observations, five detailed case reports, and publication of a peer-reviewed article. If credentialing criteria are accepted, candidates must pass a written certification examination.

American Board of Veterinary Practitioners— Shelter Medicine Practice— https://abvp.com/

The American Board of Veterinary Practitioners (ABVP) is recognized by the American Board of Veterinary Specialties to award board certification in Shelter Medicine Practice to qualified veterinarians. To become a Diplomate of the ABVP in Shelter Medicine Practice, one must graduate from veterinary school and be legally qualified to practice veterinary medicine, attain veterinary licensure, complete 6 years of clinical practice in shelter medicine or 1 year of qualifying experience plus an approved residency program of at least 2 years' duration, meet specific experiential credentialing requirements, submit record of 90–100 continuing education hours in shelter medicine topics during the 5 years prior to certification, provide three professional references, and submit a combination of clinical case reports (1–2) and/or scientific publications (0–1) in peer-reviewed, approved journals depending on certification pathway. Credentialing requirements for residency programs that directly relate to animal behavior include a minimum of two weeks of clinical behavior practice with a veterinary behaviorist and four weeks of in-shelter behavior with an approved, credentialed supervisor. If credentialing criteria are accepted, candidates must pass a written certification examination, 17% of which is composed of items related to shelter animal behavioral health. Diplomates must renew their certification every 10 years either through passing the board certification examination or documenting approved continuing professional development activities.

Applied Animal Behaviorist

Applied animal behaviorists are scientists, educators, or other animal professionals with an academic degree in an animal behavior–related field. Applied animal behaviorists may have training in fields as diverse as psychology, biology, zoology, veterinary medicine, or animal sciences.

The Animal Behavior Society (animalbehaviorsociety.org) offers certification programs for Certified Applied Animal Behaviorists (CAABs) and Associate Certified Applied Animal Behaviorists (ACAABs) (www.corecaab.org):

- Certified Applied Animal Behaviorist (CAAB). This certification requires a doctoral degree in a biological or behavioral science with an emphasis on animal behavior, including 5 years of professional experience (including two case studies or publications), or a doctoral degree in veterinary medicine, including a 2-year residency in animal behavior and 3 years of professional experience.
- Associate Certified Applied Animal Behaviorist (ACAAB). This certification requires a master's degree in a biological or behavioral science with an emphasis in animal behavior and a research-based thesis along with 2 years of professional experience (including two case studies or publications).

Applicants for both certifications must attend and present a talk or poster at an Animal Behavior Society annual meeting within 5 years of application and present a minimum of three letters of recommendation. Recertification is required every 5 years with submission of a current resume and names of three references.

Certified Professional Dog Trainer (CPDT)—www.ccpdt.org

Through the Association of Pet Dog Trainers (www.apdt.com), the Certification Council for Professional Dog Trainers (CCPDT) offers certification programs for Dog Trainers and Behavior Consultants:

- Certified Professional Dog Trainer— Knowledge Assessed (CPDT-KA®). This certification assures a broad range of knowledge and skills in ethology, learning theory, dog training technique, and instruction. Certification requires a minimum of 300 hours experience in dog training within the last 3 years; a letter of attestation from a CCPDT certificant or veterinarian indicating a positive relationship with clients and safe dog handling; adherence to CCPDT's Standards of Practice and Code of Ethics and Least Intrusive, Minimally Aversive Effective Behavior Intervention Policy; and passing a 180 multiple-choice question examination. Re-certification must occur by earning 36 continuing education units every 3 years.
- Certified Professional Dog Trainer— Knowledge and Skills Assessed (CPDT-KSA®). This certification requires current CPDT-KA credentials and assures expert training and instruction skills through hands-on exercises. In addition to the CPDT-KA® requirements, certification requires an online application and video demonstration of four assigned training exercises submitted during a three-week testing period. Re-certification must occur

by earning a minimum of 12 hands-on continuing education units and 24 hours of didactic continuing education units every 3 years.

- Certified Behavior Consultant Canine—Knowledge Assessed (CBCC-KA®). This certification requires a minimum of 300 hours experience in canine behavior consulting with an emphasis on fear, phobias, compulsive behaviors, anxiety, and aggression within the last 3 years; a letter of attestation from a CCPDT certificant or veterinarian indicating a positive relationship with clients and safe dog handling; adherence to CCPDT's Standards of Practice and Code of Ethics and Least Intrusive, Minimally Aversive Effective Behavior Intervention Policy; and passing a 180 multiple-choice question examination. Re-certification must occur by earning 36 continuing education units every 5 years.

Trainer

Pet trainers may use a number of different titles, such as "behavior counselor," "pet psychologist," and "pet therapist." The level of education and experience among this group of professionals is not standardized and varies greatly. Most learn how to work with animals through apprenticeships with established trainers, volunteering at animal shelters, attending seminars on training and behavior, and training their own animals. Some specialized training schools may offer independent certifications.

Veterinarian

Didactic training in animal behavior is not a required component of the curriculum for American Veterinary Medical Association Council on Education–accredited veterinary institutions. However, a majority of veterinary schools provide a formal course in animal behavior or ethology, and these courses are required by most of these schools.[1] Licensed veterinarians are the only professionals legally permitted to make diagnoses and use prescription medications for treatment of (medical or) behavioral conditions in animals that they do not own.

Veterinary Behaviorist— www.dacvb.org

The American College of Veterinary Behaviorists (ACVB) is recognized by the American Board of Veterinary Specialties to promote and standardize board certification in veterinary behavior. To become a Diplomate of the ACVB one must graduate from veterinary school and attain veterinary licensure, complete an internship (generally 1 year), complete an approved 2- or 3-year residency program including a minimum of 2,600 hours of primary patient care and 400 cases, publish a scientific paper describing original research in a peer-reviewed journal, write three peer-reviewed case reports, and complete a comprehensive two-day written examination. Diplomates must renew their certification every 10 years either through passing the board certification examination or documenting approved continuing professional development activities.

---

1 Shivley, C.B., Garry, F.B., Kogan, L.R., et al. (2016). Survey of animal welfare, animal behavior, and animal ethics courses in the curricula of AVMA Council on Education-Accredited Veterinary Colleges and Schools. *J. Am. Vet. Med. Assoc.* 248 (10): 1165–1170.

Index

Animal Behavior for Shelter Veterinarians and Staff, Second Edition. Edited by Brian A. DiGangi, Victoria A. Cussen,
Pamela J. Reid, and Kristen A. Collins.
© 2022 John Wiley & Sons, Inc. Published 2022 by John Wiley & Sons, Inc.
Companion website: www.wiley.com/go/digangi/animal